P9-CRX-788

Transplantation Immunology

Transplantation Immunology

Editors

Fritz H. Bach

Professor, Harvard Medical School
Sandoz Center for Immunobiology
Department of Surgery
New England Deaconess Hospital
Boston, Massachusetts

Hugh Auchincloss, Jr.

Associate Professor, Harvard Medical School
Department of Surgery
Massachusetts General Hospital
Boston, Massachusetts

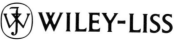 WILEY-LISS

A JOHN WILEY & SONS, INC., PUBLICATION
New York • Chichester • Brisbane • Toronto • Singapore

Address all Inquiries to the Publisher
Wiley-Liss, Inc., 605 Third Avenue, New York, NY 10158-0012

Copyright © 1995 Wiley-Liss, Inc.

Printed in the United States of America

Under the conditions stated below the owner of copyright for this book hereby grants permission to users to make photocopy reproductions of any part or all of its contents for personal or internal organizational use, or for personal or internal use of specific clients. This consent is given on the condition that the copier pay the stated per-copy fee through the Copyright Clearance Center, Incorporated, 27 Congress Street, Salem, MA 01970, as listed in the most current issue of "Permissions to Photocopy" (Publisher's Fee List, distributed by CCC, Inc.), for copying beyond that permitted by sections 107 or 108 of the US Copyright Law. This consent does not extend to other kinds of copying, such as copying for general distribution, for advertising or promotional purposes, for creating new collective works, or for resale.

Library of Congress Cataloging-in-Publication Data

Transplantation immunology / editors, Fritz H. Bach, Hugh Auchincloss,
   Jr.
      p. cm.
   ISBN 0-471-30448-4
   1. Transplantation immunology. I. Bach, Fritz H.
  II. Auchincloss, Hugh.
   [DNLM: 1. Transplantation Immunology. 2. Graft Rejection-
  -immunology. WO 680 T7714 1995]
  QR188.8.T72 1995
  617.9'5—dc20
  DNLM/DLC
  for Library of Congress   94-49601
                                                CIP

The text of this book is printed on acid-free paper.

10 9 8 7 6 5 4 3 2 1

Contents

Contributors

Hugh Auchincloss, Jr., Department of Surgery, Massachusetts General Hospital, Harvard Medical School, Boston, MA 02114 [ix,87,131,211,305]

Fritz H. Bach, Sandoz Center for Immunobiology, New England Deaconess Hospital, Harvard Medical School, Boston, MA 02215 [ix,1,105,305,347]

Clyde F. Barker, Department of Surgery, Hospital of the University of Pennsylvania, Philadelphia, PA 19104 [227]

Farid Boulad, Bone Marrow Transplantation Service, Department of Pediatrics, Memorial Sloan-Kettering Cancer Center, New York, NY 10021[161]

Luis Campos, Department of Surgery, Hospital of the University of Pennsylvania, Philadelphia, PA 19104 [227]

Stephen Cobbold, Sir William Dunn School of Pathology, University of Oxford, Oxford OX1 3RE, England [239]

Neal Flomenberg, Medical College of Wisconsin, Milwaukee, WI 53226 [53]

Paul Gores, Department of Surgery, University of Minnesota, Minneapolis, MN 55455 [147]

Rainer Gruessner, Department of Surgery, University of Minnesota, Minneapolis, MN 55455 [147]

Marc K. Jenkins, Department of Microbiology, University of Minnesota Medical School, Minneapolis, MN 55455 [295]

Robert I. Lechler, Department of Immunology, Royal Postgraduate Medical School, Hammersmith Hospital, University of London, London W12 0NN, England [1]

Joan K. Lunney, Parasite Immunology Laboratory, Agricultural Research Service, U.S. Department of Agriculture, Beltsville, MD 20705 [339]

Takashi Maki, Harvard Medical School and Division of Organ Transplantation, New England Deaconess Hospital, Boston, MA 02215 [247]

James F. Markmann, Department of Surgery, Hospital of the University of Pennsylvania, Philadelphia, PA 19104 [227]

George L. Mayo, Department of Surgery, Hospital of the University of Pennsylvania, Philadelphia, PA 19104 [227]

Richard G. Miller, Ontario Cancer Institute, and Departments of Medical Biophysics and Immunology, University of Toronto, Toronto, Ontario, Canada [267]

Anthony P. Monaco, Harvard Medical School and Division of Organ Transplantation, New England Deaconess Hospital, Boston, MA 02215 [247]

Peter J. Morris, Nuffield Department of Surgery, University of Oxford, John Radcliffe Hospital, Oxford OX3 9DU, England [277]

Randall E. Morris, Laboratory of Transplantation Immunology, Department of Cardiothoracic Surgery, Stanford University Medical School, Stanford, CA 94305-5247 [199]

Ali Naji, Department of Surgery, Hospital of the University of Pennsylvania, Philadelphia, PA 19104 [227]

John S. Odorico, Department of Surgery, Hospital of the University of Pennsylvania, Philadelphia, PA 19104 [227]

Richard J. O'Reilly, Bone Marrow Transplantation Service, Department of Pediatrics, Memorial Sloan-Kettering Cancer Center, New York, NY 10021 [161]

Esperanza Papadopoulos, Bone Marrow Transplantation Service, Department of Pediatrics, Memorial Sloan-Kettering Cancer Center, New York, NY 10021 [161]

Jeffrey L. Platt, Department of Surgery, Duke University Medical Center, Durham, NC 27710 [113]

Andrew M. Posselt, Department of Surgery, Hospital of the University of Pennsylvania, Philadelphia, PA 19104 [227]

Simon C. Robson, Sandoz Center for Immunobiology, New England Deaconess Hospital, Harvard Medical School, Boston, MA 02215 [305]

David H. Sachs, Transplantation Biology Research Center, Massachusetts General Hospital, Charlestown, MA 02129 [219,339]

Elizabeth Simpson, Transplantation Biology Group, MRC Clinical Sciences Center, Royal Postgraduate Medical School, Hammersmith Hospital, London W12 0NN, England [1]

Alfred Singer, National Institutes of Health, Bethesda, MD 20892 [105]

Jonathan Sprent, The Scripps Research Institute, La Jolla, CA 92037 [35]

David Sutherland, Department of Surgery, University of Minnesota, Minneapolis, MN 55455 [147]

Herman Waldmann, Sir William Dunn School of Pathology, University of Oxford, Oxford OX1 3RE, England [239]

Hans Winkler, Sandoz Center for Immunobiology, New England Deaconess Hospital, Harvard Medical School, Boston, MA 02215 [347]

Kathryn J. Wood, Nuffield Department of Surgery, University of Oxford, John Radcliffe Hospital, Oxford OX3 9DU, England [277]

Mary L. Wood, Harvard Medical School and Division of Organ Transplantation, New England Deaconess Hospital, Boston, MA 02215 [247]

Preface

Transplantation immunology evolved as a separate field with the recognition that rejection of a transplanted tissue or organ was mediated by immune mechanisms. Two major facets of this rejection response were studied most: the immune mechanisms that led to rejection and the antigens against which those immune responses took place.

From initial work of Medawar, Gowans, Simonsen, and others, it became apparent that lymphocytes were key mediators of rejection. At that time, and indeed even later when *in vitro* models such as the mixed leukocyte culture (MLC) test were established to study "allograft reactions" (then called homograft reactions), it was not yet appreciated that T and B lymphocytes were separate populations of cells. Following recognition of this fact from the work of Miller, Clayman, and others, it was studies of transplantation immunity that gave the impetus to the development of the field of "cellular immunology." Some of the most fundamental concepts of cellular immunology arose from studies of transplantation immunology, including the existence of class I and class II antigens as separate entities subserving different functions, and, to some extent, the interactions of helper and cytotoxic T lymphocytes; these were all discovered during the course of attempts to understand the cellular response underlying graft rejection. Indeed, the first evidence that function was associated with the H-2 I region in the mouse and HLA-D in humans (class II regions) came from studies of transplantation immunology, and only later were these regions associated with control of immune responsiveness.

Concurrent, and in fact preceding, these cellular studies, was the pioneering work of Snell, Gorer, and colleagues, who defined the transplantation–histocompatibility (H) antigens: H-2, the major histocompatibility complex and multiple minor H loci in mice, that have served as models for similar studies in many species.

It was the combining of these two areas of investigation, the cellular studies with the immunogenetics, that led to recognition of the intimate and interdependent relationship between T lymphocytes and the MHC. The antigens encoded by MHC genes were the strongest and most important in activating T cells not only for transplantation, but also for recognition of foreign antigens such as viruses, in the form of peptides of those viruses; T cells could respond to those peptides only when they were recognized together with one's own MHC-encoded antigens. The same rules obtaining for recognition of class II alloantigens preferentially by $CD4^+$ helper T cells, and class I alloantigens by $CD8^+$ cytotoxic T cells were found to apply to recognition of foreign antigens (such as the viruses just mentioned) recognized "in the context of one's own class II and class I MHC antigens."

During the course of the awarding of five Nobel prizes related to immunology, the field of transplantation immunology has become vastly complicated. The advent of molecular biology, and with it the possibilities of genetic engineering, and of the production of monoclonal antibodies, has not only provided a level of analysis of these areas that was unimaginable just a couple of decades ago, but has promised therapeutic approaches that might just serve to solve problems that have plagued the field for many years. The two areas, tolerance induction and xenotransplantation, discussed as representing the frontiers of transplantation in this volume, have both received new experimental life blood because monoclonal antibodies can be produced and the tools of molecular biology exist.

One of the most exciting aspects for workers in transplantation has been the involvement of individuals from many areas, ranging from the clinical aspects of transplantation, both surgeons and physicians, to basic biologists, now including molecular biologists, cellular immunologists, and many others. The area of vascular biology has been added to the topics recognized to be of import, bringing to students of this area new disciplines, such as complement, coagulation, and endothelial cell activation, to be studied and integrated into our overall approach to try to achieve successful transplants.

The present volume is intended as a teaching text that lays out some of the most important facts and concepts underlying all these areas while presenting the excitement and challenges facing the field. The inclusion of chapters on bone marrow transplantation and pancreas/islet transplantation was based on both the special immunological and genetic problems raised by these two forms of transplantation and our desire to have the issues associated with cellular transplants (islets and bone marrow cells) covered.

We invited authors to present their own perspectives of the areas they covered in relatively short chapters with few references, and to use primarily their own work and references to illustrate their points. Nonetheless, the presentations vary in this regard.

Tolerance induction has been the goal for transplantation since the recognition that it exists and can be induced neonatally. Today, attempts to achieve tolerance in many ways teach us as much about transplantation immunology as any other area. As such, we have included a number of chapters relating the different approaches to trying to achieve tolerance. The material included in these chapters is, to our minds, an excellent teaching exercise in the complexity of the antigens and the immune response they elicit. It is a beautiful example of how understanding at a basic level can lead to therapeutic attempts.

The severe shortage of donor organs has led to a renewal of interest in xenotransplantation. Here, more than in almost any other area of transplantation, there is optimism that genetic engineering may provide some of the answers and the therapeutic approaches needed. Use of the pig as the most likely donor species has already led to production of transgenic pigs that may blunt the action of recipient (human) complement, which plays a clear and important role in rejection of the xenotransplant. It is in this area that the disciplines not usually stressed to the student of transplantation have shown their importance. We have tried to include some of these in detail for this reason.

There are few revolutionary discoveries in scientific research. The development of molecular biology represents a distinct exception to this rule. Our increase in understanding of basic biology and the beginning of genetic engineering as a tool for therapy seem to have no scientific bound, although ethical and financial questions abound. As so often in science, the new field has introduced not only a series of new concepts but also its own language. We have included a final chapter for those readers to whom molecular biology still represents a bit of a maze. It is our purpose in that chapter to introduce the field from its most basic concepts. Many of the diagrams are our own; however, with the appearance of several textbooks covering this area in great detail, we have used, and are immensely grateful to the publishers and authors for permission to do so, many figures from other books. Our purpose was not to create new figures so much as to present the field in a relatively simple manner as it is applicable to the field of transplantation immunology. We would urge readers who are interested in greater detail to refer to those textbooks, as referenced in the last chapter.

Our reasons for introducing this text are several; perhaps the three most compelling have been these. First, both of us have not only Ph.D. students and post-Ph.D. fellows in our laboratories, but also M.D.s who want to receive basic training. The latter, and to a lesser extent the former, sometimes find it hard to gather the information that should serve as an intellectual scaffolding for their start in research in one or another aspect of this area. An introductory text, we thought, might help such students. Second, we both recognize the need for continuing education for those interested in transplantation immunology as practiced in the 1990s and beyond. Not only has this been apparent for ourselves, but in the talks we have given; clinicians must learn new basic information, and basic scientists must become familiar with what might be possible clinically. Third, while there is a vast literature in the field, and some books that deal with these problems, both the literature and the texts are given in great detail and it is hard to find a single source that is comprehensive enough in terms of covering these multiple areas and yet not so cumbersome that reading it is overwhelming.

It was our purpose to have a book that would accomplish these goals. We have divided the chapters into four sections. The first and second cover immunology, the antigens and the cellular response. The third deals with clinical aspects of transplantation, and the last with the future. We hope that our goal has been achieved.

Both of us would like to express our great gratitude to the various authors who contributed to this book. We chose those who are the authorities in their areas, realizing that for these individuals time was even harder to come by than for many. They deserve special thanks.

FRITZ H. BACH, M.D.
HUGH AUCHINCLOSS, JR., M.D.

Boston, Massachusetts

Chapter 1
Major and Minor Histocompatibility Antigens: An Introduction

Robert I. Lechler, Elizabeth Simpson, and Fritz H. Bach

THE MAJOR HISTOCOMPATIBILITY COMPLEX (MHC)

In each mammalian species studied, including mouse, rat, pig, certain nonhuman primates, and man, there is a single genetic locus that encodes the strongest transplantation antigens, referred to as the *major histocompatibility complex* (*MHC*). Matching of donor and recipient for these antigens (minimizing the number of antigens present on the donor cells that are not present in the recipient, and thus foreign to the recipient) can be of importance in determining the fate of an organ allograft, and is vitally important in bone marrow transplantation to minimize the incidence of graft-vs-host disease (see Chapter 9). *Matching* donor and recipient for HLA, the major histocompatibility complex in man, to minimize the number of foreign antigens recognized by the immune system, thus improves the likelihood of success for a transplant.

There is genetic complexity of the MHC both with regard to the extensive *allelic polymorphism* associated with most of the loci and with regard to what is known as *isotypic variation*. Allelic polymorphism refers to the existence in the population of two or more different forms of the gene present at a given locus. The different forms of the gene are referred to as alleles. The locus is polymorphic when there are several alleles in the population. For any locus that is polymorphic, a given individual can be either homozygous, having the same allele on both chromosomes (one inherited from the father and the other from the mother), or heterozygous, when the two inherited alleles are different. For highly polymorphic loci, such as several of the MHC loci, heterozygosity is common. Isotypic variation refers to the existence of multiple closely linked loci of similar structure and function along a short segment of the chromosome.

A simplified genetic map of the human MHC, the *HLA* region, is shown in Figure 1a, and a list of antigens associated with each of the loci is given in Table I. For comparison, a figure of the mouse MHC, H-2, is given in Figure 1b.

Structure of MHC Molecules

The MHC molecules are divided into two classes. The major *class I* molecules in man are *HLA-A, -B,* and *-C,* and the major *class II* molecules are *HLA-DR, -DQ,* and *-DP*. Many structural features are common to both classes of molecule. Both are transmembrane glycoprotein heterodimers (the combination of two chains that differ from each other). For the class I molecules, there is a heavy chain plus the β_2-microglobulin ($\beta2m$) light chain; in the case of the class II molecules, there are two associated chains, α and β, each of which has two domains. Thus, both class I and class II molecules have four extracellular domains; the two membrane-proximal domains are typical immunoglobulin-like structures, and the membrane-distal domains have an unique structure that is elegantly tailored to the function of the molecules, as discussed below. However, some differences exist between the two classes of molecule. The class I molecules consist of a 45,000-molecular weight

Transplantation Immunology, pages 1–34
© 1995 Wiley-Liss, Inc.

Simplified map of the HLA region

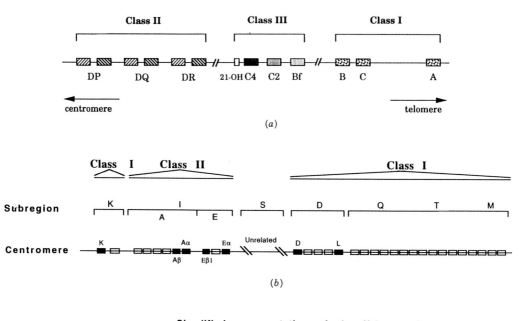

Simplified representation of the H-2 complex.
Rectangles indicate class I or II genes. Filled squares,
classical MHC genes. Distances between loci are not accurate.

Fig. 1. The arrangement of the three major regions of the HLA complex (**a**) and a simplified representation of the H-2 complex (**b**) are shown; the distances between the loci are not to scale. In the H-2 map, rectangles indicate class I or II genes; filled rectangles are the classical histocompatibility genes.

heavy chain that is inserted into the cell membrane and is encoded by a gene within the MHC. The heavy chain is complexed noncovalently with a 12,000-molecular weight protein, β2m, encoded elsewhere. The class I heavy chain is organized into three domains, the two membrane-distal α1 and α2 domains, and the α3 membrane-proximal domain. The β2m molecule contributes the second membrane-proximal domain, but is not inserted into the cell membrane. Class II molecules, in contrast, consist of two chains, referred to as α (MW approximately 32,000) and β (MW approximately 28,000), each of which has two domains (α1 and α2 plus β1 and β2); both are transmembrane molecules and both are encoded within the MHC.

Shown in Figure 2 are the primary (a) as well as the three-dimensional (b) structures of the two classes of MHC molecules. The three-dimensional structure of an MHC molecule (HLA-A2) was first solved by X-ray crystallographic analysis in 1987 (Bjorkman et al., 1987a, 1987b); the structure of two other HLA class I molecules, HLA-Aw68 (Garrett et al., 1989) and HLA-B27 (Madden et al., 1991), have since been described. Crystals of HLA class II molecules have been grown, and high resolution images of their structure have recently been obtained (Brown et al., 1993; Stern et al., 1994; Stern and Wiley, 1994). The entire molecules are approximately 70 Å in length, and at their membrane-distal portion, 50 by 40 Å across. The structures of class I and class

Table IA. Designations of HLA-A, -B, and -C Alleles

HLA alleles[a]	HLA specificity	Previous equivalents	Individual or cell line from which the sequence was derived	Accession number	References or submitting author(s)
A*0101	A1	—	LCL721, MOLT4	X55710	(31)[d]
A*0201	A2	A2.1	LCL721, JY, GM637		
A*0202	A2	A2.2F	M7		
A*0203	A203	A2.3	DK1		
A*0204	A2	—	RML, AN[b]	X57954, M86404	(32), D. Watkins
A*0205	A2	A2.2Y	WT49, AM		
A*0206	A2	A2.4a	CLA, T7527		
A*0207	A2	A2.4b	KNE		
A*0208	A2	A2.4c	KLO		
A*0209	A2	A2-OZB	OZB		
A*0210	A210	A2-LEE	XLI-ND		
A*0211	A2	A2.5	KIME, GRC 138	X60764	(33), P. Parham
A*0212	A2		KRC 033	M84378	P. Parham
A*0301	A3	A3.1	JG[b]		
A*0302	A3	A3	E1B2		
A*1101	A11	A1	CJO		
A*1102	A11	A1	CJO		
A*2301	A23(9)	—	SHJO, EL.ON	M64742	(34)
A*2401	A24(9)	—	JG[b]		
A*2402	A24(9)	—	SHJO, 32/37	M64740	(34)
A*2403	A2403	A9.3	APA, KPE	M64741	(34)
A*2501	A25(10)	—	BM92		
A*2601	A26(10)	—	GM637, O2BN5		
A*2901	A29(19)	—	JOE		
A*2902	A29(19)	A29.2	LAM[b]	X60108	(35)
A*3001	A30(19)	A30.3	LBF		
A*3002	A30(19)	A30.2	CR-B	X61702	P. Parham
A*31011[c]	A31(19)	—	JHAF		
A*31012	A31(19)	—	KRC 033, TB[b]	M84375, M86405	P. Parham, D. Watkins
A*3201	A32(19)	—	AM		
A*3301	A33(19)	Aw33.1	JOE		

(Continued)

Table IA. Designations of HLA-A, -B, and -C Alleles (Continued)

HLA alleles[a]	HLA specificity	Previous equivalents	Individual or cell line from which the sequence was derived	Accession number	References or submitting author(s)
A*3401	A34(10)	—	ENA	X61704	P. Parham
A*3402	A34(10)	—	WWAI	X61705	P. Parham
A*3601	A36	—	MASCH	X61700	P. Parham
A*4301	A43	—	CC	X61703	P. Parham
A*6601	A66(10)	—	25-1501	X61711	(36)
A*6602	A66(10)	—	CR-B	X61712	(37, 36)
A*6801	A68(28)	Aw68.1	LB		
A*6802	A68(28)	Aw68.2	PA, TO		
A*6901	A69(28)	—	IDF, ZM, BJ		
A*7401	A74(19)	—	CC, PDAV, ATUR	X61701	P. Parham
B*0701	B7	B7.1	CF		
B*0702	B7	B7.2	JY		
B*0703	B703	BPOT	POT71	X64454	P. Reekers
B*0801	B8	—	LCL721, MF, CGM1	M59841	(38)[d]
B*1301	B13	B13.1	HE		
B*1302	B13	B13.2	LBF, TO		
B*1401	B14	—	MRWC		
B*1402	B65(14)	—	BB, CGM1	M59840	(38)[d]
B*1501	B62(15)	—	MF		
B*1502	B75(15)	—	APA	M75138	(39)
B*1503	B72(70)	—	CC	X61709	P. Parham
B*1504	B62(15)	Bw62-G	GRC 138, KG[b]	M84382, M86402	P. Parham, D. Watkins
B*1801	B18	—	SGAR		
B*2701	B27	27f	LH		
B*2702	B27	27e, 27K, B27.2	BRUG		
B*2703	B27	27d, 27J	CH (CHI)[a]		
B*2704	B27	27b, 27C, B27.3	WEWAK 1		
B*2705	B27	27a, 27W, B27.1	BRUG, CD[b]		
B*2706	B27	27D, B27.4	LIE		
B*2707	B27	B27-HS	HS	M62852	(40)
B*3501	B35	—	HS[b]		

B*3502	B35	—	DL[b]	M81798	
B*3503	B35	—	C1R, HMY2	M86403	(41)
B*3504	B35		AN[b]		D. Watkins
B*3505	B35	B35-G	GRC 212	M84385	P. Parham
B*3506	B35	B35-K	KRC 103	M84381	P. Parham
B*3701	B37		KASO, MG		
B*3801	B38(16)	B16.1	Z[b]		
B*3901	B3901	B16.2	S[b]	M94052	M. Takiguchi[f]
B*3902	B3902	B39.2	YAM[b]	M94053	M. Takiguchi
B*4001	B60(40)	—	LB		
B*4002	B40	B40*	SWEIG		
B*4003	B40	B40-G1	GRC 138	M84383	P. Parham
B*4004	B40	B40-G2	GRC 212	M84384	P. Parham
B*4005	B4005	BN21	00136	M84694	P. Parham
B*4101	B41	—	SGAR		
B*4201	B42		BB		
B*4401	B44(12)	B44.1	BAU		
B*4402	B44(12)	B44.2	FMB		
B*4403	B44(12)	B44.1:New	PITOUT	X64366	(42)
B*4501	B45(12)	—	OMW	X61710	P. Parham
B*4601	B46	—	T7527		
B*4701	B47	—	PLH		
B*4801	B48	—	KRC103	M84380	P. Parham
B*4901	B49(21)	—	AM		
B*5001	B50(21)	—	SH.JO	X61706	P. Parham
B*5101	B51(5)	—	LKT-2, TO, BM92		
B*5102	B5102	B5.35	UM, 02627	M68964	M. Takiguichi, P. Parham
B*5103	B5103	BTA	30-BY3[b]	M80670	M. Takiguichi
B*5201	B52(5)	—	MT[b]		
B*5301	B53	—	AMAI, AM[b]		
B*5401	B54(22)	—	TTL	M77774	(43)
B*5501	B55(22)	—	VEN	M77778	(43)
B*5502	B55(22)	—	APA	M77777	(43)
B*5601	B56(22)	—	VOO	M77776	(43)
B*5602	B56(22)	—	ENA	M77775	(43)
B*5701	B57(17)	—	WIN, MOC, MOLT4	X55711	(44)[d]
B*5702	B57(17)	Bw57.2	3232	X61707	P. Parham

(Continued)

Table IA. Designations of HLA-A, -B, and -C Alleles (Continued)

HLA alleles[a]	HLA specificity	Previous equivalents	Individual or cell line from which the sequence was derived	Accession number	References or submitting author(s)
B*5801	B58(17)	—	WT49	X61708	P. Parham[d]
B*7801	B7801	B'SNA', Bx1	SNA, 3232	M62852	(40)
B*7901	—	B''X''-HS	HS		
Cw*0101	Cw1	Cw1.1	BRUG	M84171	(45)
Cw*0102	Cw1	Cw1.2	T7527, AP		
Cw*0201	Cw2	Cw2.1	BRUG		
Cw*02021	Cw2	Cw2.2	MVL		
Cw*02022	Cw2	Cw2.2	SWEIG		
Cw*0301	Cw3	—	JG[b]		
Cw*0302	Cw3	—	AP	M84172	(45)
Cw*0401	Cw4	—	C1R, KRC103	M84386	P. Parham
Cw*0501	Cw5	—	QBL		
Cw*0601	Cw6	—	JOE		
Cw*0701	Cw7	—	MF		
Cw*0702	Cw7	JY328	JY		
Cw*0801	Cw8	—	02627	M84174	(45)
Cw*0802	Cw8	—	CGM1, LWAGS, WT51	M59865, M84173	(38, 45)
Cw*1201	—	Cx52	AKIBA		
Cw*1202	—	Cb-2	MT[b]		
Cw*1301	—	CwBL18	TCC		
Cw*1401	—	Cb-1	LKT2		
E*0101	—	JTW15	JT,[b] YN,[b] HF[b]		
E*0102	—	HLA-6.2	LCL721		
E*0103	—	M32507	MT,[b] MH,[b] TK[b]		
E*0104	—	M32508	KS[b]		

[a] Allele names given in bold type are newly assigned.
[b] Individual from which sequence was derived.
[c] Cell line is also known by alternative name.
[d] Confirmatory sequence.
[e] This sequence has been previously assigned with a four-digit allele name.
[f] This reference is to a corrected sequence.

Tables IA–D reproduced from Bodmer et al. (1992) Eur J Immunogenet 19:327–344.

Table IB. Designations of HLA-DR Alleles

HLA alleles[a]	HLA-DR serological specificities	HLA-D-associated (T cell-defined) specificities	Previous equivalents	Individual or cell line from which the sequence was derived	Accession number	References or submitting author(s)
DRA*0101	—	—	DRα, PDR-α-2	JY, RAJI	J00194, J00196, J00203	(47, 48, 49)
DRA*0102	—	—	DR-H	—	J00201	(50)
DRB1*0101	DR1	Dw1	DR1	45.1, LG2		
DRB1*0102	DR1	Dw20	DR1-NASC	NASC		
DRB1*0103	DR103	DwBON'	DR1-CETUS, DRB1*BON	RAI, BG		
DRB1*1501	DR15(2)	Dw2	DR2B DW2	PGF		
DRB1*1502	DR15(2)	DW12	DR2B Dw12	BGE, DHO		
DRB1*1503	DR15(2)			G247*	M35159	(51)
DRB1*1601	DR16(2)	Dw21	DR2B Dw21	AZH, MN-2		
DRB1*1602	DR16(2)	Dw22	DR2B Dw22	REM (RML)[b]		
DRB1*0301	DR17(3)	Dw3		RAJI, AVL, WT49		
DRB1*0302	DR18(3)	Dw'RSH'		2041		
DRB1*0303	DR18(34)			B25	M81743	R. Apple
DRB1*0401	DR4	DW4		GM3103, WT51		
DRB1*0402	DR4	Dw10		FS		
DRB1*0403	DR4	Dw13	DR4 DW13A, 13.1	SSTO		
DRB1*0404	DR4	Dw14	DR4 DW14A, 14.1	BIN40, LS40		
DRB1*0405	DR4	Dw15		KT3		
DRB1*0406	DR4	DW'KT2'		KT2		
DRB1*0407	DR4	Dw13	DR4 Dw13B, 13.2	JHF		
DRB1*0408	DR4	Dw14	DR4-CETUS, Dw14B, 14.2	M36, RA1		
DRB1*0409	DR4	—	—	R80		
DRB1*0410	DR4	—	DR4.CB	CB, ABCC60	M81670	X. Gao[c]
DRB1*0411	DR4	—	DR4.EC	EC, HV846	M81700	X. Gao[c]
DRB1*0412	DR4	—	AB2	ABO1078	M77672	X. Gao
DRB1*1101	DR11(5)	Dw5	DRw11.1	SWEIG	M34316	(52)[d]
DRB1*11012	DR11(5)	Dw5		1180, 1249		(53)

(Continued)

Table IB. Designations of HLA-DR Alleles (Continued)

HLA alleles[a]	HLA-DR serological specificities	HLA-D-associated (T cell-defined) specificities	Previous equivalents	Individual or cell line from which the sequence was derived	Accession number	References or submitting author(s)
DRB1*1102	DR11(5)	DW'JVM'	DRw11.2	JVM		
DRB1*1103	DR11(5)		DRw11.3	UA-S2		
DRB1*11041	DR11(5)	Dw'FS'	—	FPA (FPF)[b]		(54)[d]
DRB1*11042	DR11(5)		—	2094	M34317	(53)
DRB1*1105	DR11(5)		—	DBUG	M84188	R. Apple
DRB1*1201	DR12(5)	DW'DB6'		HERLUF, FO, HK		
DRB1*1202	DR12(5)		DRw12b	KI		
DRB1*1301	DR13(6)	DW18	DRw6aI	HHKB, APD		
DRB1*1302	DR13(6)	DW19	DRw6cI	WT46		
DRB1*1303	DR13(6)	DW'HAG'	—	HAG, MRS, EGS, OSC, MGA, JRS, 1183, 2708		
DRB1*1304	DR13(6)		RB1125-14	1124, 1125		
DRB1*1305	DR13(6)		DRw6'PEV'	TA, JP, HS, BP, DES, DI		(55)[c]
DRB1*1306	DR13(6)	Dw9	DRB1*13.MW	MW	M61899	(56)
DRB1*1401	DR14(6)	Dw16	DRw6bI	4/w6, TEM		
DRB1*1402	DR14(6)			AMALA (LIA, AZL)[b]		
DRB1*1403	DR1403		JX6	MI		
DRB1*1404	DR1404		DRB1*LY10, DRw6b.2	CEPH-137502, KGU		
DRB1*1405	DR14(6)		DRB1*14c	36M, 38M		
DRB1*1406	DR14(6)		DRB1*14.GB, 14.6	GB, SAS5041, SAS9080	M63927, M74032	(56, 57)
DRB1*1407	DR14(6)		14.7	PNG141, PNG196	M74030	(57)
DRB1*1408	DR14(6)		A01, 14.8	HV178, PNG198, PNG202	M77673, M74031	(57) X. Gao
DRB1*1409	DR14(6)		AB4	1103	M77671	X. Gao
DRB1*1410	—		AB3	ABCC31	M77670	X. Gao
DRB1*0701	DR7	Dw17		BURKHARDT		
DRB1*0702	DR7	Dw'DB1'		LBF		
DRB1*0801	DR8	Dw8.1		MADURA		
DRB1*08021	DR8	Dw8.2	DRw8-SPL	SPL		
DRB1*08022	DR8	Dw8.2	DRw8b	OLL		

DRB1*08031	DR8	Dw8.3	DRw8-TAB	TAB089		
DRB1*08032	DR8	Dw8.3	—	KT°FO		
DRB1*0804	DR8	—	RB1066-1, DR8-V86	1066, PM	M84446	(58)[c]
DRB1*0805	DR8	—	DR8-A74	MS	M84357	(58)
DRB1*09011	DR9	DW23	—	ISK		
DRB1*09012	DR9	DW23	—	DKB		
DRB1*1001	DR10	—	—	RAJI		
DRB3*0101	DR52	Dw24	DR3 ■, DRw6a ■	AVL, HHKB		
DRB3*0201	DR52	Dw25	DRw6b ■	4/w6, WT49		
DRB3*0202	DR52	Dw25	pDR5b.3	SWEIG		
DRB3*0301	DR52	Dw26	—	WT46		
DRB4*0101	DR53	Dw4, Dw10, Dw13, Dw14, Dw15, Dw17, Dw23	—	LBF, DKB, BURKHARDT, KT3, FS, PRIESS, MANN		
DRB5*0101	DR51	Dw2	DR2A Dw2	PGF		
DRB5*0102	DR51	Dw12	DR2A Dw12	BGE, DHO		
DRB5*0201	DR51	Dw21	DR2A Dw21	AZH, MN-2		
DRB5*0202	DR51	Dw22	DR2A Dw22	REM (RML)[b]		
DRB6*0101	—	—	DRBo*0101, DRBX11	BAC, KAS116, MZ070782, HON, SAS6211	X53357, M83892	(16, 19) A. Kimura
DRB6*0201	—	—	DRBX21, DRBVI	PGF, DO208915, CGG E4181324	M77284, X53358, M83893	(17, 19) A. Kimura
DRB6*0202	—	—	DRBo*0201, DRBX22, DRB6III	RML, KAS011, DEM, RGM, JMI	M83204, M83894	(16, 19) A. Kimura

[a] Allele names given in bold type are newly assigned.
[b] Cell line is also known by alternative name.
[c] This reference is to a confirmatory sequence.
[d] This sequence has been previously assigned with a four-digit allele name.
[e] Individual from which the sequence was derived.

Table IC. Designations of HLA-DQ Alleles

HLA alleles[a]	HLA-DQ serological specificities	HLA-D-associated (T cell-defined) specificities	Previous equivalents	Cell line	Accession number	References or submitting author(s)
DQA1*0101	—	Dw1, w9	DQA 1.1, 1.9	LG2, BML		
DQA1*0102	—	Dw2, w21, w19	DQA 1.2, 1.19, LAZH	PGF, LB, CMCC, AZH, WT46		
DQA1*0103		Dw18, w12, w8, DW'FS'	DQA 1.3, 1.18, DRw8-DQwl	APD, TAB, FPF, WVB, 2012		
DQA1*0104	—	—	—	1183, 2013, 2012, 2708	M34314	(59)
DAQ1*0201	—	Dw7, w11	DQA 2, 3.7	LG10, BEI		
DQA1*03011	—	DW4, w10, w13, w14, w15	DQA 3, 3.1, 3.2	MMCC, JY, NIN		
DQA1*03012		Dw23	DQA 3, 3.1, 3.2, DR9-DQw3	DKB		
DQA1*0302		Dw23	DQA 3, 3.1, 3.2, DR9-DQw3	ISK		
DQA1*0401		Dw8, Dw'RSH'	DAQ 4.2, 3.8	ARC, 2041, MADURA, SPL		
DQA1*0501*		Dw3, w5, w22	DQA 4.1, 2	SWEIG		
DQA1*05011		Dw3	DQA 4.1, 2	RAJI, CMCC		
DQA1*05012		Dw5	DQA 4.1, 2	MG3		
DQA1*05013		Dw22	DQA 4.1, 2	REM(RML)[c]		
DQA1*0601		Dw8	DQA 4.3	LUY		
DQB1*0501	DQ5(1)	Dw1	DQB 1.1, DRw10-DQw1.1	LG2, 45.1, BML, MVL		
DQB1*0502	DQ5(1)	Dw21	DQB 1.2, 1.21	AZH, FJO		
DQB1*05031	DQ5(1)	Dw9	DQB 1.3, 1.9, 1.3.1	WT52, HU129, HU128		

Allele[a]	DQ	Dw	DQB	Cell	GenBank	Reference
DQB1*05032	DQ5(1)	Dw9	DQB 1.3, 1.9, 1.3.2	AP106,[b] AP109,[b] AP110,[b] AP115[b]		
DQB1*0504	—	—	DQB 1.9	DG[b]		
DQB1*0601	DQ6(1)	Dw12, w8	DQB 1.4, 1.12	DQBS4, BGE, TAB		
DQB1*0602	DQ6(1)	Dw2	DQB 1.5, 1.2	DQBS5, PGF, VYT		
DQB1*0603	DQ6(1)	Dw18, Dw'FS'	DQB 1.6, 1.18	WVB, APD, FPF, 2012		
DQB1*0604	DQ6(1)	Dw19	DQB 1.7, 1.19	CMCC, DAUDI		
DQB1*0605	DQ6(1)	Dw19	DQB 1.8, DQBSLE, 1.19b, 2013-24	CI,[b] KT,[b] MR,[b] 2013		
DQB1*0606	—	—	DQB1*WA1	LINE66	M86226	(60)
DQB1*0201	DQ2	Dw3, w7	DQB2	WT49, QBL, BURKHARDT, CMCC		
DQB1*0301	DQ7(3)	Dw4, w5, w8, w13	DQB 3.1	SWEIG, DQB37, NIN, JHA, LUY, JGL, JME		
DQB1*0302	DQ8(3)	Dw4, w10, w13, w14	DQB 3.2	DCB4, FS, BIN40, 3102		
DQB1*03031	DQ9(3)	Dw23	DQB 3.3	DKB		
DQB1*03032	DQ9(3)	Dw23, w11	DQB 3.3	DBB, KOZ		
DQB1*0304	DQ7(3)	—	DQB1*03HP, *03new	HP, RG	M74842, M83770	(61, 62)
DQB1*0401	DQ4	Dw15	DQB 4.1, Wa	KT3		
DQB1*0402	DQ4	Dw8, Dw'RSH'	DQB 4.2, Wa	ARC, OLN, 2041, SPL		

[a] Allele names given in bold type are newly assigned.

[b] Individual from which sequence was derived.

[c] Cell also known by alternative name.

[d] This reference is to a confirmatory sequence.

[e] This sequence has been previously assigned with a four-digit allele name.

[f] This sequence can only be assigned a four-digit allele name, as it is either published only as a protein or partial nucleotide sequence.

Table ID. Designations of HLA-DP Alleles

HLA alleles[a]	Associated HLA-DP specificities	Previous equivalents	Cell line	Accession number	References or submitting author(s)
DPA1*0101	—	LB14/LB24, DPA1	LB, PRIESS		
DPA1*0102	—	pSBα-318	LG2		
DPA1*0103	—	DPw4α1	BO		
DPA1*0201	—	DPA2, pDAα13B	DAUDI, AKIBA		
DPA1*02021	—	2.21	CB6B	M83906	A. Kimura
DPA1*02022	—	2.22	LKT4	M83907	A. Kimura
DPA1*0301	—	3.1	AMA1	M83908	A. Kimura
DPA1*0401	—	4.1	T7526	M83909	A. Kimura
DPB1*0101	DPw1	DPB1, DPwla	LUY, RSH, P0077	M83129	(63)[b]
DPB1*0201	DPw2	DPB2.1	JY		
DPB1*02011	DPw2	DPB2.1	LB, WJR		
DPB1*02012	DPw2	DPB2.1	45.1		
DPB1*0202	DPw2	DPB2.2	QBL, MANN		
DPB1*0301	DPw3	DPB3	SLE, PRIESS		
DPB1*0401	DPw4	DPB4.1, DPw4a	HHKB, BOP, PRIESS		
DPB1*0402	DPw4	DPB4.2, DPw4b	APD, BURKHARDT		
DPB1*0501	DPw5	DPB5	HAS		
DPB1*0601	DPw6	DPB6	JMOS		
DPB1*0801	—	DPB8	PIAZ		
DPB1*0901	—	DPB9, DP'Cp63'	TOK		
DPB1*1001	—	DPB10	BM21, SAVC	M85223	A. Kimura[b]
DPB1*1101	—	DPB11	CRK		
DBP1*1301	—	DPB13	NB		
DPB1*1401	—	DPB14	8268		
DPB1*1501	—	DPB15	PLH		

Allele[a]		Names	Cell/individual	EMBL/GenBank	Reference/contributor
DPB1*1601	—	JRA			
DPB1*1701	—	JRAB			
DPB1*1801	—	JCA			
DPB1*1901	—	CB6B			
DPB1*2001	—	Oos, DPB-JA	OOS, ARENT, CC	M58608	(64, 65, 66)
DPB1*2101	—	DPB-GM, DPB30, NewD	GM, PEI52, PEI74, C1[c]	M77659, M83915, M84621	(65) A. Begovich, A. Kimura
DPB1*2201	—	DPB1*AB1, NewH	HV152, HV385, SAS60103, SAS60106	M77674, M83919	(67) A. Kimura
DPB1*2301	—	dpB32, NewB	D0208915, UK3082, UK5496	M83913, M84014	A. Kimura, T. Eiermann
DPB1*2401	—	DPB33, NewC	UK7430	M83914	A. Kimura
DPB1*2501	—	DPB34, NewE	PEI46	M83916	A. Kimura
DPB1*2601	—	DPB31, WA2	LINE70	M86229	(68)
DPB1*2701	—	DPB23, WA3	LINE92, H033[c]	M84619, M86230	(68), A. Begovich
DPB1*2801	—	DPB21	I57,[b] I1147[c]	M84617	A. Begovich
DPB1*2901	—	DPB27, NewG	RBLB66,[c] NG105,[c] NG113,[c] PNG112, PNG117[c]	M84625, M83918	A. Begovich, A. Kimura
DPB1*3001	—	DPB28	AH1377,[c] EB5[c]	M84620	A. Begovich
DPB1*3101	—	DPB22, NewFR	168,[c] I1147,[c] 16,[c] PE108	M84618, M83917	A. Begovich, A. Kimura
DPB1*3201	—	DPB24, NewI	NG78,[c] PNG167	M84622, M85222	A. Begovich, A. Kimura
DPB1*3301	—	DPB25	HO23[c]	M84623	A. Begovich
DPB1*3401	—	DPB26	HO42,[c] DH67[c]	M84624	A. Begovich
DPB1*3501	—	DPB29	AH1450,[c] AH521[c]	M84626	A. Begovich
DPB1*3601	—	New A, SSK2	SASBE41, THM1[c]	M83912, D10479	A. Kimura, T. Juji

[a] Allele names given in bold type are newly assigned.
[b] This reference is to a corrected sequence.
[c] Individual from which the sequence was derived.

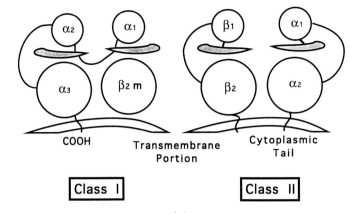

(a)

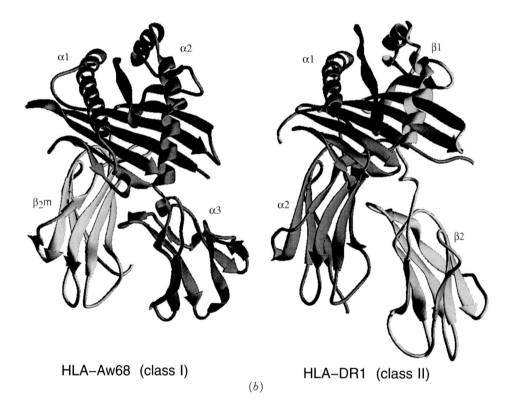

HLA–Aw68 (class I)   HLA–DR1 (class II)

(b)

Fig. 2. (a) Schematic diagram of MHC class I and class II molecules. The overall structural similarity of the two classes of molecule is illustrated. In both cases the two membrane-proximal domains have the features of immunoglobulin domains, and the membrane-distal domains are organized into a platform of anti-parallel strands on which lies a stretch of α-helical sequence. The major differences between the two classes of MHC molecule are that the domains are distributed asymmetrically in class I molecules, such that the heavy chain has three domains, coexpressed with the single domain of β-$_2$-microglobulin. In contrast, the two chains of the class II molecule both have two domains. An additional difference is that both chains of the class II molecule are inserted into the cell membrane, whereas only the heavy chain of the class I molecule spans the cell membrane. (b) Schematic of the three-dimensional structure of the class I and class II molecules as described in the text. We thank Dr. Stern for preparing these for us.

II molecules are remarkably similar, however, there are several subtle differences in the regions of the molecules that bind peptide fragments of antigen for display to T cells, as discussed below. As shown in Figure 2, the class I molecules have their two membrane-proximal domains shown at the bottom of the figure (the $\alpha 3$ domain of the heavy chain and $\beta_2 m$), and the distal domains at the top ($\alpha 1$ and $\alpha 2$). The class II molecule is shown in the same orientation.

The three-dimensional structure of the human MHC class II molecule, HLA-DR1, has recently been solved using the same approaches that were successfully applied to the analysis of class I structures (Brown et al., 1993; Stern et al., 1994). The study of the class II crystals confirmed predictions that the overall structures of class I and class II molecules were very similar. The major difference between the two classes of MHC molecule lies in their *peptide-binding clefts* (*grooves*), in that the ends of the cleft of the class II molecule are more open. This finding is entirely consistent with the parallel observations

that the peptides eluted from class II molecules were considerably longer, ranging in length from 12 to 30 amino acids (Chicz et al., 1992). It appears that peptides that are bound to class II molecules can protrude from the ends of the cleft, thus allowing greater flexibility in peptide length.

The Antigen-Binding Site

The antigen, in the form of a peptide, is firmly associated with the MHC molecule, and is located in a peptide-binding cleft or groove, which has a platform at the bottom (in terms of how the T cell receptor "looks at" the complex of peptide plus MHC molecule), and α-*helixes* above the platform on both sides of the groove. This is shown in schematic detail for a class II molecule in Figure 3. The $\alpha 1$ and $\beta 1$ domains (or in the case of the class I molecules: the $\alpha 1$ and $\alpha 2$ domains) each consists of four contiguous strands that are organized in a "Zig-Zag" manner, thereby creating a *platform* that forms the

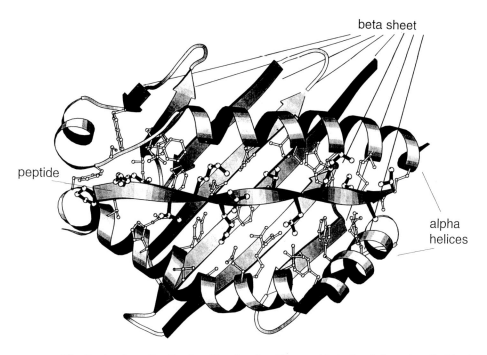

Fig. 3. A schematic of a class II molecule with a peptide in the cleft, as described in the text.

floor of the *peptide-binding site*. These strands have a β-*pleated sheet* structure, meaning that the amino acids in the strands have alternating orientations, the side chain of one pointing "up" into the peptide-binding site, and the next pointing "down" toward the membrane-proximal domains below. These strands are connected at their C-terminal ends to an α-helix of approximately 35 amino acids. The helices are non-linear, and when viewed from the side, have an arched configuration. These two domains are paired such that they form a mirror image of each other. As a consequence the four β-pleated sheets from each domain form a single platform of eight β-strands, and the α-helices are separated from one another. The folded structure creates a groove that is 25 by 10 Å in size (for the class I molecules), and is the antigen-binding site of the HLA molecule. In the course of the X-ray crystallographic studies, it was observed that this groove consistently contained electron-dense material that was not accounted for by the polypeptide structure of the HLA molecule itself. This electron-dense material represents *peptide fragments* within the binding site, which were copurified with the HLA molecule. This is shown in a model (see Fig. 3), in which a peptide is shown between the α-helixes; in this model, the platform of β-pleated sheets is not seen since it would be underneath the peptide. It is now clear that these peptides are derived from a variety of cellular proteins that are continuously being degraded during the normal life cycle of the cell.

Structural polymorphism of the antigen-binding site. When allelic sequences of the murine and human class I molecules were aligned to that of HLA-A2, the positions in the sequence that showed the greatest polymorphism were seen to be clustered around the antigen-binding site. Of the polymorphic amino acid positions on HLA-A molecules, 15 out of 17 found on HLA-A2 were located in this area. The side chains of the amino acids found at the other two positions line small pockets that lie under the α-helices, and contact the side chains of bound peptides. This lends support to the hypothesis that polymorphisms have been selected by their

functional differences, based on their ability to present peptides to T-lymphocytes. The crystallographic structure also enabled the identification of the possible contributions of particular amino acid residues to peptide binding and/or contact with the T cell antigen receptor (TcR). Residues that are on the α-helical wall of the binding site have the potential to interact with both peptides and T cell receptors, and those on the β-pleated sheet floor will predominantly interact with the peptide alone. This view correlates well with data on the effects of amino acid substitutions in the antigen-binding site of MHC molecules on T cell recognition. These have been analyzed using substitutions that occur naturally in allelic molecules, or that were generated by site-directed mutagenesis at these positions. Loss of T cell recognition as a consequence of such substitutions implies that those positions are either involved in interaction with the peptide antigen, or with the T cell receptor.

As mentioned above, crystallographic analyses have been performed on three allelic HLA class I molecules to date as described above: HLA-A*0201 and HLA-A*6801 (see Table I for explanation of HLA nomenclature), which differ by 11 amino acids at the polymorphic residues that contribute to the antigen-binding groove (Garrett et al., 1989), and HLA-B*2705 (Madden et al., 1991). Not surprisingly, all three molecules have a very similar overall structure. However, differences were seen in the shape of the peptide-binding site in all three alleles, in particular the conformation of "*pockets*" that contain polymorphic residues in the antigen-binding site. These "pockets" vary in shape and charge, and are capable of binding to a different array of peptide fragments. In HLA-Aw68, a deep negatively charged pocket formed by the presence of Asp at position 74 (compared to His in HLA-A2) can be seen, and electron density representing peptide fragments can be seen to extend into this pocket. In the B27 molecule, side chains of the amino acids of the peptide make contact with pockets that are formed by positions 45, 74, 116, 152, and 156 of the HLA molecule. The HLA molecule can therefore determine the conformation of the bound peptide on the basis of these interactions, and particular peptide sequences may bind preferentially to individual HLA alleles. This hypothesis has been confirmed by sequencing of peptide fragments eluted from murine and human class I molecules, and is discussed in more detail in a later section.

In the context of an alloresponse against transplanted tissues, the display of a wide diversity of serum and cellular peptides, bound to cell surface MHC molecules, plays an important role (Lechler et al., 1990). This is illustrated by the finding that alloreactive T cells commonly distinguish between two MHC molecules that differ only in the floor of the peptide-binding groove. Since the TcR cannot make contact with amino acids in the floor of the groove of an MHC molecule, the most likely explanation for these findings is that such anti-MHC alloreactive T cells are specific for complexes of an allogeneic MHC molecule and a bound peptide that is bound by the stimulator, but not the responder MHC molecules.

Function of MHC Molecules

The strength of immune responses that are induced by foreign MHC molecules represents the major obstacle to successful tissue transplantation. Indeed, it was in the context of experimental transplantation that the MHC molecules were first discovered. However, the immunogenicity of MHC molecules merely reflects the central role that they play in immune recognition. The function of the molecules encoded by the genes of the MHC is to present microbial antigens to the individual's own T cells. A foreign antigen can be recognized by the T cells of that individual only if it is presented in the "context" of (physically bound to) that person's own MHC molecules. Thus the MHC molecule participates in a *trimolecular complex* of T cell receptor, peptide, and MHC molecule that is shown and discussed elsewhere (Davis and Bjorkman, 1988).

In this context, it is important to note another distinction between the two classes of MHC molecule, namely in the origin of the peptides that they bind (Germain, 1986). Class I molecules bind peptides in the endoplasmic reticulum (ER), shortly after the class I molecule has been synthesized by the cell. These class I-bound peptides are derived from cytoplasmic proteins that are proteolytically cleaved into small fragments by enzymes attached to proteasome complexes in the cytosol. The peptides are then actively transported into the ER by an energy-dependent transporter complex. It is of considerable interest that the genes encoding the proteasome and transporter complexes are located within the class II region of the MHC, as discussed below. The pathway of peptide loading onto class I molecules is referred to as the endogenous pathway. As mentioned above, the peptides that occupy class I molecules have recently been characterized and shown to be of remarkably homogeneous size. The large majority are 8–9 amino acids in length, some extend to 10 or 11 residues (Falk et al., 1991). In contrast, class II molecules appear to be loaded with peptides largely, if not exclusively, in the endosomal/lysosomal compartment of the cell. Most of these peptides are derived from cell membrane and extracellular proteins that are endocytosed by class II-bearing cells, and then cleaved into small fragments by the action of proteases in endosomes and lysosomes. The peptide-binding cleft of class II molecules accommodates peptides of larger size. The pathway of peptide loading onto class II molecules is referred to as the exogenous pathway. These two pathways are represented in schematic form in Figure 4.

The molecule that plays an important role in maintaining the discreteness of these two pathways is the *invariant (Ii)* chain. The Ii chain is a conserved glycoprotein that associates with newly synthesized class II molecules in the ER, and appears to have at least two functions. The first is to prevent peptide binding to class II $\alpha\beta$ dimers until the class II dimer reaches the endosomal compartment of the cell. The second is to target the class II molecule to the endosomal compartment.

The existence of these two pathways has an appealing logic, in that the consequence is that viral antigens are presented by class I molecules only by virus-infected cells that are synthesizing viral proteins in the cytoplasm. In contrast, class II molecules present peptides derived from internalized inert proteins such as inactivated virus

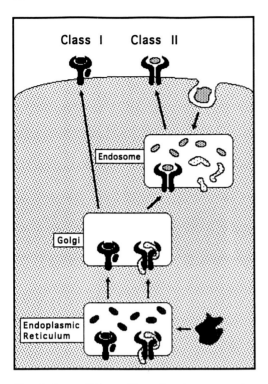

Class I   Class II

Endosome

Golgi

Endoplasmic
Reticulum

Fig. 4. Intracellular traffic and antigen processing. Different shadings have been used to represent MHC class I and class II molecules (black), invariant chain (white), exogenous antigen and fragments thereof (hatched), and endogenous antigen and fragments thereof (dotted). All elements are drawn schematically.

particles or shed viral proteins. Given that the majority of cytotoxic T cells are CD8+ and recognize antigens with MHC class I molecules, this arrangement targets their activity to virus-infected cells, leading to the eradication of such cells. Similarly the majority of helper T cells are CD4+ and recognize antigens with class II molecules, so that class II-expressing antigen-presenting cells that have internalized inert antigen are able to stimulate T cell help without becoming targets for cytotoxic T cell-mediated lysis.

Although it was known for several years that the expression of CD4 and CD8 molecules correlated with the specificity of T cell recognition for antigens with class II and class I molecules, respectively, the molecular basis of this correlation

was only established more recently. These two molecules interact with conserved sites on the membrane-proximal domains of the two classes of MHC molecule, and play an important role in the activation of T cells. It has been established recently that the CD4 and CD8 molecules are associated, intracellularly, with a tyrosine kinase enzyme, p56[lck] (Veilette et al., 1988)—see also Chapter 3. Ligation of the CD4 or CD8 molecule to class II or class I molecules leads to activation of this kinase. Together with the signals transduced as the result of TcR occupancy, this leads to phosphorylation of key elements of the CD3 complex, and the initiation of a cascade of second messengers, culminating in the transcription of genes responsible for mediating the T cell's effector function.

The Distribution of Expression of MHC Class I and II Molecules

Another important difference between the two classes of MHC molecule that has clear relevance to transplantation is that they have very different patterns of expression in the tissues of the body. HLA class I molecules are found on most somatic cells in man, although the level of expression varies from tissue to tissue. They are not detectable on the exposed surface of villous trophoblast, central nervous system neurons, corneal endothelium, and the exocrine portion of the pancreas, and only at low levels in endocrine tissue, myocardium, and skeletal muscle (Daar et al., 1984a).

The expression of class I molecules can be influenced both positively and negatively by many factors. Inflammatory mediators such as interferons, lymphokines, and cytokines increase expression of MHC class I products, and transformation of epithelial cells by viruses such as adenovirus 12 leads to decreased levels of class I expression (Andersson et al., 1985). Given the role of MHC class I molecules in the presentation of viral antigens, a virus-induced decrease in class I antigen expression may provide a mechanism for the virus to escape recognition by the host's immune system; in contrast, increased levels of class I expression may facilitate virus eradication. Increased expression of a protein at the cell surface can be due to multiple mechanisms such as increased transcription of mRNA, increased mRNA stability inside the cell, and changes in the rate of processing of mRNA following transcription. In the case of class I molecules, increased expression is usually accompanied by an increase in the amount of mRNA.

In comparison with class I molecules, the range of tissue expression of class II molecules is much more limited (Daar et al., 1984b), but on induction by cytokines, this tissue range becomes extensive. Class II molecules are present constitutively on the cell surfaces of B lymphocytes, monocytes, macrophages, and dendritic cells, which all have the common property of being antigen-presenting cells for T lymphocytes. In addition, class II molecules are also found on some vascular endothelium, various ductal epithelia (breast, gastrointestinal tract), and kidney glomeruli. The distribution of expression of the two classes of MHC molecule is summarized in Table II.

Quantitative differences in the cell surface expression of the different class II isotypes are also seen. For example, DR is generally present in much greater quantities than DQ and DP. This pattern is not always found, and cell lines derived from lymphomas and leukaemias have been shown to express DP or DQ in the absence of DR (Lee, 1989; Symington et al., 1985).

Table IIA. HLA Class I Antigens and Their Expression

Antigen	Distribution
Classical	
HLA-A	
HLA-B	Present on most nucleated cells; low expression by myocardium, and skeletal muscle; not detected on CNS neurons and villous trophoblast
HLA-C	
Nonclassical	
HLA-E	Resting peripheral T cells
HLA-F	Not known
HLA-G	Chorionic cytotrophoblast

Table IIB. Tissue Distribution of HLA-DR Antigen Expression

Constitutive expression	Induced expression
Macrophage	Vascular endothelium
B cell	Gut epithelium
Dendritic cell	Dermal fibroblasts
Thymic epithelium	Melanocytes
	Astrocytes, Schwann cells
	T cells
	Thyroid follicular epithelium
	Synovial lining cells

Expression can be augmented or induced (in the case of class II negative tissues) by cytokines and stimuli that activate cells. The best studied is interferon-γ (IFN-γ), which has been shown to induce class II expression in fibroblasts, T cells, vascular endothelium, thymic epithelium, and a range of other tissues (reviewed in Klareskog and Forsum, 1986). Tumor necrosis factor-α (TNF-α) also increases class II expression on monocytes and macrophages, and it acts synergistically with IFN-γ (Arenzana-Seisdedos et al., 1988). The increase in surface expression is parallelled by increases in the levels of mRNA transcription.

The induction of expression of class II genes by cytokines may have some relevance to the pathogenesis of autoimmune disease and to the evolution of graft rejection, as histopathological studies have demonstrated "aberrant expression" of class II molecules in many sites of disease (Bottazzo et al., 1983). These include thyroid epithelium in Grave's disease, synovial lining cells in rheumatoid arthritis, biliary duct epithelium in primary biliary cirrhosis, and renal allografts undergoing transplant rejection. Although the mechanisms responsible for the induction of expression of MHC class II genes in these tissues have not been entirely worked out, IFN-γ is presumed to play an important role.

Immune Response Gene Effects

The significance of sequence variation between allelic subtypes of MHC molecules lies in the influence that it has an immune responsiveness to individual antigenic determinants. It was first noted in the late 1960s that genetically controlled differences existed in the magnitude of immune response following the immunization of inbred strains of animals. These phenomena were observed in guinea pigs (Benacerraf et al., 1967) and in inbred mouse strains (Mitchell et al., 1972). The genes responsible for this variation were called *immune response (Ir)* genes. It was some years later that it became clear that Ir genes were, in most cases, one and the same as MHC genes. The definition of these effects in outbred human populations is much more difficult, but several HLA-linked examples have been described (Sasazuki et al., 1989; Gotch et al., 1987; Hill et al., 1991). This kind of HLA-linked immune response variation provides a very attractive mechanism to account for many HLA-linked diseases. Three major mechanisms to account for Ir gene effects have been characterized over the past 10 years. These are discussed in turn below, and will be related to disease associations in a subsequent chapter.

Determinant selection. The concept from which this term derives is that individual MHC molecules "select" the "determinants" of an antigen that are displayed to T cells restricted by that MHC molecule. The simplest way in which to visualize this selection operating is as the result of differing abilities of particular MHC types to bind and present individual antigenic peptides.

It became possible to test this theory directly when methods were developed to measure the physical association of peptides with MHC molecules. The first examples that were studied using equilibrium dialysis, as described above, demonstrated a clear correlation between the efficiency of MHC molecule/peptide association and known Ir gene effects for the peptide in question (Babbitt et al., 1985). In other words, an MHC molecule that bound the peptide under investigation efficiently was commonly used as a restriction element by T cells specific for that peptide, and the converse was equally true. The concept of allele-specific patterns of peptide binding to MHC molecules has been well supported by the definition of naturally processed peptides, as discussed above. Little overlap was seen between the peptides eluted from the various class I molecules that have been studied. The data of Hill et al. (1992) are of particular interest in this regard, in that having observed a striking overrepresentation of the HLA class I type Bw53 in Zambia, an area where malaria is prevalent, they went on to show that the immunodominant peptide derived from a sporozite protein bound preferentially to Bw53. This is an outstanding example of determinant selection having a clearcut effect on immune protection against an environmental agent.

However, there are well-documented instances in which there is no correlation between the ability of a peptide to associate with an MHC product and its recognition with that MHC molecule. This is reviewed by Buus et al. (1987). Clearly other mechanisms underlie some Ir gene effects, as discussed below.

Holes in the T cell repertoire. Bearing in mind the extensive deletion of differentiating thymocytes with self-reactive specificities, it might be predicted that "gaps" or "holes" may be created in the exported repertoire of T cells, that manifest as a failure to recognize some extrinsic antigens. It would be predicted that the dominant genetic factor leading to the presence of such gaps would be the inheritance of individual MHC alleles. Long before current concepts of the trimolecular complex of TcR, MHC molecule and peptide had evolved, Mullbacher et al. (1981) described an Ir gene effect that appeared to be best accounted for by the existence of a hole in the repertoire. They observed that in $(b \times s) F_1$ mice the cytotoxic T cell response to the male-specific minor transplantation antigen H-Y was almost entirely restricted by H-2^s class I molecules, and the H-2^b-restricted response to H-Y was barely detectable. In contrast, homozygous H-2^b mice were able to generate strong H-Y-specific responses. In other words the presence of H-2^s-encoded MHC molecules in some way caused a marked reduction in the H-2^b-restricted response to H-Y. The clue to the mechanism underlying this phenomenon was provided by studying H-2^b-restricted, H-Y-specific T cells raised from homozygous H-2^b mice. T cells with this specificity turned out to cross react strongly on allogeneic H-2^s cells in the absence of the male-specific antigen. These data suggest that H-2^s class I molecules, as expressed in the thymus, mimic H-2^b + H-Y, and that as a consequence T cells with the potential for recognizing H-2^b + H-Y are deleted in the thymus of (b × s) F_1 mice, because of autoreactivity against H-2^s class I molecules. These were very elegant experiments, however limited additional examples exist in support of holes in the repertoire as a mechanism of Ir gene effects. This probably reflects the fact that designing suitable experiments is far from easy, rather than that this is an unimportant mechanism.

T cell-mediated suppression. The third major mechanism proposed to account for MHC-linked Ir gene effects invokes active regulation of potentially reactive cells by a population of cells whose specialist function is to suppress antigen reactivity. The idea that cells existed whose function it is to suppress an immune response was first proposed by Gershon in 1974. Such cells would be the opposite of helper T cells, and would act to prevent unwanted immunity, and perhaps serve to make immune responses self-limiting. A huge literature has accumulated on the subject of "suppressor cells" over the past 20 years, and many immunologists have traveled up a number of blind alleys. Nonetheless, there are some very clearcut, and reproducible examples of genetically determined nonresponsiveness that appears to result from the action of suppressor cells with a T cell phenotype (Ts).

Some of the clearest evidence in support of the existence of specialized Ts has been derived from experimental models of organ transplantation. Several groups have reported the observation that animals carrying an established kidney or heart allograft possess Ts, which can be adoptively transferred to a naive syngeneic recipient and provide protection for a freshly transplanted graft from the same strain as the graft residing in the Ts donor (Brent et al., 1982; Marquet et al., 1982). These cells are specific for the donor strain, and have been variously reported to be of the CD4 and of the CD8 phenotype.

Although these examples provide strong support for the existence of suppressor T cells, many questions about Ts remain unresolved. The major uncertainty is about their specificity. Until stable clones of Ts are obtained that can be characterized in detail, this issue will remain unresolved. The minimalist view of suppressor phenomena is that they are mediated passively by antigen-specific T cells that have been rendered tolerant, but retain cell surface receptor expression. It has been argued that such cells have the capacity to compete for the available antigen: MHC molecule complexes, and thus deprive potentially reactive T cells from obtaining sufficient productive interactions to be activated. The attraction of this hypothesis is that imposes no requirement for a separate population of T cells with distinct specificities or effector functions.

A related perspective is that suppressor cells are simply a population of T cells with entirely overlapping specificity with conventional helper cells, but that the distinctive feature of suppressor cells is that they secrete a cocktail of lymphokines that is inhibitory to neighboring T cells. This suggestion has received support from the recent elucidation of two subpopulations of CD4$^+$ T cells that are characterized by the secretion of different cocktails of cytokines. One subpopulation, referred to as the T helper 1 (Th1) subset, secrete predominantly interleukin 2 (IL-2) and IFN-γ; the other subpopulation secretes predominantly IL-4 and IL-10 and is referred to as the Th2 subset. The relevance of these findings to the phenomena of suppression is that the cytokines secreted by these two subpopulations of cells regulate the activities of the other subpopulation. For example, IL-4 and IL-10 inhibit the secretion of IL-2, and IFN-γ inhibits the secretion of IL-4. These observations and their potential *in vivo* relevance are reviewed by Fowell and colleagues (Fowell et al., 1991).

Genetics of the HLA Region

The HLA genes that make up the MHC in humans are found on the short arm of chromosome 6 and are included within approximately three recombinational units from the most centromeric locus, DP, to the most telomeric one, HLA-A. In molecular terms, there are approximately 3700 kilobases from one end of the MHC to the other.

A simplified genetic map of the HLA system was shown in Figure 1. Indicated are the genes that encode what are known to be transplantation antigens, including both class I and class II genes. The protein products of the various genes are also indicated. For the class I genes, the HLA-A, -B, and -C loci encode the heavy chain of the class I molecules. For the class II genes, the products of the A genes of each family (DR, DQ and DP) combine with the products of the B genes of the same family to make the protein γβ heterodimers that are the class II products. (The class II genes are referred to by the suffix A or B, encoding α or β chains, respectively.)

In reality, the HLA complex, even with regard to class I and class II genes is much more complex, as shown in Figure 5 (for reviews see Trowsdale and Campbell, 1993). For our purposes, however, the genes that are expressed as cell surface molecules and that can function as transplantation antigens are the most important. (The class III genes, encoding components of the complement system, are between the class I and class II genes.)

Within the class II region the DR gene family is the most complicated in two respects. First, most haplotypes carry two expressed B genes, but only one expressed A gene. The two β chains encoded by the two DRB genes both pair with the product of the single DRA gene to give rise to two DR αβ dimers. Second, the DRB genes that are expressed on different haplotypes can be products of different loci. Thus, in haplotypes that encode the DR15 antigens, the two ex-

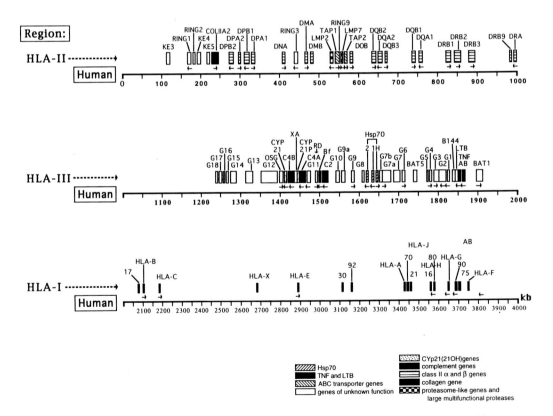

Fig. 5. A detailed map of the HLA region. From Campbell and Trowsdale (1993), with kind permission of the publisher.

pressed β chains are encoded by the DRB1 and DRB5 genes; in contrast, on the haplotypes encoding the DR3, DR11, DR12, DR13, and DR14 specificities, the DRB1 and DRB3 genes are expressed. The expression of DRB genes on different haplotypes is illustrated diagrammatically in Figure 6.

All of the class II genes, with the exception of DRA, are polymorphic, although the degree of polymorphism varies. Based largely on DNA sequence analysis, the different genes, and thus proteins, that are associated with each locus were given in Table I. An additional level of complexity is created by the possibility of the expression of haplotype- and isotype-mismatched αβ dimers. This refers to the assembly of an α chain encoded on one haplotype with the β chain from the second haplotype in a heterozygous individual (e.g., DQa2DQb7), or to the assembly of two chains encoded by the genes of two different class II loci (e.g., DRaDQb). The cell surface expression of haplotype-mismatched αβ dimers of mouse I-A and human DQ molecules has been clearly demonstrated (Beck et al., 1981; Kwok et al., 1992). In addition, the expression of an isotype-mismatched class II molecule has

been described in mice, and the same molecule has been shown to function as a restriction element *in vivo*. It is less clear whether isotype-mismatched human class II molecules are expressed at levels sufficient to influence T cell recognition. As a consequence of these pairing possibilities, the number of different expressed class II molecules in a heterozygous individual is likely to be approximately 12. The possible class II dimers that can be expressed in a heterozygous individual are shown in Figure 7.

Another important feature of the HLA region is *linkage disequilibrium* between the loci. This linkage extends from the HLA-A locus near the telomeric end of the HLA region, to the DQ locus that is near to the centromeric end. There is very little disequilibrium between all of these genes and the DP genes. The consequence of linkage disequilibrium is that given alleles of HLA-A, -B, -DR, and -DQ are found on the same haplotype significantly more often than would be predicted from the frequencies of these four genes within the study population. This leads to the inheritance of haplotypes, "en block." It is also notable that some haplotypes are highly represented in particular populations,

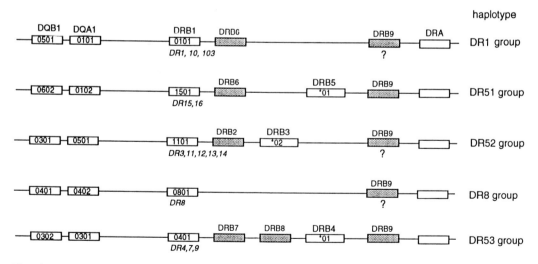

Fig. 6. Common HLA haplotypes and linkage disequilibrium between HLA-DR and -DQ alleles. The nomenclature of HLA alleles is used (Bodmer et al., 1992). The alleles of the DRB1, DQA1, and DQB1 loci are shown within the appropriate boxes. Shaded boxes indicate pseudogenes. The alleles of the other DRB loci, which are expressed on different haplotypes, are shown within the appropriates boxes. The question marks under DRB9 genes on three haplotypes indicate that its presence on these haplotypes has to be confirmed.

Haplotype-mismatched MHC class II heterodimers

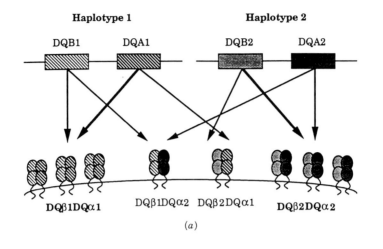

(a)

Isotype-mismatched MHC class II heterodimers

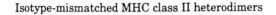
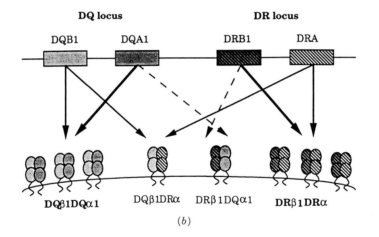

(b)

Fig. 7. (a) The four possible DQ heterodimers that can be expressed at the cell surface of a DQ heterozygous, class II positive cell are represented. As indicated by the bold arrows, and the larger number of class II dimers, *cis* pairing is favored over *trans* pairing. As discussed in the text, the extent of haplotype-mismatched assembly and expression is determined by the class II alleles carried by the two haplotypes. (**b**) The possible isotype-mismatched class II heterodimers that can arise from the α and β chains encoded at the DR and DQ loci are shown. As discussed in the text, evidence exits for the cell surface expression of DRβDQα, however, no evidence exists to suggest that the reciprocal dimer can be expressed. As for the expression of haplotype-mismatched dimers, the assembly and expression of isotype-mismatched dimers appear to be influenced by allelic polymorphism in the class II molecules.

for example, the HLA-A1, B8, and DR3 haplotypes are found in as many as 10% of Northern European caucasians, but in less than 1% of the Chinese populations. The probable explanation for such findings is that certain haplotypes conferred protection from prevalent infectious agents at some earlier point in history.

Definition of HLA Antigens—HLA Typing

Given in Table I is the current list of alleles of each of the major HLA genes, as defined by the last HLA nomenclature committee. Polymorphisms were originally defined *serologically.* This was then supplemented by *cellular* (T lymphocyte)-based methods. More recently, polymorphism is being defined by a variety of *molecular* techniques, the most detailed definition being provided by the accumulation of nucleotide sequences of HLA genes.

Serological methods. Multiparous women, who have had several children, often become immunized to antigens on cells of the fetus that are inherited from the father and foreign to the mother. Sera (containing anti-HLA antibodies) can be tested on lymphocytes of any given individual by a number of tests. Most commonly, a complement-dependent lymphocytoxicity test is used. If the serum has one or more antibodies in it that recognize(s) a given HLA antigen, then that serum, plus others recognizing the same antigen, can be used to define that antigen. By having many such sera with known anti-HLA specificity, it is possible to define HLA antigens on the cells of most individuals. As the consequence of an international cooperation over the past three decades panels of sera have been collected and analyzed that enable the definition of many of the HLA antigens on cells of white caucasian subjects; however, our ability to do so in blacks and other races is far less developed.

The class I antigens are readily defined in this manner, however, this approach has serious limitations. First, the antisera used to recognize the various antigens can actually contain several different antibodies specific for more than one HLA antigen. Second, much of the sequence variation between different MHC molecules lies in the floor of the peptide-binding cleft of the molecule, inaccessible to antibodies. As a consequence, antibodies are unable to discriminate between a considerable number of MHC types with "buried" differences. The result of these limitations is that there has been a process of "splitting" of antigens that were defined by earlier serological reagents. This has been the result of acquiring new alloantisera that discriminate between subtypes of an earlier serotype, the application of alloreactive T cells to the definition of HLA antigens, and the sequencing of large numbers of HLA alleles. Thus, what was initially considered to be a single antigenic type can now be split into several newly defined antigens.

Class I HLA molecules are present on resting T cells, and since class II antigens are not, these cells can, and are, used to test anti-class I sera, and for routine serological HLA typing. The class II antigens are much more difficult to evaluate serologically, and even in the best laboratories, the error rate is considerable. The class II antigens are present on relatively few types of cells; in clinical testing they are usually measured on peripheral B cells.

Cellular methods—assay of class II antigens.

The *mixed leukocyte culture (MLC) test* (Bach and Hirschhorn, 1964; Bain et al., 1964) (see also Chapter 5) was in part devised to measure histocompatibility between different individuals. The test was first based on mixing leukocytes of two individuals and assessing the proliferative response, as measured by incorporation of radioactive thymidine into the responding (dividing) T cells. Since it was one purpose of the test to measure the response of a potential recipient's T cells (called the responding cells) to alloantigens present on the cells of a potential donor (the stimulating cells), a one-way MLC test was developed that allowed this. Cells of the potential donor were irradiated so that they could still present their antigens and yet could not divide.

Genetic studies demonstrated that the MLC test, in terms of proliferative responses, was a measure of HLA-D incompatibility, the region of HLA that includes what we now know to be the DR, DQ, and DP antigens. While the one-way MLC test allowed the biologically meaningful quantitation of overall disparity between two individuals with regard to HLA-D, it did not allow definition of individual HLA-D antigens carried by those individuals.

To do this, cells of individuals homozygous for HLA-D were used as the stimulating cells. Groups of such *homozygous typing cells (HTCs)* were used to define a number of HLA-D region associated "antigens," which were referred to as *HLA-Dw* specificities.

Even with what was clearly a rather crude approach to definition of the class II antigens, the use of HTCs in MLC allowed the splitting of the serologically defined antigens, as described above for class I antigens. Thus, as just one example, individuals expressing the serologically defined specificity DR4 could be divided into those that expressed one of five Dw specificities associated with DR4: Dw4, 10, 13, 14, or 15. This finer dissection by T cells seemed important not only with regard to a better understanding of polymorphism of the class II genes, but also because for transplantation it was likely that the antigens recognized by T cells, which would cause rejection of a transplant, were the important ones.

Clearly these Dw specificities were really measuring the composite response against antigens associated with all the class II products, thus other tests were developed in an attempt to define individual class II antigens by the response of T cells. One of these was the primed lymphocyte (LD) typing test; a further refinement used alloreactive T cell clones directed at given class II antigens. However, with the exception of the HTC testing, none of these tests became of great use at the patient level, largely because of the technical complexities of growing, maintaining, and using T cell reagents.

The molecular basis of the T cell response to alloantigens is begin increasingly understood. It would seem that the TcR on the recipient's responding T cells actually recognizes to the complex of an alloantigen containing one of the large diversity of MHC-bound peptides derived from cellular or serum proteins. The importance of the peptide in this recognitive process was referred to above, and is discussed in more detail in Chapter 4.

Cellular methods—assay of class I antigens. As reviewed in Chapter 5, CD4$^+$ Th respond preferentially to class II antigens whereas CD8$^+$ Tc respond to class I antigens. Tc were used to measure or define class I antigens. As with Th and the class II antigens, the Tc were able to recognize subtypes of serologically defined class I antigens. Although this was of interest with regard to understanding polymorphism of the MHC loci, Tc never became reagents that were broadly applied to defining class I antigens clinically, again because of the technical difficulty of working with T cells.

Molecular methods. With the advent and more generalized usage of molecular techniques, HLA polymorphism is increasingly being defined by these methods. Three are worthy of note: restriction fragment length polymorphism analysis, sequence-specific oligomer probing, and sequence-specific oligomer amplification (see Chapter 21 for a detailed description of the molecular methods and their basis).

Restriction fragment length polymorphism analysis. The technique and rationale of *restriction fragment length polymorphism (RFLP)* analysis is discussed in Chapter 21 on molecular biology. In brief, however, RFLP typing depends on the use of restriction enzymes that cut the DNA at specific sequences. Depending on the sequences of the DNA on both sides of, and within, a given class II B gene, for instance, the length of the fragment including the B gene will vary.

Because the haplotypes on which the different class II genes are found have multiple differences in the sequences of the DNA, not only within the genes encoding the class II molecules, but also in the intervening sequences between the genes as well as in the introns within the gene in question, a given restriction enzyme may well cut at different places in the different haplotypes. The size of the DNA fragments on which a given class II gene is found in the different haplotypes, following digestion by a variety of different restriction enzymes, will vary. It is possible, by using several different restriction enzymes, to correlate the lengths of the DNA fragments on which the various class II genes are found with the particular genes.

Thus, different patterns of DNA fragments when analyzed by size on a gel, correlate with different DR and DQ specificities. This method, however, provides limited information in that many alleles, such as the subtypes of DR4, cannot be differentiated by the known restriction enzymes based on the very limited sequence variation that exists. The method thus is no longer used to any significant extent in defining HLA genes, although it may help to confirm the results of serological typing of the HLA class II alleles.

Oligomer typing. One of the major technical innovations of recent years in molecular biology has been the development of the *polymerase chain reaction (PCR)*. This allows the rapid amplification of segments of genes, without the need for the laborious process of cDNA or genomic cloning. The details of the PCR technique for DNA amplification are illustrated in Chapter 21. PCR-based techniques have been widely applied in the field of HLA class II typing, although it is likely that similar approaches will prove to be applicable to class I typing within the next few years.

Shown in Figure 8 are nucleotide and amino acid sequences of portions of several class II genes and their products, including the polymorphic variable regions (VRs). The purpose of *oligomer typing* is to synthesize nucleotide oligomers that are complementary to the VRs of the various genes and to use these to differentiate between all the known genes in the population so that the HLA genotype of any one individual can be determined. This can be achieved in two ways. The first uses oligonucleotides as sequence-specific probes (SSP) on segments of HLA class II genes that have been PCR-amplified using oligomer primers that correspond to sequences that are conserved in all the alleles of the genetic locus under investigation. A panel of radiolabeled sequence-specific oligomers is then used to "probe" the immobilized PCR-amplified DNA. Oligomers will hybridize with the PCR products that carry complementary sequence. To differentiate any one gene from all

others in the population, it is necessary in some cases to use more than a single oligomer. This is because cassettes of sequence in the polymorphic regions of the genes are shared by different HLA class II alleles. While one oligomer should differentiate between one given sequence and many others, it may be necessary to use a second probe to provide a definitive answer. The use of multiple oligomers should provide a unique pattern of hybridization for each HLA type.

The second approach involves the use of oligonucleotides as sequence-specific primers (SSP) in a PCR amplification. The basis of this technique is that a fraction of the DNA sample to be typed is placed into 20 different test tubes with two PCR oligomer primers. One of the PCR primers corresponds to a conserved stretch of sequence in the gene under examination, and this is added to all tubes. A different, sequence-specific, second oligomer is added to each tube. After allowing the PCR amplification to occur, the contents of each tube are run on a gel. An amplified product will be seen only when the sequence-specific oligomer primer corresponds to the type of the DNA sample. One of the advantages of this second technique is that a result can be obtained within a few hours. This is clearly an important consideration when typing cadaveric donors for transplantation.

Non-HLA Genes within the HLA Region

As illustrated in Figure 5, there is a very large number of genes within the HLA region, in addition to those encoding the classical class I and class II molecules, making this the most densely populated area in the mammalian genome. Several of the genes in the class III region encoding components of the complement pathway, the 21-hydroxylase enzyme and the tumor necrosis factor proteins, were mapped to this location some years ago. In the past 3 years it has become apparent that many additional genes are located in the class I and class III regions. The functions of most of these genes have not yet been identified, however several genes encoding proteins with obvious relevance to the immune response have been characterized. The gene encoding the 70-

DRB Protein Sequences

```
              1    10   20   30   40   50   60   70   80   90   100
              .    .    .    .    .    .    .    .    .    .    .
DRB1*0101   GDTRPRFLWQLKFECHFFNGTERVRLLERCIYNQEESVRFDSDVGEYRAVTELGRPDAEYWNSQKDLLEQRRAAVDTYCRHNYGVGESFTVQRRVEPKVTVY
DRB1*0102   --------------------------------------------------------------------------------AV------------------
DRB1*0103   -----------------------------------------------------------------I--DE-------------------------------
DRB1*0104   ************--------------------------------------------------------N----------V-********************
DRB1*1501   ---------P-R------------F-D-YF---------------F------------------I--A---------V---------Q------
DRB1*1502   ---------P-R------------F-D-YF---------------F------------------I--A---------V---------Q------
DRB1*1503   *****-----P-R------------F-D-HF---------------F------------------I--A---------V---------*******
DRB1*1601   ---------P-R------------F-D-YF------------------------------------F-D---------------------Q------
DRB1*1602   ---------P-R------------F-D-YF-----------------------------------D-------------------------Q------
DRB1*1603   ---------P-R------------F-D-YF-----------------------------------F-D-A---------------------Q------
DRB1*03011  -------EYSTS----------Y-D-YFH---N-----F-------------------K-GR--N------V---------H-----
DRB1*03012  ************----------Y-D-YFH---N-----F-------------------K-GR--N------V*****************
DRB1*0302   --------EYSTS----------F---YFH---N-----------------------K-GR--N------------H-----
DRB1*0303   *********YSTS----------F---YFH---N-----------------------K-GR--N------V---------*******
DRB1*0401   --------E-V-H----------F-D-YF-H---Y----------------------K----------------Y-E----
DRB1*0402   --------E-V-H----------F-D-YF-H---Y-------------------I--DE-----------V---------*******
DRB1*0403   --------E-V-H----------F-D-YF-H--Y------------------------E-----------V---------Y-E----
DRB1*0404   --------E-V-H----------F-D-YF-H--Y-----------------------------------V---------Y-E----
DRB1*0405   --------E-V-H----------F-D-YF-H--Y---------------S-----------------------------*******
DRB1*0406   --------E-V-H----------F-D-YF-H-------------------------E-----------V---------Y-E----
DRB1*0407   --------E-V-H----------F-D-YF-H--Y-------------------------E-----------------*******
DRB1*0408   ************----------F-D-YF-H--Y--------------------------------------********
DRB1*0409   **************--------F-D-YF-H--Y---------------S----------K----------********
DRB1*0410   ******--E-V-H----------F-D-YF-H--Y---------------S----------------------V---*********
DRB1*0411   ******--E-V-H----------F-D-YF-H--Y---------------S----------E-----------V---*********
DRB1*0412   ******--E-V-H----------F-D-YF-H--Y---------------S---------I--D---L------V---*********
DRB1*0413   ************H----------F-D-YF-H--Y-----------------------K----------V---*********
DRB1*0414   ************----------F-D-YF-H--Y------------------------I--DE-----------V---*********
DRB1*0415   *****---E-V-H----------F-D-YF-H--Y------E-----------F-D----------*********
DRB1*0416   ************----------F-D-YF-H--Y-----Q-----------K----------V---*********
DRB1*11011  -------EYSTS----------F-D-YF-----Y-----F-------E-----------F-D---------------H-----
DRB1*11012  -------EYSTS----------F-D-YF-----Y-----F-------E-----------F-D---------------H----*
DRB1*1102   --------EYSTS----------F-D-YF-----Y-----F-------E-----------I--DE---------------H-----
DRB1*1103   --------EYSTS----------F-D-YF-----Y-----F-------E-----------I--DE---------------H-----
DRB1*11041  --------EYSTS----------F-D-YF-----Y-----F-------E-----------F-D---------------V---*******
DRB1*11042  --------EYSTS----------F-D-YF-----Y-----F-------E-----------F-D---------------V---H-----
DRB1*1105   ****----EYSTG----------F-D-YF-----Y-----F-------E-----------F-D---------------*******
DRB1*1106   *****---EYSTS----------F-D-YF-----Y-----F-------E-----------F-D---------AV----*********
DRB1*1201   --------EYSTG--Y-------------HFH----LL-----F-------V--S------I--D---------AV------H-----
DRB1*1202   *****---EYSTG--Y-------------HFH----LL-----F-------V--S------I--D---------AV******************
DRB1*1301   --------EYSTS----------F-D-YFH---N-----F-------------------I--DE-----------V---------H-----
DRB1*1302   --------EYSTS----------F-D-YFH---N-----F-------------------I--DE-----------*********
DRB1*1303   --------EYSTS----------F-D-YF-----Y---------------S---------I--DK---------------H----*
DRB1*1304   --------EYSTS----------F-D-YF-----Y---------------S---------I--DE-----------V---------H----*
DRB1*1305   *****---EYSTS----------F-D-YFH---N-----F-------------------F-D---------------*********
DRB1*1306   **************--------F-D-YFH---N-----F-------------------I--D-----------V---*********
DRB1*1307   ******--EYSTS----------F-D-YF-----Y-------------------------I--D---------------*********
DRB1*1308   ******--EYSTS----------F-D-YFH----F-------------------------I--DE-----------V---*********
DRB1*1401   --------EYSTS----------F-D-YFH----F--------A--H---------R---E-----------V---*********
DRB1*1402   --------EYSTS----------F---YFH----N-----------------------------------------*********
DRB1*1403   --------EYSTS----------F---YFH----N--------------------------D--L------------------
DRB1*1404   *****---EYSTG--Y-------F-D-YFH----F--------A--H---------R---E-----------V---*********
DRB1*1405   ******--EYSTS--Q-------F-D-YFH----F-----------------------R---E-----------*********
DRB1*1406   ********EYSTS----------F---YFH----N-----------------------R---E-----------V---*********
DRB1*1407   ********EYSTS----------F-D-YFH----F--------A--H---------R---E-----------*********
DRB1*1408   ******--EYSTS----------F-D-YFH----F-----------------------H---------R---E-----------V---*********
DRB1*1409   ******--EYSTS----------F-D-YFH----N-----------------------H---------R---E-----------V---*********
DRB1*1410   ******--E-V-H----------F-D-YFH----F--------A--H---------R---E-----------V---*********
DRB1*1411   ********EYSTG--Y-------F-D-YFH----F-----------------------E-----------R---E-----------V*****************
DRB1*0701   ---Q------G-YK----------QF---LF-----F-----------------V--S------I--D-GQ--V-----------------H-E----
DRB1*0702   ---Q------G-YK----------QF---LF-----F-----------------V--S------I--D-GQ--V-----------------H-E----
DRB1*0801   --------EYSTG--Y-------F-D-YF-----Y---------------S---------F-D--L------------*********
DRB1*08021  --------EYSTG--Y-------F-D-YF-----Y-----------------------F-D--L---------------H-----
DRB1*08022  *****---EYSTG--Y-------F-D-YF-----Y-----------------------F-D--L---------------H-----
DRB1*08031  *****---EYSTG--Y-------F-D-YF-----Y---------------S---------I--D--L---------------H-----
DRB1*08032  --------EYSTG--Y-------F-D-YF-----Y---------------S---------I--D--L---------------*******
DRB1*0804   --------EYSTG--Y-------F-D-YF-----Y-----------------------F-D--L------V---------H----*
DRB1*0805   *****---EYSTG--Y-------F-D-YF-----Y---------------S---------F-D--L------------*********
DRB1*0806   ****----EYSTG--Y-------F-D-YF-----Y---------------S---------F-D--L------V*****************
DRB1*09011  *******************-------Y-H-G-------N-----------------V--S------F-R---E---V------------H-E----
DRB1*09012  ---Q----K-D------------Y-H-G-------N-----------------V--S------F-R---E---V------*****************
DRB1*1001   --------EEV------------RVH----YA-Y-----------------------R------------------Q------
DRB3*0101   --------ELR-S----------Y-D-YFH----FL-----------------V--S---------K-GR--N--------H-Q----
DRB3*0201   --------EL--S----------F---HFH----YA--------R----------------------K-GQ--N-------V--------H-Q----
DRB3*0202   --------EL--S----------F---HFH----YA--------R----------------------K-GQ--N-------V--------H-Q----
DRB3*0301   --------EL--S----------F---YFH----F----------------V--S----------K-GQ--N-------V--------H-Q----
DRB4*0101   ---Q----E-A-C----L------WN-I-Y-------YA-YN--L---Q---------------------R--E---------Y---V------Q------
DRB4*0102   ********************---WN-I-Y-------YA-YN--L---Q---------------------R--E-G----Y---V------*********
DRB5*0101   --------Q-D-Y----------F-H-D----DL-------------------------F-D-------------------------
DRB5*0102   --------Q-D-Y----------F-H-G-------N-----------------------F-D-------------------------
DRB5*0201   -----C--Q-D-Y----------F-H-G-------N------------------------I---A-----------AV-----
DRB5*0202   -----C--Q-D-Y----------F-H-G-------N------------------------I---A-----------AV-----
DRB5*0203   ******--Q-D-Y----------F-H-G-------N------------------------I---A-----------*********
```

kDa *heat shock protein* (*Hsp 70*) lies between the class III and class I regions. It is thought that the Hsp 70 molecule plays a role in the folding and transport of molecules inside cells, and could therefore influence the presentation of intracellular antigens.

Arguably the most interesting newly discovered genes in the HLA complex are found in a cluster between the *DNA* and *DOB* loci (see Fig. 6). Two of these genes encode a *peptide-transporter complex* that is inserted into the endoplasmic reticulum (ER) of the cell. This *TAP 1* and *2* complex is a member of a family of ATP-dependent transporters, and appears to have the function of moving peptides from the cytoplasm of the cell into the ER. This is the site at which class I molecules are loaded with peptides, as discussed in an earlier section of this chapter. The vital role played by this TAP complex is illustrated by several mutant B cell lines that are defective in their TAP complex. These cell lines have almost no cell surface class I expression, and are unable to present antigens with their class I molecules.

The other two genes in this cluster encode two components of the *proteasome complex,* low-molecular proteins (LMP) 2 and 7. The proteasomes are responsible for the degradation of intracellular proteins; and LMP 2 and 7 form part of these multisubunit complexes. There is little evidence, as yet, that the presence or absence of the LMP 2 and 7 proteins influences antigen presentation, although this may reflect the particular experimental systems that have been studied.

Particular interest has been aroused by the finding that these four genes are polymorphic. Between two and seven alleles have been described in man. There is no evidence, as yet, that the sequence variation between the human alleles is of functional significance, however two alleles of the TAP 2 gene have been defined in the rat that give rise to substantial differences in

immune recognition. The molecular basis of these differences has not yet been determined, but may reflect the ability of the two Tap alleles to load class I molecules with different peptides. The possibility that similar differences may be seen in man is of considerable interest to those interested in autoimmune and alloimmune responses.

MINOR HISTOCOMPATIBILITY ANTIGENS

In Vivo and *In Vitro* Definitions

All histocompatibility (H) antigens were originally identified by graft rejection (Snell, 1948). Once the major histocompatibility antigens eliciting the most rapid graft rejection were defined as products of the HLA locus or complex in humans and H-2 in mice (Gorer et al., 1948; Ceppellini et al., 1969), it was clear that there were many additional loci encoding other "minor" histocompatibility antigens which caused graft rejection between donor–recipient pairs matched for MHC antigens. In mice, breeding experiments allowed segregation of individual minor H loci and development of congenic strains differing single minor H loci (Bailey, 1975). Studies using these mice showed that while antigens encoded by many single loci were indeed weak, eliciting prolonged graft rejection times, differences at multiple minor loci could stimulate rejection almost as rapid as that against MHC antigens, i.e., their effects were additive or even synergistic. This is apparent in humans from the development of severe graft-versus-host (gvh) disease in recipients of bone marrow transplants from HLA identical siblings (Van Els et al., 1990a, 1990b). In such cases, there are always multiple minor H differences except between monozygotic twins. Kidney transplant patients receiving grafts from HLA-identical siblings do much better than recipients of HLA-mismatched grafts but they still require immunosuppression because of host-versus-graft (hvg) response against minor H incompatibilities.

In vivo hvg and gvh responses to histoincompatible tissue are mediated predominantly by T lymphocytes. B lymphocytes also make anti-

---

Fig. 8. Amino acid sequences of the first domain of the DRβ1 chains of different haplotypes, showing the three hypervariable regions. Dashes signify sharing of amino acids with the sequence given at the top of the figure.

bodies to MHC antigens and serological studies were of great importance in the early investigations of the genetics of the MHC and their biochemical characterization, culminating in the crystal structure (Bjorkman et al., 1987a, 1987b). T cell responses to histocompatibility antigens can also be obtained *in vitro*. Against MHC antigens, primary mixed lymphocyte reactions (MLR) occur, characterized by proliferation of CD4$^+$ T cells against MHC class II disparities and the development of CD8$^+$ cytotoxic T cells specific for class I disparities. MLR against minor H antigens can be obtained using responder T cells from individuals immunized *in vivo* by grafting or with spleen cells expressing the relevant antigen (Gordon et al., 1975; Bevan, 1975). No antibodies are made to minor H antigens. However, CD4$^+$ and CD8$^+$ T cell clones specific for components of minor H antigens can be isolated from secondary MLR: the minor H specificities defined by these T cell clones cosegregate with loci encoding minor H antigens defined by *in vivo* grafting (Loveland and Simpson, 1986). Minor H-specific T-cells, like those specific for viruses, are MHC restricted, recognizing the minor H antigen associated with a self-MHC molecule, either class I for CD8$^+$ T cells or class II for CD4$^+$ T cells (Tomonari, 1983). These T cells have been used to chromosomally map genetic regions encoding minor H antigens and trace segregation of minor H loci in experimental backcross studies (Loveland et al., 1985; Fowlis et al., 1992).

Immunogenetics of Minor H Antigens

In vivo studies in mice showed that minor H antigen genes were not MHC-linked but were scattered throughout the genome. They were chromosomally mapped in congenic and recombinant inbred strains using their linkage to previously identified markers (Bailey, 1975). The development of minor H congenic strains, each differing from the parental strain by a single minor locus, allowed investigations of *in vivo* and *in vitro* responses to isolated minor H antigens, as did the use of selected inbred strains in which the females were able to generate immune responses to cells and grafts from males of the same strain. These responses defined the male-specific minor H antigen, H-Y, encoded on the Y chromosome (Eichwald and Silmser, 1955; Simpson, 1982). The responses to H-Y, both *in vivo* and *in vitro*, demonstrated an asymmetry which is now apparent in responses to other minor H antigens. The presence of a minor H antigen thus represents a + allele and its absence a mutation resulting in loss of expression detectable by T cells, i.e., a null allele.

This explanation also accounts for the frequency of minor H antigens defined by T cell clones in human populations (Van Els et al., 1992; Schreuder et al., 1993). Some minor H antigens appear with very high frequency (> 90%), others much lower (< 10%). Each is inherited in a Mendelian fashion, transmitted by parents who from analysis of their progeny could be phenotypically positive for a particular minor H antigen either by being homozygous (+/+) or heterozygous (+/−) for the encoding gene.

Minor H antigens that are the targets of gvh and hvg responses *in vivo* must be expressed on target tissues. There is evidence for ubiquitous expression of a number of minor H antigens (Johnson, 1981).

Two Signal Requirement for Rejection of Minor H Mismatched Grafts

On close examination, it became clear that minor H "loci" consisted of a complex of closely linked genes (Roopenian, 1992). From spleen cells of mice immunized *in vivo* by grafting with skin disparate for minor H antigens such as H-Y, H-3, or H-4, one can isolate CD4$^+$ and CD8$^+$ T cell clones restricted by MHC class II and class I molecules respectively (Tomonari, 1983; Roopenian, 1992). These clones can be used to type inbred, recombinant inbred, and backcross mice (Loveland, 1985; Roopenian, 1993) for the relevant minor H antigen. Using a CD4$^+$ and a CD8$^+$ T cell clone raised between an H-3 congenic pair, Roopenian and Davis (1989) typed a number of independently derived H-3 congenic strains. The CD4$^+$ T cell clone identified an epitope encoded by a gene separate from that of the CD8$^+$ T cell clone. This was confirmed by classic backcross analysis, separating by recombination the genes encoding the two epitopes. A study of the H-4 region produced comparable results (Davis and Roopenian, 1990), and an analogous approach to the H-Y gene (Scott et al., 1991). These data and findings from transgenic mice expressing only components of minor H antigens recognized by CD8[+] T cells, whose grafts are not rejected by transgene negative littermates (Hederer R. and Antoniou A., unpublished), argue that to stimulate rejection, separate epitopes recognized by CD4[+] and CD8[+] T cells are necessary.

The Molecular Nature of Minor H Antigens

T cells specific for minor H antigens, like viral peptides, are MHC-restricted (Gordon et al., 1975; Bevan, 1975; Zinkernagel and Doherty, 1974; Townsend et al., 1986b). The crystal structure of HLA class I molecules showed an electron dense area in the peptide binding groove (Bjorkman, 1987a). It is now clear that peptide is an essential component stabilizing the structure of MHC molecules. These observations suggest that minor H antigens are endogenous peptides in the peptide binding grooves of class I and class II molecules. From knowledge of the allele- and isotype-specific peptide binding motifs, the relevant class I bound peptides will be 8–10 mers with anchor residues near each end, the class II bound peptides longer. Class I and class II bound peptides are derived from endogenous proteins and become loaded into the corresponding MHC molecule during biosynthesis. For class I molecules, this occurs in the ER but the route by which class II molecules acquire peptides from endogenously synthesised proteins may represent "leakage" of the class II pathway involving autophagy.

There is direct evidence for the peptide nature of several minor histocompatibility antigen components defined by CD8[+] T cells *in vitro*. The pioneering work of Rammensee showed that peptides separated from membrane-bound MHC class I molecules by acid elution followed by HPLC fractionation can subsequently be used to sensitize target cells expressing the appropriate MHC molecules (but not the minor H antigen in question) for lysis by minor H antigen-specific CTL clones (Rötzschke et al., 1990). T cell clones specific for a D[b]-restricted H-Y epitope and a D[b]-restricted H-4 epitope were so de-

fined (Rötzschke et al., 1990). A D[b]-restricted H-1 epitope recognized by CD8 cells has been similarly defined (Yin et al., 1994), as well as HLA class I restricted minor H epitopes recognized by CD8 T cell clones (Sekimata et al., 1992). Loveland et al. (1990) described the identification of a peptide derived from a mitochondrial genome-encoded protein, recognized by T cells in association with a non-classic MHC class I molecule, Hmt. A number of human and murine tumor-specific transplantation antigens (TSTA) defined by CD8[+] T cells have also been shown to be peptides following the cloning of genes encoding them and identification of the minimal DNA sequence specifying the peptide (De Plaen et al., 1988; Van den Eynde et al., 1991; Van der Bruggen et al., 1991).

A better understanding of how to trigger activation of effector T cells directed against TSTA and of how best to prevent activation of effector cells against the minor H antigen targets of gvh and hvg responses is now needed. The CD8 recognized epitopes alone are insufficient to cause activation: concomitant triggering of CD4[+] T cells against other epitopes are necessary. It is clear in mice and humans that certain epitopes present among many, as in responses to multiple minor H antigens, elicit a dominant effector response (Loveland and Simpson, 1986; Yin et al., 1994). The molecular basis of this potentially clinically important finding is not yet understood but can be investigated using T cell clones of known restriction and peptide specificity, peptide elution from MHC molecules and the expression cloning systems for detection using T cell clones (De Plaen et al., 1988; Rötzschke et al., 1990; Van den Eynde et al., 1991; Van der Bruggen et al., 1991; Scott et al., 1992; Sekimata et al., 1992; Hunt et al., 1992; Yin et al., 1994).

REFERENCES

Andersson M, Paabo S, Nilsson T, et al. (1985): Impaired intracellular transport to class I MHC antigens as a possible means for adenoviruses to evade immune surveillance. Cell 43:215–222.

Arenzana-Seisdedos F, Mogensen SC, Vuillier F, et al. (1988): Autocrine secretion of tumor necrosis factor under the influence of interferon-gamma amplifies HLA-DR gene induction in human monocytes. Proc Natl Acad Sci USA 85:6087–6091.

Babbit BP, Allen PM, Matsueda G, et al. (1985): Binding of immunogenic peptides to Ia histocompatibility molecules. Nature (London) 317:359–361.

Bach FH, Amos DB (1967): Hu-l: Major histocompatibility locus in man. Science 156:1506–1508.

Bach FH, Hirschhorn K (1964): Lymphocyte interaction: A potential histocompatibility test in vitro. Science 143:813–814.

Bailey DW (1975): Genetics of histocompatibility in mice I. New loci and congenic lines. Immunogenetics 2:249–256.

Bain B, Vas MR, Lowenstein L (1964): The development of large immature mononuclear cells in mixed leukocyte cultures. Blood 23:108–116.

Beck BN, Frelinger JG, Shigeta M, et al. (1982): T cell clones specific for hybrid I-A molecules. Discrimination with monoclonal anti-I-Ak antibodies. J Exp Med 156:1186–1193.

Benacerraf B, Green I, Paul WE (1967): The immune response of guinea pigs to hapten-poly-L-lysine conjugates as an example of the genetic control of the recognition of antigenicity. Cold Spring Harbor Symp Quant Biol 32:569–576.

Berumen L, Halle-Pannenko O, Festenstein H (1983): Histocompatibility effects of the Mls locus. Transplant Proc 15:213–216.

Bevan MJ (1975): The major histocompatibility complex determines susceptibility to cytotoxic T cells directed against minor histocompatibility antigens. J Exp Med 142:1349–1364.

Bjorkman PJ, Saper MA, Samraoui B, et al. (1987a): Structure of the human class I histocompatibility antigen, HLA-A2. Nature (London) 329:506–512.

Bjorkman, PJ, Saper MA, Samraoui B, et al. (1987b): The foreign antigen binding site and T cell recognition regions of class I histocompatibility antigens. Nature (London) 329:512–518.

Bodmer J, March SGE, Albert ED, et al. (1992): Nomenclature for factors of the HLA system 1989. Tissue Antigens 35:1–8.

Bottazzo GF, Pujol-Borrell R, Hanafusa T (1983): Role of aberrant HLA-DR expression and antigen presentation in induction of endocrine autoimmunity. Lancet 2:1115–1119.

Brent L, Opara SC (1979): Specific unresponsiveness to skin allografts in mice. V. synergy between donor tissue extract, procarbazine hydrochloride and antilymphocyte serum in creating a long lasting unresponsiveness mediated by suppressor T cells. Transplantation 27:120–126.

Brown JH, Jardetsky TS, Gorga JC, et al. (1993): Three-dimensional structure of the human class II histocompatibility antigen HLA-DRI. Nature (London) 364:33–39.

Buus S, Sette A, Colon SM, et al. (1987): The relation between major histocompatibility complex (MHC) restriction and the capacity of Ia to bind immunogenic peptides. Science 235:1353–1357.

Campbell RD, Trowsdale JT (1993): Map of the Human MHC. Immunol Today 14(7):349–352.

Ceppellini R, Mattiuz PL, Scudeller G, et al. (1969): Experimental allotransplantation in man I. The role of the HLA system in different genetic combinations. Transplant Proc 1:385–389.

Chicz, RM, Urban RG, Lane WS, et al. (1992): Predominant naturally processed peptides bound to HLA-DR1 are derived from MHC-related molecules and are heterogenous in size. Nature (London) 358:764–768.

Daar AS, Fuggle SV, Fabre JW, et al. (1984a): The detailed distribution of HLA–A,B,C antigens in normal human organs. Transplantation 38:287–292.

Daar AS, Fuggle SV, Fabre JW, et al. (1984b): The detailed distribution of MHC class II antigens in normal human organs. Transplantation 38:293–298.

Davis AP, Roopenian DC (1990): Complexity at the mouse minor histocompatibility locus H-4. Immunogenetics 31:7–12.

Davis M, Bjorkman PJ (1988) Nature (London) 334:395–402.

De Plaen E, Lurquin C, Van Pel A, et al. (1988): Immunogenic (tum-) variants of mouse tumor P815: Cloning of the gene of tum- antigen P91A and identification of the tum- mutation. Proc Natl Acad Sci USA 85:2274–2278.

Eichwald EJ, Silmser CR (1955): Untitled. Transplant Bull 2:148.

Falk K, Rotzschke O, Stevanovic S, et al. (1991): Allele-specific motifs revealed by sequencing of self-peptides from MHC molecules. Nature (London) 351:290–296.

Festenstein H (1973): Immunogenetic and biological aspects of in vitro lymphocyte allotransformation (MLR) in the mouse. Transplant Rev 15: 62–88.

Fowell D, McKnight AJ, Powrie F, Dyke R, Mason D (1991) Subsets of CD4+ T cells and their roles in the induction and prevention of autoimmunity. Immunol Rev 123:37–64.

Fowlis GA, Fairchild S, Tomonari K, et al. (1992): Toward identification of minor histocompatibility antigens in mouse and man. Transplant Proc 24:1689–1691.

Garrett TPJ, Saper MA, Bjorkman PJ, et al. (1989): Specificity pockets for the side chains of peptide antigens in HLA-Aw68. Nature (London) 342: 692–695.

Germain R (1986): The ins and outs of antigen processing and presentation. Nature (London) 322: 687–689.

Gershon R (1974): T-cell control of antibody production. Contemp Top Immunobiol 3:1–40.

Gordon R, Simpson E, Samelson L (1975): In vitro cell-mediated immune responses to the male specific (H-Y) antigen in mice. J Exp Med 142:1108–1120.

Gorer PA, Lyman, S, Snell GD (1948): Studies on the genetic and antigenic basis of tumour transplantation: Linkage between a histocompatibility gene and 'fused' in mice. Proc R Soc London Ser B 135:499–505.

Gotch FM, Roghbard J, Howland K, et al. (1987): Cytotoxic T lymphocytes recognize a fragment of influenza virus matrix protein in association with HLA-A2. Nature (London) 326:881–885.

Hämmerling G, Moreno J (1990): The function of the invariant chain in antigen presentation by MHC class II molecules. Immunol Today aa:337–340.

Hill AVS, Allsopp CEM, Kwiatkowski D, et al. (1991): Common West African HLA antigens are associated with protection from severe malaria. Nature (London) 352:565–600.

Hill AVS, Elvin J, Willis AC, et al. (1992): Molecular analysis of the association of HLA-B53 and resistance to severe malaria. Nature (London) 360: 434–439.

Hunt DF, Henderson RA, Shabanowitz J, et al. (1992): Characterization of peptides bound to the class I MHC molecule HLA-A2.1 by mass spectrometry. Science 255:1261–1263.

Johnson LL, Bailey DW, Mobraaten LE (1981): Genetics of histocompatibility in mice. IV. Detection of certain minor (non-H-2) H antigens in selected organs by the popliteal node test. Immunogenetics 14:63–71.

Klareskog L, Forsum U (1986): Tissue distribution of class II antigens: Presence on normal cells. In Solheim B, Moller E, Ferrone S, (eds): "HLA Class II Antigens." New York: Springer-Verlag, pp 339–348.

König R, Huang LY, Germain RN (1992): MHC class II interaction with CD4 mediated by a region analogous to the MHC class I binding site for CD8. Nature (London) 356:796–798.

Kwok WW, Schwarz D, Nepom BS, et al. (1988): HLA-DQ molecules form ab heterodimers of mixed allotype. J Immunol 141:3123–3127.

Lechler RI (1988): MHC class II molecular structure—permitted pairs? Immunol Today 9:76–78.

Lechler RI, Lombardi G, Batchelor JR, et al. (1990): The molecular basis of alloreactivity. Immunol Today 11:83–88.

Lee JS (1989): Regulation of HLA class II gene expression. In Dupont B (ed): "Immunobiology of HLA." Vol II. New York: Springer-Verlag, pp 49–61.

Loveland BE, Simpson E (1986): The non-MHC transplantation antigens reviewed: neither weak nor minor. Immunol Today 7:223–229.

Loveland BE, Sponaas A-M, Simpson E (1985): Mapping H-1 with the distal break point of chromosome 7 in Cattanach's insertion. Immunogenetics 22:503–510.

Loveland BE, Wang CR, Yonekawa H, et al. (1990): Maternally transmitted histocompatibility antigen of mice: A hydrophobic peptide of a mitochondrially encoded protein. Cell 60:971–980.

Madden DR, Gorga JC, Strominger JL, et al. (1991): The structure of HLA-B27 reveals nonamer self-peptides bound in an extended conformation. Nature (London) 353:321–325.

Marquet RL, Heyskek GA (1981): Induction of suppressor cells by donor-specific blood transfusions and heart transplantation in rats. Transplantation 31:271–274.

Mitchell GF, Grumet FC, McDevitt HO (1972): Genetic control of the immune response: The effect of thymectomy on the primary and secondary anti body response of mice to poly-l(Tyr, Glu)-poly-d, l-Ala—poly-l-Lys. J Exp Med 135:126–135.

Mullbacher A, Sheena JH, Fierz W, et al. (1981): Specific haplotype preference in congenic F1 hybrid mice in the cytotoxic T cell responses to the male specific antigen H-Y. J Immun 127(2):686–689.

Roopenian DC (1992): What are minor histocompatibility loci? A new look to an old question. Immunol Today 13:7–10.

Roopenian DC, Davis AP (1989): Responses against antigens encoded by the H-3 histocompatibility locus: Antigens stimulating class I MHC- and class II MHC-restricted T cells are encoded by separate genes. Immunogenetics 30:335–343.

Roopenian DC, Christianson GJ, Davis AP, et al. (1993): The genetic origin of minor histocompatibility antigens. Immunogenetics 38:131–140.

Rötzschke O, Falk K, Wallny, HJ, et al. (1990): Characterization of naturally occurring minor H peptides including H-4 and H-Y. Science 249:283–287.

Salter RD, Benjamin RJ, Wesley PK, et al. (1990): A binding site for the T-cell co-receptor CD8 on the alpha 3 domain of HLA-A2. Nature (London) 345:41–46.

Sasazuki T, Kikuchi I, Hirayama K, et al. (1989): HLA-linked immune suppression in humans. Immunology 2:21–24.

Schreuder GMT, Pool J, Blokland E, et al. (1993): A genetic analysis of human minor histocompatibility antigens demonstrating Mendelian segregation independent of HLA. Immunogenetics 38:98–105.

Scott D, McLaren A, Dyson PJ, et al. (1991): Variable spread of X inactivation affecting the expression of different epitopes of the Hya gene product in mouse B cell clones. Immunogenetics 33:54–61.

Scott D, Dyson PJ, Simpson E (1992): A new approach to the cloning of genes encoding T cell epitopes. Immunogenetics 36:86–94.

Sekimata M, Griem P, Egawa K, et al. (1992): Isolation of human minor histocompatibility peptides. Int Immunol 4:301–304.

Simpson E (1982): The role of H-Y as a minor transplantation antigen. Immunol Today 3:97–106.

Simpson E, Dyson PJ, Knight AM, et al. (1993): T cell receptor repertoire selection by mouse mammary tumour viruses and MHC molecules. Immunol Rev 131:93–115.

Snell GD (1948): Methods for the study of histocompatibility genes. J Genet 49:87–103.

Stern LJ, Wiley DC, (1994): Antigenic peptide binding by class I and class II histocompatibility proteins. Structure, in press.

Stern LJ, Brown JH, Jardetzky TS, Gorga JC, Urban RG, Stominger JL, Wiley DC (1994): Crystal Structure of the MHC class II protein HLA-DR1 complexed with an influenza virus peptide. Nature (London), in press.

Symington FW, Levine F, Braun M, et al. (1985): Differential Ia antigen expression by autologous human erythroid and B lymphoblastoid cell lines. J Immunol 135:1026–1032.

Tomonari K (1983): Antigen and MHC restriction specificity of two types of cloned male-specific T cell lines. J Immunol 131:1641–1645.

Townsend ARM, Rothbard J, Gotch FM, et al. (1986): The epitopes of influenza nucleoprotein recognized by cytotoxic T lymphocytes can be defined by short synthetic peptides. Cell 44:959–968.

Van den Eynde B, Lethe B, Van Pel A, et al. (1991): The gene coding for a major tumor rejection antigen of tumor P815 is identical to the normal gene of syngeneic DBA/2 mice. J Exp Med 173:1373–1384.

Van der Bruggen P, Traversari C, Chomez P, et al. (1991): A gene encoding an antigen recognized by cytolytic T lymphocytes on a human melanoma. Science 254:1643–1647.

Van Els CACM, Bakker A, Zwinderman AH, et al. (1990a): Effector mechanisms in graft versus host disease in response to minor histocompatibility antigens. I. Absence of correlation with cytotoxic effector cells. Transplantation 50:62–66.

Van Els CACM, Bakker A, Zwinderman AH, et al. (1990b): Effector mechanisms in graft versus host disease in response to minor histocompatibility antigens. I. Evidence of a possible involvement of proliferative T cells. Transplantation 50:67–71.

Van Els CACM, D'Amaro J, Pool J, et al. (1992): Immunogenetics of human minor histocompatibility antigens: Their polymorphisms and immunodominance. Immunogenetics 35:161–165.

Veillette A, Bookman MA, Horak, EM, et al. (1988): The CD4 and CD8 T cell surface antigens are associated with the internal membrane tyrosine-protein kinase p56^{lck}. Cell 55:301–308.

Yin L, Poirier G, Neth O, et al. (1994): Few peptides dominate CTL responses to single and multiple minor histocompatibility antigens. Int Immunol 5:1003–1009.

Zinkernagel RM, Doherty PC (1974): Restriction of in vitro mediated cytotoxicity in lymphocytic choriomeningitis within a syngeneic or semi-allogeneic system. Nature (London) 248:701–702.

Chapter 2
The Thymus and Self/Nonself Discrimination

Jonathan Sprent

This chapter gives a brief overview of T cell differentiation in the murine thymus and the mechanisms involved in self/nonself discrimination. As an introduction to these topics, it is important to highlight some of the unique properties of normal mature T cells and the pivotal role of major histocompatibility complex (MHC) molecules in controlling T cell specificity and function.

FEATURES OF MATURE T CELLS

Typical mature T cells are divisible into two distinct subsets on the basis of CD4 and CD8 expression (Sprent and Webb, 1987). In contrast to immature T cells in the thymus, the expression of CD4 and CD8 molecules on mature T cells is mutually exclusive. CD4 (CD4$^+$8$^-$) T cells generally outnumber CD8 (CD4$^-$8$^+$) cells by a ratio of 2 to 1 and are largely responsible for delayed-type hypersensitivity and the delivery of T cell "help" for B cells leading to antibody production. CD8 cells act as precursors of cytotoxic T cells. Both T cell subsets express T cell receptor (TCR) molecules consisting of $\alpha\beta$ heterodimers. Although CD4 and CD8 T cells account for the vast majority of mature T cells, a small proportion of T cells display a CD4$^-$8$^-$ phenotype. Some of these T cells express $\alpha\beta$ TCR molecules, but others express $\gamma\delta$ TCR molecules. The function of $\gamma\delta$ T cells is still largely a mystery (Haas et al., 1993) and in this chapter $\gamma\delta$ cells will be discussed only in passing.

Like B cells, mature CD4 and CD8 T cells reside within the recirculating lymphocyte pool (Sprent and Webb, 1987). Recirculating lym-

phocytes have a prolonged life span and move constantly from one lymphoid organ to another via the bloodstream and the central lymphatic vessels. Lymphocyte recirculation is controlled by specific homing molecules (Picker and Butcher, 1992) and enables the immune system to mobilize antigen-specific T and B cells from throughout the body and concentrate these cells in regions where foreign antigens are broken down into immunogenic moieties by phagocytes and other "antigen-presenting cells" (APCs). For T cells, presentation of antigen by APCs is largely restricted to the T-dependent areas of the secondary lymphoid tissues, i.e., the periarteriolar lymphocyte sheaths of the splenic white pulp, the paracortex of lymph nodes, and the interfollicular regions of Peyer's patches. In these areas, the interaction between antigen-specific T cells and APCs causes T cells to divide and differentiate into effector cells. These activated T cells express a new set of homing receptors that enables the cells to penetrate the walls of capillary blood vessels and thereby percolate throughout the body and mediate their effector functions.

As discussed in other chapters in this volume, the specificity of T cells is not directed to native antigens but to degraded fragments of antigen (peptides) bound to MHC molecules on APC (Germain and Margulies, 1993). MHC molecules are highly polymorphic, and peptides bind selectively to a specialized groove on the membrane-distal portion of the molecule; this applies to both class I and class II molecules. TCR binding to MHC-bound peptides is augmented by CD4 and CD8 molecules (Janeway,

Transplantation Immunology, pages 35–52
© 1995 Wiley-Liss, Inc.

1992). These molecules act as coreceptors by binding to monomorphic sites on MHC class II and class I molecules, respectively. Operationally, this means that CD4 cells have specificity for MHC class II-associated peptides whereas CD8 cells have specificity for peptides bound to class I molecules. At the level of unprimed T cells, the MHC class specificity of CD4 and CD8 cells is stringent (Sprent et al., 1986).

One of the striking features of the T cell repertoire is that the pool of mature T cells encompasses reactivity to an almost infinite variety of foreign peptides, but generally ignores self-peptides. Such self-tolerance is rather remarkable given that most cell-surface MHC molecules collectively display hundreds (perhaps thousands) of different self peptides as the result of intracellular degradation of proteins (Rammensee et al., 1993). How then does the T cell system distinguish self from nonself? This begs the question of how the T cell repertoire is formed. As discussed below, typical T cells are selected from a large pool of precursor cells in the thymus by a stringent process involving both positive and negative selection. As the result of thymic selection, the T cells released from the thymus are poised to respond strongly to foreign antigens while tolerating self-antigens.

FORMATION OF THE T CELL POOL IS THYMUS DEPENDENT

The first clear evidence that the formation of T cells requires the presence of the thymus came from the demonstration of Miller that neonatal thymectomy in mice causes profound lymphocytopenia and depression of the functions now ascribed to T cells (Miller and Osoba, 1967). Although it was initially thought that the thymus might function by releasing "thymic hormones" into the bloodstream, it soon became clear that T cells are formed within the thymus itself; thymic hormones are still discussed in clinical circles, but the evidence that such factors can promote the formation of T cells in the absence of an intact thymus is unconvincing. The notion that T cells arise in the thymus was consolidated by the subsequent discovery that T cells are rare in animals with congenital thymic aplasia, e.g., in rodents expressing the nude (*nu/nu*) mutation and patients with Di George's syndrome.

The profound T lymphocytopenia in nude and neonatally thymectomized mice is illustrated in Table I. In the experiment shown, numbers of T and B cells were quantitated by thoracic duct cannulation. This procedure causes rapid mobilization of T cells from throughout the body (ex-

Table I. Numbers of T and B Lymphocytes Collected from Thoracic Duct Lymph of Normal Mice vs. Nude and Neonatally Thymectomized Mice[a]

Source of TDL	Number of TDL collected over 24 hr ($\times 10^{-6}$)	% T cells	% B cells	Total number of T and B cells collected over 24 hr ($\times 10^{-6}$)	
				T cells	B cells
Nude	23	<1	97	1	22
Nude littermates	140	78	20	109	28
NTx CBA	29	12	65	4	18
Normal CBA	131	82	16	104	21

[a] Mean of data from 6 to 17 mice/group; mice were 8–10 weeks of age. Neonatal thymectomy (NTx) was performed within 24 hr of birth. Thoracic duct lymphocytes (TDL) were collected on ice; T and B cells were defined on the basis of Thy 1 and Fc receptor expression, respectively. Adapted from Sprent (1973).

cluding the thymus), and very large numbers of T cells can be collected in lymph over a 24-hr period, i.e., over 1×10^8 cells from normal euthymic mice. It is evident that T cell counts are extremely low ($< 5\%$ of normal) in neonatally thymectomized mice and are almost undetectable in (young) nude mice. B cell counts in these mice are near normal.

In mice, the thymus does not start to export T cells until the time of birth (Miller and Osoba, 1967). In many other species, however, the thymus is fully functional early in ontogeny, and large numbers of mature T cells are released from the thymus before birth. In such species, including man, removing the thymus at birth has relatively little effect, presumably because preexisting mature T cells undergo progressive expansion after thymectomy. Likewise, little or no evidence of T lymphocytopenia occurs when the thymus is removed in adult life. However, when adult thymectomized mice are exposed to whole body irradiation (which kills mature T cells in interphase), reconstitution of these mice with T cell-depleted bone marrow as a source of stem cells fails to reconstitute the T cell pool; B cells, by contrast, are rapidly regenerated. These "B" mice remain profoundly T-deficient almost indefinitely.

Whether *all* T cells arise in the thymus is controversial (Sprent, 1993a). Since nude mice are not totally devoid of T cells, it is often argued that T cells can be formed in sites other than the thymus, e.g., the intestines and liver. However, despite the current popularity for extrathymic differentiation of T cells, it should be emphasized that T cell formation in athymic animals is very limited indeed, especially in young life (Table I). Although old nude mice can eventually develop significant numbers of T cells, the repertoire of these cells tends to be pauciclonal, which makes it likely that these cells arise by gradual expansion of a limited number of mature precursor cells. Where these precursor cells initially arise is unknown.

The evidence that the vast majority of T cells originate in the thymus applies to the typical T cells found in spleen, LN, and Peyer's patches. The situation with T cells found in the intra-

epithelial layer of the small intestine, however, is less clear (Lefrancois, 1991). Gut intraepithelial T cells comprise a mixture of $\alpha\beta$ and $\gamma\delta$ cells, and there is increasing evidence that a sizable proportion of these cells, especially $\gamma\delta$ cells, arise *in situ* in the absence of the thymus. At present the factors controlling T cell differentiation in gut epithelium are poorly understood.

T CELL MIGRATION FROM THE THYMUS

Originally it was considered that the thymus releases immature T cells, and that maturation of these cells into functionally mature T cells occurs in the secondary lymphoid organs. This idea is no longer tenable because it is clear that the vast majority of T cells released from the thymus display most of the surface markers and functions of mature T cells (Scollay and Shortman, 1985; Shortman et al., 1990). In particular, very few of the T cells leaving the thymus have the "double-positive" ($CD4^+8^+$) phenotype of typical immature thymocytes. Recent thymic emigrants are not completely mature, but full maturation of these cells in the extrathymic environment takes only a few days and does not appear to involve cell division. In terms of total numbers, the output of cells from the thymus is quite low, i.e., only about 2×10^6 cells/day in young mice (Table II). Outputs are much lower in older mice.

ARCHITECTURE OF THE THYMUS

In sections, the thymus (which is bilobed) contains two discrete regions, the cortex and medulla (van Ewijk, 1991). These two regions are easily distinguished by light microscopy because the density of cells in the cortex is much higher than in the medulla. The cortex forms the outer portion of the thymus and constitutes about 80% of thymic tissue in young life; the vast majority of T cells in the cortex are immature $CD4^+8^+$ cells. The medulla forms the small central area of the thymus and consists largely of semimature $CD4^+8^-$ and $CD4^-8^+$ cells. The medulla also harbors blood-borne APCs such as

Table II. Outputs of T Cells from the Thymus of Mice at Different Ages[a]

Age	Total cells per thymus ($\times 10^{-7}$)	Total migrants/24 hr ($\times 10^{-6}$)	Total migrants/24 hr per 10^6 thymocytes ($\times 10^{-3}$)
6 days	3	0.1	4.7
$3^{1}/_{2}$–$5^{1}/_{2}$ weeks	20	1.9	9.5
$3^{1}/_{2}$ months	7	0.2	3.0
6 months	8	0.1	1.3

[a] Cell exit from the thymus of live mice was studied by allowing a dye (fluorescein isothiocyanate) or a DNA precursor ([³H]TdR) to penetrate a short distance into the outer cortex of the thymus of short-term anesthetized mice. The mice were then killed at intervals to search for labeled cells appearing in the peripheral lymphoid tissues. The data refer to migrants detected in blood, spleen, and lymph nodes. It is evident that maximum export of T cells from the thymus occurs in young mice, i.e., mice with a very large thymus. The authors of this study concluded that only about 4% of the total daily production of thymocytes in young mice are exported. Adapted from Scollay and Shortman (1985).

macrophages and dendritic cells; these cells are concentrated at the corticomedullary junction and play a crucial role in self-tolerance induction (see below). With the exception of scattered MHC class II⁻ macrophages, the cortex is largely free of blood-borne APC.

In addition to lymphohematopoietic cells, the thymus contains a rich network of epithelial cells (Fig. 1) (van Ewijk, 1991; Surh et al., 1992). Epithelial cells are especially prominent in the cortex, and these cells play a critical role in controlling positive selection of immature thymocytes. Epithelial cells are also found in the medulla; these cells are heterogeneous with respect to their surface markers, but the function of medullary epithelial cells is largely unknown. In many species (but not mice), medullary epithelial cells form dense aggregates termed Hassal's corpuscles.

SUBSETS OF THYMOCYTES

When the thymus is pressed through a sieve or put through a tissue grinder, the vast majority (>99%) of the intact cells that come into suspension are lymphohematopoietic cells (von Boehmer, 1988; Fowlkes and Pardoll, 1989). Of these, around 98% are T cells (Figs. 2 and 3). Typical CD4⁺8⁺ cortical thymocytes account for 80–85% of thymocyte suspensions, and

these cells express low (but significant) levels of the $\alpha\beta$ T cell receptor (TCR); "double-positive" (DP) CD4⁺8⁺ cells also express low levels of CD3 molecules (a complex of cell-surface molecules involved in T cell triggering). Most of the remaining cells in thymocyte suspensions comprise a mixture of CD4⁺8⁻ and CD4⁻8⁺ cells; these "single-positive" (SP) cells express high levels of $\alpha\beta$ TCR and CD3 molecules and are the immediate precursors of the cells destined for export from the thymus. In addition to SP and DP cells, thymocyte suspensions contain about 2% "double-negative" (DN) cells, i.e., cells lacking expression of both CD4 and CD8 molecules.

Though small in number, DN thymocytes display considerable heterogeneity. Most DN thymocytes do not express TCR molecules and these cells act as stem cells for DP cells. A small proportion of DN cells express high levels of $\alpha\beta$ TCR and CD3 molecules; most of these cells are presumed to be functionally mature T cells, which, for obscure reasons, have down-regulated both CD4 and CD8 expression after positive selection. Finally, a proportion of DN thymocytes express $\gamma\delta$ TCR molecules. A brief synopsis of $\gamma\delta$ T cell differentiation in the thymus will be presented later.

With regard to turnover, the vast majority of T cells in the thymus have a rapid rate of turnover

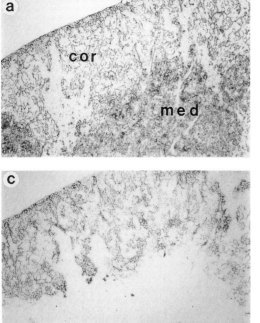
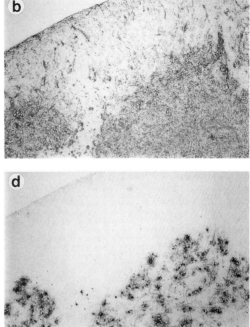

Fig. 1. Architecture of the mouse thymus. Serial cryostat sections of normal adult thymus were stained for expression of various markers using biotinylated antibodies followed by incubation with horseradish peroxidase–streptavidin and then 3-amino-9-ethyl-carbazole. (**a**) MHC class II expression: there is confluent staining of marrow-derived APC in the medulla (med) and reticular staining of epithelial cells in the cortex (cor). (**b**) MHC class I expression: except for less intense staining of the cortex, class I expression is very similar to class II expression. (**c**) Staining with 6C3 antibody: this antibody stains epithelial cells in the cortex but does not stain medullary epithelial cells or APC. (**d**) Staining with UEA-1: this fucose-specific lectin stains a subset of medullary epithelial cells; these UEA-1$^+$ epithelial cells also show strong MHC class I and II expression (not shown). The medulla also contains a separate subset of UEA-1$^-$ epithelial cells; these cells are MHC$^-$ but show dense expression of I-O molecules, a class of atypical nonpolymorphic class II molecules (not shown). Adapted from Surh et al. (1992) with permission.

(Fig. 4) (Shortman et al., 1990). It is important to emphasize, however, that relatively few cells in the thymus are in cell cycle. In fact, proliferation of thymocytes is largely limited to the small subset of TCR$^-$ DN stem cells. These cells are situated under the capsule of the thymus and divide rapidly to give rise to DP blast cells and then to typical small DP cells. Except for the minority population of blast cells, most DP cells are in interphase and >90% of these cells appear to undergo programmed cell death within a few days of their formation. SP thymocytes turn over more slowly. As discussed below, positive selection of DP cells leading to the production of SP cells does not involve cell division and most SP thymocytes remain in interphase until these cells are exported from the thymus. Based on the rate at which SP thymocytes incorporate labeled DNA precursors during repeated administration, most SP thymocytes seem to remain in the medulla as resting cells for 1–2 weeks before being exported.

ONTOGENY OF THYMOCYTE DEVELOPMENT

The thymic anlage consists largely of epithelial cells and is derived from the ectoderm and endoderm of the third and fourth pharyngeal pouches, respectively (Owen and Jenkinson,

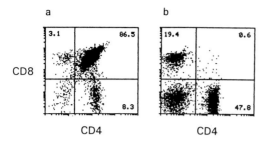

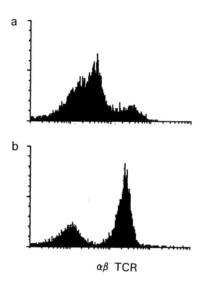

Fig. 2. CD4 and CD8 expression on normal adult thymus vs. lymph node demonstrated by flow cytometry. Using two-color staining, cell suspensions were stained with anti-CD4 and anti-CD8 antibodies and then analyzed on a FACScan. (**a**) Thymus. It is evident that most thymocytes express both CD4 and CD8 molecules. These double-positive thymocytes are situated in the cortex and express a low density of $\alpha\beta$ TCR molecules. Single-positive CD4$^+$8$^-$ and CD4$^-$8$^+$ cells comprise 10–15% of thymocytes; these cells are found largely in the medulla and express a high density of $\alpha\beta$ TCR molecules. CD4$^-$8$^-$ thymocytes are a minority population but are very heterogeneous; some CD4$^-$8$^-$ thymocytes act as stem cells for $\alpha\beta$ T cells whereas others belong to the $\gamma\delta$ lineage. (**b**) Lymph node. Nearly all of the T cells in lymph nodes are mature single-positive CD4 and CD8 cells expressing a high density of $\alpha\beta$ TCR molecules; CD4$^+$8$^+$ cells are very rare. Most of the CD4$^-$8$^-$ cells in lymph nodes are B cells; some CD4$^-$8$^-$ cells are $\gamma\delta$ cells, but these cells are a minority population (<2% of normal lymph node cells). Data kindly provided by C. D. Surh.

Fig. 3. Density of $\alpha\beta$ TCR molecules on normal thymus and lymph node cells. Cell suspensions were stained with an antibody specific for $\alpha\beta$ TCR molecules and then analyzed on a FACScan. (**a**) Thymus: $\alpha\beta$ TCR expression on thymocytes is heterogeneous. Only a small proportion of thymocytes (10–15%) are TCR^{high} cells; these cells are found largely in the medulla and comprise a mixture of mature CD4 and CD8 cells. The bulk of thymocytes express TCR molecules at a low level; most of these cells are CD4$^+$8$^+$ cortical cells. TCR expression on some cortical thymocytes is almost undetectable; these TCR$^-$ cells are presumed to be recently generated CD4$^+$8$^+$ cells. (**b**) Lymph node: Virtually all $\alpha\beta$ TCR$^+$ cells are TCR^{high} and comprise a mixture of CD4$^+$ and CD8$^+$ cells; most of the $\alpha\beta$ TCR$^-$ cells are B cells. Data kindly provided by C. D. Surh.

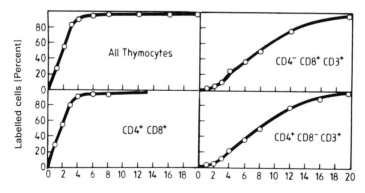

Continuous Labelling Time [Days]

Fig. 4. Turnover of thymocytes. The data show the rate at which subsets of thymocytes become radiolabeled during twice-daily injection of mice with [^{3}H]TdR (a DNA precursor). Subpopulations of thymocytes were isolated by cell sorting at the times indicated, and the frequency of labeled cells was determined by autoradiography. The data illustrate that CD4$^+$8$^+$ cells, which represent the bulk of thymocytes, turn over at a rapid rate. These cells arise from a subset of cycling CD4$^-$8$^-$ cells. The populations of mature CD4$^+$8$^-$ and CD4$^-$8$^+$ cells expressing a high density of $\alpha\beta$ TCR and CD3 molecules show a relatively slow turnover. These cells arise from a subset of CD4$^+$8$^+$ cells. Data adopted from Shortman et al. (1990) with permission.

1981). In mice, the thymic anlage descends into the anterior mediastinum on day 10 of gestation (the gestation period in mice being about 21 days). At this stage the thymus is devoid of stem cells. Lymphoid stem cells begin to appear in the mouse thymus on day 11. These cells enter from the bloodstream and are presumed to arise either from the yolk sac or the liver (the bone marrow being aplastic at this stage). Although there has been much discussion on whether thymic stem cells are precommitted to T cell development, it now seems likely that the thymus is colonized by pluripotent stem cells (Ikuta et al., 1992). Entry of stem cells into the thymus is controlled by chemotactic peptides in birds, but whether this also applies in mammals is unclear.

After entering the thymus, stem cells rapidly become committed to the T cell lineage and give rise to large numbers of DP cells expressing a low density of $\alpha\beta$ TCR molecules (Fowlkes and Pardoll, 1989). These cells are rare before day 15 but are prominent by day 16 to 17. SP cells are first evident on around day 18. By day 20 to 21—the time of birth—the thymus closely resembles the adult thymus.

TCR GENE REARRANGEMENT AND TCR EXPRESSION

The differentiation of early T cells into $\alpha\beta$ TCR$^+$ cells seems to depend initially on preventing DN stem cells from undergoing rearrangement of TCR γ-genes (Haas et al., 1993; Leiden, 1993). This involves activation of a "γ-silencer"; the cells are then committed to $\alpha\beta$ TCR expression. At this early stage, α and β TCR genes are in germ-line configuration. Expression of these genes begins with rearrangement of β-chain genes, with D to J rearrangement preceding V to DJ rearrangement. If productive, the rearranged gene is expressed on the cell surface, initially perhaps as a $\beta\beta$ homodimer and then as an $\alpha\beta$ heterodimer. The expression of β-chains initiates CD4 and CD8 expression and results in V to J rearrangement of α-chain genes. Since δ-chain genes are aligned between Vα and Jα genes, V-Jα rearrangement deletes (excises) all δ-chain gene segments, thereby precluding the possibility of $\gamma\delta$ TCR expression on $\alpha\beta$ T cells. The

expression of $\alpha\beta$ TCR molecules on thymocytes is evident at the early DP stage and remains at a low level unless the cells undergo positive selection. Low TCR expression on DP cells seems to reflect an active mechanism because rapid up-regulation of TCR expression occurs when suspensions of DP cells are placed in tissue culture (Nakayama et al., 1990).

For $\gamma\delta$ cells, the failure to activate the γ-silencer on early DN cells allows these cells to rearrange γ-chain genes (V to J) (Haas et al., 1993; Leiden, 1993). This is followed by δ-chain rearrangement (D to J, then V to DJ) and expression of $\gamma\delta$ heterodimers on the cell surface; α- and β-chain genes generally remain in germ-line configuration. Whereas TCR expression on $\alpha\beta$ cells is accompanied by rapid transition to DP cells, $\gamma\delta$ cells usually retain a DN phenotype. The paucity of $\gamma\delta$ cells in the thymus ($<2\%$ of thymocytes) presumably means that proliferation of $\gamma\delta$ precursors is very limited.

The discussion of positive selection of T cells given below is restricted to $\alpha\beta$ T cells. There is some evidence that $\gamma\delta$ T cells are subject to positive selection, but detailed evidence on thymic selection of $\gamma\delta$ cells is still rather sparse.

POSITIVE SELECTION

The notion that T cell differentiation in the thymus involves positive selection stems from the early observation that T cell responses to foreign antigens tend to be higher when antigens are presented by self rather than nonself MHC molecules (Moller, 1978; Sprent and Webb, 1987). Thus, for responses to a given foreign peptide, peptide X, T cells from strain a (MHC^a) mice generally give higher responses to MHC^a/X than to MHC^b/X (with the proviso that the responding T cells are first depleted of MHC^b alloreactivity). It was discovered, however, that allowing MHC^a T cells to differentiate in a thymus expressing MHC^b molecules enables post-thymic T cells to mount strong responses to MHC^b/X. Such "thymus learning" does not depend on the genotype of the T cells. Thus, if MHC-heterozygous ($a \times b$) F$_1$ stem cells differentiate in a strain b thymus, the F$_1$ T cells display MHC restriction to strain b, i.e., the cells respond more effectively to MHC^b/X than to MHC^a/X. Conversely, F_1 T cells differentiating in a strain a thymus display MHC^a restriction. With an $(a \times b)F_1$ thymus, both MHC^a and MHC^b restriction is observed; this does not represent cross-reactivity but the generation of separate subsets of MHC^a-restricted and MHC^b-restricted T cells.

These findings on the role of the thymus in controlling the MHC-restricted specificity of T cells came from studies on bone marrow chimeras and thymus-grafted mice. A summary of the data is shown in Table III. Collectively, the data from these early experiments indicate that the preference for mature postthymic T cells to recognize antigen presented by self-MHC molecules, e.g., MHC^a, requires prior contact with MHC^a molecules in the thymus during early ontogeny. It is now generally agreed that such "positive selection" of T cells is controlled by the MHC molecules expressed on thymic epithelial cells, specifically on cortical epithelial cells.

Table III. MHC-Restricted Specificity of T Cells Generated in Bone-Marrow Chimeras and Thymus-Grafted Mice[a]

T cell donor	MHC molecules encountered on thymic epithelial cells	Reactivity of unprimed T cells to	
		$MHC^a + X$	$MHC^b + X$
Normal strain a[b]	a	+++	+
Normal strain b	b	+	+++
Normal $(a \times b)F_1$[c]	a, b	+++	+++
$a \to (a \times b)F_1$ BMC[d]	a, b	+++	+++
$(a \times b)F_1 \to a$ BMC[e]	a	+++	+
$(a \times b)F_1 \to b$ BMC	b	+	+++
$a \to b$ BMC	b	+	+++
$(a \times b)F_1 \to$ Tx $(a \times b)F_1$	—	—	—
With $(a \times b)F_1$ TG[f]	a, b	+++	+++
With a TG	a	+++	+
With b TG	b	+	+++

[a]The results summarize the work of many different investigators in the 1970s (reviewed in Sprent and Webb, 1987). A number of points should be made. First, the quality of the data varied considerably. Some workers found very strong restriction to thymic MHC, but others observed only a rather weak preference. In general, the data were more dramatic for MHC class II restriction than for class I restriction. Second, it is important to emphasize that the data refer to *unprimed* responses. If primed responses are measured, the results depend on the conditions of priming. Thus, if primed responses are measured in $a \to b$ BMC, the donor (MHC^a) origin of the APC in these chimeras means that priming will be restricted to residual MHC^a-restricted T cells and will not involve the MHC^b-restricted T cells.

[b]Testing the specificity of strain a T cells for MHC^b/X necessitates removing (or excluding) T cells specific for MHC^b alloantigens.

[c]Various techniques have shown that the T cells generated in F_1 hybrid mice comprise separate subsets of MHC^a-restricted and MHC^b-restricted cells. In terms of their pattern of MHC restriction, $(a \times b)F_1$ T cells thus behave as a mixture of parent a and parent b T cells.

[d]Parent $\to F_1$ bone marrow chimeras (BMC) are prepared by subjecting F_1 mice to heavy irradiation (e.g., 1000 rad) and reconstituting these mice with parental-strain marrow cells depleted of mature T cells. The T cells developing in these chimeras are of parental-strain origin.

[e]$F_1 \to$ parent chimeras are prepared by reconstituting irradiated parental-strain mice with T-depleted F_1 marrow cells. The T cells developing in these chimeras are of F_1 origin.

[f]Thymus-grafting of these F_1 mice necessitates prior thymectomy (Tx) to remove the endogenous host thymus. The mice are then irradiated, reconstituted with T-depleted F_1 marrow cells, and given a thymus graft (TG), which is usually inserted under the kidney capsule. Thymus grafts are usually irradiated prior to grafting, thereby destroying preexisting T cells in the grafts.

Table IV. Positive Selection in TCR TG Mice[a]

MHC restriction of T cell clone used to make TCR TG mice	Clonotype-positive cells generated in TCR TG mice: CD4/CD8 phenotype		Generation of mature clonotype-positive cells after backcrossing TCR TG mice to		
	CD4 cells	CD8 cells	MHC[a]	MHC[b]	MHC[a × b]
MHC class I[a]	−	+	+	−	+
MHC class II[a]	+	−	+	−	+

[a]The data summarize the results obtained by a number of different investigators (von Boehmer, 1990). Generation of clonotype-positive cells in mice lacking the MHC molecules required for positive selection is usually very low (though not entirely absent); T cells are produced in these strains, but most of these cells show expression of endogenous (non-TG) α-chains.

Strong support for positive selection of T cells has come from studies with TCR transgenic mice (von Boehmer, 1990) and "knockout" mice expressing only class I and not class II molecules, or vice versa (Chan et al., 1993). With regard to TCR transgenic (TG) mice, the key finding is that the production of mature T cells is heavily influenced by the MHC molecules expressed by the TG mice (Table IV). Thus, if TCR TG mice are prepared from an MHC[a] (class I[a])-restricted CD8 T cell line, backcrossing the TG mice to an MHC[a] background generates large numbers of CD8 T cells, most of which express both chains of the TG TCR molecules. Notably, however, generation of these "clonotype-positive" cells is absent (or only very limited) when the TG mice lack MHC[a] expression, e.g., if the mice are backcrossed to MHC[b]. In this situation, clonotype-positive cells remain in the thymus as immature DP cells.

An interesting feature of TCR transgenic mice is that the CD4/CD8 phenotype of the clonotype-positive cells corresponds to the phenotype of the original donor T cells (Table IV). Thus, for TCR TG mice prepared from a class I-restricted CD8 T cell clone, the vast majority of the mature clonotype-positive cells arising in the TG mice are CD8 cells rather than CD4 cells; reciprocal findings apply to TG mice prepared from a class II-restricted CD4 T cell clone. These findings imply that the pivotal role of CD4 and CD8 molecules in determining the MHC class specificity of mature T cells is also operative during positive

selection in the thymus (see below). Direct support for this notion has come from studies on MHC "knockout" mice (Table V). Thus, if the genes for class II molecules are deleted, the T cells generated in these mice are almost exclusively CD8 cells. Conversely, nearly all of the T cells in mice lacking class I molecules are CD4 cells. In mice expressing neither class I nor class II molecules, mature T cells are almost nonexistent.

Table V. Generation of Mature T Cells in "Knockout" Mice Selectively Lacking MHC Class I or MHC Class II Molecules[a,b]

MHC expression in knockout mice		Production of mature T cell subsets	
class I	class II	CD4 cells	CD8 cells
+	+	+ + + +	+ + + +
+	−	+/−[c]	+ + + +
−	+	+ + + +	+/−[c]
−	−	−	−

[a]The data summarize the results from several different investigators (Chan et al., 1993).

[b]Knockout mice are made by homologous recombination using embryonic stem cells. Class I-deficient mice are prepared by deleting the gene for β$_2$-microglobulin. In the absence of β$_2$-microglobulin, class I molecules are very unstable and are present on the cell surface in only low concentrations.

[c]The few T cells made in this situation are only semimature, and most of these cells seem to die in the thymus.

MECHANISM OF POSITIVE SELECTION

Positive selection can be viewed as a device for skewing the mature T cell repertoire toward covert recognition of self-MHC molecules (Sprent et al., 1988; von Boehmer et al., 1989). Such "physiological" MHC reactivity is not sufficient to break self-tolerance but makes T cells hypersensitive to slight perturbations of self, i.e., to self-MHC molecules displaying foreign peptides. During selection, immature thymo-

cytes are screened for their reactivity to self MHC molecules, and only those cells displaying the requisite physiological specificity for self-MHC molecules are selected for survival. The rest of the cells—the bulk of thymocytes—are destroyed *in situ*.

Positive selection probably occurs at the DP level and reflects TCR contact with MHC molecules expressed on cortical epithelial cells (Fig. 5). Since nearly all MHC molecules are complexed to various endogenous self-peptides, pos-

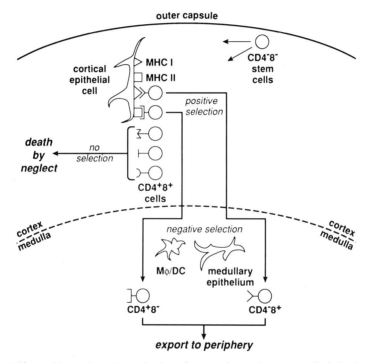

Fig. 5. A model for positive and negative selection of T cells in the thymus. As discussed in the text, small numbers of CF4⁻8⁻ stem cells under the outer capsule of the cortex proliferate extensively and generate large numbers of immature CD4⁺8⁺ cortical thymocytes. These cells are screened for self-MHC reactivity through exposure to the class I and class II molecules expressed on cortical epithelium; TCR recognition of polymorphic epitopes of class I and class II molecules (plus the self-peptides bound to these molecules) is aided by CD8 and CD4 molecules, respectively; these molecules act as coreceptors. T cells able to bind to MHC molecules on epithelial cells receive a protective signal that enables the cells to survive and move to the medulla. These positively selected T cells down-regulate the unwanted coreceptor (CD4 or CD8) and up-regulate TCR and CD3 ex-

pression to become typical single-positive CD4⁻8⁺ and CD4⁺8⁻ cells. In the medulla and the corticomedullary junction, CD4⁻8⁺ and CD4⁺8⁻ cells are screened for overt reactivity to MHC molecules expressed on bone-marrow-derived macrophages (Mφ) and dendritic cells (DC) and also on medullary epithelial cells; strong interactions with these cells causes T cells to die by apoptosis. Cells surviving negative selection are exported to the periphery via veins and lymphatics. Positive and negative selection of T cells applies to only a very small proportion (<5%) of thymocytes. Most CD4⁺8⁺ thymocytes do not have significant reactivity for the particular MHC molecules expressed in the thymus and these cells die within a few days by an unknown process. From Sprent (1993b) with permission.

itive selection is presumed to be directed to peptide/MHC complexes rather than epitopes expressed on naked MHC molecules. TCR recognition of peptide/MHC complexes also involves CD4 or CD8 molecules. By acting as coreceptors, these molecules augment TCR/MHC interaction and thereby increase the avidity of T cell binding to TEC: CD4 molecules strengthen TCR interaction with class II molecules whereas CD8 molecules augment TCR contact with class I molecules. If the avidity of T/TEC interaction is above a certain threshold, positive selection occurs and the T cells rapidly up-regulate TCR expression and down-regulate the unwanted CD4 or CD8 coreceptor molecule. Thus, positive selection to class II molecules is followed by down-regulation of CD8 but retention of CD4; conversely, positive selection to class I molecules results in down-regulation of CD4. After selection, the maturing T cells migrate to the medulla and reside there as SP cells before being exported to the periphery.

The above scheme is oversimplified and many details of positive selection remain to be resolved. Several points should be made. First, the notion that down-regulation of CD4 or CD8 molecules occurs *after* positive selection—the "instructional" model of selection—has been challenged by recent evidence favoring CD4/CD8 down-regulation *before* selection (the "stochastic" model) (Chan et al., 1993; Davis et al., 1993). Second, some workers incline to the view that positive selection is directed to unique self-peptides displayed selectively on TEC (Marrack and Kappler, 1987). Without direct evidence on the range of self-peptides expressed on TEC, it is difficult to assess this idea. Third, the intriguing question of why positive selection is controlled by TEC rather than other cell types has yet to be resolved; the least interesting explanation is that TEC are simply the predominant MHC-bearing cell in the cortex.

The signals involved in positive selection are now coming under close scrutiny. Since cell division is not involved, positive selection would appear to involve the delivery of a type of "protective" signal that rescues the cells and stimulates differentiation and maturation into SP cells (Sprent et al., 1988; von Boehmer et al., 1989).

Nonselected T cells fail to receive this protective signal and these "neglected" T cells succumb to some form of programmed cell death. Although the nature of the putative protective signal is still unknown, increasing evidence suggests that positive selection is a reflection of a covert form of intracellular signaling. The first evidence on this question came from the finding that positive selection can be blocked by cyclosporine (Fig. 6) (Gao et al., 1988; Jenkins et al., 1988); this drug inhibits calcium-dependent activation of T cells. More recently it has been found that positive selection is associated with *de novo* synthesis of certain activation antigens, e.g., CD69 and CD5 (Kaye and Ellenberger, 1992; Wallace et al., 1992; Swat et al., 1993), and requires the protein tyrosine kinase p56[lck] (Molina et al., 1992).

NEGATIVE SELECTION

To maintain self-tolerance, it has long been argued that the T cell repertoire has to be purged of cells displaying overt autoreactivity (Nossal, 1983). The first direct evidence on this question came from the discovery that mouse strains expressing endogenous superantigens show TCR Vβ-specific "holes" in the repertoire (Kappler et al., 1987, 1988; MacDonald et al., 1988). Significantly, superantigen-induced Vβ deletion is marked at the level of postthymic T cells and SP thymocytes but is relatively inconspicuous for DP thymocytes (Table VI). This crucial finding indicates that clonal deletion of autoreactive T cells takes place in the thymus during T cell ontogeny. Comparable evidence for negative selection (clonal deletion) in the thymus has come from studies with TCR TG mice (von Boehmer, 1990). Thus, if the TCR expressed in the TG line has allospecificity, e.g., for MHC[b], backcrossing the line to MHC[b] causes massive deletion of the clonotype-positive cells in the thymus. Deletion is a reflection of apoptosis, a specialized form of cell death involving activation of endogenous endonucleases.

In TCR TG mice, the stage at which T cells undergo clonal deletion in the thymus depends on the antigen studied. As in normal mice, expression of endogenous superantigens in TCR

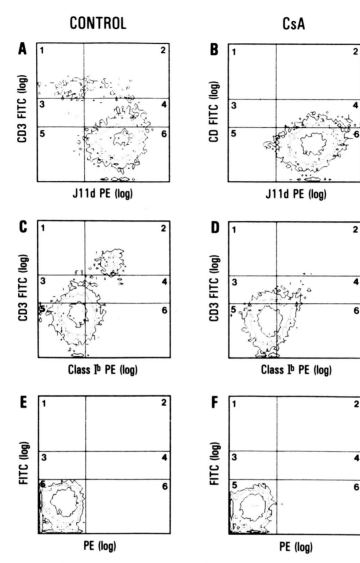

Fig. 6. Treating mice with cyclosporine (CsA) blocks positive selection in the thymus. Young mice were exposed to low-dose irradiation (600 rad) and then given daily injections of CsA (10–20 mg/kg) in olive oil for 7 weeks (**B, D, F**); control mice received olive oil alone (**A, C, E**). Using two-color fluorescence, thymocytes were stained for expression of CD3 molecules vs. either Jlld (heat-stable antigen) or MHC class I. For the control mice, it can be seen that the bulk of thymocytes (CD4+8+ cortical cells) express only a low density of CD3 and class I molecules; nearly all of these cells are Jlld+. The control thymocytes also contain a discrete population of CD3high cells (equivalent to mature SP cells); these cells are class Ihigh cells and comprise a mixture of Jlld+ (semi-mature) and Jlld− (fully mature) cells. In CsA-treated mice, thymocytes consist almost entirely of CD3−/low thymocytes, CD3high cells being conspicuously absent. In sections, the thymus of CsA-treated mice consists solely of cortical tissue, discrete regions of medulla being virtually undetectable. The capacity of CsA to block the production of mature T cells in the thymus is associated with profound T lymphocytopenia in the peripheral lymphoid tissues. From Gao et al. (1988) with permission.

Table VI. Mls[a] Endogenous Superantigens Cause Clonal Deletion of V_β6[+] T Cells in the Medulla But Not in the Cortex[a,b]

Strain studied	Expression of Mls[a] antigen	V_β expression in cortex		V_β expression in medulla	
		$V_\beta 6$	$V_\beta 8$	$V_\beta 6$	$V_\beta 8$
BALB/c	−	63	148	65	145
DBA/2	+	66	127	1	143
BALB.D2	+	59	139	1	162

[a] Endogenous superantigens are unique to mice and are encoded in the mouse genome by genes derived from mouse mammary tumor virus. In contrast to conventional antigens, superantigens appear to be recognized by T cells as native molecules; these molecules bridge T cells and APC by binding to the sides of MHC class II molecules and TCR molecules. Binding of superantigens to TCR molecules is V_β specific, which means that the precursor frequency of T cells for these antigens is very high (5–20%). Mls[a] (mtv-7) antigens are prototypical endogenous superantigens and are recognized by $V_\beta 6^+$ T cells but not by $V_\beta 8^+$ T cells; in mouse strains lacking Mls[a] antigens, e.g., BALB/c, $V_\beta 6^+$ T cells are common and display strong reactivity for APC from Mls[a] mice, e.g., for spleen cells from DBA/2 and BALB.D2 mice. The experiment illustrated shows the density of $V_\beta 6^+$ T cells in the thymus of Mls[a]-positive vs. Mls[a]-negative mice. These cells and control $V_\beta 8^+$ T cells were detected in cryostat sections of thymus with the aid of V_β-specific monoclonal antibodies. The data show the mean numbers of stained cells per test area. For the cortex, the data refer to weakly stained cells; brightly stained cells (cells expressing a high TCR density) were very rare in all three strains. Conversely, for the medulla the data refer to brightly stained cells.
[b] For T cells in the medulla, it can be seen that $V_\beta 6^+$ T cells are present in Mls[a]-negative mice but are almost undetectable in Mls[a]-positive mice. For the cortex, by contrast, there is little or no reduction of $V_\beta 6^+$ cells in Mls[a]-positive mice. This illustrates that clonal deletion of T cells to endogenous superantigens occurs at a relatively late stage of differentiation and is largely restricted to SP cells in the medulla. The lack of deletion in the cortex may reflect that endogenous superantigens are expressed only in the medulla and not the cortex; direct evidence on this question is lacking, however, because the precise tissue distribution of superantigens is unknown. An alternative possibility is that V_β deletion to these antigens is restricted to T cells expressing a high TCR density, TCR[high] cells being rare in the cortex but common in the medulla. Data adapted from Hengartner et al. (1988).

TG mice causes clonal deletion at a relatively late stage of differentiation, i.e., during the transition from DP cells to SP cells; histologically, clonal deletion is prominent only in the medulla and not in the cortex. With expression of alloantigens, by contrast, negative selection affects DP cells as well as SP cells and causes marked destruction of the cortex. This is also seen when TCR TG mice are injected with soluble antigens. Thus, if class II-restricted TCR TG mice specific for ovalbumin are injected with this antigen in peptide form, the clonotype-positive cells in the cortex die rapidly and the cortex collapses (Murphy et al., 1990). Since class II expression in the cortex is largely restricted to epithelial cells, clonal deletion by peptides in the cortex presumably reflects contact with epithelial cells rather than BM-derived APC (see below). Clonal deletion following peptide injection is much less evident in the medulla than the cortex, which illustrates that clonal deletion is restricted to immature thymocytes.

In ovalbumin-specific TCR TG mice, it is notable that clonal deletion in the cortex is seen only when antigen is given in peptide form. Thus when native ovalbumin is injected the cortex remains intact. This observation is in line with the evidence that the cortex is relatively impermeable to intact soluble proteins (Raviola and Karnovsky, 1972). How then is the immune system rendered tolerant to circulating self-proteins, e.g., albumin? The most likely explanation is that tolerance to these antigens occurs predominantly in the medulla through contact with marrow-derived APC. Unlike the cortex, the medullary region of the thymus is relatively permeable to blood-borne proteins and these molecules can be broken down *in situ* into peptides by local APC. In addition, constant migration of APC into the medulla from the periphery presumably means that many self-antigens are carried into the thymus in cell-bound form. The APC in the thymus form a dense network at the corticomedullary junction, and this ensures optimal display of self antigens to the newly formed SP T cells passing from the cortex to the medulla. Being still partly immature, the self-reactive T cells in this population then undergo clonal deletion *in situ*.

RELATIONSHIP OF POSITIVE AND NEGATIVE SELECTION

As described above, it is highly likely that self-tolerance induction (clonal deletion) to circulating self-antigens takes place largely in the medulla through T cell contact with self-antigens expressed on APC. As mentioned earlier, however, it is clear that clonal deletion can also occur in the cortex, presumably through contact with constitutive self antigens expressed on TEC. If so, one is presented with the paradox that MHC expression on cortical TEC can induce either positive or negative selection, implying that each form of selection can be controlled by the *same* set of MHC-associated self-peptides. This begs the thorny question of why all the T cells that undergo positive selection in the cortex do not subsequently (or simultaneously) undergo negative selection. What then is the relationship between positive and negative selection?

The explanation favored by this writer rests on two assumptions. First, positive and negative selection are closely related, the essential difference between these two forms of selection being the *intensity* of the TCR-mediated signals the cells experience: negative selection reflects strong signaling whereas positive selection reflects weak signaling. The second assumption is that the sensitivity of T cells to TCR-mediated signals *decreases rapidly* as the cells mature.

Assuming that immature cortical T cells are initially hypersusceptible to TCR-mediated signals, one can envisage that any cortical cells having more than minimal ("physiological") binding affinity for the MHC–peptide complexes displayed on cortical TEC are deleted *in situ* as a reflection of excessive signaling. With binding affinities at or just below this minimal level, cortical T cells receive a lower (subtolerogenic) dose of signals. This level of signaling is not sufficient to tolerize (delete) the cells but is adequate to induce the cells to begin to differentiate into mature T cells, i.e., to induce positive selection. After positive selection, the T cells start to lose their hypersensitivity to TCR signals. As a result, no TCR-mediated signaling occurs when the T cells reach the medulla (or the periphery) and reencounter the same MHC/peptide complexes that led to initial positive selection. This ensures full self-tolerance to the selecting ligands. Nevertheless the loss of hypersensitivity to TCR signals remains incomplete until the cells differentiate into fully mature T cells. Operationally, this means that the cells remain tolerance susceptible for a brief period after entering the medulla. As a result, the newly formed T cells entering the medulla can be tolerized to the various extrathymic self-antigens that enter the medulla from the bloodstream, either in soluble form or borne by APCs.

SELF-TOLERANCE TO TISSUE-SPECIFIC ANTIGENS

As discussed earlier, self-tolerance to circulating self-antigens is probably largely, and perhaps entirely, a reflection of clonal deletion in the thymus. In this respect it is virtually impossible to break self-tolerance to serum albumin and other common blood-borne proteins. These molecules are present in high concentrations and are presumed to delete even low-affinity T cells in the thymus. The situation with circulating self-antigens present in only low concentrations, e.g., certain hormones, is likely to be different. For these antigens, one can envisage that clonal deletion in the thymus is quite limited and is restricted to high-affinity T cells. Although low-affinity T cells would escape deletion, these cells would pose no danger: the low concentration of the antigen encountered in the periphery would be insufficient to cause activation of residual low-affinity T cells, and these cells would be operationally tolerant. Because the concentration of antigen required for stimulating mature T cells is substantially higher than for inducing clonal deletion in the thymus, the immune system can probably tolerate a modest elevation in the level of self-antigens, e.g., in sex hormones at the time of puberty.

Although one can make a strong case that tolerance to circulating self-antigens is a reflection of clonal deletion, the situation with tissue-specific antigens is quite different. For these antigens there is abundant evidence that self-tolerance does not involve clonal deletion. This is apparent from the finding that self-tolerance to myelin basic protein and other tissue-specific antigens can easily be broken, e.g., by injecting the antigen in soluble form in the presence of adjuvant.

To explain self-tolerance to tissue-specific antigens, many workers favor the view that tolerance to these antigens is a reflection of some form of postthymic tolerance such as anergy or suppression (Schwartz and Datta, 1989; Sinha et al., 1990). This idea has been assessed by preparing TG mice in which antigens are expressed in defined sites with the aid of tissue-specific promoters (Miller and Morahan, 1992). For example, with the insulin promoter one can express a viral protein in the β cell of the pancreas. The general finding with this model is that expression of antigen in tissue-specific sites does not lead to local autoimmune disease. The key observation, however, is that tolerance induction to the transgenic antigen is the exception rather than the rule. Some groups do see a limited degree of tolerance induction (anergy), but such tolerance is probably a reflection of minor expression of the antigen in sites other than the pancreas, e.g., the thymus. When the antigen is restricted to the pancreas, tolerance is undetectable or very limited. Interestingly, this also applies in TCR TG mice. Thus, no tolerance or signs of autoimmunity occur when TG mice expressing a viral protein in pancreatic β cells are backcrossed to a viral-protein-specific TCR TG line (Ohashi et al., 1991). In this double TG line, tolerance can easily be broken, i.e., by injecting the mice with infectious virus. Here, confrontation with antigen in the lymphoid tissues causes T cell activation followed by rapid migration of blast cells to the pancreas and local tissue destruction.

In light of the above findings, there is no necessity to postulate that tolerance to tissue-specific antigens is a reflection of postthymic tolerance. "Tolerance" is simply a reflection of segregation: tissue-specific antigens remain sequestered, and T cells with potential reactivity to these antigens remain within the confines of the recirculating lymphocyte pool. A breakdown of one or other of these barriers is probably the main precipitating event for the induction of autoimmune disease.

As argued above, tolerance to self-antigens can be explained entirely in terms of clonal deletion in the thymus combined with antigen segregation. Self/nonself discrimination is then sharply defined and the immune system is free to give unrestricted responses to foreign antigens. Despite the continuing popularity of postthymic tolerance mechanisms there is no convincing evidence that normal self/nonself discrimination involves either anergy or suppression. However, if self-tolerance breaks and autoimmune disease results, various forms of immunoregulation are probably highly important for suppressing the response of autoreactive T cells. This topic has been extensively reviewed elsewhere.

ACKNOWLEDGMENTS

This work was supported by Grants CA38355, CA25803, and AI21487 from the United States Public Health Service. Publication No. 8063-IMM from The Scripps Research Institute.

REFERENCES

Chan SH, Cogrove D, Waltzinger C, Benoist C, Mathis D (1993): Another view of thymocyte selection. Cell 73:225–236.

Davis CB, Killeen N, Casey Crooks ME, Raulet D, Littman DR (1993): Evidence for a stochastic mechanism in the differentiation of mature subsets of T lymphocytes. Cell 73:237–247.

Fowlkes BJ, Pardoll DM (1989): Molecular and cellular events of T cell development. Adv Immunol 44:207–264.

Gao E-K, Lo D, Cheney R, Kanagawa O, Sprent J (1988): Abnormal differentiation of thymocytes in mice treated with cyclosporin A. Nature (London) 336:176–179.

Germain RN, Margulies DH (1993): The biochemistry and cell biology of antigen processing and presentation. Annu Rev Immunol 11:403–450.

Haas W, Pereira P, Tonegawa S (1993): Gamma/delta cells. Annu Rev Immunol 11:637–686.

Hengartner H, Odermatt B, Schneider R, Schreyer M, Walle G, Macdonald HR, Zinkernagel RM (1988): Deletion of self-reactive T cells before entry into the thymus medulla. Nature (London) 336:388–390.

Huessmann M, Scott B, Kisielow P, von Boehmer H (1991): Kinetics and efficacy of positive selection in the thymus of normal and T cell receptor transgenic mice. Cell 66:533–540.

Ikuta K, Uchida N, Friedman J, Weissman IL. (1992): Lymphocyte development from stem cells. Annu Rev Immunol 10:759–783.

Janeway C (1992): The T cell receptor as a multicomponent signalling machine: CD4/CD8 coreceptors and CD45 in T cell activation. Annu Rev Immunol 10:645–674.

Jenkins MK, Schwartz RH, Pardoll DM (1988): Effects of cyclosporine A on T cell development and clonal deletion. Science 241:1655–1658.

Kappler JW, Roehm N, Marrack P (1987): T cell tolerance by clonal elimination in the thymus. Cell 49:273–280.

Kappler JW, Staerz U, White J, Marrack PC (1988): Self-tolerance eliminates T cells specific for Mls-modified products of the major histocompatibility complex. Nature (London) 332:35–40.

Kaye J, Ellenberger DC (1992): Differentiation of an immature T cell line: A model of thymic positive selection. Cell 71:423–435.

Lefrancois L (1991): Extrathymic differentiation of intraepithelial lymphocytes: Generation of a separate and unequal T-cell repertoire? Immunol Today 12:436–438.

Leiden JM (1993): Transcriptional regulation of T cell receptor genes. Annu Rev Immunol 11:539–570.

MacDonald HR, Schneider R, Lees RK, et al. (1988): T-cell receptor V beta use predicts reactivity and tolerance to Mls[a]-encoded antigens. Nature (London) 332:40–45.

Marrack P, Kappler J (1987): The T cell receptor. Science 238:1073–1079.

Miller JFAP, Morahan G (1992): Peripheral T cell tolerance. Annu Rev Immunol 10:51–69.

Miller JFAP, Osoba D (1967): Current concepts of the immunological function of the thymus. Physiol Rev 47:437–520.

Molina TJ, Kishihara K, Siderovski DP, VanEwijk W, Mak T (1992): Profound block in thymocyte development in mice lacking p56 lck. Nature (London) 357:161–163.

Moller G (ed) (1978): Acquisition of the T cell repertoire. Immunol Rev 42:3–270.

Murphy KM, Heimberger AB, Loh DH (1990): Induction by antigen of intrathymic apoptosis of $CD4^+$ $CD8^+$ TCR^{lo} thymocytes in vivo. Science 250:1720–1723.

Nakayama T, June CH, Munitz TI, Sheard M, McCarthy SA, Sharrow SO, Samelson LE, Singer A (1990): Inhibition of T cell receptor expression and function in immature $CD4^+8^+$ cells by CD4. Science 249:1558–1561.

Nossal GJV (1983): Cellular mechanisms of immunologic tolerance. Annu Rev Immunol 1:33–62.

Ohashi PS, Oehen S, Burki K, Pircher HP, Oshashi CT, Odermatt B, Malissen B, Zinkernagel R, Hengartner H (1991): Ablation of tolerance and induction of diabetes by virus infection in viral antigen transgenic mice. Cell 65:305–317.

Owen JJT, Jenkinson EJ (1981): Embryology of the immune system. Prog Allergy 29:1–34.

Picker LJ, Butcher EC (1992): Physiological and molecular mechanisms of lymphocyte homing. Annu Rev Immunol 10:561–591.

Rammensee H-G, Falk K, Rotzschke O (1993): Peptides naturally presented by MHC class I molecules. Annu Rev Immunol 11:213–244.

Raviola E, Karnovsky MJ (1972): Evidence for a blood-thymus barrier using electron-opaque tracers. J Exp Med 136:466–498.

Schwartz RS, Datta SK (1989): Autoimmunity and autoimmune disease. In Paul WE (ed): "Fundamental Immunology," 2nd ed. New York: Raven Press, pp 819–866.

Scollay R, Shortman K (1985): Cell traffic in the adult thymus: cell entry and exit, cell birth and death. In Watson JD, Marbrook J (eds): "Recognition and Regulation in Cell-Mediated Immunity." New York: Marcel Dekker, pp 3–30.

Sinha AA, Lopez MT, McDevitt HO (1990): Autoimmune diseases: The failure of self tolerance. Science 248:1380–1388.

Shortman K, Egerton M, Spangrude GJ, Scollay R (1990): The generation and fate of thymocytes. Semin Immunol 2:3–12.

Sprent J (1973): Circulating T and B lymphocytes of the mouse. I. Migratory properties. Cell Immunol 7:10–39.

Sprent J (1993): T lymphocytes and the thymus. In Paul, WE (ed): "Fundamental Immunology," 3rd ed. New York: Raven Press, pp 75–109.

Sprent J (1995): T cell biology and the thymus. In Frank MM, Austen KF, Claman HN, Unanue ER (eds.): "Samter's Immunological Diseases," 5th ed. Boston: Little, Brown, pp 73–85.

Sprent, J, Webb SR (1987): Function and specificity of T cell subsets in the mouse. Adv Immunol 41:39–133.

Sprent J, Lo D, Gao E-K, Ron Y (1988): T cell selection in the thymus. Immunol Rev 101:173–190.

Sprent J, Schaefer M, Lo D, Korngold R (1986): Functions of purified L3T4⁺ and Lyt-2⁺ cells in vitro and in vivo. Immunol Rev 91:195–218.

Surh CD, Gao E-K, Kosaka H, et al. (1992): Two subsets of epithelial cells in the thymic medulla. J Exp Med 176:495–506.

Swat W, Dessing M, von Boehmer H, Kisielow P (1993): CD69 expression during selection and maturation of CD4⁺8⁺ thymocytes. Eur J Immunol 23:739–746.

van Ewijk W (1991): T-cell differentiation is influenced by thymic microenvironments. Annu Rev Immunol 9:591–615.

von Boehmer H (1988): The developmental biology of T lymphocytes. Annu Rev Immunol 6:309–326.

von Boehmer H (1990): Developmental biology of T cells in T cell receptor transgenic mice. Annu Rev Immunol 8:531–556.

von Boehmer H, Teh H-S, Kisielow P (1989): The thymus selects the useful, neglects the useless and destroys the harmful. Immunol Today 10:57–61.

Wallace VA, Fung-Leung WP, Timms E, Grey D, Kishihara K, Loh DY, Penninger J, Mak TW (1992): CD45RA and CD45RBʰⁱᵍʰ expression induced by thymic selection events. J Exp Med 176:1657–1663.

NOTE ADDED IN PROOF

This chapter was written in June 1993, and a considerable amount of new information on the thymus and T cell selection has emerged in the interim. Some of the more important new data are summarized below.

In the case of early thymocyte differentiation, it is now clear that the "pre-receptor" expressed on DN cells switching to DP cells is not a ββ homodimer but a heterodimer consisting of a β chain linked to a non-polymorphic TCR chain termed gp33 (Groettrup et al., 1993; Saint-Ruf et al., 1994); the ligand for the β gp33 heterodimer is still unknown.

Positive and negative selection of αβ T cells in this article is explained in terms of different levels of signalling resulting from T cell contact with weak (positively selecting) vs strong (tolerizing) self peptides. Direct support for this affinity/avidity model of thymic selection has come from a series of recent experiments on the effects of adding defined self-peptides to fetal thymic organ cultures prepared from class I-deficient and TAP-1-negative mice (Hogquist et al., 1994; Ashton-Richardt et al., 1994; Sebzda et al., 1994). The key finding in these studies is that peptides with weak TCR affinity (antagonist peptides) induce positive selection of CD8⁺ cells at low doses but negative selection at high doses.

In the case of negative selection, direct evidence that self tolerance induction to circulating self antigens takes place largely in the medulla rather than the cortex has come from studies on TCR transgenic mice specific for C5, a serum complement component (Zal et al., 1994); in this line, deletion of C5-reactive T cells is pronounced for SP cells (CD4⁺ cells) but minimal for DP cells.

Until recently, demonstrating negative selection in the thymus has rested largely on defining holes in the repertoire at the level of DP vs SP cells by FACS analysis. It is now possible to demonstrate negative selection *in situ*, i.e., in cryostat sections, using a sensitive staining method for apoptotic cells. With this procedure, negative selection of T cells to endogenous mtv antigens in TCR transgenic models is limited to the medulla and corticomedullary junction (Surh and Sprent, 1994). In the normal thymus, however, apoptotic cells are quite rare in the medulla but prominent throughout the cortex. Studies with MHC-deficient mice suggest that apoptosis in the cortex is due largely to death by neglect (lack of positive selection) rather than negative selection. Cell death from negative selection thus seems to apply to only a very small proportion of total thymocytes.

Additional References

Ashton-Rickardt PG, Bandeira A, Delaney JR, Van Kaer L, Pircher H-P, Zinkernagel RM, Tonegawa S (1994): Evidence for an avidity model of T cell activation in the thymus. Cell 73:1041–1049.

Groettrup M, Ungewiss K, Azogui O, Palacios R, Owen MJ, Hayday AC, von Boehmer H (1993): A novel disulfide-linked heterodimer on pre-T cells consists of the T cell receptor β chain and a 33 kd glycoprotein. Cell 75:283–294.

Hogquist KA, Jameson SC, Heath WR, Howard JL, Bevan MJ, Carbone FR (1994): T cell receptor antagonist peptides induce positive selection. Cell 76:17–23.

Saint-Ruf C, Ungewiss K, Groettrup M, Bruno L, Fehling HJ, von Boehmer H (1994): Analysis and expression of a cloned pre-T cell receptor gene. Science 266:1208–1212.

Sebzda E, Wallace VA, Mayer J, Yeung RSM, Mak TW, Ohashi PS (1994): Positive and negative thymocyte selection induced by different concentrations of a single peptide. Science 263:1615–1618.

Surh CD, Sprent J (1994): T-cell apoptosis detected *in situ* during positive and negative selection in the thymus. Nature 372:100–103.

Zal T, Volkmann A, Stockinger B (1994): Mechanisms of tolerance induction in major histocompatibility complex class II-restricted T cells specific for a blood-borne self antigen. J Exp Med 180:2089–2099.

Chapter 3
Cellular Immunology

Neal Flomenberg

INTRODUCTION

The immune system's function in health and disease is largely governed by the actions of T lymphocytes. The immune system can protect or paradoxically attack the body through a number of mechanisms discussed throughout this book. T cells may play direct roles in some of these processes, but also are responsible for regulating many of the other components of the immune system (for example, providing "help" for antibody production). Thus their role in most immune responses is a central one. T lymphocytes derive their name from the fact that they are dependent on the thymus for their development. While minor subpopulations of T cells may develop in athymic animals, the major subset fails to develop in these animals, rendering them immunoincompetent (Flanagan, 1966; Pantelouris, 1968). A rare disorder in man, known as DiGeorge syndrome, is associated with failure of the thymus to develop and the consequential absence of T cells (DiGeorge, 1968; Rosen et al., 1984).

In contrast to antibodies, the molecules of humoral immunity, T cells do not interact with antigen free in solution. Indeed, for the most part, they do not interact with intact antigen at all, but rather with fragments of antigen that have been bound in the groove of MHC molecules, on the surface of another cell. The details of antigen processing and presentation are reviewed in Chapter 2. Activation of T cells leads to a number of events, including the production of lymphokines and lymphokine receptors, activation of the cytolytic machinery, and cellular proliferation. These events occur in two stages. The

first phase requires physical interaction of the T cell with the antigen-presenting cell through a variety of cell surface molecules, including the T cell receptor (TcR), which imparts specificity to the response. When appropriately signaled during this phase, the T cell proceeds through the G_1 phase of the cell cycle and expresses lymphokine receptors such as interleukin 2 (IL-2) receptors on its surface. Subsets of T cells are also induced to secrete lymphokines such as IL-2 through these cell-to-cell interactions. Binding of IL-2 to its receptor, through autocrine or paracrine mechanisms, leads to progression through S phase and cellular proliferation. The activity of the T cell is regulated as a consequence of these cell contact and cytokine-mediated events. The T cells in turn additionally regulate the activities of a wide array of immune effector cells. Production of antibodies to most though not all antigens requires help from T cells. T cell-mediated help is a complex process, which includes T cell–B cell contact events necessary for B cell activation. Additionally, T cell-mediated help reflects the secretion by the T cell of appropriate cytokines, which are necessary to support the activation, growth, and/or differentiation of B cells and which may direct such processes as antibody class switching. T cells may conversely actively suppress the humoral response. T cells often play a very direct role in the elimination of virally infected cells through cytolytic attack of the infected population. T cell-derived cytokines can modulate the activity of monocyte/macrophages, neutrophils, natural killer (NK) cells. Moreover, many of the cytokines that regulate hematopoiesis are T cell derived. Thus, as illus-

Transplantation Immunology, pages 53–86
© 1995 Wiley-Liss, Inc.

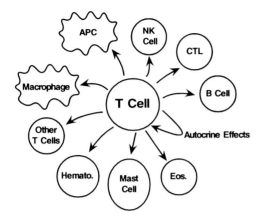

Fig. 1. The central role of T cells in the immune response is illustrated. Through the secretion of soluble mediators and contact events, T cells may facilitate or inhibit the activation, growth, differentiation, and effector functions of a variety of cellular populations. These include antigen presenting cells (APC), macrophages, hematopoietic progenitor cells (Hemato), mast cells, eosinophils (Eos), B cells, and NK cells. The activities of T cells are similarly regulated. T cells may be influenced by their own soluble mediators (autocrine effects) or by mediators produced by neighboring T cells (paracrine effects). Many cytotoxic T lymphocytes (CTL) and other populations of T cells are dependent on the mediators produced by helper T cells for their growth and differentiation.

trated in Figure 1, the T cell occupies a very central position in the body's defense network. Many of the same processes that would normally be directed toward the elimination of pathogens may also contribute to allograft rejection.

GENERATION OF T CELL DIVERSITY

The recognition of a diverse array of foreign molecules requires that T cells express a diverse array of receptor molecules. As is also the case for antibody-producing cells, a single T cell typically produces only a single functional receptor. The progeny of a single T cell (known as a clonal population) can thus be recognized through their expression of identical receptor molecules. The ability to recognize a diverse array of antigens is thus dependent on the ability to generate large numbers of T cells each expressing a unique receptor molecule.

The mechanisms through which T cells and B cells generate diversity in their receptors are similar, though not entirely identical. There are presently two recognized families of T cells in man. The predominant family, including 85–98% of circulating T cells, is defined by their use of α and β chains to generate their receptors ($\alpha\beta$ T cells) (Chien et al., 1984; Hedrick et al., 1984; Saito et al., 1984; Yanagi et al., 1984). The minor subset (1–15%) of circulating T cells utilizes γ and δ chains to generate their receptors (Brenner et al., 1988; Winoto and Baltimore, 1989). These chains are inherited as a series of discontinuous genetic elements, brought together by rearrangement of the DNA. The genetic regions encoding each of these chains consist of V (variable), J (joining), and C (constant) region gene segments. Some of these loci also include a fourth region, the D (diversity) segment between V and J (reviewed in Davis and Bjorkman, 1988). For the T cell receptor α and β loci, the number of segments presently known is as follows:

	V	D	J	C
α	50	—	50	1
β	70	2	13	2

During the process of T cell development in the thymus, DNA rearrangements will bring V (D) J and C region segments together to form α and β chains. This process is illustrated in Figure 2A. The diversity present in the germ line DNA, in different V, D, and J segments associating randomly with one another, and in different α and β chains combining with one another can lead to the production of approximately 10^7 unique T cell receptors. This, however, represents only the tip of the iceberg with regard to receptor complexity. At the joints between the various gene segments, the DNA recombinational machinery can randomly remove or insert DNA nucleotides. The net gain or loss of nucleotides must occur in multiples of 3 if the receptor gene is to remain in proper frame, but appears to be under little other constraint (Fig. 2B). This component of receptor diversity, referred to as

A.

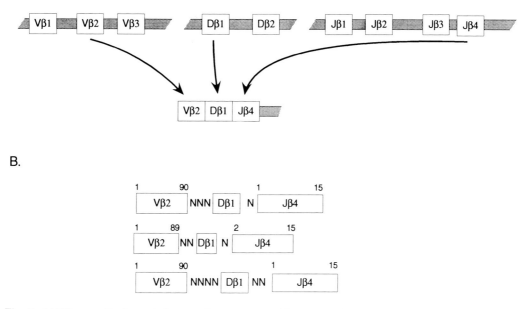

B.

Fig. 2. (**A**) The genetic elements that contribute to an individual TcR are located discontinuously in germ line DNA. During T cell differentiation, rearrangements of the DNA juxtapose these elements. V, D, and J regions are randomly brought together, leading to TcR diversity. (**B**) The process of DNA arrangement leads to the random insertion or deletion of nucleotides (N). As long as the gene remains in frame after final assembly, the rearrangement is functional. The addition and removal of nucleotides, nevertheless, contribute to TcR diversity. As illustrated, three T cell receptors, all composed of $V_\beta 2$, $D_\beta 1$, and $J_\beta 4$, are all unique because of the diversity introduced at the junctions of these genetic elements.

junctional diversity, actually accounts for more of the variation in T cell receptors than that generated by rearrangement of the germ line segments (combinational diversity). A similar process occurs in γ/δ T cells, except that junctional diversity plays an even larger role and combinational diversity an even lesser role. One present model of T cell receptor structure suggests that the areas of combinational diversity predominantly contact the α helices of the MHC molecule, while the regions of junctional diversity predominantly contact the peptide. Such a model would align the most diverse portions of the T cell receptor with the most diverse portions of the antigen–MHC complex and vice versa (reviewed in Davis and Bjorkman, 1988). Typically, the T cell will rearrange one of its two β loci. If successful, the process stops. If an aberrant nonfunctional β chain is produced through improper splicing, then the second β locus on the remaining chromosome is utilized. Thus, only one functional β chain is generated, a process known as allelic exclusion. Allelic exclusion is less absolute in rearrangements of the α gene.

THYMIC SELECTION OF T CELLS

To be functional in the periphery, a T cell must recognize a peptide fragment/self-MHC complex in the periphery. The fact that antigen and MHC are seen together imparts the characteristic of MHC restriction to T cell-mediated immunity (Zinkernagel and Doherty, 1974). Antigen/peptide does not lead to T cell activation in the absence of the appropriate MHC molecule (Doherty et al., 1976; Doherty and Zinkernagel, 1975). Random receptor generation is likely to generate many receptors that have no appreciable affinity for self-MHC + peptide. Such receptors (and such T cells) are essentially physiologically functionless. Other randomly generated receptors have the potential to recognize self-MHC + self-peptides too well, potentially producing autoimmune responses. Consequently, the T cell repertoire must be shaped by selective forces to imprint the T cell repertoire with the characteristics of MHC restriction and self-tolerance (Sha et al., 1988). These selective forces operate predominantly within the thymus, the primary site of T cell maturation. Following rearrangement of their T cell receptor genes, the cells undergo positive selection in the thymic cortex. Engagement of the T cell receptor with self-MHC within the appropriate thymic microenvironment appears to turn off cellular production of the recombinational machinery (Turka et al., 1991). Failure to engage identifies the cell as functionless and marks it for elimination. Thus MHC restriction is a consequence of positive selection (Blackman et al., 1989; Scott et al., 1989; Sha et al., 1988).

Following positive selection, T cells pass through the thymic medulla where their reactivity with self-MHC is again assessed. Those cells with an unacceptably strong interaction with self-MHC are negatively selected (Fig. 3) (Finkel et al., 1989; Kappler et al., 1987; Kisielow et al., 1988). Thymocytes appear to be eliminated in the thymus by a process termed apoptosis, wherein their DNA undergoes a characteristic pattern of fragmentation in association with cell death (McConkey et al., 1990). While clonal elimination within the thymus is an important mechanism in maintaining self-tolerance, it is by no means the sole mechanism. Other mechanisms, including induction of anergy and ongoing suppression of the immune response, are likely to contribute to maintaining self-tolerance. The relative importance of each of these processes is likely to vary depending on the nature and distribution of the self-antigen in question.

During their maturation, thymocytes undergo a series of phenotypic changes correlating with their stage of development. The earliest thymocytes lack expression of either CD4 or CD8, two molecules that define subpopulations of mature T cells. These early thymocytes, which represent less than 5% of the total thymocyte population, are referred to as "double negatives" based upon their lack of either CD4 or CD8 expression. T cell receptors are also not expressed at this stage. With progression through the maturation process, CD4 and CD8 become coexpressed leading to the "double positive" cell, which comprises 80% of thymocytes. These cells express low levels of $\alpha\beta$ T cell receptors. CD8 may actually precede CD4 expression leading to a small population of cells between these two stages, which are $CD8^+CD4^-TcR\alpha\beta^-$. The most mature thymocytes lose expression of either CD4 or CD8, express high levels of T cell receptors, and thus exhibit phenotypes similar to peripheral T cells (single positives) (Fig. 3) (Bluestone et al., 1987; Mathieson and Fowlkes, 1984; Shortman and Scollay, 1985; Sprent and Webb, 1987; von Boehmer, 1988; von Boehmer et al., 1988).

FLEXIBILITY IN T CELL ACTIVATION: MULTIPLE MOLECULES WORKING IN CONCERT

When T cells encounter an appropriate antigenic challenge, they become activated and a number of secondary events occur, which are necessary for the development of an immune response to the antigenic stimulus. These secondary events include clonal expansion of the activated cells, lymphokine secretion, activation of the cells cytolytic effector pathways, as well as other events. Thus for an immune response to develop, it is necessary that the recognition events occurring at the cell surface can transmit signals to the interior of the cell to activate the cell and initiate the subsequent cellular events. The mechanisms underlying signal transduction from the cell surface to the interior of the cell are discussed in detail in the subsequent sections.

Although the T cell repertoire is selected to exhibit appropriate reactivity toward self-MHC + peptide, not every encounter with antigen results in the same immunologic outcome. The immune system may be activated to produce an aggressive response or the cells may instead be rendered unresponsive, either transiently or permanently. Within the thymus, receptor engagement may lead to both positive and negative se-

Intrathymic Development

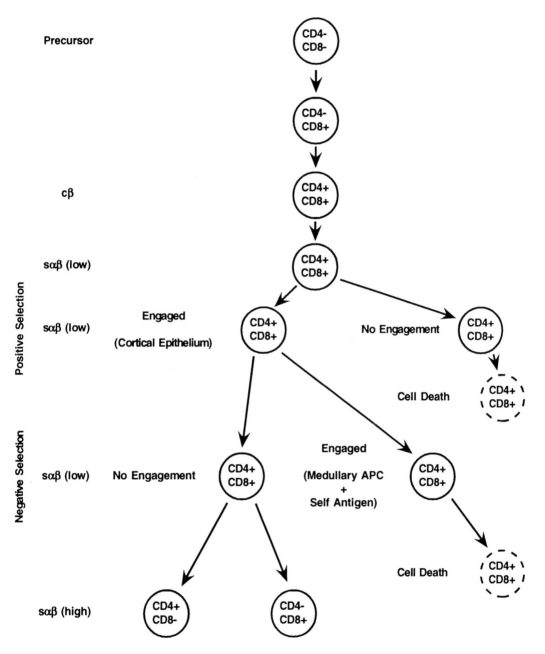

Fig. 3. The differentiation of mature T cells from precursor elements is illustrated, as well as their selection during intrathymic development. cβ, cytoplasmic β chain, denotes the presence of β chain in the cytoplasm, but not on the cell surface. With subsequent differentiation, αβ TcR dimers are expressed on the cell surface (sαβ).

lection. This presents a dilemma. Given the one cell–one receptor concept, how can multiple potential outcomes result? Other questions also arise on closer examination. The T cell receptor has a very short cytoplasmic tail that appears inadequate for transducing signals from the cell surface to the interior. How then are the signals transmitted? Additionally, the affinity/avidity of the T cell receptor for its ligand is extremely low, raising the question of how the T cell adheres to the antigen presenting cell long enough to undergo activation.

The answer to these seeming paradoxes is that the T cell receptor, while it imparts specificity to the response, is not the sole molecule through which T cells interact with their environment (see Fig. 4). The events at the cell surface begin with a nonspecific stage of adhesion, between the T cell and antigen presenting cell, which is independent of the T cell receptor. Thereafter, the T cell receptor (and other T cell surface molecules) may interact with their ligands. Many of the other interactions also provide signals to the T cells. Depending on the outcome of these inter-actions, the cells may simply detach, the T cell may become activated, or anergy may result.

Although adhesion and activation are often thought of as distinct processes, this is an over-simplification. The same molecules may sub-serve both functions. Moreover, as will be dis-cussed below, adhesion and activation can have reciprocal effects upon one another. Similarly, the traditional concept has been that when a T cell interacts with an antigen-presenting cell, the flow of information is from the antigen-presenting cell to the T cell. Rather, the process is more akin to a dialogue back and forth be-tween the two cells. An appropriate cascade of signals leads to activation of both cells, while incomplete information exchange results in fail-ure of activation, anergy, or tolerance. Thus, the encounter between a T cell and a cell expressing its antigen/MHC ligand can be either positive or negative, depending on the environment and the secondary signals received. Over 20 accessory molecules that may participate in T cell adhe-sion/activation are now known. Many of these are illustrated with their ligands in Figure 4.

SIGNALING THROUGH THE TcR: REQUIREMENTS FOR RECEPTOR CROSS-LINKING

T cell activation requires that T cell receptor molecules are both bound to their antigen–MHC ligands (receptor engagement) and drawn to-gether (receptor cross-linking) (Kaye et al., 1983; Meuer et al., 1983). Simple engagement of the receptor with an antireceptor antibody free in solution does not lead to activation (Meuer et al., 1983). In contrast, if the antibodies are cross-linked on a surface or in a matrix, activa-tion ensues. Cross-linking occurs with many an-tibodies when cells bearing Fc receptor are pre-sent (Van Wauwe et al., 1980). Binding of antibody to the TcR provides receptor engage-ment. In addition, binding of the opposite end of the antibody (the Fc region) to the Fc receptor provides the cross linking. Adding a second anti-body that recognizes the constant portion of the antireceptor antibody can also result in cross-linking. Alternatively, the antireceptor anti-bodies can be bound directly to plastic or some

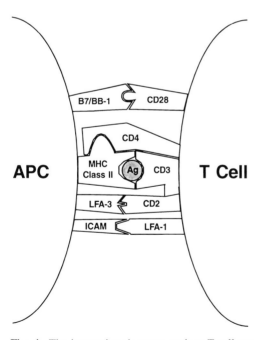

Fig. 4. The interactions between various T cell sur-face molecules and their molecular counterparts on the surface of the APC are illustrated.

other surface (Meuer et al., 1983). In all of these situations, multiple T cell receptors are engaged by artificial ligands on an opposing surface or matrix. Physiologically, the same sort of cross-linkage would occur when the receptor encounters its MHC peptide ligand on the surface of another cell. Activation of T cells has been shown to generate a rise in intracellular free calcium and activation of protein kinase C (PKC) (Imboden et al., 1985; Manger et al., 1987; Oettgen et al., 1985; Weiss et al., 1984).

THE CD3 COMPLEX

Although cross-linking the TcR can result in T cell activation, the receptor itself, which has only a tiny cytoplasmic tail, has no direct means for signal transduction (Hedrick et al., 1984; Yanagi et al., 1984). This function is mediated by CD3, one of the first human T cell surface molecules to be identified. This molecule coassociates with the T cell receptor in the cytoplasm and the entire complex moves to the cell surface as a unit. If one of the T cell receptor chains is defective such that a functional TcR cannot be formed, CD3 remains trapped in the cytoplasm (Geisler et al., 1990; Ohashi et al., 1985). CD3 is itself a complex molecule, consisting of at least five proteins in man: γ, δ, ε, ζ, and η. Note that the γ and δ chains of CD3 are distinct from γ/δ T cell receptors, though CD3 is coassociated with both α/β and γ/δ type receptors. CD3γ, δ, and ε are the products of three closely linked genes (Clevers et al., 1988). ζ and η appear to be alternate products derived from the same gene, which is structurally distinct from both the T cell receptor and the other components of the CD3 complex (Jin et al., 1990a). These molecules appear to be closely associated with the signal-transducing functions of the CD3 complex (Sussman et al., 1988). The majority of CD3 complexes (approximately 90%) contain a ζ–ζ homodimer, while the minority contain a ζ–η heterodimer (Baniyash et al., 1988a). Although CD3 is a multimeric structure, the ε chain seems to be particularly immunogenic, and the majority of antibodies recognizing human CD3 appear directed primarily or exclusively to this chain. The exact stoichiometry of the various chains in the CD3 complex has not been definitively established. It may be that two ε chains are present per CD3 complex. It has also been suggested that the γ and δ chains are not present within a single receptor, but rather are used alternatively to produce two distinct types of CD3 complexes (Fig. 5) (Konig et al., 1990;

The TcR/CD3 Complex

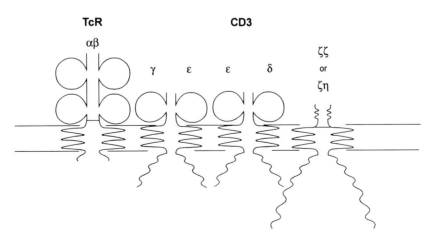

Fig. 5. A model of the organization of the TcR/CD3 complex.

Jin et al., 1990b). Antibodies to the CD3 complex exhibit many functional similarities to antibodies that recognize the TcR directly, reflecting their close functional association (Van Wauwe et al., 1980). CD3 probably does not serve as the direct signaling molecule, but is associated with p59^{fyn}, a member of the Src family of tyrosine kinases (Samelson et al., 1990). Activation of p59^{fyn} is probably responsible for transducing at least some of the signals from the TcR–CD3 complex into the cell interior.

CD4 AND CD8

For many years, T cells appeared divisible into two functional subsets, helper and cytotoxic/suppressor cells. With the advent of monoclonal antibodies that recognize T cell differentiation antigens, two subsets of T cells could be identified that appeared to correlate with these functional divisions. These two molecules, CD4 and CD8, which in general are present on reciprocal subsets of T cells, have been demonstrated to represent functional coreceptors that play an integral role in T cell activation. The ligands for CD4 and CD8 are nonpolymorphic portions of class II and class I MHC molecules, respectively (Doyle and Strominger, 1988; Norment et al., 1988). While the functional subdivisions do largely correlate with these phenotypic subsets, exceptions do exist. CD4$^+$CD8$^-$ cytotoxic T cells have been demonstrated, for example. In contrast to the more characteristic CD4$^-$CD8$^+$ cytotoxic cells, which recognize or are restricted by MHC class I molecules, the CD4$^+$ cytotoxic T cells utilize class II MHC molecules as their target or restriction element (Ball and Stastny, 1982; Biddison et al., 1982; Flomenberg et al., 1983; Krensky et al., 1982; Meuer et al., 1982). CD8 cells may produce a variety of cytokines, associated a fraction more often with CD4$^+$ helper T cells. In contrast to most CD4$^+$ helper T cells that recognize or are restricted by MHC class II molecules, the CD8$^+$ cytokine producing cells typically utilize class I MHC molecules as their target or restriction element (Flomenberg et al., 1984; Widmer and Bach, 1981). Thus the subdivision into CD4 and CD8 subsets correlates best with the type of MHC

product recognized by the T cell. Helper T cells are most often activated by specialized antigen-presenting cells that express MHC class II molecules, and thus helper T cells are often CD4$^+$. Cytotoxic T cells that might be called on to rid the body of virally infected cells more often interact with the more ubiquitous MHC class I molecules, allowing them to destroy virtually any infected cell in the body. Thus the correlation between CD4/CD8 phenotype and cellular function is actually secondary to the type of MHC molecules recognized by these two phenotypic subsets.

While CD4 and CD8 are typically expressed in a mutually exclusive fashion by peripheral blood T cells, these molecules can be coexpressed on minor populations of T cells and upon small numbers of activated T cells. As described above, they are coexpressed by most thymocytes during an intermediate stage of differentiation.

Despite their functional homology, CD4 and CD8 are structurally distinct. CD4 consists of a simple protein of 55 kDa in size (Littman, 1987). The murine CD4 molecule is commonly known as L3T4. In addition to expression on subsets of T cells and thymocytes, CD4 is also expressed at low density on other cells such as monocytes and macrophages. CD4 is the molecule to which the human immunodeficiency viruses, the etiologic agents of AIDS, attach in the course of infecting the T cell (Landau et al., 1988; Peterson and Seed, 1988).

In contrast, CD8 consists of a dimer of two smaller subunits of around 32kDa (CD8α) and 30 kDa (CD8β) in size (Littman, 1987). The exact sizes vary among species. The murine CD8 products are known as Lyt-2 and Lyt-3, respectively. CD8 can be expressed on the cell surface either as a CD8 α/α homodimer or as a CD8 α/β heterodimer. CD8 is also weakly expressed on subsets of natural killer and lymphokine-activated killer cells (Terry et al., 1990).

γ/δ T cells differ from α/β T cells in their expression of CD4 and CD8. Few γ/δ cells express CD4. About one-third express CD8, while the rest are double negatives.

A tremendous number of experiments have been performed to address the role of CD4 and

CD8 in T cell activation. Depending on the experimental systems, either agonistic or antagonistic effects have been demonstrated. The data can be summarized in simplified form as follows. During activation, CD4 or CD8 will associate with the TcR/CD3 complex on the cell surface. The T cell interacts with its MHC ligand at two levels in this supramolecular complex. The TcR contacts the α-helices and peptide at the most distal portion of the MHC molecule, while CD4 or CD8 bind to nonpolymorphic regions of MHC molecules within the α_1/β_1 domains of the MHC molecule, closer to the surface of the antigen-presenting cell (Doyle and Strominger, 1988; Norment et al., 1988). This double interaction is important for activation, as experimental manipulations that bring TcR/CD3 and CD4/CD8 together tend to produce synergistic activation effects. Conversely, manipulations that separate these molecules tend to be inhibitory (Emmrich, 1988; Ledbetter et al., 1988; Saizawa et al., 1987).

Consistent with these observations, the ability of CD4 and CD8 to augment T cell activation is dependent on expression of the appropriate class II or class I ligand on the activating antigen-presenting cell. However, the cytoplasmic tails of CD4 and CD8 are also critical. Molecularly engineered CD4 or CD8 variants without cyto-

plasmic tails do not facilitate T cell activation. This observation relates to the fact that CD4 and CD8 are also associated with another Src family tyrosine kinase, p56[lck]. This kinase appears to bind to a Cys-X-Cys-Pro motif present in the tails of CD4 and CD8α (Turner et al., 1990). Thus, interaction of the TcR/CD3/CD4–8 complex triggers the actions of at least two tyrosine kinases that contribute to initiating some of the events that activate the T cell (Fig. 6).

CD2: THE SHEEP ERYTHROCYTE RECEPTOR

Prior to the advent of monoclonal antibody technology, it was noted that human T cells could be distinguished from their B-cell counterparts by virtue of their property of forming rosettes with sheep erythrocytes (Lay et al., 1971). Subsequently, the molecule primarily responsible for sheep RBC rosette formation was shown to be CD2, another important molecule in T cell activation. In man, CD2 has a molecular weight of 55 kDa. It is expressed in virtually all stages of thymocytes (with the possible exception of the most primitive forms) (Reinherz et al., 1980). Its distribution in man is limited to thymocytes, T cells, and natural killer cells, while in other species, the distribution is broader. The ligand for

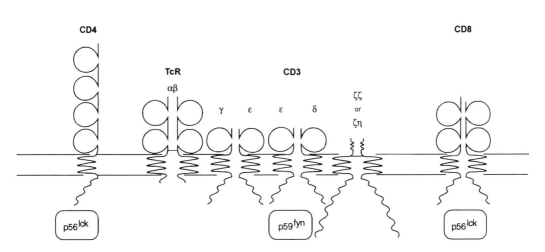

Fig. 6. Engagement of a T cell with its MHC–peptide ligand activates at least two tyrosine kinases, one associated with the TcR/CD3 complex and one associated with either CD4 or CD8.

CD2 is a molecule known as LFA-3 (CD58), a 55–70 kDa molecule with a widespread distribution (Bierer et al., 1988; Dustin et al., 1987a). Intriguingly, the genes for CD2 and LFA-3 map near one another. LFA-3 is expressed both in a transmembrane and a PI linked form. Red blood cells express only the PI linked form, while nucleated cells express both forms (Dustin et al., 1987b; Seed, 1987).

CD2 plays a complex role in both the adhesion of T cells to antigen-presenting cells and their subsequent activation. It also serves as a prototypic example of how adhesion and activation affect each other in reciprocal fashion and do not represent distinct events or processes.

A variety of antibodies recognizing distinct epitopes on the CD2 molecule have been identified. Some epitopes are expressed on resting or unperturbed T cells. Others are expressed only when the T cell has received an activation signal or when another CD2 antibody recognizing a distinct (usually resting) epitope has bound to the CD2 molecule. CD2 can participate in the activation of T cells in a number of ways. Antibodies to some CD2 epitopes, particularly those induced by an activation signal, can further augment signaling through the T cell receptor. However, stimulation of T cells through the CD2 molecule can also induce full cellular activation in the absence of stimulation of the T cell receptor. Such TcR-independent activation requires interaction with at least two distinct sites on the CD2 molecule (Brottier et al., 1985; Meuer et al., 1984). This can occur either via two distinct CD2 monoclonal antibodies or via one monoclonal antibody and binding of CD2 to its ligand, LFA-3 (Hunig et al., 1987). Activation does not occur by CD2-LFA-3 interaction alone (Dustin et al., 1989; Tiefenthaler et al., 1987), although other activation signals such as TcR engagement may be augmented by this interaction. In addition, the interaction of CD2 and LFA-3 enhances binding of the T cell to APCs. Interactions between CD2 and LFA-3 may induce IL-1 production by monocytes, which can further facilitate T cell activation (Webb et al., 1990) (see below).

Reciprocally, activation of the T cell results in increased avidity of CD2–LFA-3 binding through at least three mechanisms. Activation results in increased expression of CD2, an altered conformation of CD2 on the cell surface (including expression of activation epitopes), and a decrease in the negative change of the T cell surface reducing electrostatic repulsion (Bell et al., 1984; Wigzell and Hayry, 1974).

The engagement of CD2 and LFA-3 additionally transduces signals into the antigen-presenting cells. Antibodies binding to LFA-3 can stimulate release of interleukin 1 (IL-1) from thymic epithelial cells or monocytes. As described below, IL-1 facilitates T cell activation. Additionally, anti-LFA-3 antibodies can freeze MHC molecules rather than allowing them to move freely across the surface of the APC. This effectively increases their density at the site of engagement of APC and T cell, allowing for more effective TcR cross-linking.

CD18: THE LEUKOCYTE INTEGRIN FAMILY

LFA-1, another important molecule in T cell adhesion/activation, is a member of a large family of adhesion molecules known as integrins (Hynes, 1987; Springer, 1990). LFA-1 belongs to a subset of the integrins known as the leukocyte integrins, of which at least three members exist. These molecules exist as heterodimers of a larger α chain and smaller β chain. The β chain is common to each integrin subfamily and, in the case of the leukocyte integrins, is the β_2 chain (CD18), with a molecular weight of 95 kDa. All three α chains defined to date (CD11a, CD11b, and CD11c) exhibit homology to one another and bind divalent cations (Dransfield et al., 1992). The pairing of CD11a (180 kDa) with CD18 gives rise to the molecule known to as LFA-1. The dimer of CD11b (170 kDa) and CD18 is known as MAC-1 and represents the complement receptor 3 (CR3) molecule. CD11b$^+$CD8$^+$ T cells are associated with suppressive activity. CD11c, or complement receptor 4, is a slightly smaller molecule (150 kDa) found on monocytes and in low level on granulocytes and NK cells (Springer, 1990).

LFA-1 is a potent adhesion molecule. Antibodies to LFA-1 block binding of T cells to B cells, monocytes, fibroblasts, endothelial cells, and synovial cells (Kishimoto et al., 1989;

Springer et al., 1987). The interaction of LFA-1 with its ligands is probably one of the earliest events in T cell adhesion. However, here again, the demarcation between adhesion and activation is blurred. Some LFA-1 antibodies are capable of inducing T cell proliferation and cytokine release. As a generality, antibodies to the α chain are more likely to activate, while antibodies to the β chain are more likely to inhibit the T cell (Bednarczyk and McIntyre, 1990; Campanero et al., 1990; Gulino et al., 1990; van Kooyk et al., 1991).

LFA-1 was first shown to bind to a ligand known as ICAM-1 (intercellular adhesion molecule), a variably glycosylated molecule expressed on endothelial cells, lymphocytes, fibroblasts, and monocytes (Rothlein et al., 1986). ICAM-1 is a member of the immunoglobulin supergene family, related to neural crest adhesion molecules (NCAM) and more distantly to CD2 (Simmons et al., 1988; Staunton et al., 1988). Low basal levels of ICAM-1 are expressed on antigen-presenting cells (Dustin et al., 1986), but expression increases during T cell activation and after exposure to IL-1 and interferon-γ (Dustin and Springer, 1988; Kishimoto et al., 1989; Springer et al., 1987). In analyses of

LFA-1 mediated adhesion, it was demonstrated that antibodies to ICAM-1 did not disrupt adhesion as completely as antibodies to LFA-1. This suggested that a second ligand for LFA-1 might exist, which was subsequently confirmed (Staunton et al., 1989). The second ligand, ICAM-2, is related to ICAM-1 and belongs to the immunoglobulin supergene family. In contrast to ICAM-1, however, its expression is constitutive and is not increased by inflammatory mediators (Springer, 1990).

T cell activation alters the interaction of LFA-1 and ICAM-1, changing the avidity of the interaction from low to high. The increase occurs within minutes and may be PKC dependent (Rothlein et al., 1986; Rothlein and Springer, 1986). This finding is not unique to this particular intermolecular interaction. The avidity of other adhesion molecules such as VLA-4, VLA-5, VLA-6 (see below), and CD8 may also increase (Shimizu et al., 1990). This may help to explain how T cells attach and detach from other cellular populations. With appropriate activation, multiple molecules hold tighter to their ligands, increasing the period of contact between the cells, favoring further activation rather than detachment.

Table I. The Integrin Families[a]

Integrin β₁: VLA Family				
α_1/β_1	CD⁻/CD29	VLA-1	210/130	LM, CO
α_2/β_1	CD49b/CD29	VLA-2, gpIaIIa, ECMRII	165/130	CO
α_3/β_1	CD⁻/CD29	VLA-3, ECMRI	135/130	FN, LM, CO
α_4/β_1	CD49d/CD29	VLA-4, LPAM-1	150/130	FN
α_4/β_p	CD49d/CD⁻	LPAM-1	150/100	
α_5/β_1	CD⁻/CD29	VLA-5, FNR, gpIcIIa, ECMRVI	130/130	FN
α_6/β_1	CD49f/CD29	VLA-6, gpIcIIa		LM
α_6/β_4	CD49f/CD⁻			LM
Integrin β2: Leukocyte Integrin Family				
α_L/β_2	CD11a/CD18	LFA-1	180/95	ICAM-1, ICAM-2
α_M/β_2	CD11b/CD18	CR3, Mac-1, OKMI	170/95	C3bi, FB, FX
α_X/β_2	CD11c/CD18	p150, 95	150/95	?C3bi
Integrin β3: VNR and gpIIbIIIa				
α_{IIb}/β_3	CD41/CD61	gpIIbIIIa	130+23/105	FN, FB, VN, VWF
α_v/β_3	CD51/CD61	VNR	135+25/115	VN, FB, VWF, FN
α_v/β_5	CD51/CD⁻		165/100	VN, FN

[a]LM, laminin; CO, collagen; FN, fibronectin; FB, fibrinogen; FX, factor X; VN, vitronectin; VWF, von Willibrand factor. The first three columns represent various designations for the specific integrin molecule. The fourth column lists the molecular weights of the component chains. The last column lists the ligands.

The question can be raised as to why adhesion molecules should also subserve signaling functions. The teleologic answer is that they serve as additional eyes, telling the T cell what it is in fact interacting with. Antigen/MHC recognition by the T cell receptor is only one facet of the T cell's sampling of its surroundings. Through the large number of additional inputs from the accessory/adhesion molecules, the T cell receives more information about the nature of the opposing cell.

β1 AND β3 INTEGRINS

In addition to defining the nature of the opposing cell, it is also relevant for the T cell to sample the extracellular environment in which it exists. Input concerning the surrounding extracellular milieu is obtained, in part, through other members of the integrin families. At present, the integrins are sorted into three families based on the β chain used. Those using β_2 include LFA-1 and its family members as discussed above. The β_1 integrins include the VLA family (very late antigen), so named because the original members were identified as being expressed on T cells approximately 2 weeks after their activation (Hemler, 1990). The third family includes the vitronectin receptor and platelet glycoproteins IIb/IIIa. The integrin family members are shown in Table I. VLA-4 and VLA-5 interact with fibronectin, VLA-6 with laminin, VLA-3 and CD26, yet another adhesion molecule, with collagen (Hynes, 1987; Shimizu et al., 1990; Springer, 1990). Thus, the surroundings in which the T cell is present, or through which it has just passed, also influences its activation potential (Springer, 1990).

CD28

One of the receptor–ligand pairs that has received a great deal of attention recently is CD28-B7/BB1, which also subserves both adhesive and activation functions. CD28 is a 44 kDa molecule expressed on most CD4 and a subset of CD8 cells (Damle et al., 1983; Yamada et al., 1985). The interaction of CD28 with its ligand, B7/BB1 (Linsley et al., 1990), is thought to represent an important "second" signal to the T cell (June, 1991; June et al., 1989; Young et al., 1992), independent of the T cell receptor, which is necessary for T cells to become activated. Lack of engagement of this receptor ligand pair during T cell receptor engagement may result in T cell inactivation (reviewed in Mueller et al., 1989). At the biochemical and molecular level (as discussed below), the activation effects of CD28 are quite distinct from those initiated by many other molecular interactions including the TcR. A second potential receptor for B7/BB-1 is the CTLA-4 molecule (Linsley et al., 1991). CTLA-4 is less well characterized than many of the other lymphocyte differentiation antigens because it failed to stimulate production of monoclonal antibodies to the same extent as many of the other lymphocyte surface molecules.

RECIPROCAL FLOW OF INFORMATION BETWEEN THE T CELL AND ITS SURROUNDINGS

It is important to reiterate that the flow of signals between the T cell and its surroundings is reciprocal. Cross-linking of HLA-class II molecules (as would occur via TcR engagement) results in increased B7 expression on B cells (Koulova et al., 1991) and increased ICAM-1 expression on monocytes (Dustin and Springer, 1989; Mourad et al., 1990). It may also induce secretion of cytokines such as IL-1 and IL-6 from the APCs (Landis et al., 1991; Webb et al., 1990). All of these events facilitate subsequent steps in T cell activation. Thus, when a T cell engages an APC, nonspecific interactions such as those between LFA-1 and ICAM produce weak adhesion. Without signaling, the cells simply detach. If, however, the T cell receptor is engaged by its appropriate MHC/peptide ligand, the strength of LFA-1 binding increases. Weaker interactions such as CD2-LFA-3 come into play. IL-1 is secreted by the monocyte that promotes further events in T cell activation. Interferon-γ reciprocally may induce changes in monocytes that increase their potency in activating T cells. The result is a spiral of events facilitating tighter adhesion and activation. The concept is similar in T cell–B cell interactions though the molecules and cytokines differ slightly. Both contact events and cytokine secretion are essential for T cell activation and for the reciprocal activation of B cells and monocytes (Kawakami et al., 1989; van Seventer et al., 1991).

The complex interplay between the various adhesion molecules and the environment is not related solely to lymphocyte activation. The process is also influenced by maturation and differentiation. Memory T cells, for example, have higher levels of numerous adhesion molecules and ligands versus naive cells. Of the various β_1 integrins, some are expressed constitutively, some only after activation, and levels vary with maturation as well (reviewed in Springer, 1990). Similar interactions between adhesion molecules and the extracellular environment may influence lymphocytic trafficking. For example, the migration of T cells from blood to lymph is mediated by ligands known as vascular addressins, which are expressed on high endothelial venules (Stoolman, 1989; Yednock and Rosen, 1989). The addressins are recognized by Leu-8, CD44, β_1 integrins, and other T cell surface molecules (reviewed in Springer, 1990). Thus, although primarily studied in the context of T cell triggering, the various adhesion molecules help the T cell to take multiple samples of its surroundings, allowing it to become activated, traffic to the appropriate site, or take other actions as necessary.

BIOCHEMICAL EVENTS IN T CELL ACTIVATION

The appropriate interactions between the T cell and its surroundings trigger a number of intracellular events that, in cascading fashion, lead to cellular activation, cellular proliferation, release of cytokines, and other products such as cytotoxic effector molecules through which T cell functions are mediated. Like many other cell types, T cells utilize protein phosphorylation through the actions of a number of protein kinases and phosphatases to regulate cellular activity. Kinases are molecules that add phosphate residues to molecules, while phosphatases reciprocally remove phosphate residues. Protein kinases are typically divided into two subsets,

depending on the amino acids to which they add phosphate residues. These two subsets are the serine/threonine-directed kinases and the tyrosine-directed kinases. Depending on the particular molecules that are modified, the addition of phosphates can either enhance or reduce the activity in question. Following T cell activation, a number of phosphorylation events take place including serine phosphorylation of CD3γ, CD4, CD8α, and tyrosine phosphorylation of CD3ζ, and several of the serine/threonine and several tyrosine kinases themselves (reviewed in Weiss, 1991; van Seventer et al., 1991).

PHOSPHOLIPASE-C ACTIVATION

Biochemical analysis of T cells during activation has demonstrated that elevation in intracellular free calcium concentrations (Manger et al., 1987; Weiss et al., 1984) and activation of PKC (a serine/threonine kinase) (Imboden et al., 1985; Oettgen et al., 1985) are associated with the activation process. Indeed, combinations of pharmacologic agents that increase intracellular free calcium (e.g., ionomycin) and activate PKC [e.g., phorbol myristic acetate (PMA)] activate T cells, bypassing the membrane receptors (Truneh et al., 1985; Yamamoto et al., 1985). The physiologic mediators of calcium mobilization and PKC activation are two cleavage products of phosphatidylinositol 4,5-bisphosphate, specifically, inositol triphosphate (IP$_3$) and diacyl glycerol (DAG). Phosphatidylinositol is cleaved into these two derivatives by the actions of phospholipase C (Imboden and Stobo, 1985). IP$_3$ induces release of Ca^{2+} from the endoplasmic reticulum, as well as an influx through the plasma membrane. Activation of PKC results in its translocation from the cytosol to the cell membrane (Berridge and Irvine, 1989; Damjanovich et al., 1992). Phospholipase C is actually a family of related enzymes known as isoenzymes or isoforms rather than a single molecule. The various forms may be activated in different ways. In T cells, the actual manner in which phospholipase C is activated is still somewhat unsettled, but probably requires prior activation of a tyrosine kinase, which may directly phosphorylate and activate one of the PLC isoforms (Weiss et al., 1991). It has also been suggested that PLC activation may be regulated by guanine nucleotide binding proteins (G-proteins), a family of proteins widely involved in signal transduction (Goldsmith et al., 1989). G-proteins are active when bound to GTP, which they convert through intrinsic GTPase activity to GDP. It remains uncertain whether subsets of T cells or subsets of TcRs within the T cell utilize G-proteins rather than tyrosine kinases to couple the TcR to PLC (Imboden et al., 1986; Mustelin et al., 1986). The bulk of the data available point

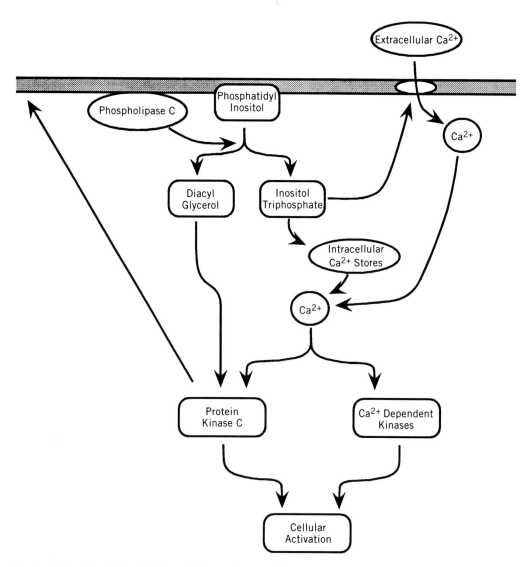

Fig. 7. Activation of phospholipase C cleaves phosphatidylinositol into diacyl glycerol and inositol triphosphate. Increases in inositol triphosphate results in elevation of intracellular concentrations of free calcium from both intracellular and extracellular sources. Increased calcium concentrations facilitate the actions of a variety of Ca^{2+}-dependent kinases and in concert with the increased concentrations of diacyl glycerol result in activation of protein kinase C. Activation of protein kinase C is associated with its translocation from the cytoplasm to the cell membrane.

to a more critical role for the tyrosine kinases. It has also been debated as to whether the TcR may be coupled to tyrosine kinases through G-protein activation or vice versa (Fig. 7).

TYROSINE KINASES AND PHOSPHATASES

The finding that tyrosine kinases are important in lymphocyte activation is not surprising, given their role in a number of other biologic systems. Receptors for a number of important hormones, such as insulin, EGF, PDGF, CSF-1, and others, contain tyrosine kinase activity in their intracytoplasmic domains. Other tyrosine kinases do not serve as receptors themselves, but instead associate with cell surface molecules with receptor functions. Roles for at least two such molecules have been defined in T cells, $p59^{fyn}$ and $p56^{lck}$. It is likely that other tyrosine kinases (such as ZAP-70) are also involved in T cell activation. Both of these molecules are members of the Src family of tyrosine kinases. $p56^{lck}$, which is expressed primarily in T cells, is associated with CD4 and CD8, recognizing a Cys-X-Cys-Pro motif in the cytoplasmic tail of CD4 and $CD8\alpha$ (Turner et al., 1990). $p59^{fyn}$ is associated with the T cell receptor/CD3 complex (Samelson et al., 1990). Fyn is present in a variety of cells types, though the form present in T cells may be unique in the way it is spliced (Cooke and Perlmutter, 1990). Following TcR activation, a number of tyrosine phosphorylation events have been documented, including the CD3 ζ chain (Baniyash et al., 1988b), p110 GAP, and the serine/threonine kinases RAF and MAP2.

Tyrosine phosphatases also serve to regulate the activation pathways. They can directly antagonize tyrosine kinases by performing the reciprocal function. In addition, they may also directly regulate the kinases themselves by altering the patterns of phosphorylation of the kinases. The best characterized tyrosine phosphatases within the lymphohematopoietic system are the CD45 family of molecules (Tonks et al., 1988), known as the leukocyte common antigens or the T-200 series of molecules (because of their high molecular weight). CD45 is responsible for 80% of the tyrosine phosphatase activity present within T cells (Altman et al., 1990). These molecules are distributed throughout the lymphoid, monocytic, and granulocytic families. The intracytoplasmic portion of the molecule containing the phosphatase activity is common to all members of the family as is much of the extracellular portion of the molecule. The variation within this family is based on the differential utilization of three optional exons (A, B, C) (Streuli et al., 1987). Within the T cell family, differences in the use of the optional exons have been correlated with differences in the functional or maturational state of the T cell (Smith et al., 1986). Originally, it was suggested that cells that activate suppressor cells (suppressor inducer cells) were predominantly found in the subset of T cells coexpressing CD4 and CD45RA (Morimoto et al., 1985). "R" refers to "restricted" or a subset of the CD45 family. "A" refers to selective case of the A exon without B or C. Cells activating helper T cells (helper inducer cells) were found predominantly in the reciprocal subset of $CD4^+$ T cells (Tedder, et al., 1985). These cells do not commonly express CD45RA, but often express the CD29 or Leu 8/TQ-1 molecules. Subsequently it was suggested that the use of CD45 isoforms correlated better with the T cell's maturational state, rather than its function. Naive cells tend to express large amounts of the CD45RA isoform. Following activation, as T cells mature into memory cells, expression of CD45RA declines and expression of CD45 R0 (which does not utilize any of the optional exons) increases (Akbar et al., 1988; Clement et al., 1988; Serra et al., 1988). Cells that lack CD45 do not generate PLC activation or a calcium flux after TcR cross-linking (Koretzky et al., 1990; Pingel and Thomas, 1989). Partial inhibition of phosphatase activity by phenyl arsine oxide augments TcR signaling while complete inactivation inhibits TcR signal transduction (Garcia-Marales et al., 1990). Thus CD45 and/or other tyrosine kinases are likely necessary to activate or maintain the activity of the tyrosine kinases themselves (reviewed in Alexander et al., 1992; Altman et al., 1990). Such studies support the concept that tyrosine phosphorylation serves as the primary regulator of PLC activation in T cells (Fig. 8).

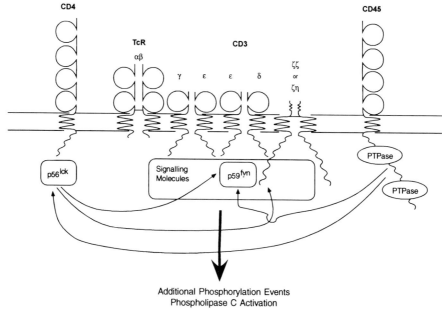

Fig. 8. Interactions between the tyrosine kinases and phosphatases associated with T cell surface molecules are critical for the activation of T cells. The kinases themselves, as well as the ζ chain of CD3, are targets for tyrosine phosphorylation. CD45 and/or other phosphatases regulate the ability of the kinases to mediate their activation effects.

ADDITIONAL SIGNALS IN THE ACTIVATION CASCADE

In addition to tyrosine kinase/phosphatase activity, Ca^{2+} flux, and PKC activation, other molecular signals may converge on these pathways or activate other pathways. Engagement of CD28 may activate a distinct tyrosine kinase (Lu et al., 1992) and may activate a distinct phospholipase C as well (Ledbetter et al., 1990). It also contributes to IL-2 gene activation through the induction of a unique transcriptional activator distinct from those induced by the T cell receptor (Fraser et al., 1991). In addition, signals transduced from the CD28 molecule serve to stabilize IL-2 mRNA (Lindsten et al., 1989). This latter phenomenon is also distinct from the activation signals provided through the T cell receptor. Many of the effects of CD28 stimulation are resistant to the immunosuppressive agent, cyclosporine-A, in contrast to those induced by TcR activation (Thompson et al., 1989).

In some experiments, a serine kinase has also been coprecipitated with the T cell receptor and other kinases such as raf-1 and microtubule associated protein 2 kinase may be activated as well, perhaps later in the activation pathway. LFA-1 cross-linking may also increase intracellular Ca^{2+}, although the mechanism is not established.

SOLUBLE MEDIATORS ACTIVATING T CELLS

In addition to the cell surface events that lead to T cell activation, soluble mediators also contribute to the first (pre-IL-2) stage of the activation process. The initial soluble mediator identified to serve as a T cell coactivator was IL-1. Initially, IL-1 was felt to be produced primarily by monocytes or macrophages. In reality, this cytokine is produced by a wide variety of cells, including keratinocytes, endothelium, renal mesangium, natural killer and dendritic cells, as well as others (Durum et al., 1986). Two forms of IL-1 have been demonstrated, IL-1α and IL-1β, encoded by two distinct genes (Auron et al., 1984; LoMedico et al., 1984). These molecules have only limited sequence homology. At least two IL-1 receptors exist as well (Solari, 1990). Despite their structural differences, both IL-1 molecules bind to the predominant receptor form with similar affinity, which probably explains their common functional properties. IL-1 has a diverse array of systemic effects. IL-1 serves as a comitogen for thymocytes. It can facilitate production of IL-2, IL-6, IFN-γ, and IL-2R as well (reviewed in Mizel, 1987).

IL-6 may also play an important role in the early activation of T cells (Garman et al., 1987). Within the immune system, the major source is again the monocyte/macrophage (Aarden et al., 1985), although T cells also produce IL-6 (Hirano et al., 1985). Fibroblasts, keratinocytes, endothelial cells, and other "nonimmune" cells also are capable of IL-6 production (Zilberstein et al., 1986). Many of the properties previously attributed to IL-1 actually reflect its induction of IL-6. IL-6 increases high affinity IL-2 receptor expression (Garman et al., 1987) and facilitates the response of thymocytes and T cells to IL-1 and IL-4. Both IL-1 and IL-6 have an array of broader effects on B cells, hematopoietic cells, and as acute phase reactants, though the effects of these two cytokines are by no means identical.

LINKING CELL MEMBRANE AND CYTOPLASMIC EVENTS TO NUCLEAR EVENTS

Following the activation of T cells, the biochemical signals described above lead to the initiation of transcription of IL-2, IL-2 receptors (IL-2R), other cytokines and receptors, cytotoxic effector molecules, and other mediators of T cell function. Additionally, levels of expression of other molecules may change as a result of activation. The predominant CD45 isoforms change. The expression of many adhesion molecules increases, and new adhesion molecules may become expressed. Of all these changes in the T cell resulting from activation, the events leading to IL-2 production are perhaps the most

precisely defined. Moreover, activation of IL-2 is under much more stringent regulation than activation of IL-2R (requiring more prolonged TcR engagement, for example). As such, it will be utilized as a model for how the cytoplasmic signals described above reach the nucleus to activate or deactivate genes essential for the immune response.

Transcription of IL-2, like that of other genes, is regulated by the binding of regulatory proteins to specific DNA sequences in the enhancer region of the gene. In the IL-2 enhancer, at least six regions have been identified in the region 50 to 500 bases 5′ to the transcription initiation site that contribute to the regulation of transcriptional activity (reviewed in Crabtree, 1989). Multiple DNA-binding proteins appear to interact with the enhancer, including AP-1, NFIL-2A (Oct-1), NFkB, AP-3, and NFAT-1. Both NFAT-1 and AP-3 appear to participate in the cyclosporine mediated sensitivity of the IL-2 enhancer. Several of the molecules binding to these regions are ubiquitous such as AP-1, NFkB, and Oct-1. The AP-1 site is probably responsible for the phorbol ester/PKC responsiveness of the enhancer (reviewed in Crabtree, 1989). AP-1 represents a heterogeneous group of molecules, including the product of the *jun* protooncogene. *jun* may form a homodimer or a heterodimer with the *fos* protooncogene product. Both complexes may bind to the AP-1 site, although the heterodimer binds with greater affinity and is a more efficient transcriptional activator. Both *jun* and *fos* are upregulated by PMA. In addition to AP-1, the DNA binding elements AP-3 and NFkB have been implicated in PMA responsiveness in other cellular systems (reviewed in Crabtree, 1989). Both AP-1 and NFkB binding sites are also present in the IL-2Rα enhancer. NFkB is typically constitutively present in an inactive form, due to an inhibitor. Activation modifies the inhibitor, probably through phosphorylation, activating NFkB.

In contrast to AP-1, NFkB, and Oct-1, several of the regulatory elements may be more restricted, such as an element induced by CD28 activation, and particularly the nuclear factor of activated T cells (NFAT-1) generated following T cell receptor stimulation. The expression of this last DNA binding protein closely parallels IL-2 production in T cells. NFAT-1 is actually a complex of 2 subunits. One subunit is T cell specific, confined to the cytoplasm, while the other is more ubiquitous, located predominantly in the nucleus and rapidly induced by PKC activation (Flanagan et al., 1991). More recent data suggest that the nuclear component may also be a member of the c-*jun* family. The effective association of these two subunits is Ca^{2+} dependent.

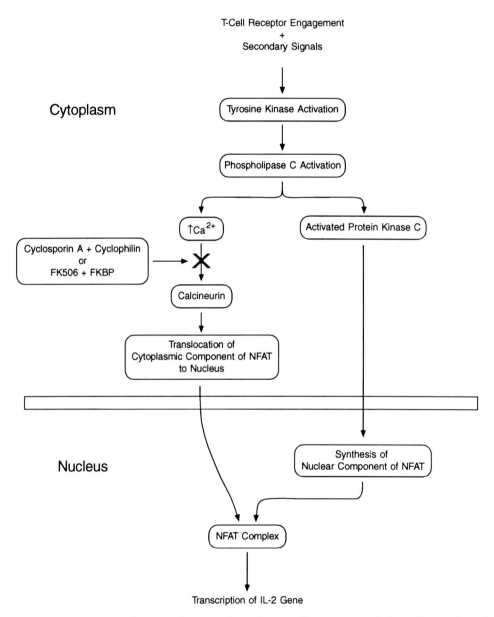

Fig. 9. T cell activation leads to translocation of a preformed cytoplasmic component of NFAT to the nucleus, as well as synthesis of the nuclear component of NFAT. The association of these two components results in an active NFAT complex, which facilitates IL-2 gene transcription. The cyclosporine–cyclophilin complex or FK506–FKBP complex inhibits activation of calcineurin, which subsequently leads to a failure of translocation of the cytoplasmic component.

An important intermediate step in the formation of NFAT-1 may be mediated by calcineurin, a phosphatase, which is Ca^{2+} dependent. Calcineurin probably represents the relevant target of the immunosuppressive drugs cyclosporine-A and FK506 (Clipstone and Crabtree, 1992). These drugs bind to distinct cytoplasmic binding proteins known as immunophilins. Cyclosporine binds to cyclophilin and FK506 binds to FK-binding protein (FKBP). Both of the immunophilins have enzymatic activity, serving as prolyl-peptidyl *cis–trans* isomerases that can regulate protein folding (Schreiber, 1991). Though functionally similar, these molecules belong to distinct families of proteins. Despite the lack of structural similarities between cyclosporine and FK506 or between their binding proteins, both sets of complexes bind to calcineurin (Clipstone and Crabtree, 1992). Inhibition of calcineurin's phosphatase activity either directly or indirectly may block progression of the cytoplasmic component of NFAT to the nucleus for assembly, thereby inhibiting IL-2 production (Flanagan et al., 1991). Thus detailed analysis of IL-2 production provides at least a partial explanation for how Ca^{2+} mobilization and PKC activation contribute to T cell activation and how some clinically useful immunosuppressive agents mediate their functions (Fig. 9).

THE IL-2R AND SUBSEQUENT EVENTS IN T CELL ACTIVATION

The receptor for IL-2 is yet another example of a multichain complex on the T cell surface. Following binding of IL-2 to its receptor, the complex is internalized and activation events ensue. The first component of the complex to be identified was the α chain (CD25), a 55 kDa molecule originally known as T cell activation antigen (TAC) (Leonard et al., 1982; Uchiyama et al., 1981). This molecule is not expressed on resting T cells, but is induced following activation. Antibodies to CD25 were indeed capable of blocking IL-2 mediated T cell proliferation and the molecule was capable of binding IL-2 (Leonard et al., 1982). However, the affinity of IL-2 binding in CD25 transfectants was far weaker than that observed in T cells, prompting for a search

for additional receptor components. Subsequently, a 75 kDaβ chain (Sharon et al., 1986) and a 64 kDaγ chain were identified (Takeshita et al., 1990, 1992). IL-2Rβ is expressed constitutively in some CD8 T cells but not in CD4 T cells, and is further induced upon activation, while the γ chain is constitutively expressed (reviewed in Taniguchi and Yasuhiro, 1993). Coexpression of the various IL-2R chains leads to an increased affinity of IL-2 binding (Sharon et al., 1986; Teshigawara et al., 1987; Tsudo et al., 1986). Unless the particular chain is specified, cells are referred to as IL-2 receptor positive based upon expression of CD25, the inducible component, which is present at highest density on the cell surface.

IL-2Rβ and IL-2Rγ belong to a new superfamily of cytokine receptors that includes the receptors for IL-3, IL-4, IL-5, and GM-CSF (Itoh et al., 1990; Taniguchi and Yasuhiro, 1993). Like other superfamilies, these molecules exhibit similarities in their structural organization that are reflected in similarities (homologies) in the DNA sequence of their genes. Members of a superfamily are presumed to have arisen from a common ancestor in evolution that originally duplicated and then diverged to generate various members of the superfamily. Expression of both IL-LRβ and IL-2Rγ is required for signal transduction from IL-2R (Arima et al., 1992; Taniguchi and Yasuhiro, 1993). Unlike previously characterized cytokine receptors (EGF, PDGF, CSF-1), the new superfamily lacks an intrinsic protein tyrosine kinase activity. However, the receptor complex is associated with p56[lck] (Hatakeyama et al., 1991; Horak et al., 1991) and, in mutant cells lacking p56[lck], with p59[fyn] or p59[lyn], other members of the Src family (Torigoe et al., 1992). Following activation, a variety of intracellular substrates are phosphorylated, including lck and S6 kinases. The substrates are largely distinct from those phosphorylated by TcR activation, although some substrates may be common to both pathways. These findings suggest either that activation of different sets of kinases and phosphatases leads to different patterns of phosphorylation or that the enzymes or substrates are compartmentalized in some way. Tyrosine kinase activity appears to be linked to the induction of p21^ras and subsequently to the activation of c-*fos* and c-*jun*. c-*myc* is also activated by IL-2/IL-2R interaction, but this appears to be tyrosine kinase independent (or perhaps dependent on other tyrosine kinases, such as Raf-1). The IL-2Rβ subunit has the longest intracytoplasmic tail, which appears to contain the regions most important for *lck* binding and *myc* activation (Taniguchi and Yasuhiro, 1993). In contrast to activation of the TcR, phosphatidylinositol-specific phospholipase C activation does not occur following IL-2/IL-2R interaction.

Intriguingly, several cases of X-linked severe combined immunodeficiency appear to be related to defects in the IL-2R γ subunit. This congenital disorder is associated with failure of T cell development. B cells may or may not be present, but even when present, they are functionally impaired (Noguchi et al., 1993).

The IL-2/IL-2R signal transduction events are the target for another important immunosuppressive agent, rapamycin. It appears that both FK506 and rapamycin bind to the same immunophilin, FKBP, with similar affinities. However, while binding of FK506 to FKBP inhibits the IL-2 generation pathway, the rapamycin/FKBP complex does not affect this pathway, acting instead as an inhibitor of IL-2-mediated effects (Bierer et al., 1990, 1991). Recent data would suggest that the phosphorylation and activation of S6 kinase are specifically blocked by rapamycin/FKBP, which may at least partially explain the effects of this agent (Fig. 10) (Kuo et al., 1992). It is not presently known whether rapamycin/FKBP blocks the activation of a kinase necessary to activate S6 kinase or, alternatively, activates a phosphatase that dephosphorylates and inactivates this molecule.

CYTOKINE SECRETION

Many of the effector functions of T-lymphocytes reflect the secretion of immunologically

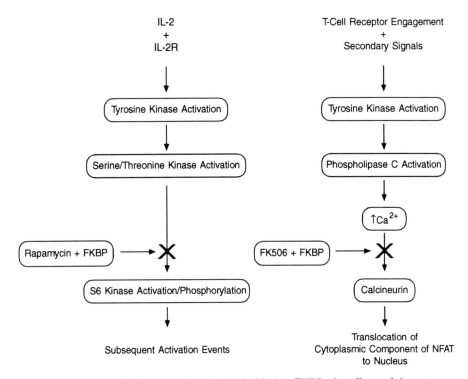

Fig. 10. Although both rapamycin and FK506 bind to FKBP, the effects of these two complexes are distinct. FK506–FKBP blocks IL-2 transcription, while rapamycin–FKBP blocks signals generated from the interaction of IL-2 with its receptor.

active hormones or cytokines. These molecules typically function within an immunologic microenvironment, although some of the systemic responses to illness such as fever, myalgias, and even cachexia may be mediated in part by immunologically induced cytokines.

The prototypic T cell produced cytokine is IL-2. This cytokine induces T cell growth in an autocrine or paracrine manner (Gillis and Smith, 1977; Morgan et al., 1976). As described above, T cell receptor stimulation leads to production of IL-2 and IL-2 receptors. It is the interaction of IL-2 with its receptor that leads to T cell growth. IL-2 is a 15–16 kDa molecule consisting of a single polypeptide chain (Robb et al., 1983). Although the molecule is glycosylated, nonglycosylated recombinant IL-2 is equipotent with natural material (Taniguchi et al., 1983).

The effects of IL-2 were initially thought to be restricted to T cells, and the molecule was originally known as T cell growth factor. However, IL-2 has subsequently been shown to serve as a growth and differentiation factor for B cells and can activate macrophages (Belosevic et al., 1990; Espinoza-Delgado et al., 1990; Hermann et al., 1989; Kovaks et al., 1989; Malkovsky et al., 1987). It also serves to support the growth of natural killer cells (Hefenider et al., 1983) and results in their activation into lymphokine-activated killer (LAK) cells (Mule et al., 1985; Rosenberg et al., 1985). These activated NK cells have a broader range of lytic activity than resting NK cells. Together with IL-2, LAK cells have been applied to the treatment of a variety of malignant disorders. Some successes have been seen in patients with melanoma and renal cell carcinoma (Rosenberg et al., 1988).

Interferon-γ (IFN-γ) is a type II interferon, produced by T cells after antigen or mitogen stimulation. Although all interferons were recognized based upon their ability to inhibit viral replication (Wheelock, 1965), IFN-γ has a broader range of activities within the immune system. IFN-γ activates macrophages, leading to expression of high affinity IgG receptors (FcRI). It increases clearance of immune complexes, phagocytosis and antibody-dependent cellular cytotoxicity, and activates oxidative metabolism. As a consequence, the activated mac-

rophages become capable of killing facultative intracellular pathogens (Chen et al., 1987; Roberts and Vasil, 1982).

Expression of both class I and class II MHC molecules is augmented by IFN-γ. This occurs in a wide range of cells, including macrophages, Langerhans cells, endothelial cells, keratinocytes, and melanoma cells. This increase in MHC expression may augment T cell activation or inhibition depending on the cell type involved and its ability to provide accessory signals to T cells (Virelizier et al., 1984).

IFN-γ can also directly influence immunologically active cells. NK activity is increased. IL-2R expression may be increased on T cells. B cells are induced to undergo terminal maturation and isotype switching to IgG_{2a} (reviewed in Coffman et al., 1988). IFN-γ may also suppress hematopoiesis.

Tumor necrosis factor (TNF) was originally identified based upon its ability to induce hemorrhagic necrosis of tumors (Carswell et al., 1975). Two molecules, TNF-α (17 kDa) and TNF-β or lymphotoxin (25 kDa), have been identified as mediating these effects. Interestingly, these molecules are encoded in the class III region of the MHC (Nedwin et al., 1985; Pennica et al., 1984). TNF-α is produced by activated macrophages, and to a lesser extent by T cells and NK cells, while TNF-β is produced only by activated T cells (reviewed in Cuturi et al., 1987; Old, 1985). The two molecules exhibit about 35% sequence homology. They produce systemic effects and cause the cachexia seen in a number of chronic illnesses (Beutler and Cerami, 1986). Endothelial cells are sensitive to these cytokines with a resultant increase in vascular permeability and up-regulation of ICAM-1. IL-2R expression on activated T cells may also be up-regulated (reviewed in Old, 1985).

Interleukin-4 (19 kDa) was previously known as B cell growth factor and B cell stimulating factor-1 (Howard et al., 1982; Paul, 1984). It has a variety of effects on B lineage cells. It serves as a costimulant for B cell proliferation induced by cross-linking surface immunoglobulin (Howard et al., 1982). It increases B cell expression of MHC class II molecules (Noelle et al., 1984) and low affinity receptors for IgE (CD23) (Kikutani et al., 1986). It induces class switching to IgG_1 and, at high concentrations, to IgE (Coffman et al., 1986; Vitetta et al., 1985). Many effects of IL-4 and IFN-γ on B cells are mutually antagonistic, particularly their effects on Ig class switching (Coffman and Carty, 1986; Snapper and Paul, 1987).

With its molecular characterization, IL-4 has been shown to have effects on a variety of immune and hematopoietic elements (Paul, 1991). IL-4 itself can act as a growth factor for T cells, particularly for TH_2 cells (see below) (Kurt-Jones et al., 1987). This effect is strikingly potentiated by IL-1 (Fernandez-Botran et al., 1988). IL-4 may induce production of IL-2 and expression of high affinity IL-2R (Fernandez-Botran et al., 1988). Production of IL-4 after T cell stimulation is markedly enhanced by the addition of IL-2. Paradoxically, IL-4 may antagonize the effects of IL-2 on some cells. IL-4 may enhance the proliferation and differentiation of cytotoxic T cell precursors into fully formed cytotoxic cells (Trenn et al., 1988; Widmer and Grabstein, 1987). IL-4 may also modulate the mast cell and hematopoietic cell growth effects of other cytokines (Brown et al., 1987; Mosmann et al., 1986; Peschel et al., 1987). IL-4 has been shown to mediate some antitumor effects. In some systems, these appear to be direct antitumor effects, while in others they appear to be immunologically mediated and T cell dependent (Forni et al., 1989; Tepper et al., 1989).

Interleukin-5 was also originally recognized for its effects on B cells (B cell growth factor II) (Yokota et al., 1987). It increases IgA production (Coffman et al., 1989; Esser and Radbruch, 1990; Finkelman et al., 1990) and can induce IL-2R expression on activated and resting B cells (Yoshimoto et al., 1990). It can similarly induce IL-2R on some thymocytes and can induce their differentiation into cytotoxic T cells. IL-5 also has profound effects on hematopoiesis, inducing eosinophilia (Warren and Moore, 1986). The IL-4 and IL-5 genes are closely linked in both mouse and man (Le Beau et al., 1988; Takahashi et al., 1989; reviewed in Sanderson et al., 1988).

Interleukin-6 has a broad range of effects. Its effects on T cell activation have been described above. This molecule is a 21–28 kDa glycoprotein. It is a hematopoietic growth factor with significant thrombopoietic effects (Wong et al., 1988). Within the B cell lineage, it induces the terminal differentiation of B cells (Hirano et al., 1985). Growth of some malignant B cells and plasma cells is supported by IL-6 (Nordan and Potter, 1986). It enhances immunoglobulin secretion of IgM, IgG, and IgA. Addition of anti-IL-6 antibodies drastically reduces Ig secretion by mitogen-activated B cells. IL-6 also has a variety of systemic inflammatory effects similar to those of IL-1 (reviewed in Van Snick, 1990).

COORDINATED PRODUCTION OF CYTOKINES

Studies of murine T cell clones have suggested that helper T cells can be divided in two groups, terminal TH_1 and TH_2, based on their profiles of cytokine production (Mosmann et al., 1986). TH_1 clones have been associated with production of IL-2, IFN-γ, and TNF-β, while TH_2 clones have been associated with products of IL-4, IL-5, and IL-6. Other cytokines such as IL-3, GM-CSF, and TNF-α are made by both cell types. TH_1 clones rely on IL-2 as their growth factor. TH_2 cells produce and respond to IL-4, but proliferate in response to IL-2 as well. TH_1 clones appear more capable of inducing delayed type hypersensitivity responses and antibody responses in which an IgE response is minimal. TH_2 clones induce antibody responses in which IgE is prominent. Certain types of infections may trigger an *in vivo* response, which is TH_1-like (most viruses), while others (helminthic parasites) produce responses that are more TH_2-like (Heinzel et al., 1989; Scott et al., 1988; reviewed in Mosmann and Coffman, 1989).

In man, it has not been possible to demonstrate distinct TH_1 and TH_2 clones as in the mouse (Del Prete et al., 1988; Romagnani et al., 1989). Even in the mouse, sharp distinction between the two does not occur immediately, but becomes more clear cut with serial propagation of the clones (Street et al., 1990). Cells with broader patterns of cytokine secretion have been referred to as TH_0 cells (Firestein et al., 1989; Kelso and Gough, 1988). The concept of TH_1 and TH_2 cells as irreversibly fixed and distinct developmental lineages may overstate the data. With the addition of appropriate mediators (such as 1,25-dihydroxyvitamin D_3 and dehydroepiandrosterone, an adrenal androgen), it has been possible to shift cytokine production from IL-2 to IL-4 and vice versa (Daynes and Araneo, 1992). In addition to the above mediators, IL-10 may alter the balance of TH_1/TH_2 cytokines. IL-10 decreases production of cytokines by activated TH_1 clones in the mouse and may decrease production of TH_1-associated cytokines by cells of broader cytokine-producing potential (Fiorentino et al., 1989). IFN-γ inhibits the response of TH_2 clones in reciprocal fashion. Teleologically, one would anticipate that under some conditions the immune system may require certain cytokines to accomplish the task at hand, while in other circumstances, production of other cytokines may be more appropriate. The concept of selective production and secretion of distinct families of cytokines is consistent with the multiplicity of responses the immune system must generate and has some support from the analysis of intact animals. Just as the multiplicity of adhesion molecules may provide the T cell with many cues as to the nature of its surroundings, it is likely that the T cell has some flexibility in tailoring its response based upon the signals it receives.

T CELL-MEDIATED CYTOTOXICITY

One of the major functions mediated by T cells is the cytotoxic response, which under physiologic circumstances would be utilized by the body to rid itself of viral infection through lysis of the infected cells. The capacity of T cells to mediate cytolysis is substantially increased following the initial activation of naive T cells and their differentiation into memory cells, a process that requires activation and cell division. T cell-mediated cytotoxicity has been associated with exocytosis of cytoplasmic granules that contain a number of mediators that participate in the lytic process (Bach et al., 1989; Gromo et al., 1987). The exocytic process is Ca^{2+} dependent, and occurs in a polarized fashion such that granule contents are released at the T cell/target cell junction. One of the major components is perforin, a 70-kDa protein that forms multimers on the target cell surface, resulting in the formation of holes or pores in the cell membrane. Perforin exhibits substantial homology to the C9 component of complement that performs a similar pore forming lytic function after antibody binding (Podack et al., 1991; Young et al., 1986). Perforin is not the sole component of the cytotoxic granules (Jenne and Tschopp, 1988). A variety of other molecules, including a number of serine esterases known as granzymes, have been identified within the cytoplasmic granules. The exact mechanism of lysis remains controversial. Although perforin and granzymes may play a role, additional events in the target cell are not explained by these molecules alone. Cell death mediated by complement, perforin, or isolated cytoplasmic granules results from osmotic lysis/necrosis. CTL-mediated cell death frequently exhibits features of apoptosis (DNA fragmentation from endonuclease activation within the target cell). This occurs rapidly (within 15 min) and is not seen following complement-mediated lysis. It appears to represent activation of endogenous endonucleases, in effect representing an induced suicide in the target cell (Duke et al., 1989; McConkey et al., 1990; Peters et al., 1990; Podack et al., 1991). Among the cytokines induced by T cell activation, TNF-β has the most pronounced intrinsic lytic capability and can induce apoptosis. However, TNF secretion does not appear to play a major role in T cell mediated cytotoxicity. TNF-mediated apoptosis occurs much more slowly and in a much more limited target spectrum than that mediated by CTL. It is presently unclear as to whether these two systems have evolved as an additive, synergistic, or redundant combination to ensure that any challenge requiring T cell-mediated lysis can be adequately met.

DELAYED-TYPE HYPERSENSITIVITY

In addition to providing help for antibody responses and generating cytotoxic T cell-mediated responses, one of the important potential consequences of T cell activation is the generation of a delayed type hypersensitivity (DTH) response. After initial sensitization to a variety of infectious agents, particularly agents capable of infecting tissue macrophages, reexposure of immunized animals to the pathogen in question produces an inflammatory response at the site of antigen that peaks in 2–3 days. The inflammation that results may, in some cases, cause tissue necrosis, but is typically followed by healing of the lesion (Zinsser, 1921). This type of immunologic reaction may play an important role in the treatment of a number of mycobacterial, fungal, and protozoal infections, and may also contribute to immunity toward bacterial and viral pathogens as well. DTH is associated with infiltration by CD4[+] helper T cells, which secrete lymphokines that attract and activate macrophages (Mackaness, 1971). These include many of the lymphokines associated with TH_1 cells (Chen et al., 1987). Interferon-γ, in particular, helps to activate macrophages (Roberts and Vasil, 1982), which in their activated state develop cytolytic activity toward a number of infected cells or tumor targets. Activated but not resting macrophages are able to destroy infected cells and infectious organisms present in these lesions. The activated macrophage is likely also responsible for much of the tissue damage that can be seen in DTH lesions. Thus the T cell imparts specificity to the response during its activation phase. The activated macrophage, responsible for the effector phase of the response, is immunologically nonspecific, being recruited to the inflammatory site and activated by the cytokines produced by the helper T cell. In selected model systems, a CD8[+] suppressor cell may prevent the generation of DTH responses (Nakamura et al., 1982). Whether a DTH response develops or not is dependent on the balance between the helper and suppressor populations recognizing the antigens in question.

SUMMARY

T cells have evolved a remarkable system for integrating a number of cell surface and cytokine-mediated signals into a composite response, appropriate for both the specific antigen and the immunologic microenvironment in which antigen recognition occurs. The response generated can vary from simple cellular disengagement to anergy to full blown activation. Even when fully activated, the array of functional programs that can be mustered by T cells is quite diverse, and can be altered, at least in part, by the immunologic environment. As the mechanisms underlying T cell signaling have become better defined, the mechanisms underlying our present drugs for modulating the immune response have also become clearer. Further definition of the events involved in T cell activation and anergy induction will hopefully allow for the development of more selective and specific agents either to turn off the immune response or to alter the response (for example, resulting in an altered pattern of cytokines secreted). Such developments are likely to fundamentally change our approaches to transplantation, as well as the treatment of autoimmunity, malignancy, and infectious disease.

REFERENCES

Aarden L, Lansdorp P, Degroot E (1985): A growth factor for B cell hybridomas produced by human monocytes. Lymphokines 10:175–185.

Akbar AN, Terry L, Timms A, Beverley PCL, Janossy G (1988): Loss of CD45R and gain of UCHL1 reactivity is a feature of primed T cells. J Immunol 140:2171–2176.

Alexander D, Shiroo M, Robinson A, Biffen M, Shivnan E (1992): The role of CD45 in T-cell activation-resolving the paradoxes? Immunol Today 13:477–481.

Altman A, Coggeshall M, Mustelin T (1990): Molecular events mediating T cell activation. Adv Immunol 48:227–360.

Arima N, Kamio M, Imada K, Hori T, Hattori T, Tsudo M, Okuma M, Uchiyama T (1992): Pseudo-high affinity interleukin-2 (IL-2) receptor lacks the third component that is essential for functional IL-2 binding and signaling. J Exp Med 176:1265–1272.

Auron PE, Webb AC, Rosenwasser LJ, Mucci SF, Rich A, Wolff SM, Dinarello CA (1984): Nucleotide sequence of human monocyte interleukin-1 precursor cDNA. Proc Natl Acad Sci USA 81: 7907–7911.

Bach FH, Geller RL, Nelson PJ, Panzer S, Gromo G, Benfield MR, Inverardi L, Podack ER, Wilson JC,

Houchins JP, Alter BJ (1989): "Minimal signal-stepwise activation" analysis of functional maturation of T lymphocytes. Immunol Rev 111:35–57.

Ball EJ, Stastny P (1982): Cell-mediated cytotoxicity against HLA-D region products expressed in monocytes and B lymphocytes. IV. Characterization of effector cells using monoclonal antibodies against human T-cell subsets. Immunogenetics 16:157–169.

Baniyash M, Garcia-Morales P, Bonifacino JS, Samelson LE, Klausner RD (1988a): Disulfide linkage of the ζ and η chains of the T cell receptor. J Biol Chem 263:9874–9878.

Baniyash M, Garcia-Morales P, Luong E, Samelson LE, Klausner RD (1988b): The T cell antigen receptor ζ chain is tyrosine phosphorylated upon activation. J Biol Chem 263:18225–18230.

Bednarczyk JL, McIntyre BW (1990): Induction of lymphocyte aggregation by mAb binding to a member of the integrin supergene family. J Immunol 144:777–784.

Bell GI, Dembo M, Bongrand P (1984): Cell adhesion. Competition between nonspecific repulsion and specific bonding. Biophys J 45:1051–1064.

Belosevic M, Finbloom DS, Meltzer MS, Nacy CA (1990): Interleukin-2: A cofactor for induction of macrophage resistance to infection. J Immunol 145:831–839.

Berridge MJ, Irvine RF (1989): Inositol phosphates and cell signaling. Nature (London) 341:197–205.

Beutler B, Cerami A (1986): Cachectin and tumor necrosis factor as two sides of the same biological coin. Nature (London) 320:584–588.

Biddison WE, Rao PE, Talle MA, Goldstein G, Shaw S (1982): Possible involvement of the OKT4 molecule in T cell recognition of class II HLA antigens. Evidence from studies of cytotoxic T lymphocytes specific for SB antigens. J Exp Med 156:1065–1076.

Bierer BE, Barbosa J, Hermann S, Burakoff SJ (1988): Interaction of CD2 with its ligand, LFA-3, in human T cell proliferation. J Immunol 140:3358–3363.

Bierer BE, Mattila PS, Standaert RF, Herzenberg LA, Burakoff SJ, Crabtree G, Schreiber SL (1990): Two distinct signal transmission pathways in T lymphocytes are inhibited by complexes formed between an immunophilin and either FK506 or rapamycin. Proc Natl Acad Sci USA 87:9231–9235.

Bierer BE, Jin YJ, Fruman DA, Calvo V, Burakoff SJ (1991): FK 506 and rapamycin: Molecular probes of T-lymphocyte activation. Transplant Proc 23:2850–2855.

Blackman MA, Marrack P, Kappler J (1989): Influence of the major histocompatibility complex on positive thymic selection of $V_\beta 17a^+$ T cells. Science 244:214–217.

Bluestone JA, Pardoll D, Sharrow SO, Fowlkes BJ (1987): Characterization of murine thymocytes with CD3 associated T cell receptor structures. Nature (London) 326:82–84.

Brenner MB, Strominger JL, Krangel MS (1988): The γδ T cell receptor. Adv Immunol 43:133–191.

Brottier P, Boumsell L, Gelin C, Bernard A (1985): T cell activation via CD2 (T, gp 50) molecules: accessory cells are required to trigger T cell activation via CD2-D66 plus CD2-9.6 T11 (sub 1) epitopes. J Immunol 135:1624–1631.

Brown MA, Pierce JH, Watson CJ, Falco J, Ihle JN, Paul WE (1987): B cell stimulatory factor-1/interleukin-4 mRNA is expressed by normal and transformed mast cells. Cell 50:809–818.

Campanero MR, Pulido R, Ursa MA, Rodriguez-Moya M, de Landazuri MO, Sanchez-Madrid F (1990): An alternative leukocyte homotypic adhesion mechanism. LFA1/ICAM-1-independent, triggered through the human VLA4 integrin. J Cell Biol 110:2157–2163.

Carswell EA, Old LJ, Kassel RL, Green S, Fiore N, Williamson B (1975): An endotoxin-induced serum factor that causes necrosis of tumors. Proc Natl Acad Sci USA 72:3666–3670.

Chen L, Suzuki Y, Wheelock EF (1987): Interferon γ synergizes with tumor necrosis factor and with interferon 1 and requires the presence of both monokines to induce antitumor cytotoxic activity in macrophages. J Immunol 139:4096–4101.

Chien Y, Becker DM, Lindsten T, Okamura M, Cohen DI, Davis MM (1984): A third type of murine T-cell receptor gene. Nature (London) 312:31–35.

Clement LT, Yamashita N, Martin AM (1988): The functionally distinct subpopulations of human helper/inducer T lymphocytes defined by anti-CD45R antibodies derive sequentially from a differentiation pathway that is regulated by activation-dependent post-thymic differentiation. J Immunol 141:1464–1470.

Clevers H, Alarcon B, Willeman T, Terhorst C (1988): The T cell receptor/CD3 complex: A dynamic protein ensemble. Annu Rev Immunol 6:29–662.

Clipstone NA, Crabtree GR (1992): Identification of calcineurin as a key signaling enzyme in T-lymphocyte activation. Nature (London) 357:695–697.

Coffman RL, Carty J (1986): A T-cell activity that enhances polyclonal IgE production and its inhibition by interferon-γ. J Immunol 136:949–954.

Coffman RL, Ohara J, Bond MW, Carty J, Zlotnick A, Paul WE (1986): B cell stimulatory factor-1 enhances the IgE response of lipopollysaccharide-activated B cells. J Immunol 136:4538–4541.

Coffman RL, Seymour BWP, Lebman DA, Hiraki DD, Christiansen JA, Shrader B, Cherwinski HM, Savelkoul HFJ, Finkelman FD, Bond MW, Mosmann TR (1988): The role of helper T cell products in mouse B cell differentiation and isotype regulation. Immunol Rev 102:5–28.

Coffman, RL, Savelkoul HE, Lebman DA (1989): Cytokine regulation of immunoglobulin isotype switching and expression. Semin Immunol 1: 55–53.

Cooke MP, Perlmutter RM (1990): Expression of a novel form of the fyn proto-oncogene in hematopoietic cells. New Biol 1:66–74.

Crabtree GR (1989): Contingent genetic regulatory events in T lymphocyte activation. Science 243: 355–361.

Cuturi MC, Murphy M, Costa-Giomi MP, Weinmann R, Perussia B, Trinchieri G (1987): Independent regulation of tumor necrosis factor and lymphotoxin production by human peripheral blood lymphocytes. J Exp Med 165:1581–1594.

Damjanovich S, Szollosi J, Tron L (1992): Transmembrane signalling in T cells. Immunol Today 13:A12–A15.

Damle NK, Mohagheghpour N, Hansen JA, Engleman EG (1983): Alloantigen-specific cytotoxic and suppression T lymphocytes are derived from phenotypically distinct precursors. J Immunol 131:2296–3300.

Davis MM, Bjorkman PJ (1988): T-cell antigen receptor genes and T-cell recognition. Nature (London) 334:395–402.

Daynes RA, Araneo BA (1992): Natural regulators of T-cell lymphokine production in vivo. J Immunother 12:174–179.

Del Prete G, Maggi E, Parronchi P, Chretien I, Tiri A, Macchia D, Ricci M, Banchereau J, DeVries J, Romagnani S (1988): IL-4 is an essential factor for the IgE synthesis induced in vitro by human T cell clones and their supernatants. J Immunol 140: 4193–4198.

DiGeorge AM (1968): Congenital absence of the thymus and its immunological consequences: concurrence with congenital hypothyroidism. Birth Defects 4:116–123.

Doherty PC, Zinkernagel RM (1975): A biological role for the major histocompatibility antigens. Lancet 1:1406–1409.

Doherty PC, Gotze D, Trinchieri G, Zinkernagel RM (1976): Models for recognition of virally modified cells by immune thymus derived lymphocytes. Immunogenetics 3:517–524.

Doyle C, Strominger JL (1988): Interaction between CD4 and class II MHC molecules mediates cell adhesion. Nature (London) 330:256–258.

Dransfield I, Cabanas C, Craig A, Hog N (1992): Divalent cation regulation of the function of the leukocyte integrin LFA-1. J Cell Biol 116:219–226.

Duke RC, Persechini PM, Chang S, Liu C-C, Cohen JJ, Young JD-E (1989): Purified perforin induces target cell lysis but not DNA fragmentation. J Exp Med 170:1451–1456.

Durum SK, Schmidt JA, Oppenheim JJ (1986): Interleukin 1: an immunological perspective. Annu Rev Immunol 3:263–287.

Dustin ML, Springer TA (1988): Lymphocyte function-associated antigen-1 (LFA-1) interaction with intercellular adhesion molecule-1 (ICAM-1) is one of at least three mechanisms for lymphocyte adhesion to cultured endothelial cells. J Cell Biol 107:321–331.

Dustin ML, Springer TA (1989): T-cell receptor cross-linking transiently stimulates adhesiveness through LFA-1. Nature (London) 341:619–624.

Dustin ML, Rothlein R, Bhan AK, Dinarello CA, Springer TA (1986): Induction by IL-1 and interferon-gamma-tissue distribution, biochemistry, and function of a natural adherence molecule (ICAM-1). J Immunol 137:245–254.

Dustin ML, Sanders ME, Shaw S, Springer TA (1987a): Purified lymphocyte function-associated antigen 3 binds to CD2 and mediates T lymphocyte adhesion. J Exp Med 165:677–692.

Dustin ML, Selvaraj P, Mattaliano RJ, Springer TA (1987b): Anchoring mechanisms for LFA-3 cell adhesion glycoprotein at membrane surface. Nature (London) 329:846–848.

Dustin ML, Olive D, Springer TA (1989): Correlation of CD2 binding and functional properties of multimeric and monomeric lymphocyte function-associated antigen 3. J Exp Med 169:503–517.

Emmrich F (1988): Cross-linking of CD4 and CD8 with the T-cell receptor complex: Quaternary complex formation and T-cell repertoire selection. Immunol Today 9:296–300.

Espinoza-Delgado I, Longo DL, Gusella GL, Varesio L (1990): Expression and role of p75 IL-2 receptor on human monocytes. J Exp Med 171:1821–1832.

Esser C, Radbruch A (1990): Immunoglobulin class switching: Molecular and cellular analysis. Annu Rev Immunol 8:717–735.

Fernandez-Botran R, Sanders VM, Mosmann TR, Vitetta ES (1988): Lymphokine-mediated regulation of the proliferative response of clones for T helper 1 and T helper 2 cells. J Exp Med 168:543–558.

Finkel TH, Cambier JC, Kubo RT, Born WK, Marrack P, Kappler JW (1989): The thymus has two functionally distinct populations of immature $\alpha\beta^+$ T cells: One population is deleted by ligation of $\alpha\beta$ TCR. Cell 58:1047–1054.

Finkelman FD, Holmes J, Katona IM, Urban JF Jr, Beckmann MP, Park LS, Schooley KA, Coffman RL, Mosmann TR, Paul WE (1990): Lymphokine control of in vivo immunoglobulin isotype selection. Annu Rev Immunol 8:303–333.

Fiorentino DF, Bond MW, Mosmann TR (1989): Two types of mouse T helper cell. IV. Th2 clones secrete a factor that inhibits cytokine production by Th1 clones. J Exp Med 170:2081–2095.

Firestein GS, Roeder WD, Laxer JA, Townsend KS, Weaver CT, Hom JT, Linton J, Torbett BE, Glasebrook AL (1989): A new murine CD4+ T cell subset with an unrestricted cytokine profile. J Immunol 143:518–525.

Flanagan SP (1966): "Nude," a new hairless gene with pleiotropic effects in the mouse. Genet Res 8:295–309.

Flanagan WM, Corthesy B, Bram RJ, Crabtree GR (1991): Nuclear association of a T-cell transcription factor blocked by FK-506 and cyclosporin A. Nature (London) 352:803–807.

Flomenberg N, Duffy E, Naito K, Dupont B (1983): Two distinct phenotypes of HLA-DR specific cytotoxic T cell lines. Immunogenetics 17:317–324.

Flomenberg N, Russo C, Ferrone S, Dupont B (1984): HLA Class I specific T lymphocyte clones with dual alloreactive functions. Immunogenetics 19:39–51.

Forni G, Giovarelli M, Bosco MC, Caretto P, Modesti A, Boraschi D (1989): Lymphokine-activated tumor inhibition: combinatory activity of a synthetic nonapeptide from interleukin-1, interleukin-2, interleukin-4, and interferon-gamma injected around tumor-draining lymph nodes. Int J Cancer Suppl 4:62–65.

Fraser JD, Irving BA, Crabtree GR, Weiss A (1991): Regulation of interleukin-2 gene enhancer activity

by the T cell accessory molecule CD28. Science 251:313–316.

Garcia-Marales P, Minami Y, Luong E, Klausner RD, Samelson LE (1990): Tyrosine phosphorylation in T cells is regulated by phosphatase activity: studies with phenylarsine oxide. Proc Natl Acad Sci USA 87:9255–9259.

Garman TD, Jacobs KA, Clark SC, Raulet DH (1987): B-cell-stimulatory factor 2 (beta $_2$ interferon) functions as a second signal for interleukin 2 production by murine T cells. Proc Natl Acad Sci USA 84:7629–7633.

Geisler C, Scholler J, Wahi M, Rubin B, Weiss A (1990): Association of the human CD3-ζ chain with $\alpha\beta$-T cell receptor/CD3 complex: clues from a T cell variant with a mutated T cell receptor-α chain. J Immunol 145:1761–1767.

Gillis S, Smith KA (1977): Long term culture of tumour-specific cytotoxic T cells. Nature (London) 268:154–156.

Goldsmith MA, Desai DM, Schultz T, Weiss A (1989): Function of a heterologous muscarinic receptor in T cell antigen receptor signal transduction mutants. J Biol Chem 264:17190–17197.

Gromo G, Geller RL, Inverardi L, Bach FH (1987): Signal requirements in the step-wise functional maturation of cytotoxic T lymphocytes. Nature (London) 327;424–426.

Gulino D, Ryckwaert JJ, Andrieux A, Rabiet MJ, Maarguerie G (1990): Identification of a monoclonal antibody against platelet gpIIb that interacts with a calcium-binding site and induces aggregation. J Biol Chem 265:9575–9581.

Hatakeyama M, Kono T, Kobayashi N, Kawahara A, Levin SD, Perlmutter RM, Taniguchi T (1991): Interaction of the IL-2 receptor with the src-family kinase p561ck: Identification of novel intermolecular association. Science 252:1523–1528.

Hedrick SM, Nielsen EA, Kavaler J, Cohen DI, Davis MM (1984): Sequence relationships between putative T-cell receptor polypeptides and immunoglobulins. Nature (London) 308:153–158.

Hefeneider SH, Conlon PJ, Henney CS, Gillis S (1983): In vivo interleukin 2 administration augments the generation of alloreactive cytolytic T lymphocytes and resident natural killer cells. J Immunol 130:222–227.

Heinzel FP, Sadick MD, Holaday BJ, Coffman RL, Locksley RM (1989): Reciprocal expression of interferon gamma or interleukin 4 during the resolution or progression of murine leishmaniasis. Evidence for expansion of distinct helper T cell subsets. J Exp Med 169:59–72.

Hemler ME (1990): VLA proteins in the integrin family: structures, functions, and their role on leukocytes. Annu Rev Immunol 8:365–400.

Hermann F, Cannistra SA, Lindemann A, Blohm D, Rambaldi A, Mertlesmann RH, Griffen JD (1989): Functional consequences of monocyte IL-2 receptor expression. Induction of IL-1β secretion by IFN and IL-2. J Immunol 142:139–145.

Hirano T, Yaga T, Nakano N, Yasakawa K, Kashiwamura S, Shimizu K, Nakajima K, Pyun K, Kishimoto T (1985): Purification to homogeneity and characterization of human B cell differentiation factor (BCDF or BSFp-2). Proc Natl Acad Sci USA 8:5490–5494.

Horak ID, Gress RE, Lucas PJ, Horak EM, Waldmann TA, Bolen JB (1991): T-lymphocyte interleukin 2-dependent tyrosine protein kinase signal transduction involves the activation of p56lck. Proc Natl Acad Sci USA 88:1996–2000.

Howard M, Farrar J, Hilfiker M, Johnson B, Takatsu K, Hamaoka T, Paul WE (1982): Identification of a T-cell derived B-cell growth factor distinct from interleukin-2. J Exp Med 155:914–923.

Hunig T, Tiefenthaler G, Meyer zum Buschenfelde KH, Meuer SC (1987): Alternative pathway activation of T cells by binding of CD2 to its cell surface ligand. Nature (London) 326:298–301.

Hynes RO (1987): Integrins: Family of cell surface receptors Cell 48:549–554.

Imboden JB, Stobo JD (1985): Transmembrane signalling by the T cell antigen receptor: Perturbation of the T3-antigen receptor complex generates inositol phosphates and releases calcium ions from intracellular stores. J Exp Med 161:446–456.

Imboden JB, Weiss A, Stobo JD (1985): The antigen receptor on a human T cell line initiates activation by increasing cytoplasmic free calcium. J Immunol 134:663–665.

Imboden JB, Shoback DM, Pattison G, Stobo JD (1986): Cholera toxin inhibits the T-cell antigen receptor-mediated increases in inositol trisphosphate and cytoplasmic free calcium. Proc Natl Acad Sci USA 83:5673–5677.

Itoh N, Yonehara S, Schreurs J, Gorman DM, Maruyama K, Ishii A, Yahara I, Arai K, Mikajima A (1990): Cloning of an interleukin-3 receptor gene: A member of distinct receptor gene family. Science 247:324–327.

Jenne DE, Tschopp J (1988): Granzymes, a family of serine proteases released from granules of cytolytic T lymphocytes upon T cell receptor stimulation. Immunol Rev 103:53–71.

Jin YI, Clayton LK, Howard FD, Koyasu S, Sieh M, Steinbrich R, Tarr GE, Reinharz EL (1990a): Molecular cloning of the CD3 eta subunit identifies a CD3 zeta-related product in thymus-derived cells. Proc Natl Acad Sci USA 87:3319–3323.

Jin YJ, Koyasu S, Moingeon P, Steinbrich R, Tarr GE, Reinherz EL (1990b): A fraction of CD3 ε subunits exists as disulfide-linked dimers in both human and murine T lymphocytes. J Biol Chem 65:15850–15853.

June CH (1991): Signal transduction in T cells. Curr Opin Immunol 3:287–293.

June CH, Ledbetter JA, Lindsten T, Thompson CB (1989): Evidence for the involvement of three distinct signals in the induction of IL-2 gene expression in human T lymphocytes. J Immunol 143:153–161.

Kappler JW, Roehm N, Marrack P (1987): T cell tolerance by clonal elimination in the thymus. Cell 49:273–280.

Kawakami K, Yamamoto Y, Kakimoto K, Onoue K (1989): Requirement for delivery of signals by physical interaction and soluble factors from accessory cells in the induction of receptor-mediated T-cell proliferation. Effectiveness of IFN gamma modulation of accessory cells for physical interaction with T cells. J Immunol 142:1818–1825.

Kaye J, Porcelli S, Tite J, Jones B, Janeway CA Jr (1983): Both a monoclonal antibody and antisera specific for determinants unique to individual cloned helper T-cell lines can substitute for antigen and antigen-presenting cells in the activation of T-cells. J Exp Med 158:836–856.

Kelso A, Gough NM (1988): Coexpression of granulocyte-macrophage colony-stimulating factor, gamma interferon, and interleukins 3 and 4 is random in murine alloreactive T-lymphocyte clones. Proc Natl Acad Sci USA 85:9189–9193.

Kikutani H, Inui S, Sato R, Barsumian E, Owaki H, Yamasaki K, Kalaho T, Uchibayashi N, Hardy R, Hirano T, Taunasawa S, Sakiyama S, Suemura M, Kishimoto T (1986): Molecular structure of human lymphocyte receptor for immunoglobulin. Cell 47:657–665.

Kishimoto TK, Larson RS, Corbi AL, Dustin ML, Staunton DR, Springer TA (1989): The leukocyte integrins. Adv Immunol 46:149–182.

Kisielow P, Bluthmann H, Staerz UD, Steinmetz M, von Boehmer H (1988): Tolerance in T-cell-receptor transgenic mice involves deletion of nonmature CD4$^+$8$^+$ thymocytes. Nature (London) 333:742–746.

Konig F, Maloy WI, Coligan JE (1990): The implications of subunit interactions for the structure of the T cell receptor-CD3 complex. Eur J Immunol 20:299–305.

Koretzky GA, Picus J, Thomas ML, Weiss A (1990): Tyrosine phosphatase CD45 is essential for coupling T-cell antigen receptor to the phosphatidyl inositol pathway. Nature (London) 346:66–68.

Kouova L, Clark EA, Shu G, Dupont B (1991): The CD28 ligand B7/BB1 provides costimulatory signal for alloactivation of CD4+ T cells. J Exp Med 173:759–562.

Kovaks J, Brock B, Varesio L, Young HA (1989): IL-2 induction of IL-1β mRNA expression in monocytes. J Immunol 143:3532–3537.

Krensky A, Reiss C, Mier J, Strominger JI, Burakoff SJ (1982): Generation of long-term human cytolytic cell lines with persistent natural killer activity. J Immunol 129:1748–1751.

Kuo CJ, Chung J, Fiorentino DF, Flanagan WM, Blenis J, Crabtree GR (1992): Rapamycin selectively inhibits interleukin-2 activation of p70 S6 kinase. Nature (London) 358:70–73.

Kurt-Jones EA, Hamberg S, Ohara J, Paul WE, Abbas AK (1987): Heterogeneity of helper/inducer T lymphocytes. I. Lymphokine production and lymphokine responsiveness. J Exp Med 166:1774–1787.

Landau NR, Warton M, Littman DR (1988): The envelope glycoprotein of the human immunodeficiency virus binds to the immunoglobulin-like domain of CD4. Nature (London) 334: 159–167.

Landis RC, Friedman ML, Fisher RI, Ellis TM (1991): Induction of human monocyte IL-1 mRNA and secretion during anti-CD3 mitogenesis requires two distinct T-cell-derived signals. J Immunol 146:128–135.

Lay WH, Mendes NF, Bianco C, Nussenzweig V (1971): Binding of sheep red blood cells to a large population of human lymphocytes. Nature (London) 230:531–532.

LeBeau MM, Lemons RS, Espinosa R III, Larson RA, Arai N, Rowley JD (1988): Interleukin-4 and interleukin-5 map to human chromosome 5 in a region encoding for growth factors and receptors and are deleted in myeloid leukemias with a del(5q). Blood 73:647–650.

Ledbetter JA, June CH, Rabinovitch PS, Grossman A, Tsu TT, Imboden JB (1988): Signal transduction through CD4 receptors: Stimulatory vs inhibitory activity is regulated by CD4 proximity to the CD3/T cell receptor. Eur J Immunol 18:525–532.

Ledbetter JA, Imboden JB, Schieven GL, Grosmaire LS, Robinovitch PS, Lindsten T, Thompson CB, June CH (1990): CD28 ligation in T cell activation: Evidence for two signal transduction pathways. Blood 75:1531–1539.

Leonard WJ, Depper JM, Uchiyama T, Smith KA, Waldmann TA, Greene WC (1982): A monoclonal antibody that appears to recognize the receptor for human T-cell growth factor; partial characterization of the receptor. Nature (London) 300:267–269.

Lindsten T, June CH, Ledbetter JA, Stella G, Thompson CB (1989): Regulation of lymphokine messenger RNA. Stability by a surface-mediated T cell activation pathway. Science 224:339–343.

Linsley PS, Clark EA, Ledbetter JA (1990): T-cell antigen CD28 mediates adhesion with B cells by interacting with activation antigen B7/BB-1. Proc Natl Acad Sci USA 87:5031–5035.

Linsley PS, Brady W, Grosmaire I, Ledbetter JA, Damle NK (1991): CTLA-4 is a second receptor for the B cell activation antigen B7. J Exp Med 174:561–570.

Littman DR (1987): The structure of the CD4 and CD8 genes. Annu Rev Immunol 5:561–584.

LoMedico PT, Gubler U, Hellmann CP, Dukowich M, Giri JG, Pan YCE, Collier K, Semonow R, Chua AO, Mizel SB (1984): Cloning and expression of murine interleukin 1 cDNA in *Escherichia coli*. Nature (London) 312:458–462.

Lu Y, Granelli-Piperno A, Bjorndahl JM, Phillips CA, Trevillyan JM. CD28-induced T cell activation: Evidence for a protein-tyrosine kinase signal transduction pathway. J Immunol 149:14–29, 1992.

Mackaness GB (1971): Delayed hypersensitivity and the mechanism of cellular resistance to infection. In Amos B (ed): "Progress in Immunology." New York: Academic Press, p 413.

Malkovsky M, Loveland B, North M, Asherson GL, Gao L, Ward P, Friers W (1987): Recombinant Interleukin-2 directly augments the cytotoxicity of human monocytes. Nature (London) 325:262–263.

Manger B, Weiss A, Imboden J, Laing T, Stobo J (1987): The role of protein kinase C in transmembrane signaling by the T cell receptor complex: Effects of stimulation with soluble or immobilized T3 antibodies. J Immunol 139:395–407.

Mathieson BJ, Fowlkes BJ (1984): Cell surface antigen expression on thymocytes: Development and phenotypic differentiation of intrathymic subsets. Immunol Rev 82:141–173.

McConkey DJ, Orrenius S, Jondal M (1990): Cellular signalling in programmed cell death (apoptosis). Immunol Today 11:120–121.

Meuer SC, Schlossman SF, Reinherz EL (1982): Clonal analysis of human cytotoxic T lymphocytes: T4+ and T8+ effector T cells recognize products of different major histocompatibility complex regions. Proc Natl Acad Sci USA 79:4395–4399.

Meuer SC, Hodgdon JC, Hussey RE, Prontentis JP, Schlossman SF, Reinherz EL (1983): Antigen-like effects of monoclonal antibodies directed at receptors on human T cell clones. J Exp Med 158:988–993.

Meuer SC, Hussey RE, Fabbi M, Fox D, Acuto O, Fitzgerald KA, Hodgdon JC, Protentis JP, Schlossman SF, Reinherz EL (1984): An alternative pathway of T cell activation: A functional role for the 50 kd T11 sheep erythrocyte receptor protein. Cell 36:897–906.

Mizel SB (1987): Interleukin 1 and T cell activation. Immunol Today 8:330.

Morgan DA, Ruscetti FW, Gallo RC (1976): Selective in vitro growth of T lymphocytes from normal human bone marrows. Science 193:1007–1008.

Morimoto C, Letvin NL, Distaso JA, Aldrich WR, Schlossman SF (1985): The isolation and characterization of the human suppressor inducer T cell subset. J Immunol 134:1508–1513.

Mosmann TR, Coffman RL (1989): Heterogeneity of cytokine secretion patterns and functions of helper T cells. Adv Immunol 46:111–147.

Mosmann TR, Bond MW, Coffman RL, Ohara J, Paul WE (1986a): T cell and mast cells respond to B cell stimulatory factor-1. Proc Natl Acad Sci USA 83:5654–5658.

Mosmann TR, Cherwinski H, Bond MW, Giedlin MA, Coffman RL (1986b): Two types of murine helper T cell clone. I Definition according to profiles of lymphokine activities and secreted proteins. J Immunol 136:2348–2357.

Mourad W, Geha RS, Chatila T (1990): Engagement of major histocompatibility complex class II molecules induces sustained, lymphocyte function-associated molecule 1-dependent cell adhesion. J Exp Med 172:1513–1516.

Mueller DL, Jenkins MK, Schwartz RH (1989): Clonal expansion versus functional clonal inactivation: A costimulatory signalling pathway determines the outcome of T cell antigen receptor occupancy. Annu Rev Immunol 7:445–480.

Mule JJ, Shu S, Rosenberg SA (1985): The anti-tumor efficacy of lymphokine-activated killer cells and recombinant interleukin-2 in vivo. J Immunol 135:646–652.

Mustelin T, Poso H, Andersson LC (1986): Role of G-proteins in T cell activation non-hydrolysable GTP analogues induce early ornithine decarboxylase activity in human T lymphocytes. EMBO J 6:3287–3290

Nakamura RM, Tanaka H, Tokunaga T (1982): In vitro induction of suppressor T-cells in delayed-type hypersensitivity to BCG and an essential role of I-J positive accessory cells. Immunol Lett 4:295–299.

Nedwin GW, Naylor SL, Sakaguchi AY, Smith D, Jarrett-Nedwin J, Pennica D, Goeddel DV, Gray PW (1985): Human lymphotoxin and tumor necrosis factor genes: Structure, homology and chromosomal localization. Nucleic Acids Res 13:6361–6371.

Noelle R, Krammer PH, Ohara J, Uhr JW, Vitetta ES (1984): Increased expression of Ia antigens on resting B cells: A new role for B cell growth factor. Proc Natl Acad Sci USA 81:6149–6153.

Noguchi M, Yi H, Rosenblatt HM, Filipovich AH, Adelstein S, Modi WS, McBride OW, Leonard WJ (1993): Interleukin-2 receptor γ chain mutation results in X-linked severe combined immunodeficiency in humans. Cell 73:147–157.

Nordan RP, Potter M (1986): Macrophage-derived factor required by plasma cytomas for survival and proliferation in vitro. Science 233:566–569.

Norment AM, Salter RD, Parham P, Engelhard VH, Littman DR (1988): Cell-cell adhesion mediated by CD8 and MHC class 1 molecules. Nature (London) 336:79–81.

Oettgen HC, Terhorst C, Cantley LC, Rosoff PM (1985): Stimulation of the T3-T cell receptor complex induces a membrane-potential-sensitive calcium influx. Cell 40:583–590.

Ohashi PS, Mak TW, Van den Elsen P, Yanagi Y, Yoshikai Y, Calman AF, Terhorst C, Stobo JD, Weiss A (1985): Reconstitution of an active surface T3/T-cell antigen receptor by DNA transfer. Nature (London) 316:606–609.

Old LJ (1985): Tumor necrosis factor (TNF). Science 30:630–632.

Pantelouris EM (1968): Absence of thymus in a mouse mutant. Nature (London) 217:370–371.

Paul WE (1984): Nomenclature of lymphokines which regulate B-lymphocytes. Mol Immunol 21:343.

Paul WE (1991): Interleukin-4: A prototype immunoregulatory lymphokine. Blood 77:1859–1870.

Pennica D, Nedwin GE, Hayflick JS, Seeburg PH, Derynck R, Palladino MA, Kohr WJ, Aggarwal BB, Goeddel DV (1984): Human tumour necrosis factor: Precursor structure, expression and homology to lymphotoxin. Nature (London) 312:724–729.

Peschel C, Paul WE, Ohara J, Green I (1987): Effects of B-cell stimulatory factor-1/interleukin-4 on hematopoietic progenitor cells. Blood 70:254–263.

Peters PJ, Geuze HJ, van der Donk HA, Borst J (1990): A new model for lethal hit delivery by cytotoxic T lymphocytes. Immunol Today 11:28–32.

Peterson A, Seed B (1988): Genetic analysis of monoclonal antibody and HIV binding sites on the human lymphocyte antigen CD4. Cell 54:65–72.

Pingel JT, Thomas ML (1989): Evidence that the leukocyte-common antigen is required for antigen-induced T lymphocyte proliferation. Cell 58:1055–1065.

Podack ER, Hengartner H, Lichtenfeld MR (1991). A central role of perforin in cytolysis? Annu Rev Immunol 9:129–157.

Reinherz EL, Kung PC, Goldstein, G. Levey RH, Schlossman SF (1980): Discrete stages of human intrathymic differentiation: Analysis of normal thymocytes and leukemic lymphoblasts of T cell lineage. Proc Natl Acad Sci USA 77:1588–1592.

Robb RJ, Kutny RM, Chowdhry V (1983): Purification and partial sequence analysis of human T-cell growth factor. Proc Natl Acad Sci USA 80:5990–5994.

Roberts WK, Vasil A (1982): Evidence for the identity of murine gamma interferon and macrophage activating factor. J Interferon Res 2:519–532.

Romagnani S, Maggi E, Del Prete GF, Parronchi P, Macchia D, Tiri A, Ricci M (1989): Role of interleukin 4 and gamma interferon in the regulation of human IgE synthesis: Possible alterations in atopic patients. Int Arch Allergy Appl Immunol 88:111–113.

Rosen FS, Cooper MD, Wedgwood RJP (1984): The primary immunodeficiencies. Part I. N Engl J Med 311:235–242.

Rosenberg SA, Mule JJ, Spiess PJ, Reichart CM, Schwarz SL (1985): Regression of established pulmonary metastases and subcutaneous tumor mediated by the systemic administrations of high-dose recombinant interleukin-2 J Exp Med 161:1169–1188.

Rosenberg SA, Packard BS, Aebersold PM, Solomon D, Topalian S, Toy ST, Simon P, Lotze MT, Yang JC, Seipp CA, Simpson C, Carter C, Bock S, Schwartzentruber D, Wei JP, White DE (1988): Use of tumor infiltrating lymphocytes and interleukin-2 in the immunotherapy of patients with metastatic melanoma. A preliminary report. N Engl J Med 319:1676–1680.

Rothlein R, Springer TA (1986): The requirement for lymphocyte function-associated antigen 1 in homotypic leukocyte adhesion stimulated by phorbol ester. J Exp Med 163:1132–1149.

Rothlein R, Dustin ML, Marlin SD, Springer TA (1986): A human intercellular adhesion molecule (ICAM-1) distinct from LFA-1. J Immunol 17:1270–1274.

Saito H, Kranz D, Takagaki Y, Hayday AC, Eisen HN, Tonegawa S (1984): A third rearranged and expressed gene in a clone of cytotoxic T lymphocytes. Nature (London) 312:36–40.

Saizawa K, Rojo J, Janeway CA (1987): Evidence for a physical association of CD4 and the CD3: $\alpha:\beta$ T-cell receptor. Nature (London) 328:260–263.

Samelson LE, Phillips AF, Luong ET, Klausner RD (1990): Association of the fyn protein-kinase with the T cell antigen receptor. Proc Natl Acad Sci USA 87:4358–4362.

Sanderson CJ, Campbell HD, Young IG (1988): Molecular and cellular biology of eosinophil differentiation factor (IL-5) and its effects on human and mouse B cells. Immunol Rev 102:29–50.

Schreiber SL (1991): Chemistry and biology of the immunophilins and their immunosuppressive ligands. Science 251:283–287.

Scott B, Bluthmann H, Teh HS, von Boehmer H (1989): The generation of mature T cells requires interaction of the $\alpha\beta$ T-cell receptor with major histocompatibility antigens. Nature (London) 338:591–593.

Scott P, Natovitz P, Coffman RL, Pearce E, Sher A (1988): Immunoregulation of cutaneous leishmaniasis. T cell lines that transfer protective immunity or exacerbation belong to different T helper subsets and respond to distinct parasite antigens. J Exp Med 168:1675–1684.

Seed B (1987): An LFA-3 cDNA encodes a phospholipid-linked membrane protein homologous to its receptor CD2. Nature (London) 329:840–842.

Serra HM, Krowka JF, Ledbetter JA, Pilarski LM (1988): Loss of CD45R (Lp220) represents a post-thymic T cell differentiation event. J Immunol 140:1441–1445.

Sha WC, Nelson CA, Newberry RD, Kranz DM, Russell JH, Loh DY (1988): Positive and negative selection of an antigen receptor on T cells in transgenic mice. Nature (London) 336:73–76.

Sharon M, Klausner RD, Cullen BR, Chizzonite R, Leonard WJ (1986): Novel interleukin-2 receptor subunit detected by cross-linking under high-affinity conditions. Science 234:859–863.

Shimizu Y, van Seventer GA, Horgan KJ, Shaw S (1990): Roles of adhesion molecules in T-cell recognition: Fundamental similarities between four integrins on resting human T cells (LFA-1, VLA-4, VLA-5, VLA-6) in expression, binding, and costimulation. Immunol Rev 90:109–143.

Shortman K, Scollay R (1985): Cortical and medullary thymocytes. In Watson JD, Marbrook J (eds): "Recognition and Regulation in Cell-Mediated Immunity." New York: Marcell Dekker, pp 31–60.

Simmons D, Makgoba MW, Seed B (1988): ICAM, an adhesion ligand of LFA-1, is homologous to the neural cell adhesion molecule, NCAM. Nature (London) 331:624–627.

Smith SH, Brown MH, Rowe D, Callard RE, Beverley PCL (1986): Functional subsets of human helper-inducer cells defined by a new monoclonal antibody, UCHL1. Immunology 58:63–70.

Snapper CM, Paul WE (1987): Interferon gamma and B cell stimulatory factor-1 reciprocally regulate Ig isotype production. Science 236:944–947.

Solari R (1990): Identification and distribution of two forms of this interleukin 1 receptor. Cytokine 2:21–28.

Sprent J, Webb SR (1987): Function and specificity of T cell subsets in the mouse. Adv Immunol 41:39–133.

Springer TA (1990): Adhesion receptors of the immune system. Nature (London) 346:425–434.

Springer TA, Dustin ML, Kishimoto TK, Marlin SD (1987): The lymphocyte function-associated LFA-1, CD2, and LFA-3 molecules: Cell adhesion receptors of the immune system. Annu Rev Immunol 5:223–252.

Staunton DE, Marlin SD, Stratowa C, Dustin ML, Springer TA (1988): Primary structure of ICAM-1 demonstrates interaction between members of the immunoglobulin integrin supergene families. Cell 52:925–933.

Staunton DE, Dustin ML, Springer TA (1989): Functional cloning of ICAM-2, a cell adhesion ligand for LFA-1 homologous to ICAM-1. Nature (London) 339:61–64.

Stoolman LM (1989): Adhesion molecules controlling lymphocyte migration. Cell 56:907–910.

Street NE, Schumacher JH, Fong TA, Bass H, Fiorentino DF, Leverah JA, Mosmann TR (1990): Heterogeneity of mouse helper T cells. Evidence from bulk cultures and limiting dilution cloning for precursors of Th1 and Th2 cells. J Immunol 144:1629–1639.

Streuli M, Hall LR, Saga Y, Schlossman SF, Saito H (1987): Differential use of three exons generates at least five different mRNAs encoding human leukocyte common antigens. J Exp Med 166:1548–1566.

Sussman JJ, Bonifacino JS, Lippincott-Schwartz J, Weissman AM, Saito T, Klausner RD, Ashwell JD (1988): Failure to synthesize the T-cell CD3-zeta chain: Structure and function of a partial T cell receptor complex. Cell 52:85–95.

Takahashi M, Yoshida MC, Satoh H, Hilgers J, Taoita Y, Honjo T (1989): Chromosomal mapping of the mouse IL-4 and human IL-5 genes. Genomics 4:47–52.

Takeshita T, Asao H, Suzuki J, Sugamura K (1990): An associated molecule, p64, with high-affinity interleukin 2 receptor. Int Immunol 2:447–480.

Takeshita T, Ohtani K, Asao H, Kumaki S, Nakamura M, Sugamura K (1992): An associated molecule, p64, with IL-2 receptor β chain: Its possible involvement in the formation of the functional intermediate-affinity IL-2 receptor complex. J Immunol 148:2154–2158.

Taniguchi T, Yasuhiro M (1993): The IL-2/IL-2 receptor system: A current overview. Cell 73:5–8.

Taniguchi T, Matsui H, Gajita T, Tyakaoka C, Kashima N, Yoshimoto R, Hamuro J (1983): Structure and expression of a cloned cDNA for human interleukin-2. Nature (London) 302:305–310.

Tedder TF, Cooper MD, Clement LT (1985): Human lymphocyte differentiation antigens HB-10 and HB-11. II. Differential production of B cell growth and differentiation factors by distinct helper T cell subpopulations. J Immunol 134:2989–2994.

Tepper RI, Pattengale PK, Leder P (1989): Murine interleukin-4 displays potent anti-tumor activity in vivo. Cell 57:503–512.

Terry LA, DiSanto JP, Small TN, Flomenberg N (1990): Differential expression and regulation of the human CD8α and CD8β chains. Tissue Antigens 35:82–91.

Teshigawara K, Wang H-M, Kato D, Smith KA (1987): Interleukin 2 high-affinity receptor expression requires two distinct binding proteins. J Exp Med 165:223–238.

Thompson CB, Lindsten T, Ledbetter JA, Kunkel SL, Young HA, Emerson SG, Leiden JM, June CH (1989): CD28 activation pathway regulates the production of multiple T-cell derived lymphokines/cytokines. Proc Natl Acad Sci USA 86: 1333–1337.

Tiefenthaler G, Hunig T, Dustin ML, Springer TA, Meuer SC (1987): Purified lymphocyte function-associated antigen-3 and T11 target structure and actions in CD2-mediated T cell stimulation. Eur J Immunol 17:1847–1850.

Tonks NK, Charbonneau H, Diltz CD, Fischer EH, Walsh KA (1988): Demonstration that the leukocyte common antigen CD45 is a protein tyrosine phosphatase. Biochemistry 27:8695–8701.

Torigoe T, Saragovi HU, Reed JC (1992): Interleukin-2 regulates the activity of the lyn protein-tyrosinase kinase in a B-cell line. Proc Natl Acad Sci USA 89:2674–2678.

Trenn G, Takayama H, Hu-Li J, Paul WE, Sitkovsky MV (1988): B cell stimulatory factor 1 (IL-4) enhances the development of cytotoxic T cells from Lyt-2+ resting murine T lymphocytes. J Immunol 140:1101–1106.

Truneh A, Albert F, Golstein P, Schmitt-Verhulst AM (1985): Early steps of lymphocyte activation bypassed by synergy between calcium ionophores and phorbol ester. Nature (London) 313:318–320.

Tsudo M, Kozak RW, Goldman CK, Waldmann TA (1986): Demonstration of a non-Tac peptide that binds interleukin-2: A potential participant in a multichain interleukin 2 receptor complex. Proc Natl Acad Sci USA 83:9694–9698.

Turka LA, Schatz DG, Oettinger MA, Chun JJ, Gorka C, Lee K, McCormack WT, Thompson CB (1991): Thymocyte expression of RAG-1 and RAG-2: Termination by T cell receptor crosslinking. Science 253:778–781.

Turner JM, Brodsky MH, Irving BA, Levin SD, Perlmutter RM, Littman DR (1990): Interaction of the unique N-terminal region of tyrosine kinase p56lck with cytoplasmic domains of CD4 and CD8 mediated by cysteine motifs. Cell 60:755–765.

Uchiyama T, Broder S, Waldmann TA (1981): A monoclonal antibody (anti-Tac) reactive with activated and functionally mature human T cells. I. Production of anti-Tac monoclonal antibody and distribution of Tac (+) cells. J Immunol 126: 1393–1397.

van Kooyk Y, Weder P, Hogervorst F, Verhoeven AJ, van Seventer G, te Velde A, Borst J, Keizer GD,

Figdor CG (1991): Activation of LFA-1 through a Ca^{2+}-dependent epitope stimulates lymphocyte adhesion. J Cell Biol 112:345–354.

van Seventer GA, Shimizu Y, Shaw S (1991): Roles of multiple accessory molecules in T-cell activation. Curr Opin Immunol 3:294–303.

Van Snick J (1990): Interleukin-6: An overview. Annu Rev Immunol 8:253–278.

Van Wauwe JP, DeMey JR, Goossens JG (1980): OKT3: A monoclonal anti-human T lymphocyte antibody with potent mitogenic properties. J Immunol 124:2708–2713.

Virelizer JL, Perez N, Arenzana-Seisdedos F, Devos R (1984): Pure interferon gamma enhances class II HLA antigens on human monocyte cell lines. Eur J Immunol 14:106–108.

Vitetta ES, Ohara J, Myers C, Layton J, Krammer PH, Paul WE (1985): Serologic, biochemical and functional identity of B cell stimulatory factor-1 and B cell differentiation factor for IgG_1. J Exp Med 162:1726–1731.

von Boehmer H (1988): The developmental biology of T lymphocytes. Annu Rev Immunol 6:309–326.

von Boehmer H, Karjalainen K, Pelkonen J, Borgulya P, Rammensee H-G (1988): The T-cell receptor for antigen in T-cell development and repertoire selection. Immunol Rev 101:21–37.

Warren DJ, Moore MAS (1986): Synergism among interleukin 1, interleukin 3, and interleukin 5 in the production of eosinophils from primitive hematopoietic stem cells. J Immunol 140:94–99.

Webb DS, Shimizu Y, van Seventer GA, Shaw S, Gerrard TL (1990): LFA-3, CD44 and CD45: Physiologic triggers of human monocyte TNF and IL-1 release. Science 249:1295–1297.

Weiss A (1991): Molecular and genetic insights into T cell antigen receptor structure and function. Annu Rev Genet 25:487–510.

Weiss A, Imboden J, Shoback D, Stobo J (1984): Role of T3 surface molecules in human T-cell activation: T3-dependent activation results in an increase in cytoplasmic free calcium. Proc Natl Acad Sci USA 81:4169–4173.

Weiss A, Koretzky G, Schatzman R, Kadlecek T (1991): Functional stimulation of the T cell antigen receptor induces tyrosine phosphorylation of phospholipase C γ. Proc Natl Acad Sci USA 88:5484–5488.

Wheelock EF (1965): Interferon-like virus-inhibitor induced in human leukocytes by cytohemagglutinin. Science 149:310–311.

Widmer MB, Bach FH (1981): Antigen-driven helper cell-independent cloned cytolytic T lymphocytes. Nature (London) 294:750–752.

Widmer MB, Grabstein KH (1987): Regulation of cytolytic T-lymphocyte generation by B-cell stimulatory factor. Nature (London) 326:795–798.

Wigzell H, Hayry P (1974): Specific fractionation of immunocompetent cells; application in the analysis of effector cells involved in cell mediated lysis. Curr Topics Microbiol Immunol 67:1–42.

Winoto A, Baltimore D (1989): Separate lineages of T cells expressing the $\alpha\beta$ and $\gamma\delta$ receptors. Nature (London) 338:430–432.

Wong GG, Witek-Giannotti JS, Temple PA, Kriz R, Frenz C, Hewick RM, Clark SC, Ikebuchi K, Ogawa M (1988): Stimulation of murine hematopoietic colony formation by human IL-6. J Immunol 140:3040–3044.

Yamada H, Martin PJ, Bean MA, Braun MP, Beatty PG, Sadamoto K, Hansen JA (1985): Monoclonal antibody 9.3 and anti-CD11 antibodies define reciprocal subsets of lymphocytes. Eur J Immunol 15:1164–1168.

Yamamoto Y, Ohmura T, Fujimoto K, Onoue K (1985): Interleukin 2 mRNA induction in human lymphocytes: Analysis of the synergistic effect of a calcium ionophore A23187 and a phorbol ester. J Immunol 15:1204–1208.

Yanagi Y, Yoshikai Y, Leggett K, Clark SP, Aleksander I, Mak TW (1984): A human T cell-specific cDNA clone encodes a protein having extensive homology to immunoglobulin chains. Nature (London) 308:145–149.

Yednock TA, Rosen SD (1989): Lymphocyte homing. Adv Immunol 44:313–378.

Yokota T, Coffman RL, Hagiwara H, Rennick DM, Takebe Y, Yokota K, Gemmell L, Schrader B, Yang G, Meyerson P, Luh J, Hoy P, Pene J, Briere F, Spits H, Bancherau J, deVries J, Lee FD, Arai N, Arai K (1987): Isolation and characterization of lymphokine cDNA clones encoding mouse and human IgA-enhancing factor and eosinophil colony-stimulating factor activities: Relationship to interleukin 5. Proc Natl Acad Sci USA 84:7388–7392.

Yoshimoto T, Nakanishi K, Matsui K, Hirose S, Hiroshi K, Tanaka T, Hada T, Hamaoka T, Higashino K (1990): IL-5 upregulates but IL-4 downregulates IL-2R expression on a cloned B lymphoma line. J Immunol 144:183–190.

Young JD-E, Hengartner H, Podack ER, Cohn ZA (1986): Purification and characterization of a cytolytic pore-forming protein from granules of cloned lymphocytes with natural killer activity. Cell 44:849–859.

Young JW, Koulova L, Soergel SA, Clark EA, Steinman RM, Dupont B (1992): The B7/BB1 antigen provides one of several costimulatory signals for the activation of CD4+ T lymphocytes by human blood dendritic cells in vitro. J Clin Invest 90:229–237.

Zilberstein A, Ruggieri R, Korn JH, Revel M (1986): Structure and expression of cDNA and genes for human interferon-beta-2, a distinct species inducible by growth-stimulatory cytokines. EMBO J 5:2529–2537.

Zinkernagel RM, Doherty PC (1974): Immunological surveillance against altered self components by sensitised T lymphocytes in lymphocytic choriomeningitis. Nature (London) 251:547–548.

Zinsser H (1921): Studies on the tuberculin reaction and on specific hypersensitiveness in bacterial infection. J Exp Med 34:495–522.

FOR FURTHER READING

Alexander D, Shiroo M, Robinson A, Biffen M, Shivnan E (1992): The role of CD45 in T-cell activation-resolving the paradoxes? Immunol Today 13:477–481.

Clevers H, Alarcon B, Willeman T, Terhorst C (1988): The T cell receptor/CD3 complex: a dynamic protein ensemble. Annu Rev Immunol 6:629–662.

Cohen JJ, Duke RC (1992): Apoptosis and programmed cell death in immunity. Annu Rev Immunol 10:267–293.

Davis MM, Bjorkman PJ (1988): T-cell antigen receptor genes and T-cell recognition. Nature (London) 334:395–402.

Geppert TD, Davis LS, Gur H, Wacholtz MC, Lipsky PE (1990): Accessory cell signals involved in T-cell activation. Immunol Rev 117:5–66.

June CH (1991): Signal transduction in T cells. Curr Opin Immunol 3:287–293.

Springer TA (1990): Adhesion receptors of the immune system. Nature (London) 346:425–434.

Taniguchi T, Yasuhiro M (1993): The IL-2/IL-2 receptor system: a current overview. Cell 73:5–8.

van Seventer GA, Shimizu Y, Shaw S (1991): Roles of multiple accessory molecules in T-cell activation. Curr Opin Immunol 3:294–303.

Weiss A (1991): Molecular and genetic insights into T cell antigen receptor structure and function. Annu Rev Genet 25:487–510.

Chapter 4
Antigen Presentation

Hugh Auchincloss, Jr.

INTRODUCTION

The subject of antigen presentation stems from the fundamental phenomenon in cellular immunology that T cells cannot be stimulated by soluble foreign antigens in their environment but rather require that antigens be presented to them in a particular way, by cells with specialized functions. The particular way in which antigens must be presented involves the breakdown of foreign proteins into peptides that are then associated with MHC molecules on the cell surface. T cell receptors can then interact with a determinant formed by a complex of the MHC molecule and the foreign peptide. The specialized functions of the cells that present antigen involve both their ability to process and present the foreign peptides and also to bind and activate T cells whose receptors can interact with the MHC/peptide determinant. Cells that have these specialized functions are called "antigen-presenting cells," generally referred to as "APCs."

Both *in vitro* and *in vivo* evidence has demonstrated the importance of APCs in cellular immunology. *In vitro*, APCs must be present along with T cells in order to obtain a proliferative response from the T cell mitogens, phytohemagglutinin (PHA) and concanavalin A (Con A). In addition, the mixed lymphocyte response (MLR) requires the presence of APCs from either the respondor or the stimulator population for proliferation to occur. *In vivo*, depletion of APCs from some types of endocrine tissues allows prolonged survival of these tissues when transplanted to normal recipients.

This chapter describes APCs and their specialized functions. It then outlines the cellular mechanisms that provide for antigen presentation. Finally, it considers the unique aspects of antigen presentation in the case of alloreactivity, where two sets of APCs are available, those of the donor and those of the recipient.

TYPES OF ANTIGEN-PRESENTING CELLS

Several different types of cells have APC function, all of which are derived from bone marrow progenitors. The protype of the APC is the dendritic cell, which appears to be the most potent stimulator of T cells on a per cell basis. The concentration of dendritic cells in different tissues appears to depend on how likely that tissue is of encountering foreign pathogens and on its role in generating an immune response. Therefore, dendritic cells are plentiful in skin, intestine, liver, lymph nodes, and spleen. The dendritic cells in these different tissues have different names, such as Langerhans cells in the skin and Kuppfer cells in the liver. Other bone marrow-derived cells can also function as APCs. Macrophages and B cells can do so, although with less potency than dendritic cells. The APC function of B cells is increased if they are activated. T cells in some species and some circumstances have also been found to have APC function.

One of the common features of the APCs is that they express class II MHC antigens "constitutively," meaning that they do so at all times regardless of the presence of exogenous lymphokines. This is reasonable since APCs most often stimulate CD4$^+$ cells, which respond to antigen presented in association with class II molecules.

Transplantation Immunology, pages 87–103
© 1995 Wiley-Liss, Inc.

Class II antigen expression is not an absolute requirement for APCs, however, and cells with APC function for CD8$^+$ T cells have been found that do not express MHC class II antigens. Indeed, there is an open question whether CD8$^+$ T cells have quite the same stringent requirement for APCs to achieve activation that CD4$^+$ cells have (Kosaka et al., 1992).

THE FUNCTIONS OF ANTIGEN-PRESENTING CELLS

There are basically four functions of antigen presenting cells in stimulating T cell responses (Table I). First, they provide a platform on which foreign antigens are presented in association with MHC molecules. Second, they provide a vehicle for transporting the foreign antigens to the T cells. Third, they provide a set of linking molecules that hold passing T cells in order that they may inspect the antigens on the platform. Finally, they provide a set of signals required for T cell activation.

APCs as a Platform for Presenting Antigen: The Principle of Associative Recognition

The first function of an antigen-presenting cell is required because T cell receptors cannot engage soluble antigens, nor even cell surface molecules, unless they are presented in association with MHC molecules. This is referred to as associative recognition. Because of the central importance of this antigen-presenting function of APCs in cellular immunology, several aspects of associative recognition, especially with respect to transplantation immunology, are considered here in some detail.

Table I. Functions of Antigen-Presenting Cells

1. Presentation of foreign antigen in association with MHC molecules
2. Transportation of foreign antigen to draining lymph nodes
3. Nonspecific binding of T cells
4. Costimulation of T cells

The original experiments that demonstrated this principle were performed during the late 1970s (Doherty and Zinkernagel, 1975; Zinkernagel et al., 1978). As diagrammed in Figure 1, a typical experiment involves an (A × B)F$_1$ animal, challenged in vivo with a virus, or other antigen, X, then stimulated in vitro with virally infected A cells (A + X). T cells from these cultures can lyse infected A cells (A + X), but not infected B cells (B + X). Thus it appeared that recognition of antigen X required that some property of the stimulating cell be shared by the target cell. Further experiments with congenic-resistant strains demonstrated that the crucial feature was sharing of the MHC antigens.

Since the basic observation from these experiments was that recognition of an antigen by T cells was restricted to those target cells sharing MHC antigens with the stimulating cells, the phenomenon was often referred to as *MHC restriction*. Many more experiments were required during the 1980s, as well as a better understanding of the structure of T cell receptors and MHC molecules, before it became clear that MHC restriction was the result of the physical association of antigen X with an MHC molecule. Thus the term *associative recognition* is more commonly used today.

The biologic mechanism of associative recognition. The mechanism of "associative" recognition requires (1) that foreign antigens be able to associate with MHC molecules, (2) that T cell receptors be able to see both X and the self-MHC molecule, and (3) that mature T cells be limited so that their receptors can only recognize X with an MHC molecule. Each of these elements of associative recognition is discussed in detail elsewhere in this book and only briefly mentioned here.

The capacity of MHC molecules to present peptides was revealed dramatically by the demonstration of the three-dimensional structure by crystallography. MHC molecules turn out to have a "cleft," formed by the outer two domains of the molecule, which is perfectly suited to present peptides of foreign antigens to T cell receptors (see Chapter 1).

Primary In Vivo Challenge with Virus X	Secondary In Vitro Challenge with Cells Expressing Virus X	Target Cell Lysis	
	A Cells	A + X	No
		B + X	No
	B Cells	A + X	No
(AxB)F1 Mouse		B + X	No
	A Cells + X	A + X	Yes
		B + X	No
	B Cells + X	A + X	No
		B + X	Yes

Fig. 1. Experimental evidence for the principle of "associative recognition." After *in vivo* priming and secondary stimulation with virus X, T cells cannot recognize the virus X independently, but must instead see X in association with the same MHC antigens expressed by the APCs that first stimulated the T cells.

One early idea to explain how T cells could see both X and self-MHC molecules was that T cells had two receptors, one for foreign antigens and another for self-MHC molecules. It is now clear that this is not the case and that a single T cell receptor can recognize a complex formed by X and an MHC molecule (see Chapter 3). The T cell receptor is made up of two chains, called α and β, and while a few studies have suggested that the α chain is more involved in recognition of the MHC molecule, and the β chain is more involved in the recognition of X, most of the evidence suggests that the two chains together provide the combining site for the complex of X plus MHC.

Finally, the third crucial element was the finding that T cells are selected in the thymus to mature only if their receptors have affinity for modified MHC molecules (see Chapter 2) (Sprent et al., 1988). This process, called "positive selection" or "thymic education," allows only a small portion of the potential T cells that enter the thymus to mature and enter the periphery. Those selected are the ones with receptors that have affinity for self-MHC molecules mod-

ified by the presence of a new peptide in the cleft of the MHC molecule.

The teleologic basis for associative recognition. After it became clear that T cells were restricted to recognizing foreign antigens in association with MHC molecules, the question was why this restriction was useful. The answer is speculative, of course, but it seems likely that the purpose is to focus the T cell response against targets suitable for a cell-mediated response. If T cells could respond to all foreign antigens without restriction, then every tiny virus would trigger T cell activation. The enormous, complex machinery of the T cell would then be wasted on each tiny viral particle, and the huge number of viral particles would overwhelm the relatively small numbers of T cells responsive to them. The immune system has a different mechanism to deal with small molecules, in the form of antibodies produced in abundance by individual B cells. The response of T cells, on the other hand, is best suited for targets more of their own size, such as cells that have been infected and damaged by viruses or tumor transformation. The restriction that T cell receptors recognize foreign antigens only after they have been presented in association with MHC molecules focuses the T cell response on these appropriate cellular targets.

Difficulties in experimental demonstration of associative recognition. Although the basic experiment outlined above easily demonstrates the principle of associative recognition, several hazards can confuse some experiments testing this principle. First, the experiment must be performed with purified cell populations *in vitro*. If all of the APCs are not removed from F_1 T cells before stimulating them with A + X, then the T cells might be stimulated by B + X in addition to A + X, if the antigen X is presented by the F_1 APCs. This would hide the phenomenon of associative recognition. Second, APCs with the appropriate MHC antigens must be available *in vivo* at the time of priming. For example, the use of chimeras in these experiments produced confusing results, such as the finding that (A→B) bone marrow chimeras, infected with antigen X, cannot respond to B + X targets, even after *in vitro* stimulation with B + X cells. This is because (A→B) chimeras have only A bone marrow progenitors and hence only A APCs *in vivo*. Thus (A→B) chimeras, infected with X, are only primed *in vivo* to recognize X in association with A MHC molecules. Third, the phenomenon of alloreactivity can mask MHC restriction. A animals infected with X can respond to B + X after stimulation *in vitro* with B + X, even though they have not been primed *in vivo* with B + X. This is because A T cells can respond to B cells alone, making the participation of the X antigen impossible to determine. Finally, the requirement for thymic education also confuses experiments seeking to demonstrate MHC restriction. Bone marrow chimeras constructed by placing (A × B)F_1 marrow into A recipients have APCs expressing MHC antigens of both A and B, and they are tolerant to both sets of antigens. However, they can be primed to respond only to X presented in association with A MHC antigens and not to antigens presented in association with B MHC molecules. This is because the

chimera has only an A thymus to positively select T cells during their development.

Although these scenarios seem complicated, it actually takes only three steps to predict the outcome of T cell priming according to the principle of associative recognition. (1) Consider the available APCs at each stage during the stimulation, (2) recognize the alloreactive T cells will respond to foreign MHC antigens whether they are presenting X or not, unless tolerance has been induced to these MHC antigens, and (3) remember that tolerant T cells can respond to a particular MHC antigen plus X only if that MHC antigen was expressed in the thymus where the T cell matured.

The problem of associative recognition after organ transplantation. Although these rules for understanding associative recognition in experimental immunology are relatively simple, the phenomenon nonetheless provides complicated issues to consider in real-life clinical transplantation. Consider the case of a patient A who receives a liver from a donor B and who also suffers from a viral infection X. T cells from the patient stimulated by X plus self-MHC antigens (A) should be able to eliminate infected cells from recipient tissues expressing A + X. However, they will not be able to respond to virally infected cells in the donor liver, which express B + X. On the other hand, T cells responsive to B + X will be stimulated by the alloreactive response to B MHC antigens alone. These B-reactive T cells, however, are the same ones that must be suppressed to prevent graft rejection. One might consider, in addition, what would happen if tolerance to the donor MHC antigens were somehow achieved: the patient would presumably also lose both B − and B + X-reactive T cells, since there would be no positive selection mechanism for modified B MHC antigens in the recipient's thymus. It would also make a difference in these scenarios whether the infection was introduced by the donor organ, when donor APCs were plentiful, or later in the clinical course, when they had been replaced by recipients APCs. The more one considers the clinical scenario, the more complicated it becomes.

At this point the actual consequences of associative recognition for clinical transplantation are too subtle for us to predict, especially when we are using exogenous immunosuppression that so powerfully affects all the immune responses. It is important to be aware of the issues and to wonder how the requirement for associative recognition is affecting what we are now doing, or what we might do with new strategies for transplantation.

APCs as Vehicles to Transport Antigen

After performing their first function (to present foreign antigen in association with MHC molecules), APCs have a second function to transport the foreign antigen to sites where T cells commonly exist. It is as if the platform provided by APCs had wheels to provide mobility.

A particular example of the transporting function of APCs has been demonstrated in the case of Langerhans cells in the skin. These APCs encounter foreign antigen entering via the skin and process the antigen into peptides to be presented in association with the MHC molecules. The Langerhans cells then undergo a change and begin to travel. These modified cells have been called "veiled" cells. The same cells then appear in draining lymph nodes where they are described as "interdigitating cells" as they insert themselves among the lymphocytes of the lymph nodes, offering their modified MHC antigens to the T cells that pass through (Steinman, 1991).

This function of APCs, as vehicles, is important because the statistical likelihood of a naive T cell encountering its particular antigen at remote sites in the periphery is very small. It would therefore be inefficient to have every T cell traveling to every portion of the body in search of foreign antigens. It is more sensible to keep naive T cells in the relatively confined spaces of the lymphatic system and to bring foreign antigens to these places.

The circulation of cells of the immune system.
The changes in T cell surface antigens that govern their circulation through the body are considered in more detail in Chapter 18. In general, naive T cells express adhesion molecules that cause them to exit the vascular bed in the post capillary, "high endothelial" venules (Gallatin et al., 1983; Butcher, 1991). From here they travel to lymph nodes and return to the vascular circulation via the thoracic duct. Activated T cells express a different set of adhesion molecules that cause them to enter peripheral tissues, especially in the kind of tissue in which the antigens that first triggered them are located (Dustin and Springer, 1991).

Since antigen-presenting cells also circulate, in this case from the peripheral tissues to their draining lymph nodes and other lymphoid organs, they must be constantly replaced from bone marrow progenitors. When bone marrow or other tissues are transplanted, it is possible to demonstrate the APCs of a particular organ being replaced over time. The turnover begins almost immediately for some organs, such as the liver, where most of the APCs seem to be replaced within several weeks. In other tissues, such as the skin, substantial replacement of APCs may take many months or longer.

The consequences of APC mobility in organ transplantation.
The function of APCs as vehicles to transport antigen has two important consequences in organ transplantation. First, it raises the issue where sensitization of alloreactive T cells actually occurs, in the donor tissue or in the recipient lymphatic system. Second, it suggests that the nature of the APCs in a transplanted organ is likely to be different over time.

Experiments by Barker and Billingham during the 1960s suggested that the primary site of sensitization to donor antigens was in the recipient's lymphatic system (Barker and Billingham, 1967). They transplanted skin by anastamosing a vascular pedicle directly to the recipients blood vessels. The pedicle was cleaned of all lymphatics and the transplanted tissue was separated from the recipient by a plastic barrier. These transplanted tissues survived for prolonged periods without immunosuppression, and they failed to sensitize the recipient to donor antigens. On the other hand, if "normal" skin was transplanted simultaneously to the same recipient, then both the normal graft and the alymphatic tissue were rejected rapidly. These results suggested that lymphatic drainage is required to allow antigen presentation and sensitization of recipient T cells in the recipient's lymphatic system. On the other hand, once sensitization has occurred, effector T cells responsible for graft destruction can enter foreign tissue via the vascular circulation.

In contrast to these early studies, more recent experiments with sponge matrix allografts and studies of the T cells that enter vascularized tissues have suggested that some naive T cells that enter the allografts can be sensitized in this peripheral site. Given the abundance of donor antigens in transplanted organs, it is not surprising that the less efficient peripheral sensitization of T cells can also occur to some degree in organ transplantation.

Immediately after transplantation, all of the APCs draining from a foreign organ will be of donor origin. These donor APCs can be detected in lymph nodes and the spleens of recipients in significant numbers shortly thereafter. These APCs will present donor MHC antigens and the peptides of other donor proteins in association with donor MHC antigens. They will also provide a source of donor proteins that may be processed and presented by recipient APCs. Over time, however, the number of donor APCs draining from a transplanted organ will diminish as they are replaced by recipient APCs. These recipient antigen-presenting cells will not present intact donor MHC antigens and will present the peptides of donor proteins only in association with recipient MHC molecules. It is likely, therefore, that the nature of the antigenic stimulus associated with organ transplantation changes over time.

Adhesion Molecules: APCs as a Sticky Surface for Passing T Cells

The third function of antigen-presenting cells is to attract and hold passing T cells long enough for them to sample the particular MHC/peptide complexes expressed on their surface. This function of APCs is accomplished by their expression of adhesion molecules that have corresponding receptors on T cells.

The best known adhesion molecule on APCs is ICAM-1, which is the ligand for LFA-3 on T cells. ICAM-2 and probably ICAM-3 are closely related molecules that bind the same receptor (Springer, 1990). Other molecules also promote the adhesion between T cells and APCs including the interaction between CD2, on T cells, and LFA-1, on APCs. These adhesion molecules are expressed constitutively on antigen-presenting cells, but the level of their expression increases when T cell activation takes place. Therefore, APCs can attract and hold passing T cells even better when they are presenting a foreign antigen.

The adhesion molecules expressed on APCs are similar, and in some cases identical, to those expressed on other cells in the body that have different purposes. For example, vascular endothelial cells express similar molecules that are responsible for directing the pattern of circulation of T cells, keeping naive T cells in the lymphatic system, and sending memory T cells into the periphery and activated cells into sites of inflammation. In addition, cytotoxic T cells use adhesion molecules to adhere to their targets at the time of cell lysis. There may also be differences in the types of adhesion molecules expressed by different APCs so that they tend to attract different kinds of T cells. However, the description of subsets of APCs on this basis is not yet well defined.

Antibodies against adhesion molecules have been used *in vivo* to attempt to prevent immune responses to transplanted organs. However, since the adhesion molecules have several different functions in the immune system, it is difficult to predict where in the system such blocking antibodies might have their effect. In the case of mice, a combination of antibodies against ICAM-1 and LFA-3 has been used to prevent T cell sensitization, whereas primates, treated with anti-ICAM-1 antibodies, appear to have sensitized T cells as well as infiltrating cells in the graft, but nonetheless show delayed graft rejection.

Costimulation: APCs Have a Signaling Function

After processing and presenting foreign antigens on their cell surface, traveling to sites of T cell congregation, and attracting passing T cells to examine their surface antigens, the fourth function of antigen-presenting cells is to communicate with T cells, providing them with signals that contribute to T cell activation (see Fig. 1). This communication is probably a two-way process in that T cells can also alter the function of APCs through the secretion of lymphokines such as interferron-γ (IFN-γ).

The molecules used by APCs to communicate with T cells include secreted lymphokines, such as IL-1, and cell surface molecules that have corresponding receptors on T cells. The best known surface molecule is B7, also referred to as BB1. This molecule binds to CD28 on T cells or the closely related molecule, CTLA-4 (Linsley et al., 1991). These T cell molecules are referred to as a coreceptors, to indicate that along with a T cell's antigen-specific receptor, binding of these structures is necessary to stimulate T cell activation. There are probably other surface molecules on APCs besides B7 that bind to coreceptors.

It is possible that different kinds of APCs express different costimulatory molecules and therefore stimulate different T cell functions. The data supporting this notion are not yet precise, but there is evidence that some types of stimulation activate Th1 cells while others activate Th2 cells.

It is not easy to distinguish between adhesion and costimulatory molecules on APCs since both are necessary for T cell activation. Functionally, the distinction can be made on the basis of what happens when T cells are exposed to APCs after the function of a particular molecule is inhibited. Blocking the adhesion molecules simply diminishes the T cell response to foreign antigen, whereas inhibition of the function of the costimulatory molecules not only prevents T cell activation but also alters T cells so that they are less responsive to the same antigen stimulation in the future (Harding et al., 1992). This downregulated state of T cells is referred to as "anergy" and is discussed elsewhere in this volume.

THE CELLULAR BIOLOGY OF ANTIGEN PRESENTATION

The process by which antigen-presenting cells encounter foreign proteins and present their peptides in association with MHC molecules is complex, involving internal mechanisms of the cell. The processes are different for class I versus class II MHC molecules.

Class I Antigen Presentation

The capacity to present peptides in association with MHC class I molecules is not limited to antigen-presenting cells. Other cells must also have this capacity so that they may be targets for T cell-mediated lysis.

The peptides that fill the cleft of MHC class I heavy chains are brought into contact with these molecules shortly after their assembly in the endoplasmic reticulum (Lorenz and Allen, 1988). Not all peptides gain access to the class I molecules, however, and the association is controlled by the function of "transporter" molecules that carry peptides to the class I molecules. At least two such transporter molecules, TAP-1 and TAP-2, have been identified, both of which are necessary for the proper assembly of MHC class I/peptide complexes. It is interesting that the genes encoding the transporter molecules are located with the MHC complex, although the reasons for this linkage are unclear.

The peptides that fit into the cleft of MHC class I molecules are trimmed either before, or possibly just after their association with the class I molecule, to be just the right size for this cleft. In the case of MHC class I, the peptide length is quite precise, being optimally nine amino acids long, although peptides as short as seven amino acids can be bound in the cleft (Monaco, 1992). For each particular MHC molecule, several of the amino acids of the peptide are especially important in determining its ability to fit into the grove. These amino acids need to have the right orientation and charge on their side chains to allow their association with the class I molecule.

In the case of MHC class I molecules, the cleft that binds peptides is formed entirely by the heavy chain of the molecule. β_2-Microglobulin associates with the heavy chain and probably has some effect on the conformation of the cleft. More importantly, class I MHC molecules that do not associate with β_2-microglobulin are inefficiently transported to the surface of the cell.

Therefore, mice lacking β_2-microglobulin have a severe deficiency in MHC class I antigen expression, although those few heavy chains that do reach the cell surface do seem capable of presenting peptides.

MHC molecules that do not associate with peptides also have a difficult time reaching the cell surface. Furthermore, the physical association of the MHC molecule with its peptide is sufficiently tight that there does not appear to be substantial loss or exchange of peptides by surface MHC molecules. As a result there are not many "empty" MHC molecules on the surface of the cell. Animals that lack the transporter proteins also have a severe deficiency in their expression of MHC molecules.

Although particular features are required of the peptides that associate with class I MHC molecules, it still turns out that many hundreds, and possibly thousands, of such peptides are generated in each cell. Therefore, the surface of the cell has hundreds of different MHC/peptide complexes. There does not appear to be any requirement that the peptides brought into association with MHC class I molecules be foreign, and thus the vast majority of surface MHC/peptide complexes represent self-antigens to which circulating T cells are tolerant. When foreign peptides are presented, following, for example, a viral infection, the number of foreign MHC/peptide complexes expressed on the surface of the cell is probably only a tiny fraction of the thousands of MHC molecules present there. T cells, however, appear to require the expression of several hundred particular MHC/peptide complexes to stimulate their antigen receptors (Christinck et al., 1991).

From the point of view of transplantation immunology, one of the most important features of class I/peptide association is that the peptides that gain access to MHC class I molecules tend to be those that are encoded and synthesized internally. For example, viruses that have been incorporated into the genome of the cell can generate proteins whose peptides are easily incorporated into the cleft of class I molecules, whereas foreign proteins elsewhere in the environment tend to be excluded from class I presentation. This exclusion does not appear to be absolute, however, and allogeneic peptides are able to be presented by self-APCs in association with class I molecules.

Another important feature for transplantation is that many of the peptides that are associated with MHC class I molecules are actually derived from MHC proteins (Benichou et al., 1992; Kievits and Ivanyi, 1991; Roetzschke et al., 1991). It is not surprising that some of the peptides have this origin since MHC proteins are internally synthesized and class I proteins are obviously present in the right physical location for their peptides to have easy access to associate with the class I molecule. Nonetheless, it does seem surprising that as many as half of the peptides that have been isolated and characterized from MHC class I molecules were derived from MHC proteins. It is not yet known whether allogeneic MHC proteins would also generate peptides that would be especially well suited for presentation by self MHC molecules.

Class II Antigen Presentation

In contrast to the presentation of peptides by class I MHC molecules, the peptides presented by class II molecules tend to be derived from proteins in the surrounding environment. These proteins are first engulfed into the APC and degraded partly in endocytic vesicles. These vesicles then bring peptides of the proteins into physical contact with MHC class II molecules as they emerge from the endoplasmic reticulum.

The cleft of MHC class II molecules is formed by the junction of two chains, called α and β (Glimcher and Kara, 1992; Neefjes and Ploegh, 1992). Recent evidence has provided a tentative model for how foreign peptides gain access to class II dimers. As the two class II chains join, the cleft they form is initially prevented from picking up a peptide by the presence of a third molecule called the *invariant chain*. When the class II molecules come in contact with the peptides generated in the endocytic vesicles, then the invariant chain dissociates from the $\alpha\beta$ dimer, allowing the foreign peptides to associate with the MHC class II molecule. The MHC/peptide complex is then allowed to travel to the cell surface. The actual mechanisms of peptide/

MHC association are probably more complex then this simple model and there is evidence, for example, that two β chains are associated with a single α chain at the time of peptide association. In addition, recent crytallographic evidence has suggested that two MHC class II molecules are associated together on the cell surface at the time of antigen presentation to T cells. It is very likely, therefore, that the mechanism of class II/peptide association and antigen presentation will turn out to be more complicated than we currently realize.

The peptides presented by class II molecules are slightly longer than those presented by class I molecules (being up to 14 amino acids long) and the requirements for particular side chains on the amino acids are less stringent (Rudensky et al., 1991). Nonetheless, characteristic motifs for the peptides presented by particular class II antigens are apparent. Peptides of MHC proteins are again very frequent among the peptides that have been isolated from the cleft of class II molecules. In this case, these peptides are probably derived from external MHC molecules, although it is even less clear than in the case of class I peptide presentation why MHC peptides should be so commonly represented in the cleft of class II molecules. Although class II molecules tend to present peptides of external proteins, they presumably have access to the full range of self-proteins through the death and degradation of self-cells throughout the body.

SPECIAL FEATURES OF ANTIGEN-PRESENTING CELL FUNCTION IN TRANSPLANTATION

The four functions of antigen-presenting cells are central to the process of T cell activation in cellular immunology. These functions are therefore critical in transplantation immunology as well. In the case of transplantation, however, there are two distinct features of antigen-presenting cell function that make allogeneic T cell responses unique. First, allogeneic MHC antigens expressed on the APCs of donor tissues are extraordinarily powerful in stimulating T cell responses. Second, transplantation represents the only situation in which two different sets of antigen-presenting cells (those of the donor and those of the recipient) are available to stimulate an immune response. Without these two features, the field of transplantation immunology would not exist, since the response to donor antigens would be just an example of an ordinary immune response. The remainder of this chapter, therefore, considers these two special features of antigen-presenting cell function in tissue transplantation.

The Extraordinary Strength of T Cell Responses to Allogeneic MHC Antigens

The extraordinary strength of T cell responses to allogeneic MHC antigens can be seen first in the observation that *in vivo* priming is not required in order to generate primary *in vitro* T cell proliferation and cytotoxicity to cells bearing allogeneic MHC antigens. In addition, measurements of the precursor frequency of T cells specific for allogeneic MHC antigens show that roughly two-per-hundred T cells can respond to a particular foreign MHC antigen, whereas more like one-per-ten thousand T cells can respond to common environmental pathogens (Fischer-Lindahl and Wilson, 1977). This several hundred-fold increase in precursor frequency exists even when the allogeneic MHC antigen differs from self MHC antigens by only a single amino acid and even though there is no known physiologic purpose for an allogeneic T cell response. Although the strength of the allogeneic response is obviously of tremendous importance in transplantation immunology, only recently have we learned enough about antigen presentation in cellular immunology to explain this accidental phenomenon.

The presence of an alloreactive repertoire.
The first key to understanding the strength of alloreactivity lies in the observation that T cells can recognize allogeneic MHC antigens as intact molecules without the requirement that they be broken into peptides and presented in association with self-MHC molecules. This makes allogeneic MHC antigens almost unique among the foreign antigens that stimulate T cell responses. At one time it was thought that the genes encoding T cell receptors provided this

alloreactive repertoire by encoding only MHC-specific receptors. It is now clear, however, that the ability of mature T cells to recognize intact allogeneic MHC antigens stems primarily from the positive selection process in the thymus. This process selects only those T cells for maturation that are reactive with modified self MHC antigens. It turns out that T cells reactive with modified self-MHC antigens can also respond to allogeneic MHC antigens because the determinants in each case look sufficiently alike (Heber-Katz et al., 1982). In shorthand terminology, this phenomenon has been described as Allo = Self + X.

Although the ability of T cells to recognize intact allogeneic MHC antigens is important for the strength of alloreactivity, this, by itself, does not explain why the frequency of T cells responding to allogeneic MHC antigens should be so much higher than the frequency of cells responding to modified self-MHC antigens. The second key to understanding this phenomenon lies in the manner in which these allo MHC antigens are presented by APCs. Two slightly different theories have been proposed to explain the high frequency.

The "determinant density" hypothesis. The first theory, called the *determinant density* hypothesis, suggests that allogeneic MHC antigens are expressed on the surface of allogeneic APCs in much larger numbers than modified self-MHC antigens are expressed on the surface of self APCs (Bevan, 1984). Consider the process of presenting a peptide X. As discussed above, this peptide is only one of hundreds, perhaps thousands, of peptides being processed and presented by MHC molecules. Therefore, the expression of the particular Self + X determinant is relatively rare on the surface of the APC. In the case of an allogeneic APC, however, every MHC molecule on the surface of the cell represents the foreign determinant recognized by a T cell. The density of this determinant on the cell surface would thus be much higher than that of the modified self-MHC molecule. The determinant density hypothesis suggests that the actual frequency of T cells responding to Allo is probably not

really different from that of cells responding to Self + X, but that the stimulus to activate these alloreactive T cells is much larger. Therefore, more T cells (with lower affinity) are stimulated by allogeneic MHC antigens.

The "determinant frequency" hypothesis. The second hypothesis to explain the strength of alloreactivity is called the *determinant frequency* hypothesis (Matzinger and Bevan, 1977). This theory is based on the realization that T cells probably rarely encounter MHC antigens that do not have some peptide in their cleft and that the determinant on allogeneic MHC molecules recognized by T cells is actually formed by some combination of the MHC molecule itself and whatever peptide is present there. In the shorthand terminology mentioned above, this is described as Allo = Allo + X. Most of the peptides presented by APCs are derived from self proteins giving rise to a large number of Xs (X_1, X_2, X_3, . . . X_n). Therefore, the MHC molecules expressed on the surface of an allogeneic APC provide many different determinants (Allo + X_1, Allo + X_2, etc.) each able to stimulate a T cell of different specificity. Of course self-APCs also express MHC molecules presenting many different peptides of self proteins (Self + X_1, Self + X_2, etc.) but in this case the T cells are tolerant to these modified self-determinants. The set of Xs available in allogeneic APCs is probably somewhat different from the set of Xs generated in self-APCs. Even if they were identical, however, the combination of Allo + X will form a new determinant for T cells even when these T cells were tolerant to Self + X. The determinant frequency hypothesis suggests that there truly is a higher frequency of alloreactive T cells because a single allogeneic MHC molecule can generate so many different new determinants.

The evidence that few empty MHC molecules exist on the cell surface and that alloreactive T cells are influenced by the nature of the peptides presented in the cleft of MHC molecules has led many to favor the determinant frequency explanation for the great strength of alloreactivity. The two theories are not mutually exclusive, however, and it is possible that both explanations are true. The important thing to recognize is that according to both theories, the extraordinary strength of alloreactivity can exist only because intact allogeneic MHC antigens can be recognized by T cells without the requirement that they be processed and presented by self-MHC molecules. As mentioned above, allogeneic MHC molecules can also be recognized after their peptides are presented by self-MHC molecules. The theories to explain the strength of alloreactivity do not suggest, however, that this form of allo-MHC recognition would be any stronger than the recognition of any other peptide from a non-MHC protein presented by a self-MHC molecule.

The unusual strength of alloreactivity gives rise to unusual types of T cell responses. The most important consequence of the unusual strength of alloreactive T cell responses is obviously that it makes cellular rejection of transplanted organs so strong. A second consequence is that it enables unusual types of T cell responses to become an important part of transplant rejection. Ordinarily, the typical T cells encountered in the response to environmental pathogens include CD4+ helper T cells, responding to modified self-class II antigens, and CD8+ cytotoxic T cells, responding to modified self-class I antigens. In transplantation, CD4+ helper cells can respond to allogeneic MHC class II molecules and CD8+ cytotoxic cells can respond to allogeneic MHC class I molecules, as would be expected. In addition, however, some CD8+ T cells can generate their own help in response to allogeneic MHC class I antigens, CD8+ cytotoxic cells have been identified that recognize allogeneic MHC class II molecules, and CD4+ T cells have been found that are cytotoxic in response to allogeneic class II stimulation and in some cases even to allogeneic class I stimulation (Rosenberg et al., 1987). The ability to detect these unusual T cell responses is probably the result of the strength of the stimulus provided by allogeneic MHC antigens, which magnifies types of T cell responses that are ordinarily trivial. With these unusual T cell responses available, there are multiple potential pathways

of T cell reactivity to transplanted organs, making the T cell response to transplanted organs far more complicated than to ordinary antigens.

Two Sets of Antigen-Presenting Cells

The second unique feature of transplantation immunology is that tissue transplantation provides the only setting in which there are two different sets of antigen-presenting cells available to stimulate the immune response. The APCs of the donor may differ from those of the recipient in the MHC antigens they express and in the collection of proteins that are generated internally in the cell as opposed to being obtained exogenously. The T cell responses to these different sets of APCs may therefore be quite different.

"Direct" versus "indirect" recognition. Transplantation immunologists have developed a terminology to describe the stimulation arising from the two different sets of APCs. *Direct* recognition refers to the stimulation of T cells by APCs derived from the donor while *indirect* recognition refers to stimulation by peptides of donor proteins presented by self-MHC antigens on APCs of the recipient (Fig. 2). This terminology has the advantage that the term "direct" describes the critical feature that T cells can recognize intact allogeneic MHC molecules without the requirement that they be processed and presented by self-MHC molecules. Allo MHC antigens are recognized "directly." The terminology has the disadvantage that the word "indirect" suggests that there is something less physiologic about the process of presenting peptides of foreign antigens in association with self-MHC molecules. Actually, of course, "indirect" recognition is the physiologic T cell response.

One source of confusion that arises about the terminology is the idea that the term "indirect" refers to the process of protein degradation and peptide presentation. Thus, some have described the recognition of peptides of donor proteins presented by donor MHC antigens as being "indirect," especially when the peptides they are discussing are derived from the donor MHC proteins themselves. This use of the term "indi-

DIRECT VS. INDIRECT
RECOGNITION

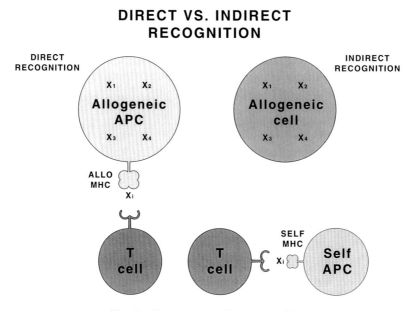

Fig. 2. Direct versus indirect recognition.

rect" to describe the feature that Allo = Allo + Y is incorrect. The terms "indirect" versus "direct" should be used to describe the source of the APCs that are stimulating the T cells, not the mechanism by which all APCs generate new determinants.

There is evidence that both direct and indirect immune responses occur at the time of graft rejection. In the case of direct recognition, the evidence comes from the importance of MHC antigens in causing rapid graft rejection. Since indirect presentation of MHC peptides would not be expected to cause a more powerful response than the indirect presentation of the peptides of minor histocompatibility antigens, the faster rejection of MHC-disparate grafts suggests that direct recognition is important. In the case of indirect recognition, the evidence comes from *in vitro* experiments showing that recipient T cells are primed to donor antigens presented in association with recipient MHC antigens (Shreffler et al., 1974). For example, (A × B)F$_1$ female mice, rejecting male skin grafts from male A donors, show *in vitro* T cell reactivity to male B cells. This phenomenon, known as "crosspriming," must arise from the indirect presenta-

tion of the donor male, H-Y antigen in association with the recipient's B MHC antigens.

Although it has been clear that both direct and indirect immune responses occur during graft rejection, the greater strength of the direct response has made it difficult to determine whether the indirect response can actually play any role in the destruction of foreign tissue. Recently, experiments using peptides of donor antigens to prime for faster graft rejection or using donor tissues that lack some of the MHC antigens needed to stimulate direct responses have suggested that indirect recognition is effective in causing graft rejection (Fangmann et al., 1992; Auchincloss et al., 1993).

Special Considerations Arising from the Presence of Two Sets of APCs

The presence of two sets of APCs capable of stimulating the T cell response to foreign tissues gives rise to several special considerations in transplantation immunology that would not arise in standard immune responses. Although we understand the nature of many of these issues, we do not yet know the resolution of some of them.

They represent some of the important un-answered questions in the field of transplantation immunology.

The diminishing presence of donor APCs. Although direct recognition of donor antigens is thought to be responsible for the special strength of early graft rejection, the importance of direct antigen presentation may diminish over time if a graft is kept in place by exogenous immunosup-pression. Since donor APCs are gradually re-placed by recipient cells, the number of donor APCs available to stimulate direct responses will gradually be fewer. The effect of this change may be small if T cell sensitization to donor anti-gens occurs while donor APCs are plentiful, since memory T cells may be susceptible to re-stimulation by cells of the donor graft that are not formally APCs. However the effect may be large, if early sensitization does not occur, and might account for the lower doses of immu-nosuppression that are generally required late af-ter clinical transplantation.

Indirect presentation provides the wrong de-terminants compared to those expressed on the donor graft. Although peptides of donor proteins presented by recipient MHC antigens generate determinants that stimulate T cell re-sponses, these determinants will not be the same as those expressed by the cells of the donor graft. This may seem in conflict with the earlier state-ment that Allo + Y = Self + X in the discussion describing the presence of a strong alloreactive T cell repertoire. However, the notion that T cell receptors can recognize allogeneic MHC anti-gens directly (because they were selected by a wide variety of modified self-MHC antigens) does not suggest that every particular X pre-sented by a self-MHC molecule will generate a determinant similar to a particular set of Allo + Y determinants. Cross-reactive T cell recogni-tion of donor MHC antigens may occasionally occur following sensitization to peptides pre-sented by self-MHC molecules, but in general T cells sensitized by indirect presentation will not recognize the antigens expressed on donor tissue.

The feature that indirect presentation gener-ates the wrong determinants creates a problem in transplantation immunology if one assumes that the T cells responsible for graft destruction must be specific for the particular antigens expressed on donor cells. Cytotoxic T cells, for example, could lyse cells of a transplanted organ only if they were sensitized to the donor antigens. This feature creates less of a problem if the process of graft destruction is less specific, requiring only that T cells be activated by any non-self-determinant.

The concern that indirect presentation gener-ates the wrong determinants disappears in those situations where there is matching between the MHC antigens of the donor and recipient. Pep-tides of donor proteins presented by recipient APCs will generate the same MHC + X determi-nant on these self-APCs as are expressed by the cells of the graft. Thus one might expect that the importance of indirect presentation would be greater in the rejection of MHC-matched grafts, although the high clinical success of such trans-plants suggests that the stimulus generated this way must be relatively susceptible to exogenous immunosuppression.

The problem of T cell communication when two different sets of APCs are available. T cell-dependent immune responses often involve communication between activated T cells (usu-ally CD4$^+$ cells) and other lymphocytes (such as CD8$^+$ T cells or B cells). In the case of transplan-tation immune responses, this communication is complicated by the possibility that one type of lymphocyte may be activated by antigens on one set of APCs while the other type of lymphocyte may be activated by antigens on the other set of APCs.

The communication between lymphocyte populations is partly in the form of lymphokine secretion, including IL-2 and IL-4, produced by one set of lymphocytes that stimulates another set through surface receptors for these mole-cules. *In vitro,* these lymphokines can be added in sufficient concentrations to replace the func-tion of the secreting lymphocyte subpopulation. However, as a general rule, the lymphokines tend to function *in vivo* more like neurotransmit-ters, working only over very short distances, than like hormones, working throughout the body (Paul, 1987). Therefore, physiologic replacement of lymphokine function by exogenous administration does not tend to be effective. Instead, the effect of pharmacologic doses of exogenous lymphokines, such as IL-2, tends to stimulate unusual populations of lymphocytes. This limitation on the physiologic function of the lymphokines makes sense teleologically since activation of an immune response is not supposed to be a general phenomenon but rather should be directed at the particular site of foreign antigen. We would not want a viral sinusitis to stimulate enhanced immunity in the distal bowel.

Since the function of lymphokines *in vivo* is limited over distance, it is generally important in generating immune responses that the relevant lymphocyte subsets be brought physically together, a process that can be facilitated by antigen-presenting cells. For example, a typical model for CD4+ helper function assisting B cells responding to allogeneic MHC antigens pictures a donor APC presenting the intact allogeneic MHC antigen to the B cell receptor and also presenting peptides of donor proteins in association with the donor's class II MHC molecules to stimulate CD4+ T cells. The presentation of two sets of determinants by the donor APC brings the APC, the CD4+ T cell, and the B cell together in a three-cell cluster. Alternatively, physical association of T and B cells might be achieved if donor cells present intact MHC antigens to stimulate B cell receptors, and the B cell itself functions as an APC for the CD4+ helper T cell, presenting peptides of donor antigens in association with its own class II MHC molecules to stimulate the T cells.

Cellular immune responses also involve communication between lymphocytes, such as the CD4+ helper function often required to generate mature CD8+ cytotoxic cells. There is evidence in cases of graft rejection that this communication also requires the physical association of the two types of T cells. For example, there are several examples of donor antigenic determinants that can stimulate CD8+ T cells but only if help is provided by CD4+ cells responding to different determinants. Under these circumstances it seems to be a requirement that both the cytotoxic

and the helper determinants be expressed on the same allogeneic tissue and it is not sufficient that one donor graft expresses the helper determinant to provide help for the CD8+ cytotoxic cells that are stimulated by the cytotoxic determinant on a different donor graft placed elsewhere on the same recipient (Rosenberg et al., 1987). As diagrammed in Figure 2, these findings are consistent with the idea that one APC must present both the helper and cytotoxic determinants in order to bring the CD4+ and CD8+ T cells into a three-cell cluster.

The suggestion that a physical association of helper and cytotoxic T cells is required to generate some alloreactive cellular responses creates a problem when considering graft rejection because of the presence of two different sets of antigen-presenting cells. In the case of MHC-mismatched grafts, only the donor APCs will present determinants to cytotoxic T cells that are also expressed on the other cells of the donor tissue. The issue then is whether helper cells stimulated by the indirect presentation of donor peptides on recipient APCs can effectively assist the relevant cytotoxic cells that are being stimulated elsewhere. Despite these theoretical concerns, however, there is evidence that indirect presentation can effectively initiate graft rejection. How the necessary communication between the different T cells takes place under these circumstances remains one of the unresolved issues in transplantation immunology.

Why is donor APC depletion sometimes effective in allowing prolonged allograft survival? The ability of donor antigens to initiate graft rejection through their indirect presentation by recipient APCs seems to be in conflict with the observation that depletion of donor antigen-presenting cells can sometimes allow allogeneic tissues to survive after transplantation without any immunosuppression. This finding was reported by Lafferty and described as the need to deplete "passenger leukocytes" (Lafferty et al., 1983). Several types of endocrine tissues, including thyroid and pancreatic islets, were found to show prolonged survival after APC depletion, although the precise conditions under which the technique is successful remain controversial.

Further experimental work indicated that the important leukocytes were actually those with APC function, providing some of the early evidence that APCs are critical in stimulating T cell responses to allogeneic tissue.

There are at least two possible explanations for the effectiveness of donor-APC depletion despite the availability of recipient APCs to stimulate graft rejection. First, indirect presentation of donor antigens may be effective in stimulating only the CD4$^+$ helper cells involved in graft rejection while the APCs of the donor may be essential to provide the determinants recognized directly by cytotoxic T cells. If so, then donor-APC depletion would not prolong graft survival if the donor were MHC class I antigen-matched with the recipient since then the cytotoxic determinants expressed on the two sets of APCs would be the same. Second, donor APCs may be necessary as the vehicles for transporting donor antigens to recipient APCs. This is one of the recognized functions of antigen-presenting cells although one might expect the death and degradation of ordinary donor cells to provide ample supplies of donor antigens in the recipients reticuloendothelial system. The reasons for and limitations on the effectiveness of donor-APC depletion are among the unresolved issues in transplantation immunology.

The consequences of indirect presentation for efforts to induce tolerance. Tolerance induction will be discussed later in this book, with descriptions of depletion, suppression, and anergy as mechanisms by which donor-specific nonresponsiveness might be achieved. The presence of the indirect pathway for presentation of donor antigens has important consequences when considering the role of anergy for transplantation tolerance.

The principal feature of anergy is that T cells stimulated by antigens in the absence of the costimulatory signals provided by APCs become nonresponsive to those antigens. The state of anergy is unstable, however, and can be broken by several manipulations, including absence of the antigens or provision of sufficient IL-2 (Jenkins and Schwartz, 1987). As discussed later, there are several strategies for anergy induc-

tion in transplantation, including the elimination of donor APCs or treatment designed to prevent the delivery of costimulatory signals by either donor or recipient APCs. No clinically applicable strategy, however, can hope to block the function of recipient APCs permanently since they must remain functional in the long run to present environmental pathogens to recipient T cells.

These considerations suggest that strategies depending on anergy for tolerance induction must inevitably face the challenge of long-term indirect presentation of donor antigens. While anergic T cells may ordinarily not respond to this stimulation, it is easy to imagine that unusual perturbations of the system (for example, a large outpouring of donor antigens caused by some nonimmunologic injury of the graft or a powerful immunologic stimulus caused by some unrelated environmental antigen) might break the anergy to donor antigens. Such a process might be analogous to that giving rise to autoimmune disease, but in the case of transplantation, the instability of anergy may be magnified by the large number of novel antigens present in a foreign organ. Although strategies to achieve tolerance by anergy induction have become popular recently, the consequences of the indirect presentation of donor antigens by recipient APCs have not yet been carefully considered.

CONCLUSION

Antigen-presenting function is crucial for stimulating immune responses to transplanted tissues just as it is in all cellular immunology. This function is provided by antigen-presenting cells that offer a platform for the expression of foreign antigens in association with MHC molecules, a vehicle for bringing these antigens to T cells, a linkage system to attract passing T cells, and a signaling system to help activate those T cells whose receptors recognize the donor antigens.

Compared to other immune responses, transplantation immunology is unique because it involves the function of two different sets of APCs, those of the donor, providing direct antigen presentation, and those of the recipient, providing indirect antigen presentation. Direct presentation of alloantigens is responsible for the unusual strength of alloreactivity and probably also for the unusual types of T cell responses to allogeneic antigens. Indirect presentation provides an alternative pathway of T cell stimulation with several important consequences for transplantation immunology. Thus the unusual features of antigen presentation in transplantation are at the heart of what makes transplantation immunology special and these features provide many of the unanswered questions in this field.

REFERENCES

Auchincloss H Jr, Lee R, Shea S, Markowitz JS, Grusby MJ, Glimcher LH (1993): The role of "indirect" recognition in initiating rejection of skin grafts from major histocompatibility complex class II-deficient mice. Proc Natl Acad Sci 90:3373–3377.

Barker CF, Billingham RE (1967): The role of regional lymphatics in the skin homograft response. Transplantation 5:962.

Benichou G, Takizawa PA, Olson CA, McMillan M, Sercarz EE (1992): Donor major histocompatibility complex (MHC) peptides are presented by recipient MHC molecules during graft rejection. J Exp Med 175:918–924.

Bevan MJ (1984): High determinant density may explain the phenomenon of alloreactivity. Immunol Today 5:128–130.

Butcher EC (1991): Leukocyte-endothelial cell recognition: Three (or more) steps to specificity and diversity. Cell 67:1033–1036.

Christinck RE, Luscher MA, Barber BH, Williams DB (1991): Peptide binding to class I MHC on living cells and quantitation of complexes required for CTL lysis. Nature (London) 352:67–69.

Doherty PC, Zinkernagel RM (1975): H-2 compatibility is required for T-cell-mediated lysis of target cells infected with lymphocytic choriomeningitis virus. J Exp Med 141:502.

Dustin ML, Springer TA (1991): Role of lymphocyte adhesion receptors in transient interactions and cell locomotion. Annu Rev Immunol 9:27–66.

Fangmann J, Dalchau R, Fabre JW (1992): Rejection of skin allografts by indirect allorecognition of donor class I major histocompatibility complex peptides. J Exp Med 175:1521–1529.

Fischer-Lindahl K, Wilson DB (1977): Histocompatibility antigen-activated cytotoxic T lymphocytes II. Estimates of frequency and specificity of precursors. J Exp Med 145:508–522.

Gallatin WM, Weissman IL, Butcher EC (1983): A cell surface molecule involved in organ specific homing of lymphocytes. Nature (London) 304:30.

Glimcher LH, Kara CJ (1992): Sequences and factors: A guide to MHC class-II transcription. Annu Rev Immunol 10:13–49.

Harding FA, McArthur JG, Gross JA, Raulet DH, Allison JP (1992): CD28-mediated signaling co-stimulates murine T cells and prevents induction of anergy in T-cell clones. Nature (London) 356:607–609.

Heber-Katz E, Schwartz RH, Matis LA, Hannum C, Fairwell T, Appella E, Hansburg D (1982): Contribution of antigen-presenting cell major histocompatibility complex gene products to the specificity of antigen-induced T cell activation. J Exp Med 155:1086–1099.

Jenkins MK, Schwartz RH (1987): Antigen presentation by chemically modified splenocytes induces antigen-specific T cell unresponsiveness in vitro and in vivo. J Exp Med 165:302.

Kievits F, Ivanyi P (1991): A subpopulation of mouse cytotoxic T lymphocytes recognizes allogenic H-2 class I antigens in the context of other H-2 class I molecules. J Exp Med 174:15–19.

Kosaka H, Surh CD, Sprent J (1992): Stimulation of mature unprimed CD8+ T cells by semiprofessional antigen-presenting cells in vivo. J Exp Med 176:1291–1302.

Lafferty K, Prowse S, Simeonovic C, Warren HS (1983): Immunobiology of tissue transplantation: A return to the passenger leucocyte concept. In Paul WE, Fathman CG, Metzgar H, (eds.): "Annual Review of Immunology." Palo Alto, CA: Annual Reviews, pp 143–173.

Linsley PS, Brady W, Urnes M, Grosmaire LS, Damle NK, Ledbetter JA (1991): CTLA-4 is a second receptor for the B cell activation antigen B7. J Exp Med 174:561–569.

Lorenz R, Allen PM (1988): Processing and presentation of self proteins. Immunol Rev 106:115–127.

Matzinger P, Bevan MJ (1977): Why do so many lymphocytes respond to major histocompatibility complex antigens? Cell Immunol 29:1.

Monaco JJ (1992): A molecular model of MHC class-I-restricted antigen processing. Immunol Today 13:173–178.

Neefjes JJ, Ploegh HL (1992): Intracellular transport of MHC class II molecules. Immunol Today 13:179–183.

Paul WE (1987): Between two centuries: Specificity and regulation in immunology. J Immunol 139: 1–6.

Roetzschke O, Falk K, Faath S, Rammensee H-G (1991): On the nature of peptides involved in T cell alloreactivity. J Exp Med 174:1059–1071.

Rosenberg AS, Mizuochi T, Sharrow SO, Singer A (1987): Phenotype, specificity, and function of T cell subsets and T cell interactions involved in skin allograft rejection. J Exp Med 165:1296.

Rudensky AY, Preston-Hurlburt P, Hong SC, Barlow A, Janeway CA Jr. (1991): Sequence analysis of peptides bound to MHC class II molecules. Nature (London) 353:622–627.

Shreffler D, David C, Gotze D, Klein J, McDevitt H, Sachs DH (1974): Genetic nomenclature for new lymphocyte antigens controlled by the Ir region of the H-2 complex. Immunogenetics 1:189–190.

Sprent J, Lo D, Gao EK, Ron Y (1988): T cell selection in the thymus. Immunol Rev 101:173–190.

Springer TA (1990): Adhesion receptors of the immune system. Nature (London) 346:425–434.

Steinman RM (ed) (1991): "The Dendritic Cell System and Its Role in Immunogenicity." Palo Alto, CA: Annual Reviews.

Zinkernagel RM, Callahan GN, Cooper AS, Klein PA, Klein J (1978): On the thymus in the differentiation of "H-2 self-recognition" by T cells: Evidence for dual recognition. J Exp Med 147:882.

Chapter 5
Allograft Immunity: *In Vitro* and *In Vivo* Studies

Alfred Singer and Fritz H. Bach

Foreign tissue allografts are rejected because the *histocompatibility antigens* they express *stimulate a response from the host's immune system*. The predominant cell type involved in tissue rejection responses is the *T lymphocyte*, as depletion or suppression of T cell function results in prolonged survival of the transplanted organ. However, the precise mechanisms by which T cells recognize and reject foreign tissue allografts remain controversial.

The controversies regarding mechanisms of allograft rejection reflect the complexity of *in vivo* rejection responses. One complicating factor is that allografts from different tissues consist of different cell types that express different surface antigens and so stimulate different kinds of immune responses. *In vivo* rejection responses are further complicated by the fact that immunocompetent T cells are not a homogeneous population of cells, but rather are heterogeneous with regard to (1) function, (2) phenotype, and (3) MHC recognition specificities (see also Chapter 3). Despite these complexities, careful analyses of *in vitro* immune reactions and *in vivo* rejection responses have led to unifying principles that have significantly enhanced our understanding of the *in vivo* immune response against tissue allografts.

FUNCTIONAL HETEROGENEITY AMONG T CELLS

Immune responses involving T cells are initiated by activation of *antigen-specific T cells* in response to their recognition of foreign antigenic peptides present on the surface of antigen presenting cells (see also Chapter 4). As a consequence of their recognition of foreign antigens, the *helper T cells (Th)* are stimulated to secrete a variety of *"helper" lymphokines,* such as interleukins 2 and 4 (IL-2, IL-4) and interferon-γ (IFN-γ). Such helper lymphokines promote a variety of cellular functions, including (1) *growth,* causing antigen-stimulated T lymphocytes to expand in number, (2) *differentiation,* promoting the transformation of antigen-reactive prekiller cells into antigen-specific cytotoxic cells and promoting the differentiation of antigen-specific B lymphocytes into antibody secreting plasma cells, and (3) *recruitment,* attracting antigen-nonspecific inflammatory cells. Because their secreted lymphokines help other cells to grow, differentiate, and function, initiating T cells are referred to as "helper" cells.

In contrast to helper cells, *effector cells* function to remove foreign antigens from the organism. For example, *B cells* are effector cells that secrete antibodies that bind to foreign antigens, causing their removal by the reticuloendothelial system or their destruction by complement-mediated lysis. However, T cells can also be effector cells as *cytotoxic T cells (Tc)* kill other cells bearing antigens that they recognize as foreign. The cytotoxic function of T cells appears to have evolved as a mechanism to clear the organism of intracellular parasites such as viruses by identifying and destroying cells that harbor them. Thus, with the help of T-helper cells,

Transplantation Immunology, pages 105–111
© 1995 Wiley-Liss, Inc.

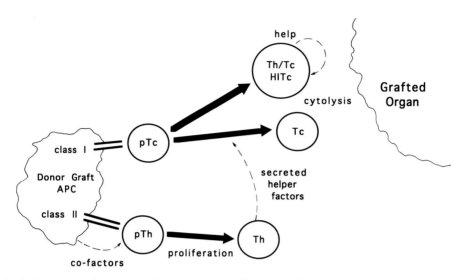

Fig. 1. Antigen-presenting cells (APC) of the donor graft present foreign allogeneic MHC-encoded class I and class II antigens to the T cells of the potential recipient (host). Precursor helper T cells (pTh) respond preferentially to allogeneic class II antigens and proliferate as well as secreting cytokines in response to those antigens. Precursor cytotoxic (killer) T cells (pTc) recognize and respond preferentially to the allogeneic class I antigens. The antigenic stimulus to the pTc plus the cytokines produced by the responding Th (for greater detail see Chapter 3) allow the cytotoxic cells to proliferate and acquire the killer phenotype. In addition to the response of these two cell populations, there is a T cell that can both secrete helper cytokines and develop killer potential, referred to as a dual function T cell, or a helper-independent cytotoxic T cell (HITc). Both class I and class II responsive cells can fall into this latter category. Adapted from Bach et al. (1976) and Rosenberg and Singer (1992).

T-killer cells arise specifically in response to cell bound foreign antigens. Because histocompatibility antigens are also cell-bound and so resemble viral antigens, histocompatibility antigens also stimulate the generation of T-killer cells. T cells can thus be grouped into two functional categories: T-helper cells and T-killer cells (Fig. 1).

PHENOTYPIC HETEROGENEITY AMONG T CELLS

Immunocompetent T cells can also be subdivided based upon their expression of the coreceptor molecules *CD4* and *CD8*. Approximately two-thirds of T cells in peripheral organs are CD4+ and approximately one-third are CD8+. Both CD4+ and CD8+ T cells derive from a common precursor cell in the thymus that expresses both CD4 and CD8 and so is a CD4+CD8+ thymocyte. Whether an individual CD4+CD8+ thymocyte differentiates into a mature CD4+ T cell or a mature CD8+ T cell depends upon the MHC molecules with which it interacts in the thymus. That is, interaction of CD4+CD8+ thymocytes with MHC class II molecules in the thymus induces them to become CD4+ T cells, whereas interaction with MHC class I molecules induces them to become CD8+ T cells. As a consequence, the phenotype that T cells express reveals the class of MHC molecule with which their T cell antigen receptors are likely to interact: CD4+ T cells have antigen receptors that primarily focus on MHC class II molecules and CD8+ T cells have antigen receptors that primarily focus on MHC class I molecules. This correlation between T cell phenotype and MHC class specificity is generally correct but, because of receptor cross reactions, is not always strictly correct. The major exception to the correlation between T cell phenotype and MHC class specificity is that a fraction of CD8+ T cells can react against MHC class II alloantigens.

RECEPTOR HETEROGENEITY AMONG T CELLS

All immunocompetent T cells express antigen receptors that focus on MHC molecules. This remarkable feature of their antigen receptors derives from the central role that interaction with MHC plays during the differentiation of mature T cells in the thymus. MHC molecules fall into two classes that vary importantly in their tissue distribution and in their function (see Chapter 1).

MHC class I molecules are present on nearly all cell types and function to present peptides of intracellular proteins. Thus, surface MHC class I molecules present peptide representations of the intracellular proteins that are present in the cells on which they are expressed.

In contrast, the cellular distribution of MHC class II molecules is far more restricted than that of MHC class I molecules. Unlike MHC class I molecules that are present on nearly all cell types, MHC class II molecules are present primarily on immunocompetent hematopoietic cells such as B cells, dendritic cells, and selective populations of epithelial cells such as those in the thymus. In addition, MHC class II molecules primarily present peptides of exogenous proteins that have been taken up by the cell, whereas MHC class I molecules present peptides of self-proteins contained within the cell.

Thus, T cells expressing receptors focused on MHC class I molecules will primarily encounter peptides of self-proteins, whereas T cells expressing receptors focused on MHC class II molecules will primarily encounter peptides of exogenous proteins.

RELATIONSHIP AMONG FUNCTION, PHENOTYPE, AND RECEPTOR SPECIFICITY IN MATURE T CELLS

Despite their marked heterogeneity, there are strong relationships regarding function, phenotype, and receptor specificities among T cells. Thus, most T-helper cells are CD4$^+$ recognizing MHC class II antigens, and most T-killer cells are CD8$^+$-interacting with MHC class I molecules. However, these relationships are only general ones with many exceptions that are relevant for *in vivo* rejection responses (see also discussion in Chapters 3 and 4). For example, T cells that secrete helper lymphokines are most frequently CD4$^+$ and focused on MHC class II molecules, but there are lymphokine-secreting T cells important in *in vivo* and *in vitro* responses that are CD8$^+$ and focused on MHC class I molecules. In a similar vein, most T-killer cells are CD8$^+$ and focused on MHC class I molecules, but there are also T-killer cells that are CD4$^+$ and focused on MHC class II molecules.

It is important to emphasize that for both *in vivo* rejection responses and for the *in vitro* models thereof, it is necessary to determine directly the function, phenotype, and receptor specificities of the T cells involved, and not to presume function or phenotype from receptor specificities. We review below *in vitro* and *in vivo* studies that analyze T cell responses to alloantigens encoded by the MHC, called HLA in humans and H-2 in mice.

IN VIVO REJECTION RESPONSES

The phenotypes of T cells that are involved in rejection of skin allografts (Rosenberg and Singer, 1992) across various histocompatibility differences have been determined by two different experimental protocols: a *cellular depletion* protocol and a *cellular reconstitution* protocol. The cellular depletion protocol depletes normal mice of either CD4$^+$ or CD8$^+$ T cells by *in vivo* injection of antibodies that are specific for either CD4 or CD8, followed by placement of a tissue allograft. Results are most clearcut in this experimental system when treated animals are also surgically thymectomized so that new T cells cannot arise to replace those that are depleted by the injected antibody. The cellular reconstitution protocol involves the adoptive transfer of isolated CD4$^+$ or CD8$^+$ T cells into T cell-deficient mice that have been engrafted with a tissue allograft. Importantly, both experimental procedures yield a consistent result: both CD4$^+$ T cells and CD8$^+$ T cells are capable of rejecting skin allografts, so that the ability to reject tissue allografts is not a function limited to one phenotypic subset of T cells.

Because most CD4$^+$ T cells function as T-helper cells, the ability of CD4$^+$ T cells to effect graft rejection was initially thought to indicate that T-helper lymphokine secretion was sufficient to mediate graft rejection. On the other hand, because most CD8$^+$ T cells function as T-killer cells, the ability of CD8$^+$ T cells function as T-killer cells, the ability of CD8$^+$ T cells to effect graft rejection was initially thought to indicate that T-killer cells were sufficient to mediate graft rejection.

However, the use of donor and host combinations across very defined antigen differences, such as combinations differing only by MHC class I or MHC class II antigens, revealed that isolated populations of CD4$^+$ and CD8$^+$ T cells could not reject the same skin allografts across the same antigenic differences. Skin allografts across an isolated MHC class I difference could be rejected by CD8$^+$ T cell populations, whereas skin allografts across an isolated MHC class II difference could be rejected by CD4$^+$ T cell populations. Skin allografts across minor histocompatibility differences were generally found to require both CD4$^+$ and CD8$^+$ T cells.

In vitro analyses of T cells present in the host that were reactive against the MHC or minor H antigens expressed by the tissue allograft revealed a striking finding: skin allografts were rejected only by T cell populations that contained BOTH lymphokine-secreting T-helper cells AND lymphokine-responsive T-killer cells that were reactive against graft antigens. T cell populations that contained only T-helper cells or only T-killer cells did not induce rejection of skin allografts. The clear implication of these findings is that *in vivo* rejection responses against skin allografts require *in vivo* activation of both T-helper cells and T-killer cells by antigens of the graft. *In vivo* experiments examining the functional T cell populations that are involved in skin allograft rejection are consistent with the concept that both lymphokine-secreting T-helper cells and lymphokine-responsive T-killer cells are necessary for rejection of skin allografts.

The evidence that T-killer cells are necessary to effect the rejection of skin allografts was first shown by Mintz and Silvers (1967). In their classic experiments, donor mice were experimentally constructed whose tissues consisted of a mixture of cells that were either genetically derived from parent 1 or parent 2 but not both; such mice were called "allophenic" or "tetraparental" mice. The skin tissues of such A ↔ B allophenic mice consisted of cells that were genetically either A or B but not both. Skin from such A ↔ B allophenic mice were grafted onto normal A mice, provoking a vigorous rejection response. However, the rejection response destroyed only a fraction of the allophenic skin graft, namely those cells in the graft that were genetically of allogeneic strain B origin; syngeneic strain A donor skin cells remained intact. These results demonstrated that the rejection response destroyed individual cells based on each cell's expression of foreign antigens, sparing cells that did not express foreign antigens. This degree of specificity, distinguishing individual cells within a single graft, is indicative of T-killer cells.

The evidence that T-helper cells are also necessary for *in vivo* rejection responses comes from experiments in which the presence of T-killer cells is insufficient to effect skin allograft rejection. For example, skin allografts across certain defined antigenic differences are not rejected and fail to activate T-helper cells. However, their rejection is effected by the addition of so-called "inducer" skin grafts that express third party antigens that activate T-helper cells. Thus, activation of T-helper cells, even against third party antigens, provides helper-lymphokines for activation of antigen-specific T-killer cells. Adoptive transfer experiments with isolated populations of CD4$^+$ and CD8$^+$ T cells provide additional evidence for a requirement for both T-helper and T-killer cells in *in vivo* rejection responses. In these experiments, the presence of CD8$^+$ T cells containing T-killer cells against minor H antigens, such as against the male antigen H-Y, is not sufficient to induce rejection; nor is the presence of CD4$^+$ T cells containing T-helper cells against H-Y sufficient to induce the rejection of male skin grafts. Rather, *in vivo* rejection of skin allografts across an H-Y antigenic difference requires the presence *in vivo* of both CD4$^+$ T-helper cells and CD8$^+$ T-killer cells.

The results of these *in vivo* experiments demonstrate that skin allograft rejection responses require activation of T-helper cell function and activation of T-killer cell function. These two T cell functions can be mediated by interacting cell populations, or, in certain circumstances, can be mediated by a single "dual-function" cell, a cell referred to as a helper T cell independent killer T cells, i.e., CD8$^+$ cytotoxic cells that produce their own help and thus do not require CD4$^+$ helper cells (Widmer and Bach, 1981). The interacting T-helper cells and T-killer cells do not need to be of the same phenotype and do not need to be reactive against the same foreign antigen, although their interactions are most efficient if both helper and killer antigens are expressed in the same tissue allograft. With regard to dual function T cells, the rejection of skin allografts by CD8$^+$ T cells across a class I MHC antigenic difference is the best example of dual function T cells effecting an *in vivo* rejection response. But it is important to appreciate that even for rejection responses mediated by a single population of dual function T cells, the rejection response required both T-helper function in the form of helper lymphokines and the generation of T-killer cell potential.

IN VITRO ASSAYS

In vitro assays of host T cell reactivity against antigens of the donor are convenient and in many instances relatively useful predictors of *in vivo* allograft rejection. These assays measure the presence of antigen-reactive T-helper cells and antigen-specific T-killer cells. However, several caveats, discussed below, must be kept in mind when interpreting the *in vitro* results.

Mixed lymphocyte culture (MLC) reactions, also referred to as MLR, were initially described (Bach and Hirschhorn, 1964; Bain et al., 1964) to measure the proliferation of host (responder) T cells in response to antigens expressed on leukocytes obtained from the donor. Later, it was recognized that one could generate host cytotoxic T lymphocytes against antigens of the donor (Hayry and Defendi, 1970; Solliday and Bach, 1970) in an MLC. The assay in which cytotoxic cells are generated is referred to as the *cell-mediated lympholysis (CML)* test. Host (responding) helper T cells reacted to class II antigens on the donor antigen-presenting cells, and host killer T cells responded to class I antigens.

In addition to constituting the majority of the proliferating cells in an MLC between two unrelated individuals, the CD4$^+$ T helper cells secreted cytokines that enabled the T-killer cells to undergo functional maturation to possessing killer activity, i.e., collaboration between CD4$^+$ Th and CD8$^+$ Tc (Bach et al., 1976).

The *in vitro* combined MLC and CML tests in some measure reflect similar responses of these cells *in vivo;* in fact, our appreciation of the relationship of CD4$^+$ Th responding to class II antigens and CD8$^+$ Tc to class I came from these *in vitro* studies. To which extent collaboration between the two subpopulations of cells, as occurs *in vitro,* contributes to rejection under various circumstances *in vivo* is not clearly established, although the involvement of both populations in some *in vivo* responses, as discussed above, is consistent with such a model. The degree of proliferation in the MLC is a convenient assay for predicting transplantation incompatibilities between hosts and donors (see Chapter 1).

An extension of, and improvement on, traditional MLC and CML assays is the ability directly to measure certain *in vitro* T cell functions that are thought to be important for *in vivo* rejection responses. That is, it is possible to isolate CD4$^+$ and CD8$^+$ T cells, and to assay the elaboration of helper lymphokines from T-helper cells reactive against donor antigens. The accuracy of such lymphokine secretion assays depends upon preventing the cultured cells from consuming the lymphokines that are produced during the assay, which can be accomplished by addition of blocking antibodies that are specific for lymphokine receptors. In addition, it is possible to isolate CD4$^+$ and CD8$^+$ T cells and to assess the generation of antigen-reactive T-killer cells under conditions in which helper lymphokines are not limiting by adding them exogenously into the CML cultures. These steps have the virtue of measuring directly and independently the presence in the host of donor-reactive T-helper cells and donor-reactive T-killer cells.

While these *in vitro* tests have proved useful for recognizing the association of class II alloantigen recognition by helper T cells, the recognition of class I antigens by cytotoxic T cells, and the collaboration between these two subsets *in vitro,* there are three limitations of any *in vitro* assay with respect to transplant rejection responses *in vivo*. The first is that *in vitro* assays measure host reactivity against antigens expressed on donor lymphoid cells, whereas *in vivo* rejection responses are directed against donor antigens expressed on cells of the grafted tissue. Consequently, *in vitro* reactions against donor lymphoid cells would not efficiently detect responses against antigens that are expressed primarily on cells of the grafted tissue. Indeed, since the density of antigens expressed on all cell types such as MHC class I antigens can vary from tissue to tissue, the intensity of *in vitro* reactions does not necessarily reflect the intensity of *in vivo* rejection responses. Second, in *in vitro* assays, cells are placed in close approximation with one another in a plastic well, efficiently promoting antigen transfer and cellular interactions that might not occur *in vivo*. Whereas the elaboration of small amounts of helper-lymphokines in a culture vessel might be efficient at generating T-killer cells, that amount of helper-lymphokine might be insufficient *in vivo*. Third, *in vitro* assays are performed over a relatively short time span (3–7 days), so that infrequent clones of T cells that would clonally expand *in vivo* in response to graft antigens fail to sufficiently expand *in vitro* during the assay. For example, it is very difficult to generate immune responses by lymphocytes from unprimed mice against minor H antigens, even though the same mice will efficiently mount *in vivo* rejection responses against skin grafts expressing the same minor H antigens. Similarly, unless the *in vitro* CML cultures are supplemented with exogenous helper lymphokines, it is difficult to detect the generation of T-killer cells against either MHC class II antigens or minor H antigens.

HETEROGENEITY OF REJECTION RESPONSES AGAINST DIFFERENT TISSUES

In vivo rejection responses against skin allografts are among the most potent and have been the most thoroughly studied. We have outlined the current concept that *in vivo* rejection responses against skin allografts require elicitation of both T-helper and T-killer cell functions. However, the phenotypes of the T-helper and

T-killer cells activated by a particular skin allograft depend upon the antigenic differences that the graft expresses.

While unifying principles are important and should not be modified lightly, it is also important to appreciate that not all *in vivo* rejection responses may require both T-helper and T-killer cell function. For example, certain tissues, such as endocrine tissues, appear to be sensitive to destruction by antigen-nonspecific inflammatory cells that can be attracted by lymphokines secreted by T-helper cells (Gill et al., 1989). Consequently, rejection responses against allografts consisting of endocrine tissue may require activation of only lymphokine-secreting T cells and may be independent of T-killer cell function.

SUMMARY

We have attempted to overview the *in vitro* and *in vivo* data on alloreactivity and rejection of allografts. The overall data are consistent with a requisite role for cytotoxic T cells in rejection of most types of grafts, with an additional amplification or other role (sometimes essential) for CD4[+] helper T cells.

REFERENCES

Bach FH, Hirschhorn K (1964): Lymphocyte interaction: A potential histocompatibility test in vitro. Science 143:813–814.

Bach FH, Bach ML, Sondel PM (1976): Differential function of major histocompatibility complex antigens in T lymphocyte activation. Nature (London) 259:273–281.

Bain B, Vas MR, Lowenstein L (1964): The development of large immature mononuclear cells in mixed leukocyte cultures. Blood 23:108–116.

Gill RG, Rosenberg AS, Lafferty KJ, Singer L (1989): Characterization of primary T cell subsets mediating rejection of pancreatic islet grafts. I Immunol 143:2176–2178.

Hayry P, Defendi (1970): Mixed lymphocyte cultures produce effector cells: Model in vitro for allograft rejection. Science 168:133–135.

Mintz B, Silvers WK, (1967): "Intrinsic" immunological tolerance in allophenic mice. Science 158:1484–1487.

Rosenberg AS, Singer A (1992): Cellular Basis of skin allograft rejection: An in vivo model of immune mediated tissue destruction. Annu Rev Immunol 10:333–358.

Solliday S, Bach FH, (1970): Cytotoxicity: Specificity after in vitro sensitization. Science 170:1406–1409.

Widmer MB, Bach FH (1981): Antigen driven helper cell-independent cloned cytolytic T lymphocytes. Nature (London) 294:750–752.

Chapter 6
Antibodies in Graft Rejection

Jeffrey L. Platt

INTRODUCTION

The reaction of recipient antibodies with a vascularized organ graft is associated with a spectrum of clinical and pathologic syndromes. Although a relationship between humoral immunity and graft rejection has been known for 65 years, the mechanisms linking humoral immunity to graft rejection are still incompletely understood. In some cases a humoral immune response against the donor organ has consequences so devastating that the presence of antidonor antibodies in the serum of a potential recipient is considered an absolute contraindication to transplantation. In other cases, antidonor antibodies appear to confer protection against cell-mediated rejection and indeed potential recipients are exposed to donor blood cells with the objective of generating such antibodies. This chapter will describe some of the clinical syndromes thought to be mediated by antidonor antibodies and explore the pathogenesis of antibody-mediated rejection. In this context current and future approaches to prevention and therapy will be discussed.

CLINICAL CONDITIONS ASSOCIATED WITH ANTIDONOR ANTIBODIES

Anti-Blood Group Antibodies

Incompatibility of blood serotypes has been considered a potential mechanism of allograft failure since the 1920s. While the basis of such incompatibility was not completely understood, the early literature on allograft acceptance makes frequent reference to the possible connection between the compatibility of blood and of organs. Although cellular immunity was clearly demonstrated to mediate allograft rejection, there existed an appreciation as early as the 1950s that early organ graft failure might be attributed in some cases to blood group incompatibility. During the early 1960s, when renal transplantation became an accepted therapy for uremia, it was widely believed that the donor and recipient should be of compatible blood types. However, as the broader clinical application of renal transplantation engendered a shortage of donor organs made worse by the absolute requirement for blood group compatibility, some investigators undertook transplants across blood group barriers. Analysis of these cases and of the occasional cases in which kidneys were inadvertently transplanted across blood group barriers provides insight into the risks associated with humoral barriers in allotransplantation.

The outcome of 24 renal transplants from donors of A or B blood group into recipients with isohemagglutinins against those antigens was analyzed by Gleason and Murray in 1967. Eleven of the transplants (45%) never functioned whereas only ~ 8% of a large number of ABO-compatible combinations failed to function.

The results of 12 kidney transplants in recipients who had isohemagglutinins against donor A and/or B antigens were reported by Wilbrandt et al. in 1969. Three of the kidneys never functioned and were thought to have been immediately rejected. Six kidneys were rejected within 3 months. Three kidneys were rejected 10 to 19 months after transplantation. The pathology of the 9 kidneys rejected within 3 months of

Transplantation Immunology, pages 113–129
© 1995 Wiley-Liss, Inc.

transplantation revealed "arterial thrombosis and parenchymal necrosis." Vascular lesions were also observed in two of the three organs that survived longer than 3 months. Based on an observation made several years before, that blood group antigens are expressed in blood vessel walls, the binding of recipient antibodies to donor blood vessels was considered a likely cause of graft injury. These results and earlier cases reported by Terasaki et al. (1965) thus underscored the risk involved in transplanting organs across humoral barriers, and suggested that the interaction of recipient antibodies with donor blood vessels might be responsible for rejection.

Subsequent studies showed that while cardiac allografts are also susceptible to hyperacute rejection, liver grafts are not. Furthermore, the risk of transplanting organs across blood group barriers is not absolute, as the transplantation of blood group A_2 kidneys into blood group O recipients does not entail a significantly increased risk of graft loss, perhaps because the A_2 antigen is less able to bind anti-A antibodies (Brynger et al., 1984).

The possibility of bridging the ABO barrier was suggested by the work of Alexandre et al. (1987) and Bannett et al. (1987). These investigators demonstrated that if isohemagglutinins were removed from the circulation of a patient, an ABO-incompatible kidney might be transplanted into that patient without a substantial risk of early graft failure. Studies by the author and colleagues demonstrated that after ABO-incompatible grafts were carried out in this way, the blood group antigens would continue to be expressed by endothelial cells in the donor organ and isohemagglutinins would return to the circulation of the recipient and yet rejection would not occur (Chopek et al., 1987). This phenomenon, in which temporary depletion of antidonor antibodies allows "permanent" engraftment of an incompatible organ, was later referred to as accommodation (Platt et al., 1990b).

Thus, early surveys illuminated several important facets of antibody-mediated rejection. First, the presence in a recipient of antidonor antibodies at the time of organ transplantation confers a very substantial risk of rejection. In approximately 25% of cases in ABO-incompatible

transplants, rejection is immediate or hyperacute; in approximately 50% of cases the cause of graft failure is accelerated cellular or acute vascular rejection and in up to 25% chronic vascular rejection will be observed. Second, the pathology of the rejecting organs—especially the prominent evidence of thrombosis—suggests that tissue injury results from the interaction of antidonor antibodies with graft blood vessels. Third, humoral rejection usually does not respond to immunosuppression. Fourth, humoral rejection can be avoided by temporary depletion of antidonor antibodies and perhaps other conditioning regimens. Why, given a relatively uniform combination of antibody and antigen, the tempo and manifestations of humoral rejection vary so greatly will be discussed in the sections on the pathogenesis and treatment of humoral rejection.

Anti-HLA Antibodies

At the same time that the risks of transplanting organs across humoral blood group barriers became known, another incompatibility was recognized. Kissmeyer-Nielson et al. (1966) described the hyperacute rejection of kidneys transplanted into recipients who were matched for ABO, but who had circulating antibodies against donor lymphocytes and kidney tissue. It was soon recognized that the target of the anti-lymphocyte antibodies was donor HLA (the reader is referred to Chapter 8 for further discussion).

Hyperacute rejection is observed in up to 80% of the kidneys transplanted into recipients with antidonor, lymphocytotoxic antibodies (Patel and Terasaki, 1969). Although the relative risk of hyperacute rejection depends on the "cross-match" assay used and, to a certain extent, on the titer of antibodies, a positive cross-match against donor lymphocytes—suggesting the presence of anti-HLA antibodies—is generally viewed as an absolute contraindication to transplantation.

If anti-HLA antibodies pose such a considerable risk, what happens to recipients who develop such antibodies after transplantation? The development of anti-HLA antibodies subsequent to transplantation has been associated with cellular rejection, acute vascular rejection, and chronic rejection. In one study, 40% of patients with acute rejection of kidney grafts could be shown to have antidonor antibodies detected by flow cytometry, whereas only 9% of patients without rejection were found to have such antibodies (Scornik et al., 1989). Another survey, focusing on anti-HLA antibodies, found such antibodies in the serum of 57% of patients with chronic rejection but in only 2–4% of patients with grafts surviving 4 or more years (Suciu-Foca et al., 1991).

Studies on serologic changes after transplantation such as those described here may help identify those patients at risk for rejection and point to a potential role of humoral immunity in various forms of rejection. However, several limitations must be considered. First, because the transplanted organ may absorb substantial amounts of antibody, the absence of antidonor antibody in the circulation does not exclude humoral graft injury. Second, the antibodies in the circulation of a recipient may not represent the antibodies bound to the graft. Third, because antibodies bound to endothelium may be taken up and processed, the absence of antibody in a pathological study cannot be interpreted as definitive evidence excluding humoral injury.

Other Antigens

While anti-ABO and anti-HLA antibodies have received the greatest attention, other humoral antigen systems have been described. Paul et al. (1979) described the hyperacute rejection of a kidney in a cross-match negative recipient. Antibodies in the rejecting organ were specific for donor endothelium and for donor monocytes but were not directed against ABO or HLA antigens. Brasile et al. (1986) reported that such antibodies could cause the accelerated rejection of a graft from a related HLA-identical donor. Some cases of humoral rejection may reflect incompatibility of antigens expressed on endothelium but not on circulating cells (Jordan et al., 1988). Until these antigen systems are more completely defined, it will be difficult to assess their importance as humoral barriers.

The development of antibodies against extracellular antigens may cause some devastating forms of tissue injury. Individuals with Alport syndrome, an hereditary disease associated with hearing loss and renal failure, lack a portion of the noncollagenous domain of basement membrane type IV collagen. After transplantation, some patients with the Alport syndrome develop antibodies against this antigen, which in turn causes rapid, unremitting decline in renal function. The "rejected" organ is found to contain recipient immunoglobulin and complement along glomerular basement membranes in a pattern resembling the classical appearance of the Goodpasture syndrome. In another rare clinical syndrome, the generation of antibodies against tubular basement membranes has been associated with severe acidosis due to functional abnormality of the overlying tubular epithelial cells. Although these humoral responses are observed only rarely, they illustrate the potential impact of the location and physiologic function of the target antigen in the humoral reaction to an allogeneic organ graft.

ANTIBODY-MEDIATED REJECTION OF ALLOGRAFTS

Hyperacute Rejection

Clinical features. The rejection of an organ graft within 24 hours of transplantation is referred to as "hyperacute rejection." The very rapid onset of the rejection reaction suggests that rejection is mediated by "natural" immunity or by immunity previously acquired by exposure to donor antigens. Although cases of "hyperacute" cellular rejection have been described, most cases of hyperacute rejection are mediated by humoral mechanisms, and, unless indicated, the use of the term hyperacute implies an humoral mechanism.

Clinical evidence of hyperacute rejection is often observed immediately upon reperfusion of the organ graft (Platt, 1994). The graft, perhaps initially taking on a normal color, rapidly develops a mottled or beefy red appearance and swells. In concert with changes in coloration, the blood flow to the transplanted organ declines dramatically and attempts to demonstrate blood flow radiographically may fail. The graft may have momentary function that declines over a period of minutes to hours, or the graft may never manifest function. In the case of renal grafts, the absence of graft function, which is more commonly caused by acute tubular necrosis and rarely by arterial thrombosis, may pose a diagnostic challenge. Cardiac grafts may be observed to beat more rapidly but weakly for a period of time and then to cease function entirely.

Hyperacute rejection is thought to occur in approximately 0.4% of renal allografts. Since the diagnosis of hyperacute rejection requires analysis of graft pathology and since biopsy samples are rarely obtained during the first days after transplantation, the incidence of hyperacute rejection is likely underestimated. Consistent with this view was an analysis by Iwaki and Terasaki (1987) of "primary renal graft nonfunction." Deducting the rate of technical graft failures from the rate of primary nonfunction, it was concluded that up to 6% of first grafts and

12% of second grafts undergo hyperacute rejection.

Pathology. The histopathology of hyperacute rejection varies more with the time course of rejection than with the type of organ undergoing rejection (Platt, 1994). Hyperacute rejection of the kidney or heart is usually characterized by the early appearance of platelet aggregates followed by interstitial hemorrhage, edema, and later by formation of fibrin thrombi (Fig. 1). In some cases, but not all, neutrophils are found to be attached to the lumenal aspect of graft endothelium and to be infiltrating the interstitium.

Ultrastructural study of tissues from organs undergoing hyperacute rejection reveals a collapsing of small blood vessels leading to the trapping of erythrocytes, aggregation and degranulation of platelets, and adherence of platelets to endothelial walls (Fig. 2). A distortion of endothelium, particularly in the vicinity of tight junctions, creates channels connecting the lumen with the extravascular spaces. Endothelial cell injury is suggested by such findings as cell membrane blebs, aberrant contour of endothelial cell

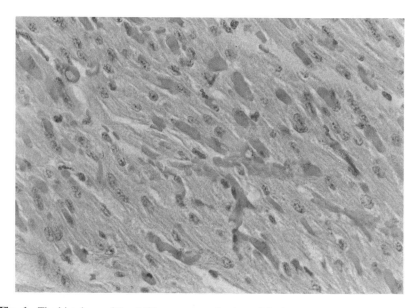

Fig. 1. The histology of "early" hyperacute rejection of the heart. Diffuse microvascular thrombosis is evident $1/2$ hr after reperfusion of a pig to nonhuman primate xenograft. Immunopathology revealed antibody and complement along endothelial cells and numerous platelet thrombin (not shown).

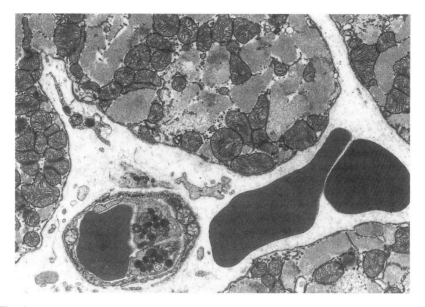

Fig. 2. Early lesion of hyperacute rejection evaluated by transmission electron microscopy. Increased interstitial fluid and hemorrhage are seen. A capillary is collapsed around an erythrocyte. The capillary contains an aggregate of 2 platelets that have not yet undergone degranulation.

surfaces, and separation of endothelium from underlying matrix and from pericytes; however, the lysis or loss of endothelium is not usually a prominent early feature.

Immunopathologic analysis reveals deposits of immunoglobulin and complement along the micro- and macrovasculature (Platt et al., 1991a). A loss of vascular integrity leading to the egress of plasma proteins including IgG from the blood vessels in the graft gives rise to diffuse extravascular reactivity for IgG. Early in the course of hyperacute rejection, fibrin is seen to be deposited along the lumenal aspect of small blood vessels. Subsequently, fibrin plugs are found to occlude blood vessels.

Immunologic mechanisms. It is widely believed that hyperacute rejection is initiated by the binding of antidonor antibodies to graft blood vessels. Antibody binding triggers activation of the complement cascade, which in turn mediates tissue injury. While there is no reason to question these long held views, instances in which lesions that resemble hyperacute rejection are encountered in the absence of apparent immune reaction and instances in which antidonor antibodies in a graft recipient fails to generate hyperacute rejection suggest that other factors may have an impact on the initiation and outcome of the rejection process.

Antidonor antibodies. The involvement of antibody in initiating the hyperacute rejection is suggested by the association between circulating antidonor antibodies and the susceptibility to hyperacute rejection, the prominent evidence of immunoglobulin and complement in rejecting tissues, and from the observation in clinical and experimental systems that depletion of antidonor antibodies may prevent hyperacute rejection. Immediate onset of hyperacute rejection precludes the eliciting of an immune response; thus, the rejection reaction must be mediated by "natural" immunity or by a secondary immune response.

"Natural" antibodies mediate rejection in ABO-incompatible allografts and xenogenetic grafts (Platt, 1994). Such natural antibodies always include donor-reactive IgM and may or may not include donor-reactive IgG.

Most cases of hyperacute rejection occur in recipients previously sensitized to donor HLA antigens. The isotype of Ig involved in these cases is usually thought to be IgG; however, IgM antibodies have been shown to mediate some cases of rejection of clinical and experimental allografts.

The events most commonly associated with sensitization are blood transfusion, prior allotransplantation, and pregnancy. Although prior exposure to donor HLA antigens increases the risk of hyperacute rejection, "third party" stimulation may also lead to the synthesis of antidonor antibodies capable of mediating hyperacute rejection.

Recent findings in xenogeneic systems suggest that the antigens recognized by natural antibodies are not merely passive targets, but may deliver signals to the target endothelial cell (Platt and Holzknecht, 1994). While it is unlikely that binding of antibodies to HLA antigens would have such a physiologic impact, there exists the possibility that anti-ABO or anti-endothelial cell-monocyte antibodies could perturb endothelial cell functions. Variation in the plasma levels of antidonor antibodies in the cir-

culation of the recipient (Wilbrandt et al., 1969), in the level of antigen expression (Wrenshall et al., 1991), and in the physiologic condition of the organ in which the antibody–antigen reaction occurs may also influence whether hyperacute rejection occurs.

Complement. An essential step in the pathogenesis of hyperacute rejection is the activation of complement. [The reader is referred to a paper by Frank (1994) for a comprehensive review of the activation and control of the complement system and to a diagrammatic summary in Fig. 3.]

Two lines of evidence demonstrate the importance of complement in hyperacute rejection. Complement components become depleted from the blood and accumulate rapidly in grafts undergoing hyperacute rejection. Inactivation of complement by agents such as soluble complement receptor type 1 (sCR1 serves as a cofactor for factor I-mediated cleave of C3 and C4 and dissociates C3 convertases) or depletion of complement with agents such as cobra venom factor (cobra venom factor activates the alternative pathway C3 convertase and causes consumption

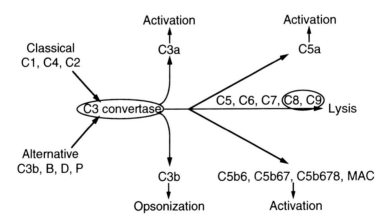

Fig. 3. The pathways of complement activation. Complement is activated by the classical pathway through fixation of C1q or the alternative pathway involving the spontaneous formation of C3b. C3 convertase formed by these pathways is the enzyme complex that drives subsequent reactions leading to formation of (1) the membrane attack complex, (2) the

anaphylotoxins C3a and C5a, and (3) biologically active oligomers such as C5b67, C5b678, and the membrane attack complex. C3bi, the major opsonin of the complement system, is formed by cleavage of C3b. Control of complement activation focuses on C3 convertase and C8/C9.

of complement complements) prevents hyper-acute rejection.

Much has been learned in recent years about how complement might become activated in a graft and, once activated, how complement contributes to graft injury. In most cases, complement is activated through the classical pathway, antibody causing the fixation of C1q, which triggers activation of the complement cascade through the classical pathway C3 convertase (Fig. 3), IgM and IgA may also trigger the alternative pathway of complement as discussed below and in a recent review (Platt and Bach, 1991).

Although most cases of hyperacute allograft rejection are initiated by recipient antibodies, there is clinical and experimental evidence that some cases may be caused by the direct activation of complement on the surface of disparate cells (Leventhal et al., 1993). This mechanism triggers a particularly rapid (10–20 min) hyperacute rejection reaction in guinea pig-to-rat xenografts. The activation of complement on xenogeneic cell surfaces independent of antibody binding is generally attributed to the alternative complement pathway (Miyagawa et al., 1988).

The alternative pathway C3 convertase is an enzyme complex the formation of which is initiated by the cleavage of C3 to yield C3b. C3b combines with serum factor B to form C3b–factor B complexes. Factor B in such complexes is cleaved by serum factor D to yield factor Bb, which in association with C3b (C3bBb) comprises the alternative pathway C3 convertase, which is stabilized by properdin (factor P). C3 convertase cleaves C3 to yield C3b, which in turn is recruited to form additional C3 convertase or which is further degraded to yield iC3b, the major opsonin of the complement system.

The alternative pathway of complement is continuously activated by the spontaneous generation of biochemically active C3b fragments. This allows the complement system to remain poised to deposit C3b on the surface of invasive organisms. Complement alternative pathway C3 activity is regulated by plasma glycoproteins that inhibit C3 activation on homologous cells. Of particular importance are the plasma factor H

and factor I. Factor H inhibits the association of C3b with factor B; factor I, in the presence of a suitable cofactor, cleaves C3b to yield iC3b and iC3b to yield the biologically inert C3d. Activation of complement in this setting probably reflects the failure of the plasma complement regulatory proteins (Horstmann et al., 1985). Complement activation might also occur through the classical pathway by the direct attachment of C1q to the graft (Cooper, 1985).

How could the alternative pathway of complement initiate graft injury independent of antibody binding to the graft? Activation of complement in the fluid phase (i.e., in the plasma) promotes the generation of alternative pathway C3 convertase on the cell surface. One stimulus for fluid phase activation of complement might be infectious microorganisms in the blood. Perhaps a more common stimulus is extracorporeal circulation of blood. Injury of an organ during harvesting and reperfusion also activates the alternative pathway of complement and may activate cell-associated proteases or phospholipases, which would cause release from the endothelium of complement regulatory proteins such as decay accelerating factor, membrane cofactor protein, or CD59. While complement activation through these mechanisms has not been demonstrated to be a singular cause of hyperacute rejection, neither has it been excluded. Given the frequent use of extracorporeal circuits, the augmentation of complement activity should be considered a potential cause of initial nonfunction of organs.

Other factors mediating "hyperacute rejection." Although hyperacute rejection is generally viewed as a manifestation of humoral immunity, other mechanisms of tissue injury may cause immediate loss of graft function. Prior to the development of currently used methods for organ preservation, a number of investigators reported that prolonged perfusion of organs between the time of harvesting and the time of transplantation might cause lesions pathologically similar to hyperacute rejection (Spector et al., 1976; Cerra et al., 1977). In some cases these lesions were attributed to high perfusion pressures and in others to the presence of antibodies in the preservation solution. Other reports described hyperacute rejection in the apparent absence of antidonor antibody and complement (Starzl et al., 1968). It is possible that the failure to identify the underlying immune mechanism reflected the limitations of the methods available at that time; however, that some cases of primary graft nonfunction might reflect organ injury through nonimmunologic mechanisms cannot be excluded.

Occasionally the onset of cellular rejection in a presensitized recipient is so rapid that authors have referred to accelerated cellular rejection as hyperacute cellular rejection. In some systems, particularly bone marrow allografts, the interaction of recipient natural killer cells with a graft is associated with immediate nonfunction of the graft. A similar phenomenon, mediated by T cells and macrophages, may impair the function of transplanted allogeneic islets (Kaufman et al., 1990).

The Pathogenesis of Tissue Injury in Hyperacute Rejection

What events might link the binding of antibody to the graft and activation of complement with the very rapid progression of tissue injury and loss of graft function that is observed in hyperacute rejection? The pathologic findings of hemorrhage, edema, and thrombosis in hyperacute rejection suggest that the pathogenesis involves the dysfunction of small blood vessels. We have postulated that these pathologic changes result from injury to endothelial cells, leading to loss of the barrier and anticoagulant properties of endothelium (Platt et al., 1990b).

The humoral rejection of an organ graft may begin during the harvesting and preservation of the organ. Already mentioned are observations suggesting that pathologic changes similar to those of hyperacute rejection may be seen in organs with severe preservation injury; tissue injury in these cases may be caused by toxic oxygen species such as superoxide anion and direct injury to endothelium. As a potential mechanism, we recently demonstrated that oxidant stress increases the susceptibility of endothelial cells to

the cytotoxic effects of antibody and complement (Magee et al., 1994).

The next step in the development of tissue lesions involves the activation of complement. Complement activation leading to formation of the membrane attack may cause the lysis of donor endothelium leading to thrombosis and interstitial hemorrhage, the pathological hallmarks of hyperacute rejection. However, in many cases endothelial cell lysis is not observed; thus, it is likely that complement activation, perhaps with the pathophysiologic consequences of antibody binding, causes a change in the functioning of endothelium that allows the rejection process to proceed in a rapid and inexorable course. Complement activation also generates anaphylotoxins such as C5a, which may activate neutrophils and thus contribute to oxidant-mediated injury.

One noncytotoxic effect of complement that may contribute to the rejection process is a rapid change in the shape of endothelial cells. Saadi and Platt (1995) have shown that exposure of cultured endothelial cells to antiendothelial cell antibodies and complement leads to the rapid development of transient gaps in the monolayer. Such gaps might also create pores through which blood cells and plasma proteins could exit and provide a nidus for the adhesion of platelets. The gaps are not related to cytotoxic changes and appear to be associated with changes in cyclic nucleotide levels in the affected cells.

Another mechanism that might contribute to the pathogenesis of hyperacute rejection involves the metabolism of heparan sulfate proteoglycan. Heparan sulfate proteoglycan promotes the functional and structural integrity of blood vessels by inhibiting the passage of blood cells and plasma proteins through blood vessel walls, by cementing endothelial cells to the extracellular matrix, and by mediating the activation and attachment of antithrombin III, a major anticoagulant, to endothelial surfaces (Marcum et al., 1987; Ihrcke et al., 1993). Thus a loss of heparan sulfate proteoglycan from the microvascular endothelium might contribute significantly to the pathological features of hyperacute rejection (Platt et al., 1990c).

Testing that hypothesis, we found that exposure of porcine aortic endothelial cell monolayers to human serum results in the rapid cleavage and loss from the cells of up to 50% of cell-associated heparan sulfate (Platt et al., 1990c). The loss of heparan sulfate depends on the binding to the endothelial cells of naturally occurring anti-pig antibodies and on the activation of complement (Platt et al., 1991b). Recent *in vivo* experiments have demonstrated that endothelial cell heparan sulfate is lost within 5 min of establishing circulation through a cardiac xenograft and that measures that limit the loss of heparan sulfate prolong graft survival (Stevens et al., 1993).

Early reports on clinical cases of hyperacute rejection stressed the potential importance of neutrophils in mediating tissue injury. Neutrophils, activated by complement anaphylotoxins, might interact with platelet activating factor and/or attach to C3bi formed on endothelial cell surfaces, causing significant tissue injury. Arguing against this idea are experimental studies demonstrating that neutrophil depletion does not extended the survival of allografts in presensitized, experimental animals (Forbes et al., 1976). However, while the experimental models show that neutrophils are not be essential in all circumstances, they do not exclude the importance of this mechanism of graft injury in the clinical setting in which humoral injury is superimposed on preservation/reperfusion injury.

Other factors that contribute to the rejection process clearly include the aggregation of platelets and the formation of fibrin thrombi. Platelet aggregation is one of the earliest pathologic events in hyperacute rejection. Platelet aggregation may be stimulated by inflammatory mediators such as platelet-activating factor released from injured endothelium, thrombin generated by endothelial cell injury, or collagen or other extracellular matrix components exposed by the retraction endothelial cells. The activated platelets stimulate thrombin generation, providing a nidus for the formation of fibrin thrombi. Because the stimuli for platelet aggregation and thrombosis are multifaceted, the use of agents that inhibit a single pathway such as platelet-

activating factor antagonists yields only modest improvement in the survival of organ grafts in presensitized recipients (Makowka et al., 1990).

Acute Vascular Rejection

Acute vascular rejection occurs days to months after transplantation of a vascularized organ. The clinical picture at onset is very similar to that of cellular rejection; however, unlike cellular rejection, acute vascular rejection responds very poorly or not at all to immunosuppressive therapy.

Acute vascular rejection is characterized by prominent changes in the pathology of capillaries and arterioles (Fig. 4). The immunopathology of acute vascular rejection varies with the clinical setting. Deposits of antibody and complement along endothelial cell surfaces in some cases of acute vascular rejection, closely resembling the picture of hyperacute rejection, suggest the pathogenesis may be related to that of hyperacute rejection (Platt et al., 1991a). However, the prominent swelling of endothelial cells, extensive infiltration of blood vessel walls by neutrophils and mononuclear cells, and extensive deposition of fibrin in vascular plugs and extravascular spaces seen in acute vascular rejection differ from the characteristic lesions of hyperacute rejection. In some cases, a prominent infiltration of mononuclear cells below the endothelium, called endothelialitis, suggests that cell-mediated immunity may have a pathogenic role in acute vascular rejection.

Immunologic mechanisms. The potential mechanisms contributing to the development of acute vascular rejection are shown in Figure 5. Lesions pathologically similar to those observed in acute vascular rejection may be caused by such nonimmunologic processes as "hyperperfusion" or nutritional changes; however, acute vascular rejection is very likely mediated by immune mechanisms since it is not seen in experimental or clinical isografts. The infiltration of T cells into some blood vessel walls observed in acute vascular rejection has led some to postulate that that form of rejection results from cellular immunity. However, the observation that acute

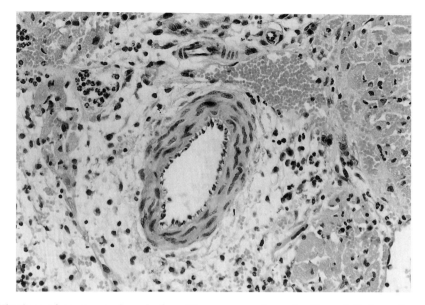

Fig. 4. Histology of acute vascular rejection. The histology of severe acute vascular rejection lesion is characterized by interstitial hemorrhage and edema and prominent infiltrate consisting of neutrophils and mononuclear cells. The endothelium of an arteriole is damaged; a few neutrophils can be seen adherent to and infiltrating the vessel wall.

vascular rejection frequently resists even the most aggressive immunosuppressive regimens raises the possibility that other mechanisms, particularly humoral immune mechanisms, play a critical role. Consistent with that view is the observation that some cases of acute vascular rejection are associated with the deposition of antiendothelial cell antibodies and complement along the walls of affected blood vessels.

Pathogenesis of acute vascular rejection.
Very little is known about the pathogenesis of acute vascular rejection. The pathology of acute

vascular rejection may include prominent evidence of thrombosis and interstitial hemorrhage, features characteristic of hyperacute rejection. These finding raise the possibility that acute vascular rejection, like hyperacute rejection, might be mediated by the binding of antibodies to endothelium and the activation of complement. One argument against this idea is that acute vascular rejection is commonly seen in experimental settings in which hyperacute rejection is inhibited by the depletion of complement (Leventhal et al., 1993). On the other hand, the prolonged period between the implantation of

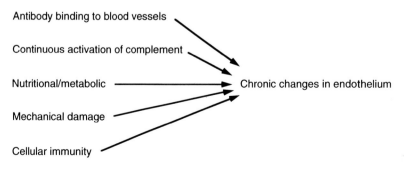

Fig. 5. Pathogenesis of acute vascular rejection.

the graft and the development of acute vascular rejection provides time for metabolic changes precluded by the time course of hyperacute rejection. With this difference in mind we hypothesized that acute vascular rejection might be the consequence of activation of endothelial cells in a vascularized graft (Leventhal et al., 1993). Stimulated by antidonor antibodies, cytokines, oxidants, etc., endothelial cells in an affected organ may undergo functional changes resulting in loss of barrier properties stimulation of coagulation and enhanced adhesiveness for platelets and neutrophils and mononuclear cells (Nawroth and Stern, 1986; Brett et al., 1989). The conversion of endothelium from being anticoagulant to procoagulant results in part from the loss of anticoagulant molecules such as thrombomodulin, and in part from the elaboration of molecules such as tissue factor, which serves as a cofactor for factor VIIa and plasminogen activator inhibitor, which retards thrombolysis (Schleef et al., 1988). Activated endothelial cells also express adhesion receptors such as E-selectin and P-selectin for circulating mononuclear leukocytes and neutrophils (Pober and Cotran, 1990). Although endothelial cell activation may occur in acute vascular rejection, whether that process is essential to the pathogenesis of acute vascular rejection is not yet known.

Accelerated Cellular Rejection

The presence of antidonor antibodies in the circulation of the recipient does not necessarily lead to hyperacute rejection or to definite pathologic evidence of acute vascular rejection. What may occur instead is an accelerated cellular rejection. This form of cellular rejection is especially resistant to immunosuppressive therapy. The mechanisms by which antibody reactivity with graft endothelium or with other cells might hasten or amplify cellular responses are not well defined. The target antigen is probably unimportant because accelerated cellular rejection is observed in HLA- and ABO-incompatible allografts as well as in some xenogeneic organ grafts.

Some investigators have suggested that the presence of antidonor antibody on donor cells promotes antibody-dependent cell-mediated cytotoxicity. While this mechanism may contribute to accelerated rejection of organ grafts in individuals with IgG antidonor antibodies, it does not account for such responses in recipients with IgM antidonor antibodies.

Another potential mechanism by which humoral immunity might accelerate and/or amplify a cellular immune response may involve inflammatory mediators. The potential impact of this mechanism is suggested by the amplification of delayed-type hypersensitivity observed when antigen is introduced together with an irritant. C5a generated by activation of the complement cascade and heparan sulfate released from graft endothelium may activate macrophages or other antigen-presenting cells in the graft leading to an augmentation of T cell responses (Ihrcke et al., 1993; Wrenshall et al., 1994). These antigen-presenting cells or endothelial cells shed into the circulation as a consequence of the humoral reaction may be carried to local lymph nodes, hastening the sensitization of the recipient.

Accommodation

In some cases the temporary depletion of antidonor antibodies from the circulation of a graft recipient and perhaps other manipulations allows the prolonged survival of a vascularized graft even after the antibodies return to the circulation and the complement system is restored. We have called this condition "accommodation" (Platt et al., 1990b). Accommodation was first observed in the transplantation of ABO-incompatible kidney allografts (Chopek et al., 1987; Alexandre et al., 1987). The temporary depletion of anti-A or anti-B antibodies from a recipient allowed engraftment of kidneys bearing A or B blood group antigens, and in many instances, vascular rejection did not occur after isohemagglutinins returned to the circulation. Accommodation has been observed in some presensitized recipients of allografts from whom antidonor antibodies were depleted using protein A columns (Palmer et al., 1989). The mechanism underlying accommodation is not known; it may involve a change in antibodies directed against the donor organs, a change in antigen expression, or a change in the graft allowing it to withstand humoral injury. Certainly the recovery from preservation-reperfusion injury would enhance the resistance to injury. The mechanism responsible for accommodation is an issue of importance in allotransplantation and potentially in the clinical application of xenotransplantation. If accommodation can be achieved, then continuous immunodepletion or other manipulations of a recipient might be avoided.

Enhancement. In some experimental systems, particularly in rodents, the development of antibodies directed against the donor does not stimulate rejection, but rather inhibits the development of a cellular immune response. The inhibition of cellular responses by antidonor antibodies is called enhancement. The reader is referred to chapters on tolerance for discussion of this phenomenon.

Assay of Antidonor Antibodies

A critical consideration in the study of antibody-mediated rejection is the method used for measuring antidonor antibodies. Antibodies directed against donor HLA antigens are most commonly detected by a lymphocytotoxicity "cross-match." In this assay, described more fully elsewhere in the text, recipient serum is diluted serially and combined with donor lymphocytes or with lymphocytes from a standard series of subjects. Complement is added and lysis of the lymphocytes ascertained. The presence of lymphocytotoxicity is associated with an increased risk of hyperacute rejection or accelerated cellular rejection. Consequently, the presence of such antibodies in recipient serum is considered a contraindication to transplantation. Individuals with the highest titers of antidonor antibodies appear to be at the highest risk for hyperacute rejection; however, many cases can be found in which recipients with high antibody titers do not hyperacutely reject an organ graft and recipients with very low titers do. Thus, factors other than antibody titer must be important in determining graft outcome. Some investigators have used assays that measure binding of antibodies to cultured endothelial cells (Platt et al., 1990a). These assays are appealing from a conceptual perspective since endothelial cells are the target of the humoral response; however,

obtaining suitable endothelial cells from prospective donors limits applicability of this method. Some have proposed the use of tissue sections that might be obtained from donor skin biopsy as a target for the measurement of antidonor endothelial cell antibodies. This method is simple and rapid; however, it cannot distinguish the binding of antibodies to antigens on the external surface of endothelial cells from binding to cytoplasmic antigens or antigens located along the inner face of the cell membrane. With further understanding of humoral alloantigen barriers, it may be possible to use purified antigens to evaluate recipient sera.

PREVENTION AND TREATMENT OF ANTIBODY-MEDIATED REJECTION

Various approaches have been used to prolong the survival of organs transplanted across a humoral immune barrier. These approaches were recently reviewed (Magee and Platt, 1994).

Splenectomy

Although, by itself, it has no impact on the outcome of grafts transplanted across humoral barriers, splenectomy is commonly performed prior to the transplantation of organs across an humoral barrier (Alexandre et al., 1987, 1989). The basis for performing the procedure is largely anecdotal. One rationale is that splenectomy significantly decreases the total number of B cells capable of synthesizing antibody as part of a secondary response. Thus, splenectomy and the administration of cytotoxic agents constitute a reasonable approach to limiting antibody production in presensitized patients. To the extent that splenectomy inhibits cellular immune responses, it may also help inhibit primary humoral responses.

Nonspecific Depletion of Antidonor Antibodies by Plasma Exchange or Plasmapheresis

Plasma exchange or plasmapheresis is the prototypic method for the nonspecific depletion of antibody from the circulation (Bach et al., 1991). Plasmapheresis has been used extensively to treat such conditions as myasthenia gravis, thrombotic thrombocytopenic purpura, and Waldenstrom's macroglobinemia. Plasma exchange has been used to remove isohemagglutinins, allowing transplantation of ABO-incompatible renal grafts (Chopek et al., 1987).

One major issue in the use of plasma exchange is the selection of the plasma replacement solution. Because all circulating proteins are removed, the recipient may be susceptible to the development of a dilutional coagulopathy, or infectious complications. Also, potentially beneficial molecules such as antithrombin III are depleted. The depletion of immunoglobulin by plasmapheresis may promote a "rebound effect" (Terman et al., 1978).

Plasmapheresis could be made semiselective by filtration of the plasma through a membrane to remove large proteins such as IgM or by extracorporeal immunoabsorption of Ig followed by reinfusion of the residual plasma components. Plasmapheresis has been combined with affinity absorption of IgG using staphylococcus protein A columns. Palmer and co-workers (1989) used such columns to remove anti-HLA antibodies in highly sensitized patients with renal failure followed by successful renal transplantation. Both total IgG levels and anti-HLA titers were effectively lowered.

Specific Depletion of Antidonor Antibodies

To avoid the shortcomings associated with the nonspecific depletion of immunoglobulins, more specific strategies are being developed (Platt, 1995). Immunoadsorption using synthetic carbohydrate antigens immobilized on solid phase columns has been successfully applied in ABO-incompatible living related renal transplantation (Bannett et al., 1987).

Blocking of Antidonor Antibodies by Administration of Soluble Antigen

Administration of soluble antigen has been used in experimental and clinical studies aimed at blocking the interaction between antidonor antibodies and a vascularized organ graft. Perper and Najarian first attempted this approach in 1966 when they administered saline extracts of porcine kidney homogenate to a dog prior to porcine renal xenotransplantation. Anti-pig erythro-cyte antibody titers decreased 4-fold following injection of the homogenate, but no increase in graft survival was noted. Linn and co-workers (1968) injected soluble antigen derived from pig erythrocyte stroma prior to xenografting pig kidneys into dogs. Anti-pig erythrocyte antibody titers decreased by 90% and xenograft survival was extended 10- to 20-fold beyond the survival of the controls.

Various studies on transplantation of organs across ABO barriers have used administration of soluble antigen as one part of an overall strategy. Using plasma as a source of soluble blood group antigen, investigators at several centers have infused type-specific plasma after antibody depletion as a way of inhibiting the reaction of isohemagglutinins with a graft. Synthetic blood group A antigen has been used clinically to treat hemolytic disease of the newborn due to ABO incompatibility. Cooper and co-workers (1992) have used intravenously administered synthetic A and B trisaccharides to perform heterotopic cardiac transplantation across the ABO barrier in presensitized baboons. In two animals treated with high dose immunosuppression and continuous trisaccharide administration for 8 and 13 days, graft survival was 17 days and greater than 30 days, respectively.

While administration of soluble antigen is an appealing technique, it may be complicated by immune complex formation, anaphylaxis, and the potential for an acceleration of an elicited humoral or cellular response against the graft. For example, the dog in study by Perper and Najarian (1966) developed circulatory shock requiring catacholamine support. Additionally, high concentrations of soluble antigen would be needed to block all potential antigen-binding sites on the IgM molecule. One other disadvantage of this approach is that low-molecular-weight antigens would be subject to rapid clearance by the kidneys and require continuous intravenous infusion (Cooper et al., 1992).

Immunosuppression

Immunosuppression regimens including combinations of cytotoxic agents have been used successfully to inhibit elicited responses to protein antigens. These regimens have not been applied in transplantation but might be considered for use in conjunction with antibody depletion.

Work in several experimental models suggests that immunosuppression might be used to inhibit humoral responses. Terman et al. (1978) suggested that administration of immunosuppressive therapy attenuates the return of circulating immunoglobulins after immunoabsorbtion. The combination of FK 506 and 15-deoxyspergualin was recently shown to significantly increase the survival of hamster-to-rat cardiac xenograft, the rejection of which is thought to be mediated in part by a humoral response (Carobbi et al., 1992). Strategies aimed at depleting B cells using monoclonal antibodies and immunotoxins have met with limited success in clinical trials and experimental models; however, use in clinical transplant recipients has not been evaluated.

Humoral Tolerance

Various strategies might be used to induce humoral tolerance. The reader is referred to chapters on tolerance for detailed consideration of this topic. Administration of antigen plus cytotoxic drugs has shown promise in experimental models and, to a limited extent, in the clinic. Lenschow et al. (1992) recently showed that administration of a CTLA-4 Ig fusion protein with the aim of inhibiting the binding of CD28 to B7 allowed the prolonged inhibition of the humoral response to xenogeneic tissue and significantly extended the survival of xenogeneic islet tissue. Promising results have been achieved by Sykes, who combined sublethal irradiation, administration of monoclonal antibodies directed against recipient T cells and NK cells, and administration of donor bone marrow (Aksentijevich et al., 1992).

Inhibition of Complement Activation

Agents that inhibit complement activation prevent hyperacute rejection. Cobra venom factor, which causes consumption of complement by activating the alternative pathway, has been used most extensively for this purpose (Gewurz et al., 1967).

Although purified cobra venom factor is well tolerated by primates, its use might be limited by an elicited humoral response to the foreign protein. Another complement inhibitory protein is soluble complement receptor type 1 (sCR1). Soluble CR1 is a recombinant protein that functions as a cofactor for factor I-mediated cleavage of C3 and C4, and that causes dissociation of C3 convertase complexes leading to inhibition of the classical and alternative pathways (Weisman et al., 1990). Soluble CR1 was used by Pruitt et al. (1994) to prevent hyperacute rejection in rodents and in a pig-to-primate xenograft model.

While inhibition of complement activation effectively prolongs xenograft survival, there is concern that recipients may be susceptible to overwhelming infection. Given the pivotal role of the classical pathway in hyperacute rejection, but its lesser role in host defense, more specific therapies might be directed at the classical pathway leaving the alternative pathway intact to defend the recipient against infectious agents. For example, the function of the classical pathway C1qrs complex is inhibited by C1 inh. Dalmasso and Platt (1994) recently showed that C1 inh abrogates porcine endothelial cell activation in response to human natural antibody and complement and proposed use of C1 inh in xenotransplantation.

Other complement activation products appear to be capable of causing endothelial cell dysfunction (Stevens and Platt, 1992), and could likewise be targeted therapeutically. For example, to the extent that neutrophils participate in xenograft rejection, antibodies directed against C5 or C3bi block neutrophil involvement and minimize subsequent tissue injury.

ACKNOWLEDGMENTS

Supported by NIH Grants HL46810, HL50985, DK38108, and HL52297.

REFERENCES

Aksentijevich I, Sachs DH, Sykes M (1992): Humoral tolerance in xenogeneic BMT recipients conditioned by a nonmyeloablative regimen. Transplantation 53:1108–1114.

Alexandre GPJ, Squifflet JP, De Bruyere M, et al. (1987): Present experiences in a series of 26 ABO-incompatible living donor renal allografts. Transplant Proc 19:4538–4542.

Alexandre GPJ, Gianello P, Latinne D, Carlier M, Dewaele A, Van Obbergh L, Moriau M, Marbaix E, Lambotte JL, Lambotte L and Squifflet JP (1989): Plasmapheresis and splenectomy in experimental renal xenotransplantation. In: Hardy MA (eds): "Xenograft 25." New York: Elsevier Science Publishers, pp 259–266.

Bach FH, Platt J, Cooper DKC (1991): Accomodation: The role of natural antibody and complement in discordant xenograft rejection. In: Cooper DKC, Kemp E, Reemtsma K, White DJG (eds): "Xenotransplantation. The transplantation of Organs and Tissues between Species" New York: Springer-Verlag, pp 81–99

Bannett AD, McAlack RF, Raja R, Baquero A, Morris M (1987): Experiences with known ABO-mismatched renal transplants. Transplant Proc 19:4543–4546.

Brasile L, Rodman E, Shield III, CF Clarke J, Cerilli J (1986): The association of antivascular endothelial cell antibody with hyperacute rejection: A case report. Surgery 99:637–640.

Brett J, Gerlach H, Nawroth P, Steinberg S, Godman G and Stern D (1989): Tumor necrosis factor/cachectin increases permeability of endothelial cell monolayers by a mechanism involving regulatory G proteins. J Exp Med 169:1977–1991.

Brynger H, Rydberg L, Samuelsson BE, Sandberg L (1984): Experience with 14 renal transplants with kidneys from blood group A (subgroup A_2) to O recipients. Transplant Proc 16:1175.

Carobbi A, Araneda D, Quarantillo P, Thomas JM, Thomas FT (1992): Synergism of splenectomy and immunosuppresive drugs in prolongation of cardiac xenograft survival. Transplant Proc 24:527.

Cerra FB, Raza S, Andres GA, Siegel JH (1977): The endothelial damage of pulsatile renal preservation and its relationship to perfusion pressure and colloid osmotic pressure. Surgery 81:534–541.

Chopek MW, Simmons RL, and Platt JL (1987): ABO incompatible renal transplantation: Initial immunopathologic evaluation. Transplant Proc 19:4553–4557.

Cooper DKC, Ye Y, Kehoe M, et al. (1992): A novel approach to neutralization" of preformed antibodies: cardiac allotransplantation across the ABO blood group barrier as a paradigm of discordant transplantation. Transplant Proc 24:566–571

Cooper NR (1985): The classical complement pathway: Activation and regulation of the first complement component. Adv Immunol 37:151–216.

Dalmasso AP, Platt JL (1994): C1 inhibitor prevents complement-mediated activation of xenogeneic endothelial cells in an in vitro model of xenograft hyperacute rejection. Transplantation (in press).

Forbes RDC, Guttmann RD, Kuramochi T, Klassen J, Knaack J (1976): Nonessential role of neutrophils as mediators of hyperacute cardiac allograft rejection in the rat. Lab Invest 34:229–234.

Frank MM (1994): Complement. In Frank MM, Austen KF, Claman HN, Unanue ER (eds): "Samter's Immunological Diseases," 5th ed. Boston, MA: Little, Brown, in press).

Gewurz H, Clark DS, Cooper MD, Varco RL, Good RA (1967): Effect of cobra venom-induced inhibition of complement activity on allograft and xenograft rejection reactions. Transplantation 5:1296–1303.

Gleason RE, Murray JE (1967): Report from kidney transplant registry: Analysis of variables in the function of human kidney transplants. Transplantation 5:343–359.

Horstmann RD, Pangburn MK, Müller-Eberhard HJ (1985): Species specificity of recognition by the alternative pathway of complement. J Immunol 134:1101–1104.

Ihrcke NS, Wrenshall LE, Lindman BJ, Platt JL (1993): Role of heparan sulfate in immune system-blood vessel interactions. Immunol Today 14:500–505.

Iwaki Y, Terasaki PI (1987): Primary nonfunction in human cadaver kidney transplantation: Evidence for hidden hyperacute rejection. Clin Transplant 1:125–131.

Jordan SC, Yap HK, Sakai RS, Alfonso P, Fitchman M (1988): Hyperacute allograft rejection mediated by anti-vascular endothelial cell antibodies with a negative monocyte crossmatch. Transplantation 46:585–602.

Kaufman DB, Platt JL, Rabe FL, Stock PG, Sutherland DER (1990): The immunological basis of islet allograft primary non-function. J Exp Med 172:291–302.

Kissmeyer-Nielsen F, Olsen S, Petersen VP, Fjeldborg O (1966): Hyperacute rejection of kidney allografts, associated with preexisting humoral antibodies against donor cells. Lancet II:662–665.

Lenschow DJ, Zeng Y, Thistlethwaite JR, et al. (1992): Long-term survival of xenogeneic pancreatic islet grafts induced by CTLA4Ig. Science 257:789–792.

Leventhal JR, Matas AJ, Sun LH, et al. (1993): The immunopathology of cardiac xenograft rejection in the guinea pig to rat model. Transplantation 56: 1–8.

Linn BS, Jensen JA, Portal P, Snyder GB (1968): Renal xenograft prolongation by suppression of natural antibody. J Surg Res 8:211–213.

Magee JC, Platt JL (1994): Xenograft rejection: molecular mechanisms and therapeutic implications. Therapeutic Immunol (in press).

Magee JC, Platt JL, Oldham KT, Guice KS (1994): Oxidant stress increases susceptibility of porcine endothelial cells to injury by xenoreactive antibodies and complement. Transplant Proc (in press).

Makowka L, Chapman FA, Cramer DV, Qian S, Sun H, Strazl TE (1990): Platelet-activating factor and hyperacute rejection. Transplantation 50:359–365.

Marcum JA, Reilly CF, Rosenberg RD (1987): Heparan sulfate species and blood vessel wall function. In Wight TN, Mecham RP (eds): "Biology of Proteoglycans." Orlando, FL: Academic Press, pp 301–343.

Miyagawa S, Hirose H, Shirakura R, et al. (1988): The mechanism of discordant xenograft rejection. Transplantation 46:825–830.

Nawroth PP, Stern DM (1986): Modulation of endothelial cell hemostatic properties by tumor necrosis factor. J Exp Med 163:740–745.

Palmer A, Welsh K, Gjorstrup P, Taube D, Bewick M, Thick M (1989): Removal of anti-HLA antibodies by extracorporeal immunoadsorption to enable renal transplantation. Lancet 1:10–12.

Patel R, Terasaki PI (1969): Significance of the positive crossmatch test in kidney transplantation. N Engl J Med 280:735–739.

Paul LC, Claas FHJ, van Es LA, Kalff MW, de Graeff J (1979): Accelerated rejection of a renal allograft associated with pretransplantation antibodies directed against donor antigens on endothelium and monocytes. New Engl J Med 300:1258–1260.

Perper RJ, Najarian JS (1966): Experimental renal heterotransplantation: In widely divergent species. 1. In widely divergent species. Transplantation 4:377–388.

Platt JL, Bach FH (1991): The barrier to xenotransplantation. Transplantation 52:937–947.

Platt JL, Holzknecht ZE (1994): Porcine platelet antigens recognized by human xenoreactive natural antibodies. Transplantation 57:327–335.

Platt JL, Turman MA, Noreen HJ, Fischel RJ, Bolman RM, Bach FH (1990a): An ELISA assay for xenoreactive natural antibodies. Transplantation 49:1000–1001.

Platt JL, Vercellotti GM, Dalmasso AP, et al. (1990b):

Transplantation of discordant xenografts: a review of progress. Immunol Today 11:450–456.

Platt JL, Vercellotti GM, Lindman BJ, Oegema TR,Jr., Bach FH, and Dalmasso AP (1990c): Release of heparan sulfate from endothelial cells: Implications for pathogenesis of hyperacute rejection. J Exp Med 171:1363–1368.

Platt JL, Fischel RJ, Matas AJ, Reif SA, Bolman RM, Bach FH (1991a): Immunopathology of hyperacute xenograft rejection in a swine-to-primate model. Transplantation 52:214–220.

Platt JL, Lindman BJ, Geller RL, et al. (1991b): The role of natural antibodies in the activation of xenogenic endothelial cells. Transplantation 52:1037–1043.

Pober JS, Cotran RS (1990): The role of endothelial cells in inflammation. Transplantation 50:537–544.

Pruitt SK, Kirk AD, Bollinger RR, et al. (1994): The effect of soluble complement receptor type 1 on hyperacute rejection of porcine xenografts. Transplantation 57:363–370.

Saadi S, Platt JL (1995): Transient perturbation of endothelial integrity induced by antibodies and complement. J Exp Med (in press).

Schleef RR, Bevilacqua MP, Sawdey M, Gimbrone MAJr., Loskutoff DJ (1988): Cytokine activation of vascular endothelium. Effects on tissue-type plasminogen activator and type 1 plasminogen activator inhibitor. J Biol Chem 263:5797–5803.

Scornik JC, Salomon DR, Lim PB, Howard RJ, Pfaff WW (1989): Posttransplant antidonor antibodies and graft rejection. Transplantation 47:287–290.

Spector D, Limas C, Frost JL, et al. (1976): Perfusion nephropathy in human transplants. N Engl J Med 295:1217–1221.

Starzl TE, Lerner RA, Dixon FJ, Groth CG, Brettschneider L, Terasaki PI (1968): Schwartzman reaction after human renal homotransplantation. N Engl J Med 278:642–648.

Stevens RB, Platt JL (1992): Physiology and cell biology update: The pathogenesis of hyperacute xenograft rejection. Am J Kidney Dis 20:414–421.

Stevens RB, Wang YL, Kaji H, et al. (1993): Administration of nonanticoagulant heparin inhibits the loss of glycosaminoglycans from xenogeneic cardiac grafts and prolongs graft survival. Transplant Proc 25:382.

Suciu-Foca N, Reed E, D'Agati VD, et al. (1991): Soluble HLA antigens, anti-HLA antibodies, and antiidiotypic antibodies in the circulation of renal transplant recipients. Transplantation 51:593–601.

Terasaki PI, Marchioro TL, Starzl TE (1965): Serotyping of human lymphocyte antigens: Preliminary trials on long-term kidney homograft survivors. In Russell PS (ed): "Histocompatibility Testing." Washington, D.C.: National Research Council, pp 83–96.

Terman DS, Garcia-Rinaldi R, Dannemann B, et al. (1978): Specific suppression of antibody rebound after extracorporeal immunoadsorbtion. Clin Exp Immunol 34:32–41.

Weisman HF, Bartow T, Leppo MK, et al. (1990): Soluble human complement receptor type 1: In vivo inhibitor of complement suppressing post-ischemic myocardial inflammation and necrosis. Science 249:146–151.

Wilbrandt R, Tung KSK, Deodhar SD, Nakamoto S, Kolff WJ (1969): ABO blood group incompatibility in human renal homotransplantation. Am J Clin Pathol 51:15–23.

Wrenshall LE, Platt JL, Chopek MW, Fischel R, Matas AJ (1991): ABO incompatible transplantation in pigtail macaque monkeys. Transplant Proc 23:703–704.

Wrenshall LE, Carlson A, Cerra FB, Platt JL (1994): Modulation of cytolytic T cell responses by heparan sulfate. Transplantation 57:1087–1094.

KEY REFERENCES

Frank MM (1994): Complement. In Frank MM, Austen KF, Claman HN, Unanue ER (eds): "Samter's Immunological Diseases," 5th ed. Boston, MA: Little, Brown, (in press).

Kissmeyer-Nielsen F, Olsen S, Petersen VP, Fjeldborg O (1966): Hyperacute rejection of kidney allografts, associated with pre-existing humoral antibodies against donor cells. Lancet II: 662–665.

Magee JC, Platt JL (1994): Xenograft rejection: Molecular mechanisms and therapeutic implications. Therapeutic Immunol 1:45–58.

Patel R, Terasaki PI (1969): Significance of the positive crossmatch test in kidney transplantation. N Engl J Med 280:735–739.

Platt JL (1994): "Hyperacute Xenograft Rejection." Austin, TX: RG Landes (in press).

Chapter 7
Immunologic Issues in Clinical Transplantation

Hugh Auchincloss, Jr.

INTRODUCTION

This book is about the science of transplantation immunology and not about the artful practice of clinical transplantation. Sometimes the two fields coincide, although perhaps not as often as we would like. To a remarkable degree, one can care successfully for transplantation patients with little knowledge of immunology and, alternatively, excellent immunologists would find it impossible to manage a clinical service. There are some clinical issues, however, which are understood best by understanding the scientific principles behind them, and there are many that present complex immunologic problems that scientists are most likely to solve. This chapter discusses some of those issues.

ANTIGEN MATCHING

The issue of antigen matching refers to the degree to which MHC antigens of the donor are the same as the MHC antigens of the recipient. The questions involved in this issue are whether better matching of MHC antigens leads to better graft survival, whether organs should be distributed according to the degree of antigen matching, and whether recipients will be better or less well able to respond to viral infections in the donor organ if its MHC antigens are better or less well matched. These questions have been the source of intense controversy and are often hotly debated, with the implication that the value or irrelevance of science (and the scientist) depends on the conclusion. Actually, the questions involved, when properly formulated, do not pose such fundamental issues and the differing answers usually represent matters of degree.

As discussed earlier, identification of the MHC antigens of donors and recipients is performed in "tissue typing" laboratories using several different techniques. Traditionally, laboratories have used serologic methods, while more recently, some laboratories have started using one of several different molecular biologic approaches. The different techniques provide different degrees of accuracy, but none of them routinely characterizes all of the MHC antigens of a given individual. Thus, when the "six" MHC antigens of transplant patients are discussed (two from the A locus, two from the B locus, and two from the DR locus) it should be clear that these represent only half of all the classical MHC antigens we know about. Furthermore, depending on the circumstances and the techniques being used, even these may be imprecisely characterized. Part of the controversy regarding antigen matching, therefore, derives from the incomplete information available in the real world.

Does Better MHC Matching Lead to Better Graft Survival?

MHC antigens were originally identified partly because of the powerful graft rejection they cause. Grafts mismatched for their MHC, but matched for everything else, are rejected much faster than grafts mismatched for any other single histocompatibility locus. In clinical transplantation also, kidney transplants from MHC-identical

Transplantation Immunology, pages 131–145
© 1995 Wiley-Liss, Inc.

siblings suffer less rejection and survive better than transplants from MHC-mismatched siblings. Thus, there is little argument that complete MHC matching leads to better graft survival.

There is also experimental evidence that matching for some, but not all, MHC antigens improves kidney graft survival. This has been demonstrated best in pigs, where genetic MHC class II antigen matching, without matching for minor or class I MHC antigens, often leads to indefinite kidney graft survival even without immunosuppression. This never occurs in class II mismatched animals (Pescovitz et al., 1984). In clinical transplantation, the value of partial matching is demonstrated by living-related donors who share one, but not both, MHC haplotypes with the recipient. Transplants from these donors survive better than from unmatched cadaver donors. There is also clinical evidence that organ survival from cadaver donors is improved by MHC class II antigen matching and that matching for particular class I antigens may also be useful (Middleton et al., 1985; Sanfilippo et al., 1984). Finally, the data in large national and international kidney transplant registries indicate that both 1-year and long-term graft survival is statistically correlated with the degree of MHC antigen matching. Thus there is substantial evidence that better MHC matching leads to better kidney graft survival.

There is ongoing uncertainty over why the effect of MHC antigen matching for cadaver donors is not more striking and whether the value of MHC class II antigen matching, in particular, would not be more obvious if the techniques for typing were more complete and precise. Efforts to improve the correlation by the use of new technologies are, therefore, being investigated.

Should Organs Be Distributed According to the Degree of Antigen Matching?

While the conclusion that better antigen matching provides a better outcome may be generally accepted, it is an entirely different question whether the level of antigen matching should be used to determine the distribution of cadaver organs. This question involves matters of degree and a balance between the amount of the benefit and the disadvantages of the effort to match MHC antigens. The size of the benefits is not simple to determine. For kidneys, they represent around 10% better 1-year graft survival for "six antigen matched" organs compared to those distributed randomly, but they are probably larger differences over 5 or 10 years (Opelz and Terasaki, 1982). On the other hand, the costs of distributing organs by antigen match are significant, including not only the financial ones, associated with identifying the MHC antigens and the long transport distances often required, but also those associated with longer ischemic times and with the inequities for the patients forced to wait longer for cadaver organs. With so many variables involved, each so difficult to evaluate, it is not surprising that disagreements exist regarding the proper role to assign antigen matching in the distribution of cadaver organs.

At present, practical issues prevent MHC antigen matching from playing a role in the distribution of the solid organs except for kidneys and sometimes pancreases. Most solid organs cannot survive the time required to perform tissue typing and pancreases can be distributed according to MHC matching only if typing is performed before organ procurement. Kidneys, however, can still function after 1 to 2 days of cold ischemia, allowing time for MHC typing to be performed and for the organs to be sent to distant locations. At present, however, MHC antigen matching is generally used in the United States for the allocation of kidneys only when all six of the commonly typed MHC antigens are found to be shared by a recipient. Some people believe even this effort at antigen matching is not cost effective, while others believe that still greater efforts to achieve better antigen matching would be worth the effort.

In contrast to the distribution of solid organs, the selection of bone marrow donors is guided almost entirely by the results of MHC antigen matching. In this case the practical issues of time and distance are of relatively little concern, whereas the measurable benefit of antigen matching is enormous. In fact, successful bone marrow transplantation with any but a perfectly matched donor is unusual. This dominant importance of MHC antigen matching in bone marrow transplantation is now the primary justification for maintaining tissue typing laboratories and for developing new techniques to identify MHC antigens more precisely.

MHC Antigen Matching and the Response to Viral Pathogens

While the issue of MHC antigen matching is usually debated in terms of its effect on rejection, antigen matching may also play a role in the ability of the immune system to recognize viral pathogens expressed in the allogeneic organ. At least three different aspects of this issue may be relevant, and at this time it is unclear which of them have clinical importance: (1) Can T cells selected in a recipient's thymus to recognize modified self-MHC antigens, recognize viruses presented in association with allogeneic MHC antigens? (2) Can T cells sensitized (either before or after transplantation) to recognize viral peptides presented by self-APCs eliminate virally infected cells in the donor organ? and (3) Will recipients who have originally suffered organ damage because they were unable to cope with virally infected cells be better off receiving organs that are MHC mismatched to avoid recapitulating this process?

T cell responses to viral peptides presented by allogeneic APCs. For as long as donor APCs are present after transplantation, viral antigens can presumably be presented by these APCs as peptides in association with allogeneic MHC antigens. One of the basic principles of immunology, however, is that T cells are selected to see peptides in association with self-MHC molecules, thus suggesting that they might not be able to see peptides with allo-MHC antigens. Actually, however, the principle is more complicated. The positive selection of T cells occurs along with the elimination of self-reactive T cells, but the process leaves intact the T cells that recognize allogeneic MHC antigens, including allo-MHC antigens presenting peptides. The experiments that demonstrated a preference for peptides presented by self-MHC molecules were possible only after alloreactive T cells had been eliminated by techniques that did not include the

positive selection process. Thus, it is the elimination of alloreactivity, without a positive selection step, that leaves a T cell repertoire unable to recognize allo + X. Since alloreactivity does remain after normal T cell development in the thymus, the response to allogeneic MHC antigens presenting viral peptides also remains.

Although recipient T cells should maintain the capacity to respond to viral antigens presented by donor MHC antigens, it is essential that alloreactive T cells be suppressed to prevent graft rejection. There is, however, no way for our immunosuppressive drugs to distinguish the alloreactive cells that would reject the normal cells of the organ from those that would reject the virally infected cells of the organ. In the eyes of a T cell, an allogeneic MHC antigen presenting peptide X is no different from an allogeneic MHC antigen presenting peptide Y, where Y happens to be derived from a virus. Both determinants look equally allogeneic. Therefore, the notion that T cells cannot see viral antigens presented by allogeneic MHC antigens is wrong, except that in clinical transplantation we are constantly suppressing the very T cells that recognize these determinants.

This problem becomes worse to the degree that the presence of the organ itself induces tolerance or that we use other tolerance-inducing strategies. Complete elimination of an allogeneic response would also eliminate completely the response to the allo-MHC antigens plus virus, unless a positive selection event were added to the tolerance-inducing strategy. Since none of the commonly proposed strategies to achieve tolerance includes a mechanism for positive selection, all of them would make the recipient incapable of eliminating virally infected cells from a donor organ.

Can T cells sensitized to virus presented by self-APCs respond to virally infected cells of the donor organ? Over time, donor antigen-presenting cells that come with a new organ are replaced by bone marrow-derived APCs from the recipient. Therefore, new viral infections that occur after transplantation will increasingly stimulate an immune response exclusively through presentation in association with recipient MHC antigens. In addition, any immune response that was stimulated before the transplant would also be directed at peptides of the pathogen presented by self-MHC antigens. In either case, according to the principle of associative recognition, these T cells should be unable to recognize peptides of the same pathogen presented by MHC antigens of the donor organ if there is no matching of donor and recipient MHC molecules. Therefore, the principle of associative recognition suggests that both previous immunity, and new immune responses occurring late after transplantation, will be ineffective in generating responses directed at pathogens within the donor organ, at least to the degree that the donor and recipient are MHC mismatched.

Might MHC matching be harmful for generating antiviral responses in some cases? The principle of associative recognition suggests that MHC matching might be useful to allow old and new T cell immunity to respond to viral infections in the transplanted organ. Under some circumstances, however, this might not be a good thing. Liver transplantation, for example, is often performed on patients who have suffered liver damage as a result of chronic viral infection. These patients are only a subpopulation of all people who suffer such viral infections, however, suggesting that there was something about their immune response to the viral infection that allowed liver destruction to continue. Perhaps the particular MHC antigens of these individuals present the peptides of these viral pathogens poorly. Alternatively, perhaps they present these peptides extremely well and it is the immune response to the virus that causes liver damage. Whatever the cause of irreparable liver damage in these individuals, it might be that MHC matching of their donor organ will allow a recurrence of the very process that brought them to liver transplantation in the first place.

It should be clear from this discussion of the issue of MHC matching and viral infection that our understanding of the actual process of viral immunity and its role in the pathogenesis of organ failure is not yet sophisticated enough to allow accurate predictions about the benefits or disadvantages of MHC matching in this regard.

It is interesting to use these considerations to speculate about immunologic reasons for the startling finding by some investigators that MHC matching for some types of organ transplantation, especially liver transplantation, actually seems to lead to a worse outcome. The primary message from this discussion, however, should be that much more needs to be learned about the immune response to viral pathogens before the science of immunology can be used to make rational clinical decisions on this basis.

THE CROSS-MATCH

Although antigen matching and the "cross-match" sound alike, they are actually very different. Whereas antigen matching compares the MHC antigens of the donor and recipient, and is marginally important for some types of solid organ transplantation (and not used at all for others), the cross-match determines whether recipients have *performed antibodies* reactive with donor antigens, and is critically important for several types of solid organ transplants.

The cross-match assay is generally performed by mixing serum from the recipient with cells from the donor and then adding a source of complement to lyse cells that have bound antibodies from the recipient's serum. The cross-match is said to be *positive* if lysis occurs. Therefore, if an organ is susceptible to hyperacute rejection, a transplant should not be performed if the cross-match is positive and can be performed if it is negative. Kidney transplants are frequently performed when there is a negative cross-match and poor antigen matching, but never performed if there is a positive cross-match even with good antigen matching.

Cross-Match Techniques

As with any assay, there are variations in the way a cross-match can be performed and thresholds that must be determined for judging when the results will be deemed "positive." One modification is to add an *antihuman antibody* after the serum from the patient has been mixed with the donor cells. This will augment the amount of antibody bound to each cell and ensure that a complement-fixing isotype is present on the cell surface. This modification increases the sensitivity of the assay. Another variation is to determine the binding of a patient's antibodies by adding fluoresceinated antihuman antibodies and then testing the cells by FACS analysis. This modification also increases the sensitivity of the assay and enables the identification of the isotypes present in the patient's serum if the fluoresceinated antibodies are isotype specific. Another modification is to vary the types of cells used in the assay. T cells express few class II antigens and therefore test primarily for anti-class I antibodies, whereas B cells can be used to test for additional anti-class II antibodies. In addition, the assay can be performed at different temperatures, which alters the sensitivity for detecting different types of antibodies, and the patient's serum can be treated with DTT, or other reducing agents, which selectively destroy antibodies of IgM isotype.

Despite the importance of the cross-match in renal transplantation, there is no universal agreement on how the assay should be performed nor on what to do with some of the results. Most laboratories use the antihuman antibody-augmented, complement-mediated lysis of T cells and consider detectable lysis, even at very low dilutions, to be positive. Others also perform a B cell cross-match, and reject transplants with a positive outcome. The standards currently used are very effective in preventing hyperacute rejection (which is rarely observed in clinical transplantation), but the issue remains whether some patients are being excluded from transplantation because the cross-match and its interpretation are too stringent. On the other hand, it is also possible that even more stringent criteria (while not likely to avoid many episodes of hyperacute rejection) might improve long-term results of transplantation if a weakly positive cross-match correlates with other important elements of the rejection process.

The Cross-Match for Nonrenal Transplantation

Although some form of cross-match is universally agreed to be important for kidney trans-plantation, the assay is often not used for many other types of organ transplantation. Part of the reason for this discrepancy is practical, since the shorter preservation times available for hearts and lungs make it difficult to perform a cross-match after organ procurement. Therefore, to avoid long delays before procuring these organs, patients with few preformed antibodies often receive transplants without a prospective cross-match. More interesting for immunologists, *some organs can be transplanted without suffering hyperacute rejection,* even if preformed antibodies reactive with their antigens are present. The liver is the most obvious example. Although evidence suggests that humoral injury to the liver, including by preformed antibody, can occur (Gordon et al., 1986), it is much less obvious and clinically important than for kidney transplants.

Uncertainties of the Cross-Match

From an immunologist's point of view, uncertainty over the cross-match even for kidney transplantation stems first from the evidence that some types of preformed antibodies do not cause hyperacute rejection and may even be beneficial for preventing rejection. One type of irrelevant antibody is a *patient's autoantibodies* that may sometimes be present. These can usually be identified by their broad reactivity and IgM isotype. More important, some preformed anti-class II antibodies, perhaps of particular isotypes or with specificity for particular epitopes, appear to cause better, not worse, graft survival. It is not clear, however, exactly what features identify such beneficial antibodies and, thus, how to perform assays that allow transplantation in the face of these positive cross-match results. Another source of confusion is that the level of preformed antibodies in a patient's serum may change over time. Thus, it is possible for patients to have a negative cross-match with a prospective donor, using their most recent serum sample, but a positive cross-match using sera from earlier times. Successful transplantation despite "historical" positive cross-matches has often been performed and, in some cases, it may even lead to better outcomes than in unsensitized patients. One possibility is that the best outcomes occur when the decline in the level of particular preformed antibodies is due to the development of antiidiotypic antibodies by the recipient. However, the putative benefit of antiidiotypic antibodies is controversial.

The second important immunologic issue is how the cross-match, testing for preformed antibodies, might correlate with other elements of transplant rejection. Weakly positive cross-matches, for example, may detect antibodies that would not be present in sufficient quantities to cause hyperacute rejection, but predict an early, vigorous humoral response to donor antigens. In addition, weakly positive cross-matches (a B cell response) may correlate with T cell sensitization to the same antigens and thus predict more vigorous cell-mediated rejection. It is not clear, however, that humoral and cellular mechanisms of graft rejection always occur together. In fact, if sensitization of B cell responses develops because T helper cells have been stimulated toward Th2 types of responses, then the Th1 responses (associated with cell-mediated rejection) might actually be weaker in patients with positive cross-matches.

Beyond the immunologic issues, there are also ethical and practical clinical issues associated with the cross-match. For example, what risks to the recipient are appropriate in trying to provide a transplant for a highly sensitized patient who has been stuck on dialysis for many years, and is it reasonable to "waste" some organs as a result of hyperacute rejection, trying to help these patients, when others could perhaps obtain a better long-term survival?

SENSITIZED PATIENTS

The term "sensitized" patient has a particular meaning in clinical transplantation that sometimes confuses immunologists. Whereas immunologic sensitization refers to previous T or B cell activation with the development of memory cells, sensitization of patients awaiting transplants refers particularly to *B cell responses* as measured by the range of HLA antigens to which preformed antibodies are detectable. To determine the level of sensitization, serum from a transplant candidate is regularly tested by the cross-match technique against a panel of cells that has been selected because together they express a wide range of human HLA antigens. Sera from unsensitized patients will not lyse any of these target cells whereas sera from patients with preformed antibodies may kill some or even all of the panel cells. A rough quantitative assessment of the degree of sensitization for a patient is expressed by the percentage of cells in the panel that are killed. This is referred to as the *PRA* or panel reactive antibody. Sera from some patients may lyse all of the cells in the panel and thus suggest that these patients are "100% sensitized." This does not imply that they have preformed antibodies to all HLA antigens, but rather that they have antibodies that react with at least one HLA antigen on every cell in that particular panel. Such patients would not have antibodies to their own HLA antigens and probably not to other antigens as well. Thus, they are not truly 100% sensitized and the quantitative assessment is only a rough indicator of the range of anti-HLA antibodies that is present.

The degree of sensitization of a transplant candidate predicts the difficulty that patient will have in finding a donor that is cross-match negative. Some highly sensitized patients wait for many years to receive a transplant and others may never find a suitable donor. Therefore, it is common to give special priority to highly sensitized patients in organ allocation schemes.

One of the ways in which immunologists have contributed to clinical transplantation has been to characterize the anti-HLA antibodies that have been formed in highly sensitized patients. Such individuals might have many different types of anti-HLA antibodies or they might have a few different types that are broadly cross-reactive with many different HLA antigens. In most cases, it turns out, even highly sensitized individuals have relatively few different antibodies that are reactive with so-called *public epitopes*. Furthermore, by absorbing the antibodies with cells expressing particular epitopes or by testing the a patient's serum against carefully selected target cells expressing known epitopes, it is possible to characterize the antibodies in the serum quite precisely. This information can then be used to predict which HLA antigens, in addition to a patient's own, are "safe" antigens and which are likely to cause a positive cross-match. Thus it is possible to search for donors expressing permissible HLA phenotypes for highly sensitized patients without the time and expense of performing hundreds of cross-matches. Some have argued that the real benefit of HLA typing for kidney transplantation is not to achieve better antigen matching per se, but rather to find cross-match negative donors for highly sensitized recipients.

BLOOD TRANSFUSIONS

Highly sensitized recipients are at a disadvantage compared to unsensitized ones in the process of obtaining cross-match negative donors. There are three ways that patients become sensitized, each causing exposure to allogeneic human HLA antigens: (1) by prior organ transplantation, (2) by pregnancy, and (3) by blood transfusions. Of the three, only future blood transfusions are under the control of the physician. Therefore, to minimize the risk of sensitizing a transplant recipient, avoiding blood transfusions is important. This logic was so apparent to transplant physicians in the 1960s that they sometimes went to extraordinary lengths to avoid blood transfusions for their kidney transplant candidates. Some dialysis patients struggled with hematocrits less than 10%, while waiting for a transplant.

The Benefit of Pretransplant Blood Transfusions

It was, therefore, something of a shock when it was reported during the 1970s that the outcome of kidney transplantation was better for those patients who had received blood transfusions prior to their transplant than for those who had not (Opelz and Terasaki, 1980). The issue was tested repeatedly by many investigators over the next 10 years and was verified more consistently than almost any finding in the medical literature. Over 60 different studies showed a benefit from pretransplant blood transfusions. On the basis of this information, transplant physicians reversed their previous policies and began transfusing al-

most all candidates for kidney transplantation whether they needed it or not. This was done despite the risk of sensitizing recipients, a risk of 10–25%, depending on how the blood transfusions were prepared and the prior history of the transplant candidate.

The reasons for the beneficial effect of blood transfusions are still not entirely clear. There may be several factors, including (1) blood transfusions may carry immunosuppressive viruses, (2) blood transfusions may cause a subclinical graft-versus-host response that is immunosuppressive, (3) blood transfusions may sensitize patients to those HLA antigens to which they are most responsive, causing a positive cross-match to donors with these antigens and preventing transplantation of the organs that are most likely to elicit powerful rejection, and (4) blood transfusions may cause specific downregulation of the immune response. There is evidence supporting each of these possibilities.

The Apparent Loss of the Beneficial Effect

Whatever the reasons for the beneficial effect, the value of pretransplant blood transfusions was so well accepted that it was again stunning when some of the same investigators who had first identified the benefit reported in 1986 that the benefit had become negligible in more recent transplant recipients (Opelz, 1987). How could such a well-demonstrated phenomenon disappear over the course of 10 years? Actually, careful analysis of the data suggested that the effect had not disappeared entirely, only that it was not much less obvious than it had been before. The reason for the change was probably that the outcome of organ transplantation for all patients was better than it had been, regardless of whether blood transfusions had been given or not. The use of powerful new immunosuppressive drugs, such as cyclosporine and OKT3, had masked the biologic effect of blood transfusions. This is not the same as saying that the biologic effect had ceased to exist.

Intentional transfusions of transplant candidates would probably have continued to be the standard practice for transplant physicians were it not that the potential harmful effects of transfusions, particularly from viral infections, were more widely recognized at just the time that the diminished beneficial effect was identified. Patients themselves, fearing AIDS, often refused blood transfusions when their hematocrits were normal. Currently, the availability of erythropoietin for dialysis patients has again made pretransplant blood transfusions less common.

Donor-Specific Transfusions

Although the clinical use of intentional blood transfusions has come full circle over the past 30 years, the suggestion that pretransplant administration of blood might be immunologically useful has led to many experimental efforts to examine the basis for this effect. Some of this experimental work has been discussed in the section on tolerance induction. Obviously, the use of blood transfusions to induce tolerance requires that the blood administered come from the same donor as for the transplanted organ. Thus, this form of blood transfusion is referred to as "donor-specific transfusion."

The use of donor-specific transfusions in clinical transplantation has been met with substantial resistance. This is because donor-specific transfusions before transplantation have usually been used primarily for living-related donors. Since the outcome of transplantation from these donors is already so excellent, physicians have been reluctant to risk sensitizing their patients by intentional transfusions (and thereby commit their patients to years of dialysis) in order to gain the uncertain, but definitely small benefits of transfusions. To meet this resistance, newer protocols for donor-specific transfusion often attempt to provide the transfusions just at the time of transplantation, thereby avoiding the problem of sensitization and making the protocols potentially applicable to cadaver-donor transplantation. In addition, as discussed in the tolerance section, strategies aimed at selecting and transfusing only the beneficial elements in blood are under investigation.

MONOCLONAL ANTIBODY THERAPY

Probably the area in which transplantation immunology has contributed most directly to clini-

cal transplantation has been in the development of anti-T cell antibody therapy to treat and prevent rejection. The idea of limiting cellular immunity by treatment with antibodies began in the 1950s with antilymphocyte serum used in mice. It was applied to humans, again with polyclonal antisera raised in horses or rabbits, during the 1960s and 1970s (Cosimi et al., 1976). In the 1980s the technique was refined by introducing monoclonal anti-T cell antibodies, first as OKT3 (an anti-CD3 antibody) and, subsequently, as a wide variety of antibodies of different specificity and isotype. Testing modifications and new types of monoclonal antibodies is one of the most active areas of clinical research in transplantation today, raising several issues of interest to immunologists.

The Effect of Monoclonal Antibodies on the Target Cell Population

The binding of antibodies to cell surface antigens can have a number of different effects on the target population. First, if the antigen is capable of providing an activation signal, binding of the antibody may trigger a response. Second, an antibody can bind to a cell surface antigen and thereby *block* the function of that molecule. Third, the target cell can lose expression of the relevant surface antigen, a phenomenon referred to as *modulation*. Finally, cells expressing the target antigen can be *depleted* from circulation or even from the immune system as a whole.

Which effect antibody treatment will have seems to depend on many different factors, including the nature of the surface antigen, the particular epitope and the density of the antigen that binds the antibody, and the isotype of the antibody itself. These factors are not yet well enough understood, however, to allow accurate predictions of the effect for any new antibody. In particular, the role of antibody isotype is confusing. Although it is often assumed that complement lysis is responsible for cell depletion, the actual mechanism probably involves *opsonization* and removal of target cells in the reticuloendothelial system. Nonetheless, experimental studies have shown that different antibodies, having identical isotypes, may deplete the target cell population in some cases, but simply coat the surface antigens without depleting the cells in others. In some cases, a single antibody can have more than one effect over time. For example, the first event after treatment with OKT3 appears to be T cell activation, manifested by the release of several cytokines. This occurs because the CD3 antigen is part of the T cell receptor's signaling apparatus. T cell activation accounts for the early systemic side-effects of OKT3 therapy, including high fevers and difficulty breathing. Within minutes, the OKT3 antibody causes depletion of circulating T cells from the peripheral blood, which can be detected by FACS analysis showing an absence of cells expressing CD3 as well CD4 and CD8 antigens. Over several days, repeat FACS analysis often shows a return to the circulation of cells expressing CD4 or CD8 but not the CD3 antigen. In the case of OKT3, these modulated cells are probably unable to function, since they lack a critical structure for their activation. Eventually, when OKT3 therapy is stopped or ceases to be effective, normal T cells return to the circulation with all of their antigens.

The Recipient's Immune Response to Monoclonal Antibody Therapy

Most monoclonal antibodies are originally produced in mice. Therefore, their use in humans represents the introduction of a foreign protein that can, itself, stimulate an immune response. Antibodies formed against these monoclonal antibodies are frequently observed in patients undergoing treatment. Some of the antiantibodies are directed at species-specific determinants of the murine protein, others at isotypic determinants, and still others at unique determinants associated with the antigen combining site of the therapeutic antibody. These last are called *antiidiotypic* antibodies.

Despite the possibility that antigen–antibody complexes might be formed, it is unusual to see any toxic effects from this immune response. On the other hand, antibody formation against the monoclonal antibodies often blocks their therapeutic effect. The most important antiantibodies that do this are those that are antiidiotypic. However, antibodies directed at constant region determinants may shorten the serum half-life of the therapeutic monoclonal antibody and the formation of antiidiotypic antibodies is enhanced by the presence of additional species-specific determinants on the constant region of the molecule. In clinical practice, the appearance of antibodies against OKT3 can be detected in ELISA assays or by noting the reappearance of CD3 cells by FACS analysis. In addition, patients may begin having side effects similar to those associated with their first dose of OKT3, when later doses are given, if CD3 cells have returned to the circulation. In clinical practice the neutralizing effect of the antiantibody response can often be overcome by simply increasing the dose of the monoclonal antibody.

Manufacturing Better Monoclonal Antibodies

Since particular monoclonal antibodies sometimes fail to produce the desired effect (e.g., cell depletion) and since monoclonal antibodies from a different species elicit a neutralizing antiantibody response by the recipient, there is considerable interest in designing better antibodies for therapeutic use. The technology to do this often uses techniques of molecular biology to splice together portions of genes encoding different antibodies to make a novel product. The portions responsible for the specificity of the antibody are taken from the murine gene encoding the original monoclonal antibody, while other portions are usually taken from human genes encoding particular isotypes. These antibodies have been referred to as *CDR-grafted antibodies* (complementarity determining region). The difficulty in this process is that it is still not clear exactly which human isotypes will produce the most effective therapeutic antibodies and the best choice may be different for antibodies with different specificities. It may also be necessary to change natural human isotypes slightly so that they perform one function (such as cell depletion) but fail to trigger another function (such as cell activation). Furthermore, the idiotypic portion of even the CDR-grafted antibodies is still xenogeneic in origin and hence likely to elicit an antiidiotypic response by the recipient. Nonetheless, the formation of antiidiotypes by patients is probably slower when the remainder of the therapeutic antibody is syngeneic and the serum half-life of the "designer" antibodies is frequently longer than for their murine counterparts.

Another approach for designing better therapeutic antibodies has been to attach additional molecules to the antibodies, usually to provide more potent destruction of the target cell. Ricin, diphtheria toxin, and several radioactive substances have been used for this purpose. Problems with antiantibody responses and unwanted effector functions still exist for these altered antibodies and they also have the potential for nonspecific effects resulting from their toxic moiety. Whether they can be used to accomplish more effective cell depletion than ordinary antibodies has not yet been established.

A variation on the therapeutic monoclonal antibody theme is to block the function of cell surface molecules or of cytokines by administering *soluble receptors* for these ligands. Like designer antibodies, these can be generated by techniques of molecular biology, splicing the extra-membrane portion of a receptor to a portion of an immunoglobulin molecule. These soluble receptors generally have much higher affinities for their target molecules than do antibodies and are therefore especially useful when persistent binding to block function is important as opposed to target cell depletion.

THE DIAGNOSIS OF REJECTION

One of the most important immunologic issues in clinical transplantation is determining which rejection of a transplanted organ is occurring. Since there are many causes of graft dysfunction (including infection, ischemia, and toxic side effects of drugs) in addition to rejection, it would obviously be useful to know which of these is involved and to know this in relatively simple, noninvasive ways. The distinction can sometimes be of dramatic clinical importance. Although this issue would seem to be at the heart of transplantation immunology, the scientific field has contributed almost nothing to solving this problem.

The best determination of rejection is the clinical intuition of the physician based on patterns of changing organ function, the timing of the event, the presence of nonimmunologic factors, and a few, unreliable clinical signs including fever and graft tenderness. The next step often involves brief therapeutic trials to see how the organ dysfunction responds to antirejection therapy or lower doses of potentially toxic drugs.

In difficult cases, the "gold standard" for diagnosing rejection in clinical transplantation is a biopsy of the organ. Even biopsies, however, may be difficult to interpret. In the setting of acute rejection, experienced pathologists can sometimes detect evidence for immune-mediated tissue destruction, usually in the form of endothelial cell inflammation, or *endothelialitis*. In many cases, however, definitive evidence of rejection is not present and the biopsy can only be interpreted as consistent with rejection and without evidence of other causes of organ dysfunction. In chronic cases, pathologists can rarely state definitively that the cause of the problem is immunologic.

One of the problems with histologic examination of allogeneic tissue is that a *lymphoid infiltrate*, often interpreted by the inexperienced observer as evidence of rejection, does not correlate well with actual organ dysfunction. Studies using scheduled, protocol biopsies, regardless of organ function, often reveal intense lymphoid infiltrates that do not seem to be causing any damage to the organ (Solez et al., 1986). Furthermore, experimental studies have shown that such lymphoid infiltrates can appear, and then disappear over time, without any immunosuppressive treatment, even in animals that go on to develop tolerance to the antigens of their organ donor. Clearly, the immunologic events responsible for these infiltrates and for triggering (or sometimes preventing) organ destruction are not understood sufficiently to interpret these histologic findings.

Numerous efforts have been made to find particular features of biopsy specimens that predict clinical rejection responses. Many correlations have been identified, such as the frequent association of IL-5 transcripts or of intense eosinophilia with severe clinical rejection. None of them, however, has so far proven sufficiently sensitive and specific to be useful for clinical purposes. Recently, the strong correlation of staining for *perforin* granules in cytotoxic T cells has been suggested as a marker of both clinical importance and of value in understanding the biologic mechanisms of graft destruction.

Given the difficulty in determining rejection even from tissue of the donor organ, it is not surprising that assays of systemic immunologic function have also been disappointing. Many efforts have been made to correlate the results of simple blood tests with rejection activity, measuring, for example, the level of interleukin 2 (IL-2) or of soluble IL-2 receptors. These efforts have frequently indicated encouraging correlations, but not results sufficiently precise to allow management of individual patients. The problem with these assays is that they tend to measure general immunologic activity rather than donor-specific responses and hence they are as likely to be positive in the face of significant viral infection as with the onset of rejection. This is exactly the distinction that is frequently needed in clinical medicine. On the other hand, *in vitro* assays of donor-specific reactivity are usually limited by the strength of the alloreactive response. T cells will respond to allogeneic stimulating cells *in vitro* even before a transplant is performed and, thus, the finding that they respond after transplantation is not of predictive value.

TESTING TO MONITOR ANTIDONOR IMMUNOREACTIVITY

Just as it is difficult to make a definitive diagnosis of rejection at the time of organ dysfunction, so too immunologists have failed to provide a reliable way of testing the likelihood of future rejection activity or of determining whether a recipient has become tolerant to their donor's antigens. In clinical transplantation, the amount of immunosuppression given a particular patient over time is again determined largely by clinical intuition and by protocols that make relatively few adjustments for individual patients.

Numerous efforts to provide immunologic assays of donor-specific responsiveness have been described, often providing good correlations

with clinical outcomes. For example, the ability to withdraw steroids from patients with stable allograft function without inducing rejection can be statistically predicted by the absence of donor-specific MLR responses. But while such assays provide good correlations, they are associated with too many exceptions in individual patients to be clinically reliable. Similarly, a recently reported biological test of the overall level of immunosuppression, provided by testing recipient responses to mitogens, to recall antigens (such as tetanus toxoid), and to third-party allogeneic stimulators, offers a useful way to judge the effectiveness of the exogenous immunosuppression, but not a means of judging donor-specific reactivity (Muluk et al., 1991). It has also recently been suggested that the ability to detect microchimerism in various tissues of the recipient indicates that tolerance to donor antigens has been induced (Starzl et al., 1992). It is not yet clear, however, whether this ability to detect surviving donor cells is simply a marker for good survival of the allograft itself or actually a marker (or even the cause) of donor-specific nonreactivity.

There are several possible reasons why *in vitro* assays might fail to predict present or future *in vivo* antidonor reactivity. First, *in vitro* assays may not be adequately sensitive to detect the level of *in vivo* responsiveness that can cause allograft rejection. Alternatively, the *in vitro* assays may not measure the immunologic function that is involved in *in vivo* graft rejection. Second, *in vitro* assays generally make use of lymphoid cells from the donor that may not express all of the tissue-specific peptides that are present in the donor organ. Therefore, a recipient might be nonresponsive in an *in vitro* MLR, but still able to respond to other determinants expressed in the allograft itself. Third, the state of immunologic responsiveness measured *in vitro* may not always be stable over time. For example, if donor nonreactivity is due to anergy of responding T cells, these T cells may escape from their nonresponsive state under some conditions. Determining how to predict clinical immunologic reactivity is one of the important contributions that immunologists could make to the practice of clinical transplantation.

IMMUNOLOGIC ISSUES ASSOCIATED WITH PARTICULAR TYPES OF ORGAN TRANSPLANTS

Much of what has been said about transplantation immunology in this book applies to any tissue or organ. There are, however, some features associated with transplanting particular organs that are of interest to immunologists.

Skin Grafts

Allogeneic and even xenogeneic skin grafts have sometimes been used in clinical practice to cover large defects caused by burns. These have even been temporarily kept in place with exogenous immunosuppression on the theory that coverage of large wounds, even on an immunosuppressed patient, was better than open wounds. For the most part, however, skin transplantation is an experimental technique used to examine the immunologic properties of rejection. It can be done rapidly on large numbers of animals and with high rates of technical success.

Two properties of skin graft rejection are unusual. First, skin grafts are extremely resistant to antibody-mediated rejection (Baldamus et al., 1973). They can survive in the face of preformed antibody and huge quantities of exogenous antibody must be given after about the tenth day to cause tissue destruction. This is probably because the vessels of the donor graft are not immediately connected to those of the recipient and it takes about a week for these connections to form. The resistance of skin grafts to humoral rejection makes them ideal for studying the cell-mediated aspects of rejection. Second, skin grafts elicit especially powerful immune responses. Therefore, the analysis of rejection mechanisms for skin often suggests a role for alloreactive responses (such as those involving CD8$^+$ cells without help from CD4$^+$ cells) that may not be available for the rejection of other organs. In addition, the amount of immunosuppression needed to prolong skin graft survival is greater than for other organs and tolerance to skin grafts is harder to induce than for many other tissues. These differences probably reflect the high density of antigen-presenting cells within skin that produces a stronger immunogenic challenge and a corresponding weaker down-regulating stimulus by parenchymal cells that lack APC function. These features may limit the generalizations about graft rejection that can be drawn from skin graft experiments, but they also suggest that skin transplantation can provide a more stringent test of immunosuppressive or tolerance-inducing strategies than can be provided by other tissues.

Kidney Transplantation

Clinical transplantation of the kidney is the prototype of organ transplantation, not only by history, but also because so many immunologic issues are relevant in this case. Since kidney recipients are usually clinically stable and the kidney transplant operation is relatively straightforward, technical failures usually do not cause the loss of renal allografts. Thus the results of kidney transplantation tend to reflect the limits imposed by immunologic factors. Since humans have two kidneys, living-related donation of kidneys is commonly undertaken. Since renal allografts are susceptible to hyperacute rejection, all of the issues connected with sensitization and cross-matching are important. Finally, since the kidneys can withstand relatively long cold ischemic times, the question of antigen matching is important as well.

One important feature of kidney transplantation is that relatively slight degrees of renal dysfunction can be detected by simple blood tests. This allows detection of rejection activity before the organ is irreversibly destroyed. It is now common practice to treat and *reverse* rejection by added immunosuppression, a possibility that was not recognized from early skin transplantation experiments, where the manifestations of rejection were not visible until the late stages of graft destruction. Furthermore, the easy detection of mild renal dysfunction has shown that clinical transplant rejection tends to occur as discrete events, referred to as *rejection episodes*. Experimental studies of kidney transplantation have also shown that rejection activity can spontaneously reverse without treatment, sometimes inducing a tolerant state. Thus the immunologists' view of rejection as an ongoing process, once it is initiated, does not adequately describe the process revealed by kidney transplantation.

Liver Transplantation

Liver transplantation is probably the most complex type of organ transplantation technically and it often involves extremely ill patients. These factors tend to dominate clinical liver transplantation. There are, however, some interesting immunologic issues associated with liver transplantation.

The liver is unusually *resistant to antibody-mediated rejection.* Despite the finding that liver endothelium does bind blood group and anti-HLA antibodies, hyperacute rejection of the liver is very rare and the outcome of liver transplantation is only slightly, if at all, worse when it is performed across blood group barriers or in the face of a positive cross-match. It is not clear whether this resistance is caused by the large size of the liver (thus distributing antibody binding at a subthreshold density), to the rapid modulation of antigens that bind antibodies, or to some other property of the liver.

The liver is also the organ for which antigen matching appears to be least beneficial and perhaps even harmful. This may reflect the importance of viruses as a cause of liver dysfunction as discussed earlier.

On the other hand, the liver, more than most other solid organs used in transplantation, carries with it substantial elements of the donor's immune system. Therefore, the liver can cause *graft-versus-host (GvH) reactions,* usually seen as hemolytic anemia when the blood group of the recipient is incompatible with that of the donor. Such GvH events are almost always self-limited, probably because the donor's immunologic elements are not replenished.

Although the short-term outcome of liver transplantation is less good than for some other organs (reflecting the technical demands and the illness of these patients), the long-term outcome for those patients who survive for 1 year is quite favorable. Very few patients loose their organs to chronic rejection and even patients who suffer several rejection episodes usually do not suffer

long-term damage to their liver. In part, this may reflect the unusual ability of the liver to repair itself after injury. It may also reflect a greater tolerance-inducing ability of liver allografts compared to other organs. Experimental liver transplantation can be performed successfully in rodents without any immunosuppression, even across MHC and minor histocompatibility barriers, and the recipients become tolerant to the donor antigens. This outcome has occasionally been achieved even in larger animals. In humans, several types of organ transplantation seem to have better outcomes when performed in conjunction with liver transplantation.

Pancreas Transplantation

Transplantation of the pancreas for treatment of diabetes mellitus lagged behind other types of organ transplantation for several reasons, including the technical difficulties of whole organ pancreas transplantation, the difficulty in detecting early rejection episodes affecting the pancreas, and the reluctance to substitute immunosuppressive therapy for insulin as treatment for diabetic patients. These issues were solved by improved technical approaches and especially by combining pancreas transplantation with kidney transplantation for patients suffering from diabetic nephropathy. The need for kidney transplantation in these patients justified the use of immunosuppression and the simultaneous presence of the donor kidney provided a way to detect rejection activity by changes in renal function. The results of whole organ pancreas combined with kidney transplantation are now nearly as good as for kidney transplantation alone.

A key immunologic assumption behind this strategy is that rejection activity affecting the kidney will reflect rejection affecting the pancreas. The better survival of pancreases transplanted with kidneys, rather than alone, supports this assumption. However, a few patients who have received both organs have lost one to rejection while maintaining function in the other. This outcome suggests that immunologic rejection may sometimes be directed at *tissue-specific antigens.* On the other hand, differences in organ survival may simply reflect different amounts of reserve function. While loss of 90% of kidney function may require a return to dialysis, loss of 90% of islets may still allow adequate blood sugar control.

The most intriguing feature of pancreas transplantation is the possibility that just *islet cells,* rather than the whole organ, might be used for insulin production. Such cell transplants could potentially be manipulated in several ways that are less applicable to whole organs, such as by depletion of donor APCs or by pretreatment with monoclonal antibodies. Cell transplants, like skin grafts that are not immediately vascularized, may also be less susceptible to preformed antibody-mediated rejection. Despite the encouraging success of islet transplantation in rodents, however, few successful transplants of pancreatic islets have been performed in humans.

Small Bowel Transplantation

The small bowel has proven to be one of the most difficult organs to transplant successfully and it is one of the organs that has shown the most benefit from simultaneous transplantation in conjunction with the liver. Whether the difficulty stems from a greater immunogenicity of the tissue or from a greater susceptibility to mild forms of rejection is not clear. From an immunologist's point of view, the organ is especially interesting because of the large amount of donor lymphoid tissue that is transplanted with the bowel. Although small bowel transplants can induce a GvH reaction, this response is self-limited and has not proven to be the primary obstacle to successful clinical transplantation.

Heart and Lung Transplantation

Hearts, hearts with lungs, and lungs alone are all now transplanted with high rates of success in human patients. Successful lung transplantation took longer to achieve primarily because the high doses of steroids in early immunosuppressive protocols were especially damaging to the tenuous bronchial anastomosis involved in lung transplantation. Thus transplantation of the lung benefited especially from the availability of cy-

closporine and other reagents that minimized the need for steroids.

As with combined kidney and pancreas transplantation, heart–lung transplants provide the opportunity to detect rejection of one organ that does not involve the other from the same donor. In this case, biopsies of both tissues can be obtained relatively easily and these have sometimes provided histologic evidence of *dysynchronous rejection.*

Lymphoid cells can be obtained from lung transplants by bronchial washings at regular intervals. Thus, for the immunologist, these transplants have provided an opportunity to monitor the types, reactivities, and specificities of the cells entering transplanted tissues. Studies of these cells, however, have so far not identified a well-characterized pattern that predicts rejection activity or severity.

A significant problem in heart transplantation is the development of *accelerated coronary artery disease* in the donor organ. In the case of lung transplantation, an analogous problem is the occurrence of *bronchiolitis obliterans.* It is widely believed that both conditions are manifestations of chronic rejection in these organs, but their immunologic origins and whether they are particularly related to humoral or cellular immune responses remain open to question. Some investigators suspect these lesions actually reflect chronic viral infections.

Bone Marrow Transplantation

Bone marrow transplantation is discussed in detail elsewhere in this book. In the context of this discussion of other organs, there are three important features to emphasize. First, unlike its marginal importance for solid organ transplantation, *HLA antigen matching* is the critical issue in bone marrow transplantation. Even the standard serologic methods of determining the HLA phenotype of patients is not sufficient to obtain the best clinical results. This has been the primary stimulus for new molecular techniques of tissue typing. Second, whereas GvH disease is an immunologically interesting, but clinically small, problem in organ transplantation, it is a very important part of bone marrow transplantation, often causing severe morbidity and even mortality. Third, the immunologic mechanisms of both host-versus-graft responses and of graft-versus-host disease associated with bone marrow transplantation are not precisely the same as those involved in nonlymphoid tissue transplantation. Natural killer cells, especially, play a prominent role in bone marrow transplantation, but have not been shown to participate in the rejection of solid organs.

CONCLUSION

This discussion should again highlight the many unanswered questions in the field of transplantation. Although the issues discussed in this chapter arise in clinical medicine, the answers are not likely to be found in studies of patient care. Rather these questions indicate the many important areas in which the science of immunology may be able to contribute to better clinical medicine.

REFERENCES

Baldamus CA, McKenzie IFC, Winn HJ, Russell PS (1973): Acute destruction by humoral antibody of rat skin grafted to mice. J Immunol 110:1532–1541.

Cosimi AB, Wortis H, Delmonico F, Russell PS (1976): Randomized clinical trial of antitymocyte globulin in cadaver renal allograft recipients. Surgery 80:155–161.

Gordon RD, Fung JJ, Markus B, Fox I, Iwatsuki S, Esquivel CO, Tzakis A, Todo S, Starzl TE (1986):

The antibody crossmatch in liver transplantation. Surgery 100:705–15.

Middleton D, Gillespie EL, Doherty CC, Douglas JF, McGeown MG (1985): The influence of HLA-A,B, and DR matching on graft survival in primary cadaveric renal transplantation in Belfast. Transplantation 39:608–610.

Muluk SC, Clerici M, Via CS, Weir MR, Kimmel PL, Shearer GM (1991): Correlation of in vitro CD4+ T helper cell function with clinical graft status in immunosuppressed kidney transplant recipients. Transplantation 52:284–291.

Opelz G (1987): Improved kidney graft survival in nontransfused recipients. Trans Proc 19:149–52.

Opelz G, Terasaki PI (1980): Dominant effect of transfusion on kidney graft survival. Transplantation 29:153.

Opelz G, Terasaki PI (1982): International study of histocompatibility in renal transplantation. Transplantation 33:87.

Pescovitz MD, Thistlethwaite JR Jr., Auchincloss H Jr, Ildstad ST, Sharp TG, Terrill R, Sachs DH (1984): Effect of class II antigen matching of renal allograft survival in miniature swine. J Exp Med 160:1495–1508.

Sanfilippo F, Vaughn WK, Spees EK, Heise ER, LeFor WM (1984): The effect of HLA-A,-B matching on cadaver renal allograft rejection comparing public and private specificities. Transplantation 38:483–489.

Solez K, McGraw DJ, Beschorner WE, Burdick JF (1986): Pathology of "acute tubular necrosis" and acute rejection: Observations on early systematic renal transplant biopsies. In Williams GM, Burdick JF, Solez K (eds): "Kidney Transplant Rejection." New York: Marcel Dekker, pp 207–224.

Starzl TE, Demetris AJ, Murase N, Ildstad S, Ricordi C, Trucco M (1992): Cell migration, chimerism, and graft acceptance. Lancet 339:1579–82.

Chapter 8
Pancreas and Islet Cell Transplantation

David Sutherland, Rainer Gruessner, and Paul Gores

INTRODUCTION

Pancreas and islet transplantation is the only treatment of type I diabetes that can establish an insulin-independent state (Sutherland, 1992). The success rate with pancreas transplantation is high relative to that with islets (Sutherland, 1993). Of pancreas transplants done in the past several years, > 70% of the recipients are insulin independent at 1 year after the procedure (Sutherland et al., 1994), while with islet allografts, even in the 1990s, long-term insulin independence has occurred in < 10% (Hering et al., 1993). Many problems remain to be overcome before islet allotransplantation will be as successful as pancreas transplants (Sutherland, 1992), and these will be discussed at the end of this review.

PANCREAS TRANSPLANTS

After a successful pancreas transplant euglycemia is constant and glycosylated hemoglobin levels are normalized as long as the graft is not rejected or afflicted by recurrence of disease (Morel et al., 1991a; Sutherland et al., 1989b). The penalty for achieving such a state is the need for immunosuppression (Sutherland, 1991). Thus most pancreas transplants are performed in diabetic patients with nephropathy who are obligated to immunosuppression because of a kidney transplant (Sollinger et al., 1988; Sutherland et al., 1993b). Nonuremic patients whose problems of diabetes are or predictably will be more serious than the potential side effects of antirejection drugs (cyclosporine, aza-

thioprine, corticosteroids) are also candidates for a pancreas transplant (Sutherland et al., 1988), but the proportion of pancreas transplant recipients in this category has been small to date (Sutherland et al., 1993b).

In uremic diabetic patients retinopathy and neuropathy are usually far advanced. Although eye function may stabilize over the long term (Ramsay et al., 1988) and nerve function may even improve (Kennedy et al., 1990), the main immediate value of adding a pancreas to a kidney transplant is the improved quality of life that comes with being insulin independent as well as being dialysis free (Gross and Zehrer, 1993). A successful pancreas transplant also prevents recurrence of diabetic nephropathy in the new kidney, an additional benefit for the long-term survivor (Bilous et al., 1989).

In nonuremic patients the potential to influence the appearance or progression of secondary complications exists, but because the penalties associated with immunosuppression or the specific side effects of the antirejection drugs may be greater in an individual patient than the complications of diabetes that were otherwise destined to appear, pancreas transplants are not usually done for this reason alone. This may change in the future as antirejection strategies with fewer side effects are developed; indeed, new drugs are currently being tested in clinical trials involving other organs. For now, however, pancreas transplants alone are primarily reserved for the nonuremic patient whose diabetes is extremely labile no matter what insulin regimen is tried and whose day-to-day living is severely compromised for this reason alone.

Transplantation Immunology, pages 147–160
© 1995 Wiley-Liss, Inc.

The most extensive experience with pancreas transplantation in nonuremic diabetic patients is at the University of Minnesota (Sutherland et al., 1993a). Even though extreme lability is a main indication, most patients have had diabetes for many years and have complications. Autonomic neuropathy in this group is common and usually is associated with gastroenteropathy with erratic food absorption, defective glucose counter-regulatory mechanisms, and hypoglycemic un-awareness, making calculations of doses diffi-cult and any method of exogenous insulin administration unsatisfactory or even hazardous.

The recipient of a pancreas transplant alone may or may not have other complications, such as retinopathy or nephropathy. Cyclosporine is nephrotoxic, and this can be a problem in some patients. Patients with a creatinine clearance rate greater than 60 ml/min usually tolerate the dos-age of cyclosporine necessary to prevent rejec-tion of the pancreas (Morel et al., 1991b). How-ever, if the creatinine clearance rate is less, the

functional deterioration already in progress from the underlying kidney disease may continue. At the University of Minnesota, approximately 80% of the recipients of pancreas transplants alone have had normal or nearly normal renal function, whereas in approximately 20% ne-phropathy was moderately advanced at the time of the transplant (Wang et al., 1993).

Graft Functional Survival Rates

Worldwide, more than 5000 transplants had been reported to the International Pancreas Transplant Registry (IPTR) by the end of 1993 (Sutherland et al., 1994), including more than 3000 in the United States (Fig. 1). Since October 1987 it has been mandatory to report outcome on cases in the United States to the IPTR through the United Network for Organ Sharing (UNOS), the organization that operates the Organ Pro-curement and Transplant Network in the United States under the auspices of the Department of

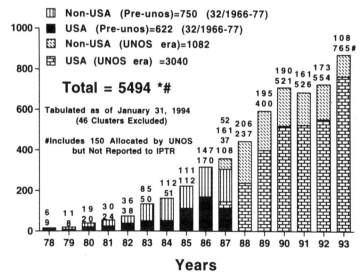

Fig. 1. Number of pancreas transplants tabulated by the International Pancreas Transplant Registry (IPTR) for 1966 to 1993 before and after the advent of the United Network of Organ Sharing (UNOS). The re-porting for 1993 is incomplete. The total number of cases for the United States (USA) was 3662 (45 clus-ters) and for the non-USA was 1832 (1 cluster). The world total with cluster cases included was 5540 (Sutherland et al., 1994).

Health and Human Services (Sutherland et al., 1994).

Of approximately 2500 U.S. pancreas transplants in the UNOS/IPTR data base for analysis as of November 1993, about 94% were in patients who also received a kidney transplant, either simultaneously ($\sim$ 2100) or prior ($\sim$ 200) to the pancreas transplant. With success defined as insulin independence, the best results have been with simultaneous pancreas and kidney (SPK) transplants with a 1 year pancreas functional survival rate of over 75%, compared to approximately 50% in the pancreas after kidney (PAK) and pancreas transplant alone (PTA) categories (Fig. 2). The recipients can return to exogenous insulin therapy if the pancreas graft fails, and patient survival rates at 1 year have been greater than 90% in all categories (Fig. 3).

The higher pancreas graft functional survival rate in the SPK category appears to be related to the ability to use the kidney graft as a monitor for rejection episodes, the physiologic manifestations of rejection appearing earlier in the kidney (increase in creatinine) than in the pancreas. In addition, uremia itself may blunt the immune response.

The UNOS Registry as well as the U.S. Renal Data System (USRDS) have calculated kidney and patient survival rates in recipients of SPK versus diabetic recipients of cadaveric kidney transplants alone (KTA) (Sutherland et al., 1993b; United States Renal Disease System, 1992). In the slightly older USRDS database the patient and kidney survival rates were similar in the two groups, whereas in the UNOS analysis kidney graft survival rates were significantly higher in the SPK group (82% at 1 year) than in the KTA group (78% at 1 year). This difference may reflect the selection of uremic diabetic patients in better physiologic condition for the SPK than the KTA procedure, because analyses at individual centers have shown higher incidence of rejection episodes and surgical complications in SPK than in KTA recipients (Sutherland, 1992; Cheung et al., 1992).

Most pancreas transplants are currently per-

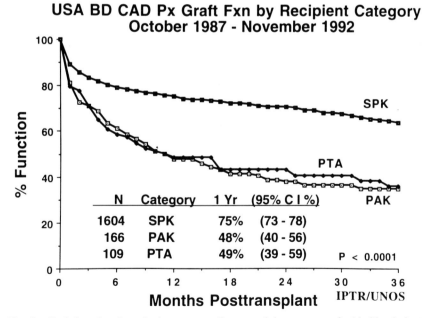

Fig. 2. Graft functional survival rates according to recipient category for bladder drained (BD) cadaveric pancreas transplants reported to IPTR/UNOS 1987–1992. SPK = simultaneous pancreas/kidney transplant, PAK = pancreas after kidney transplant, and PTA = pancreas transplant alone. (Sutherland et al., 1993b.)

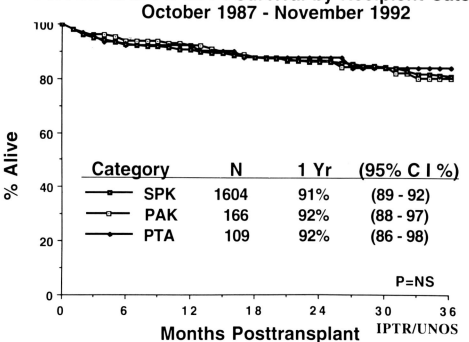

USA BD CAD Px Tx Pt Survival by Recipient Category
October 1987 - November 1992

Category	N	1 Yr	(95% C I %)
SPK	1604	91%	(89 - 92)
PAK	166	92%	(88 - 97)
PTA	109	92%	(86 - 98)

P=NS

Fig. 3. Patient survival rates according to recipient category for bladder drained (BD) cadaveric pancreas transplants reported to IPTR/UNOS 1987–1992. SPK = simultaneous pancreas/kidney transplant, PAK = pancreas after kidney transplant, and PTA = pancreas transplant alone. (Sutherland et al., 1993b.)

formed with the exocrine secretions drained into the bladder, allowing the level of urine amylase to be monitored; a decline in this level is a manifestation and a marker of rejection (Prieto et al., 1987). In SPK recipients an elevation of the level of serum creatinine usually precedes a decrease in exocrine or endocrine function during rejection episodes, making monitoring of urine amylase largely superfluous for this group. In PTA recipients, however, serum creatinine cannot be used as a monitor for rejection. Fortuitously, a decline in exocrine function (decreased urine amylase) almost always precedes a decline in endocrine function (increased blood sugar) as a manifestation of rejection. Thus the possibility exists to improve the results of PTA procedures by treating rejection episodes based on a decline in urine amylase before endocrine dysfunction occurs.

At the University of Minnesota such an approach (early treatment of solitary pancreas re-

jection episodes based on a decline in urine amylase) was taken beginning in 1988 (Sutherland et al., 1989a). In addition, it was also noted that results of solitary pancreas transplants were better in recipients of grafts from donors who were well matched to recipients with respect to HLA antigens. Of 133 solitary bladder-drained cadaver pancreas transplants performed at the University of Minnesota between November 1984 and 1991 (Sutherland et al., 1992), the actuarial 1 year insulin-independent (graft-function) rates were 80% for those mismatched for none or only one HLA, A, B, DR antigens ($n = 15$) versus 56% for those mismatched for two to three antigens ($n = 44$) and 44% for those mismatched for four to six antigens ($n = 74$). Thus beginning in 1988 emphasis was also placed on doing the best matches possible for recipients of solitary pancreas transplants.

In the subgroup of PAK patients between 1988 to 1991 who received the kidney from a related donor followed by a primary bladder-drained pancreas from a cadaver donor ($n = 17$), the 1 year insulin-independent rate was 72% (Cheung et al., 1993).

For uremic diabetic patients referred to the University of Minnesota Hospital, emphasis is placed on pursuing strategies that maximize the probability of long-term kidney function (Sutherland et al., 1993a). Thus, for patients who have a willing family member, we recommend a kidney transplant from a living related donor with the option of subsequently receiving a pancreas transplant. Only if there is no living related donor for a kidney transplant do we recommend a simultaneous PAK transplant from a cadaver donor. Over a decade, the rejection rates are much lower for kidneys from living related than from cadaver donors. Thus, by pursuing this strategy, the maximum number of patients can be rendered dialysis free for a life time. Furthermore, the insulin-independent rates with PAK transplants now approach those achieved with SPK transplants (United States Renal Disease System, 1992). Thus, the incentive to defer a pancreas transplant to achieve the advantage of a living donor kidney is even greater than before.

Effect on Complications

Studies on the effect of pancreas transplantation on secondary diabetic complications have been mixed. Advanced retinopathy is present preoperatively in most patients, and progression has been observed in up to 30% of recipients during the first 3 years posttransplantation whether the pancreas graft was successful or not: however, after 3 years retinopathy in the patients with functioning pancreas grafts has been observed to stabilize, whereas deterioration has continued to occur in those in whom grafts have failed (Ramsay et al., 1988).

In regard to neuropathy, improvement in nerve conduction velocities and stabilization of evoked muscle action potentials and of autonomic neuropathy have occurred in recipients of successful pancreas grafts, whereas deterioration has continued in those in whom grafts have failed (Kennedy et al., 1990; Solders et al., 1992). Indeed, in diabetic patients with severe neuropathy, those who undergo a successful pancreas

transplant have a significantly higher probability of survival than those in whom transplantation is not done or is unsuccessful (Bilous et al., 1987).

In regard to nephropathy, microscopic lesions of diabetes in the native kidneys of recipients with successful PTA procedures may stabilize or regress, but new lesions from cyclosporine can appear (Fioretto et al., 1993). Nevertheless, after an initial decline, renal function usually plateaus. In recipients of kidney transplants, a successful pancreas transplant can definitely prevent recurrence of diabetic nephropathy (Bilous et al., 1989).

Effect on Quality of Life

Many studies have been conducted on metabolism in patients following pancreas transplantation, and these are of great interest to endocrinologists (Diem et al., 1990). For patients and their physicians, however, the main question is what effect a successful pancreas transplant has on quality of life. Several studies have been published in this regard, and they are nearly unanimous in reporting that patients with successful transplants rate their quality of life to be better after than before procedure (Zehrer and Gross, 1991; Gross and Zehrer, 1992, 1993; Nakache et al., 1991). Pancreas transplants in patients with hyperlabile diabetes and extreme difficulty with metabolic control improve quality of life simply by inducing insulin independence (Zehrer and Gross, 1991; Bolinder et al., 1991). In uremic patients kidney transplants alone can improve quality of life by obviating the need for dialysis (Jacobson et al., 1988). Some lability is not uncommon in uremic patents, and in such patients the effect of a double transplant can be dramatic; two difficult clinical problems are corrected for as long as rejection is prevented by immunosuppression (Gross and Zehrer, 1993; Nakache et al., 1991).

For patients without nephropathy who undergo a PTA procedure, the price to rid themselves of diabetes is the same, that is, chronic immunosuppression. The natural question to ask is whether the benefit is worth the price. Recipients of pancreas transplants have emphatically stated that it is (Harmer, 1990; Loseke, 1990). In the largest study to date (Gross and Zehrer, 1992,

1993), 131 patients were analyzed 1 to 10 years posttransplantation; half had functioning grafts ($n = 65$), and half had grafts that ultimately failed ($n = 66$). Overall, 92% felt that managing immunosuppression was easier than managing diabetes (Gross and Zehrer, 1993). When asked which was more demanding of their family's time and energy, 63% felt that the diabetes was more demanding, 29% felt the two were equal, and 9% felt that the transplant was more demanding. Of the 65 patients with functioning grafts, 89% stated that they were more healthy than before the transplant. Indices of well-being as quantified by standard tests were significantly higher in patients with functioning grafts than in those without. Virtually 100% of the patients with continuing graft function and 85% of those whose graft ultimately failed said they would encourage others with similar complications of diabetes to consider pancreas transplantation. In addition, most of the patients with failed graft desired retransplantation, and those with functioning grafts said they would undergo a retransplant if their current graft failed.

Cost

Benefits must be weighed against the cost of the procedure (Evans et al., 1993). Many U.S. Transplant Centers routinely offer pancreas transplants to uremic diabetic recipients of renal allografts. In many instances the determining factor as to whether a pancreas transplant is added to the kidney depends on whether financial coverage is available. Kidney transplants are routinely covered by Medicare or private insurance, but coverage of the pancreas transplant is highly variable. Approximately 50 insurance companies have covered pancreas transplants. The average hospital charges for cadaveric pancreas/kidney transplants is approximately $40,000 more than those associated with a kidney transplant alone, with $16,000 being for the organ procurement and $24,000 for the additional care required. For recipients of a pancreas transplant performed as a solitary procedure (nonuremic patients or nephropathic patients with a previous kidney transplant), the average hospitalization cost is $65,000. Following the transplant, there

are also the ongoing costs of the immunosuppressive drugs. Patients who have also had a kidney transplant have this expense even without pancreas transplantation. However, for the nonuremic recipient the costs of these drugs are assumed solely for maintenance of the pancreas, and this can amount to several thousand dollars per year.

Thus, in uremic diabetic patients who receive a kidney, the only additional costs of adding a pancreas are those associated with the initial hospitalization. In nonuremic patients all the costs associated with pancreas transplantation are directly related to treatment of diabetes.

It is more expensive to treat diabetes with a pancreas transplant than with insulin injections. If secondary complications are ameliorated, health care costs over a lifetime may be less than if the recipient remained diabetic, but individual variations are considerable. Although more expensive, the enhanced quality of life that ensues following a pancreas transplant in patients with hyperlabile diabetes makes the procedure worth the cost. Furthermore, in these patients medical costs are high. Even though exogenous insulin itself is cheap, the need for hospitalizations and close monitoring by physicians and other health care personnel can approach the intensity of follow-up needed for posttransplant patients. This consideration is apart from the potential for amelioration of secondary complications, which may occur following a pancreas transplant; this benefit may translate into a financial one for individuals who were otherwise destined to develop such problems.

ISLET CELL TRANSPLANTS

Islet allografts, either purified or in the form of dispersed pancreatic tissue, is very successful in experimental rodent models, but it is much less so in large animals and man. Only 11 fully documented cases of insulin independence have occurred in the 139 attempts of clinical islet allotransplantation since 1974 (Federlin et al., 1993). Slow progress is, however, being made (Fig. 4). When the achievement of a basal C-peptide level in excess of 1 ng/ml at 1 month is used in place of the more rigorous endpoint of

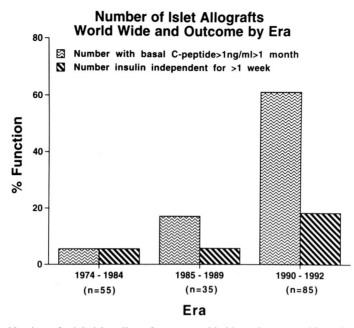

Fig. 4. Number of adult islet allograft cases worldwide and percent able to be insulin independent and with basal C-peptide after transplantation by era up to December 31, 1992. From Hering et al. (1993).

insulin independence, steady improvement in clinical results has occurred. Analysis of International Islet Transplant Registry data shows that in the era of 1974–1984 only 3 of 55 (5%) cases achieved this endpoint in contrast to 6 of 35 (17%) in 1985–1989, and 52 of 85 (61%) in 1990–1992.

The problems preventing the stable engraftment of a sufficient number of islets to achieve a state of insulin independence may be broadly classified into four categories: (1) transplantation of an insufficient mass of viable islets, (2) immune-mediated destruction of transplanted islet tissue, (3) drug toxicity, and (4) metabolic exhaustion.

Transplantation of Insufficient Islet Mass

The precise number of transplanted islets required to render a Type 1 diabetic patient insulin independent is not known. The relevant quantity is the amount of islet tissue effectively engrafted rather than the number of islets transplanted. The percentage of islets transplanted that are actually

engrafted is likely to vary considerably according to the site chosen for transplantation. Most clinical islet transplants have utilized the portal circulation as the site of implantation.

Data from clinical studies of islet autotransplantation in patients undergoing total duodenopancreatectomy show that 3,500 islets/kg are able to maintain fasting normoglycemia and normal glycosylated hemoglobin levels (Farney et al., 1991; Pyzdrowski et al., 1992). In Type 1 diabetic patient, islet engraftment may be adversely affected by the presence of long-standing microangiopathy, long-term engraftment may be hampered by the presence of autoimmunity, and insulin resistance may be present (Rayman et al., 1986; Cuthbertson et al., 1988; Moller and Flier, 1991).

The normal human pancreas contains on average approximately 1,000,000 islets of 150 mm equivalent diameter (I.E.) (Hellman, 1959; Saito et al., 1978). However, the number is quite variable with the range varying by a factor of 5. The number of islets that are recovered after intraductal collagenase digestion of the gland and subsequent density gradient centrifugation is also extremely variable.

Currently islet yields are calculated by manually counting the number of islets (as identified by dithazone staining) in an aliquot of the preparation (Ricordi et al., 1990). This type of quantification is based on crude morphology and does not give an accurate determination of the number of the *viable* islets present. Islets may be irreversibly damaged during the period of collagenase digestion, or while undergoing centrifugation on hyperosmolar gradients.

The use of multiple donors poses certain logistical problems and is not desirable from an immunologic point of view. The survival of immediately vascularized pancreas allografts is enhanced by good HLA matching and the use of multiple donors precludes good matching (Gores et al., 1992).

A practical alternative to the use of multiple donors is the use of unpurified dispersed pancreatic tissue prepared from 1 cadaver donor (Gores et al., 1993). This increases the islet yield approximately 2-fold, and since the tissue is not subjected to hyperosmolar density gradients, the yield of the viable islets is probably enhanced even more.

Little experimental work has addressed the question of the relative immunogenicity of exocrine and endocrine tissue. In a congenic mouse model a hand picked preparation consisting of 60% islets and 40% exocrine tissue survives just as well as a clean hand-picked preparation (Gores et al., 1986). However, if donor strain splenocytes are added to either of the preparations, the islet allografts are in all cases readily rejected. Gotoh et al. (1986) conducted a similar experiment on an inbred rat model. They observed that purified hand-picked islets survived significantly longer than a crude preparation consisting of islets exocrine tissue and contaminating lymphoid cells. They also demonstrated that purified islets would be uniformly rapidly rejected if donor strain splenocytes were simultaneously injected intravenously. Taken together, these studies demonstrate that lymphoid and not acinar contamination significantly increases the immunogenicity of islet allografts.

However, it must be emphasized that the results above are relative. Purified islets are rejected and when examined *in vitro* in a mixed lymphocyte/islet coculture system, they elicit an immune response, albeit less than that evoked by crude islet preparations (Stock et al., 1991; Ulrichs and Muller-Ruchholtz, 1990). Even rigorously purified β cells evoke an immune response *in vitro* unless responder (as well as simulator) antigen-presenting cells are removed from the system (Stock et al., 1991).

Since at present in large animal models systemic immunosuppression of the recipient cannot be avoided, a reasonable strategy is to utilize unpurified dispersed pancreatic tissue, thereby dramatically increasing the yield of viable islets and enhancing the probability of successful islet transplantation utilizing islets from a single cadaver donor. Since pancreatic ductal cells function as the stem cell for islet neogenesis (Bonner-Weir et al., 1993), this strategy also theoretically leaves open the possibility of expansion of the β cell mass over time.

Immune Mediated Destruction

Allogeneic islet tissue may be destroyed by nonspecific inflammatory damage, antigen-specific T cell-mediated cytolosis, or the recurrence of autoimmunity.

Nonspecific inflammatory damage. The cytokines interleukin 1 (IL-1), interleukin 6 (IL-6), and tumor necrosis factor-α (TNF-α) interact synergistically in their regulation of inflammation (Arai et al., 1990). Il-1 is a potent modulator of insulin secretion and at high concentrations is cytodestructive to pancreatic islet β and α cells (Bendtzen et al., 1986; Ling et al., 1993).

Macrophages infiltrate freshly transplanted islet grafts and predominate in grafts exhibiting poor initial function after transplantation (Kaufman et al., 1990). Most clinical attempts at islet transplantation utilize the portal circulation as the site of implantation. The islets become lodged in the presinusoidal space lined by Kupffer cells. When activated, these hepatic macrophages produce a variety of β cell toxic molecules (Nathan, 1987). Thus they may play an important role in the early destruction of transplanted islet tissue. In rodents this early destruction is inhibited by the macrophage toxin silica (Kaufman et al., 1990), as well as the novel immunosuppressive agent 15-deoxyspergualin (Kaufman et al., 1992), which has antimacrophage (Walter et al., 1987) as well as anti-T cell effects. In addition, administration of a specific nitric oxide inhibitor (N-monomethyl-L-arginine) improves the early function of rodent isografts (Stevens et al., 1994) as does injection of soluble TNF receptor (Farney et al., 1993).

Antigen-specific T cell-mediated rejection. As is the case with all allogeneic tissue, islet grafts are susceptible to classic T cell-mediated rejection. A major impediment to the successful application of islet transplantation in humans has been lack of a suitable means to detect a rejection response soon after its initiation. Currently, the only means of monitoring islet allograft function is determination of serum glucose and C-peptide levels. By the time the serum glucose level is elevated, the majority of the graft has been destroyed and it is too late to initiate effective antirejection therapy. C-peptide levels are cumbersome; the assay is not readily available in the community and requires several days before results are known. In addition, in the prebladder drainage era of pancreas transplantation, C-peptides were not found useful as a means of early detection of rejection in vascularized pancreatic allografts (Sutherland et al., 1984). Thus, at the present time, the best chance of success is when islets from only 1 donor are used and the kidney from the same cadaver donor is transplanted simultaneously so that serum creatinine can be used to monitor the presence of a rejection against donor tissue.

The successful application of islet transplantation in patients with previously transplanted functioning kidney allografts (IAK) or islet transplantation alone (ITA) in preuremic patients requires the development of a rejection-free protocol. Currently no such protocol exists for solid organ transplantation. However, 60% of patients receiving a renal allograft from a cadaver donor never experience rejection (Frey et al., 1992).

Therefore, with current immunosuppressive protocols one might expect that if sufficient islets survived the initial generalized inflammatory reaction and stably engraft, 60% of these patients would experience long-term islet allograft function.

A variety of protocols utilizing culture (Simeonovic et al., 1980), antibody (Faustman et al., 1981) or deoxyguanosine pretreatment (Al-Abdullah et al., 1991), or irradiation (Lau et al., 1984), often in combination with a brief course of systemic immunosuppression, have been successful in rodent models. These protocols have been tried in large animal models but either no benefit or only slight prolongation of islet graft function has been observed (Stegall et al., 1989; Kenyon et al., 1990).

A final approach worth mentioning that is successful in rodent models is intrathymic injection of donor antigen (islets or bone marrow) (Posselt et al., 1990, 1992) in conjunction with a short course of immunosuppression prior to islet transplantation in the periphery. This appears to result in donor-specific transplantation tolerance; however, to date this approach has not been successful in large animal models.

Drug Toxicity

After human islet transplantation, we are invariably dealing with a mass of viable islet cells that is at best marginally adequate to maintain a normal metabolic state. The immunosuppressive therapy used after islet transplantation is based on the protocols that have been developed for solid organ transplantation. Many of these agents are diabetogenic, and when used in combination, are even more so (Boudreaux et al., 1987). For example, 19% of previously nondiabetic kidney transplant recipients develop altered glucose metabolism after being placed on the combination of cyclosporine, azathioprine, and prednisone (Boudreaux et al., 1987).

Corticosteroids are known to induce insulin resistance in experimental animals and in man (Kahn et al., 1987; Cigolini and Smith, 1979). It is unlikely that islet transplantation will achieve significant levels of success as long as immunosuppressive regimens remain corticosteroid based. To maintain normoglycemia, nondiabetic kidney transplant recipients on triple immunotherapy must increase insulin secretion (as measured by C-peptide) $2^1/_2$ times (Scharp et al., 1991). When one considers that even with the use of unpurified islets, approximately half of the islet mass is lost during digestion, and invariably more is lost during the process of transplantation and engraftment, it is not surprising that single donor islet transplants rarely result in levels of insulin secretion sufficient to overcome the toxic effects of the drug used to prevent rejection.

Of the new agents currently being tested, FK506 is frankly diabetogenic (Mieles et al., 1991), however, 15-deoxyspergualin does not impair glucose-induced insulin secretion from either normal human or rat islets, and does not lead to insulin resistance in intact rats (Xenos et al., 1993). Furthermore, in clinical studies to date, no evidence of a diabetogenic tendency has emerged. RS-61443 does not appear to disturb glucose metabolism *in vivo* (Platz et al., 1991), although it may reduce glucose-mediated insulin secretion *in vitro* (Sandberg and Anderson, 1993). Rapamycin, when used in high dose, has been associated with the development of diabetes (Morris, 1992).

Metabolic Exhaustion

Sustained hyperglycemia renders β cells glucose unresponsive and if hyperglycemia is severe and prolonged, leads to direct β cell destruction (Dohan and Lukens, 1947; Leahy et al., 1992). The toxic effect is reversible if hyperglycemia is of short duration, however, prolonged exposure to hyperglycemia results in irreversible damage. Transplantation of insufficient islet number to maintain normoglycemia leads to a continuous decline in β cell mass (Montana et al., 1993).

Furthermore, hyperglycemia itself has been shown both *in vitro* (Garvey et al., 1987) and *in vivo* (Kahn et al., 1991) to lead to insulin resistance, which further exacerbates the hyperglycemia. Thus a vicious cycle occurs where the toxic effects of immunosuppressive drugs lead to

hyperglycemia, which itself causes further insulin resistance and β cell dysfunction. Fortunately, control of hyperglycemia by exogenous administration of insulin is able to reverse these effects (Zeng et al., 1993; Korsgren et al., 1989), with the hope being that insulin therapy may be withdrawn once the doses of immunosuppressive agents are lowered to baseline.

SUMMARY

Pancreas transplantation is currently a routine therapy in diabetic renal allograft recipients. It is also used to treat selected nonuremic patients with extremely labile diabetes or other diabetic problems that are not well-served by the alternative. Further expansion will depend upon advanced in specific immunosuppression and upon donor availability.

Transplantation of islets separately from the pancreas as free grafts has been successful in a few patients who also received kidney grafts (Gores et al., 1993) but there are many failures as well (Hering et al., 1993). Islet transplantation is clearly more difficult to apply clinically than pancreas transplants. From a recipient view point, it is a much simpler procedure, but from the viewpoint of a transplanter, everything but the surgery is more difficult. Nevertheless, success has been achieved, with long-term insulin independence now in a handful of patients. In those who still need insulin, but also have detectable C-peptide, diabetes management is easier and it is possible to normalize glycohemoglobin, something rarely achieved by insulin alone. However, immunosuppression is still needed and the indications for islet transplants at present are much less broad than for pancreas transplantation.

All of the problems with islet transplantation enumerated above are solvable. We would expect islet transplantation to replace pancreas transplantation in the future, first for cadaver donors with a kidney and later as a solitary procedure.

For now the only treatment that can "cure" diabetes today with a high success rate is pancreas transplantation. It is applicable to virtually all diabetic recipients of kidney transplants, and to selected nonuremic patients with difficult control problems.

REFERENCES

Al-Abdullah IH, Kumar AM, Al-Adnani MS, Abouna GM (1991): Prolongation of allograft survival in diabetic rats treated with cyclosporine by deoxyguanosine pretreatment of pancreatic islets of Langerhans. Transplantation 51:967–971.

Arai KE, Lee F, Mijajima A, Myatake S, Arai N, Yokota T (1990): Cytokines: Coordinators of immune and inflammatory responses. Annu Rev Biochem 59:783–836.

Bendtzen K, Mandrup-Poulsen T, Nerup J, Nielsen JH, Dinarello CA, Svenson M (1986): Cytotoxicity of human pl 7 interleukin-1 for pancreatic islets of Langerhans. Science 232:1545–1547.

Bilous RW, Mauer SM, Sutherland DER, Steffes MW (1987): Glomerular structure and function following successful pancreas transplantation for insulin-dependent diabetes mellitus. Diabetes 36:43A.

Bilous RW, Mauer SM, Sutherland DER, Najarian JS, Goetz FC, Steffes MW (1989): The effects of pancreas transplantation on the glomerular structure of renal allografts in patients with insulin-dependent diabetes. N Engl J Med 321:80–85.

Bonner-Weir S, Baxter LA, Schuppin GT, Smith FE (1993): A second pathway for regeneration of adult exocrine and edocrine pancreas: A possible recapitulation of embryonic development. Diabetes 42:1715–1720.

Boudreaux JP, McHugh L, Canafax DM (1987): The impact of cyclosporine and combination immunosuppression on the incidence of posttransplant diabetes in renal allograft recipients. Transplantation 44:376–381.

Cheung AHS, Sutherland DER, Gillingham KJ, McHugh LE, Moudry-Munns KC, Dunn DL, Najarian JS, Matas AJ (1992): Simultaneous pancreas-kidney (SPK) transplant versus kidney transplant alone (KTA) in diabetic patients. Kidney Int 41:924–929.

Cheung AHS, Matas AJ, Gruessner RWG, Dunn DL, Moudry-Munns KC, Najarian JS, Sutherland DER (1993): Should uremic diabetic patients who want a pancreas transplant receive a simultaneous cadaver kidney-pancreas transplant or a living related donor kidney first followed by cadaver pancreas transplant? Transplant Proc 25:1184–1185.

Cigolini M, Smith U (1979): Human adipose tissue in culture VIII. Studies on the insulin-antagonistic effect of glucocorticoids. Metabolism 28:502.

Cuthbertson RA, Koulmanda M, Mandel TE (1988): Detrimental effect of chronic diabetes on growth and function of fetal islet isografts in mice. Transplantation 46:650–654.

Diem P, Redmon JB, Abid M, Moran A, Sutherland DER, Halter JB, Robertson RP (1990): Glucagon, catecholamine and pancreatic polypeptide secretion in type I diabetic recipients of pancreas allografts. J Clin Invest 86:2008–2013.

Dohan FC, Lukens FEW (1947): Lesions of the pancreatic islets produced in cats by administration of glucose. Science 105:183.

Evans RW, Manninen DL, Dong FB (1993): An economic analysis of pancreas transplantation: Costs, insurance coverage, and reimbursement. Clin Transplant 7:166–174.

Farney AC, Najarian JS, Nakhleh RE, Lloveras G, Field MJ, Gores PF, Sutherland DER (1991): Autotransplantation of dispersed pancreatic islet tissue combined with total or near-total pancreatectomy for treatment of chronic pancreatitis. Surgery 110:427–439.

Farney AC, Xenos ES, Sutherland DER (1993): Inhibition of pancreatic islet beta cell function by tumor necrosis factor is blocked by a soluble tumor necrosis factor receptor. Transplant Proc 25:865–866.

Faustman D, Hauptfeld V, Lacy P, Davie J (1981): Prolongation of murine allograft survival by pretreatment of islets with antibody directed to Ia determinants. Proc Natl Acad Sci USA 78:5156.

Federlin KF, Bretzel RG, Hering BJ (1993): International islet transplant registry. Newletter 4(3).

Fioretto P, Mauer SM, Bilous RW, Goetz FC, Sutherland DER, Steffes MW (1993): Effects of pancreas transplantation on glomerulo structure in insulin-dependent diabetic patients with their own kidneys. Lancet 342:1193–1196.

Frey DJ, Matas AJ, Gillingham KJ (1992): Sequential therapy—A prospective randomized trial of MALG versus OKT3 for prophylactic immunosuppression in cadaver renal allograft recipients. Transplantation 54:50–56.

Garvey WT, Olefsky JM, Matthaei S, Marshall S (1987): Glucose and insulin coregulate the glucose transport system in primary cultured adiopocytes: A new mechanism of insulin resistance. J Biol Chem 262:189–197.

Gores PF, Mayoral JL, Field MJ, Sutherland DER (1986): Comparison of the immunogenicity of purified and unpurified murine islet allografts. Transplantation 41:529–531.

Gores PF, Gillingham KJ, Dunn DL, Moudry-Munns KC, Najarian JS, Sutherland DER (1992): Donor hyperglycemia as a minor risk factor and immunologic variables as major risk factors for pancreas allograft loss in a multivariate analysis of a single institutions's experience. Ann Surg 215:217–230.

Gores PF, Najarian JS, Stephanian E, Lloveras JJ, Kelley SL, Sutherland DER (1993): Insulin independence in type I diabetes after transplantation of unpurified islets from a single donor using 15-deoxyspergualin. Lancet 341:19–21.

Gotoh M, Maki T, Satomi S, Porter J, Monaco AP (1986): Immunological characteristics of purified pancreatic islet grafts. Transplantation 42:387–390.

Gross CR, Zehrer CL (1992): Health-related quality of life outcomes of pancreas transplant recipients. Clin Transplant 6:165–171.

Gross CR, Zehrer CL (1993): Impact of the addition of a pancreas to quality of life in uremic diabetic recipients of kidney transplants. Transplant Proc 25:1293–1295.

Harmer N (1990): Nonuremic pancreas transplantation (Letter). Diabetes Care 13:452–450.

Hellman B (1959): The frequency distribution of the number and volume of the islets of Langerhans in man. Acta Soc Med Upsalien 64:432.

Hering BJ, Browatzki CC, Schultz A, Bretzel RG, Federlin KF (1993): Clinical islet transplantation —registry report, accomplishments in the past and future research needs. Cell Transplant 2:269–282.

Jacobson SH, Fryd DS, Sutherland DER, Kjellstrand CM (1988): Treatment of the diabetic patient with end-stage renal failure. Diabetes Metab Rev 4:191–200.

Kahn BB, Shulman GI, Defronzo RA, Cushman SW, Rossetti L (1991): Normalization of blood glucose in diabetic rats with phlorizin treatment reverses insulin-resistant glucose transport in adipose cells without restoring glucose transporter gene expression. J Clin Invest 87:561–570.

Kahn CR, Goldfine ID, Neville DM, Demeyts P (1987): Alteration in insulin binding induced by changes in vivo in the levels of glucocorticoids and growth hormone. Endocrinology 103:1054.

Kaufman DB, Platt J, Rabe FL, Dunn DL, Bach FH, Sutherland DER (1990): Differential roles of Mac-1+ cells, and CD4+ and CD8+ T lymphocytes in primary nonfunction and classic rejection of islet allografts. J Exp Med 172:291–302.

Kaufman DB, Field MJ, Gruber SA, Farney AC, Stephanian E, Gores PF, Sutherland DER (1992): Extended functional survival of murine islet allograft with 15-deoxyspergualin. Transplant Proc 24:1045–1047.

Kennedy WR, Navarro X, Goetz FC, Sutherland DER, Najarian JS (1990): Effects of pancreatic transplantation on diabetic neuropathy. N Engl J Med 322:1031–1037.

Kenyon NS, Strasser S, Alejandro R (1990): Ultraviolet light immunomodulation of canine islets for prolongation of allograft survival. Diabetes 39:305–311.

Korsgren O, Jansson L, Andersson A (1989): Effects of hyperglycemia on function of isolated mouse pancreatic islets transplanted under kidney capsule. Diabetes 38:510–515.

Lau H, Reemtsma K, Hardy MA (1984): Prolongation of rat islet allograft survival by direct ultraviolet irradiation of the graft. Science 223:607–609.

Leahy JL, Bonner-Weir S, Weir GC (1992): Beta-cell dysfunction induced by chronic hyperglycemia. Current ideas on mechanism of impaired glucose-induced insulin secretion. Diabetes Care 15:442.

Ling Z, Veld PA, Pipeleers DG (1993): Interaction of interleukin-1 with islet B-cells. Distinction between indirect, aspecific cytotoxicity and direct, specific functional suppression. Diabetes 42:56–65.

Loseke C (1990): Quality of life after transplantation (Letter). Diabetes Care 13:541.

Mieles L, Gordon RD, Mintz D, Toussaint RM, Imventarza O, Starzl TE (1991): Glycaemia and insulin need following FK506 rescue therapy in liver recipients. Transplant Proc 23:949–953.

Moller DE, Flier JS (1991): Insulin-resistance—mechanisms, syndromes, and implications. N Engl J Med 325:938.

Montana E, Bonner-Weir S, Weir GC (1993): Beta cell mass and growth after syngeneic islet cell transplantation in normal and streptozocin diabetic C57BL/6 mice. J Clin Invest 91:780–787.

Morel P, Goetz FC, Moudry-Munns KC, Freier EF, Sutherland DER (1991a): Long term glucose control in patients with pancreatic transplants. Ann Intern Med 115:694–699.

Morel P, Sutherland DER, Almond PS, Stöblen F, Matas AJ, Najarian JS, Dunn DL (1991b): Assessment of renal function in type I diabetic patients after kidney, pancreas or combined kidney-pancreas transplantation. Transplantation 51:1184–1189.

Morris RE (1992): Rapamycins: Antifungal, antitumor, antiproliferative and immunosuppressive macrolides. Transplant Proc 6:39–87.

Nakache R, Tyden G, Groth CG (1991): Quality of life in diabetic patients after combined pancreas-kidney or kidney transplantation. Diabetes 39:802–806.

Nathan CF (1987): Secretory products of macrophages. J Clin Invest 79:319–326.

Platz KP, Sollinger HW, Mullett DA, Eckhoff DE, Eugui EM, Allison AC (1991): RS-61443—A new potent immunosuppressive agent. Transplantation 51:27–31.

Posselt AM, Barker CF, Tomaszewski JE, Marmann JF, Choti MA, Naji H (1990): Induction of donor-specific unresponsiveness by intrathymic islet transplantation. Science 249:1293–1295.

Posselt AM, Odorico JS, Barker CF, Naji A (1992): Promotion of pancreatic islet allograft survival by intrathymic transplantation of bone marrow. Diabetes 41:771–775.

Prieto M, Sutherland DER, Fernandez-Cruz L, Heil JE, Najarian JS (1987): Experimental and clinical experience with urine amylase monitoring for early diagnosis of rejection in pancreas transplantation. Transplantation 43:71–79.

Pyzdrowski KL, Kendall DM, Halter JB, Nakhleh RE, Sutherland DER, Robertson RP (1992): Preserved insulin secretion and insulin independence in recipients of islet autografts. N Engl J Med 327(4):220–226.

Ramsay RC, Goetz FC, Sutherland DER, Mauer SM, Robinson LL, Cantrill HL, Knobloch WH, Najarian JS (1988): Progression of diabetic retinopathy after pancreas transplantation for insulin-dependent diabetes mellitus. N Engl J Med 318:208–214.

Rayman G, Williams SA, Spencer PD, Smaje LH, Wise PH, Tooke JE (1986): Impaired microvascular hyperaemic responses to minor skin trauma in type I diabetes. Br Med J 292:1295–1298.

Ricordi C, Gray DWR, Hering BJ (1990): Islet isolation assessment in man and large animals. Acta Diabetol Lat 27:185–195.

Saito K, Iwama N, Takahashi T (1978): Morphometrical analysis on topographical difference in size distribution, number and volume of islets in the human pancreas. Tohoku J Exp Med 124:177.

Sandberg SS, Anderson A (1993): Exposure of rat pancreatic islets to RS-61443 inhibits B-cell function. International Congress on Pancreas and Islet Transplantation Amsterdam (abstract).

Scharp DW, Lacy PE, Santiago JV (1991): Results of our first nine intraportal islet allografts in type I,

insulin-dependent diabetic patients. Transplantation 51:76–85.

Simeonovic CJ, Bowen KM, Kotlausk I, Lafferty KJ (1980): Modulation of tissue immunogenicity by organ culture. Comparison of adult islets and fetal pancreas. Transplantation 30:174.

Solders G, Tydén G, Persson A, Groth CG (1992): Improvement of nerve conduction in diabetic neuropathy: A follow-up study 4 years after combined pancreatic and renal transplantation. Diabetes 41:946–951.

Sollinger H, Stratta RJ, D'Alessandro AM, Kalayoglu M, Pirsch JD, Belzer FO (1988): Experience with simultaneous pancreas-kidney transplantation. Ann Surg 208:748–483.

Stegall MD, Chabot J, Weber C, Reemtsma K, Hardy MA (1989): Pancreatic islet transplantation in cynomolgus monkeys. Initial studies and evidence that cyclosporine impairs glucose tolerance in normal monkeys. Transplantation 48:751–755.

Stevens RB, Ansite JD, Lokeh A (1994): The role of nitric oxide (NO) in the pathogenisis of early pancreatic islet dysfunction during rat and human intraportal (IP) islet transplantation. Transplant Proc 26(2):692.

Stock PG, Ascher NL, Chen S, Field J, Bach FH, Sutherland DER (1991): Evidence for direct and indirect pathways in the generation of the alloimmune response against pancreatic islets. Transplant Proc 52:704–709.

Sutherland DER (1991): Immunosuppression for clinical pancreas transplantation. Clin Transplant 5:549–553.

Sutherland DER (1992): Pancreatic transplantation: State of the art. Transplant Proc 24:762–766.

Sutherland DER (1993): Pancreatic transplantation: An update. Diabetes Rev 1(2):152–165.

Sutherland DER, Sibley RK, Xu XZ, Michael AF, Srikanta S, Taub F, Najarian JS, Goetz FC (1984): Twin-to-twin pancreas transplantation: Reversal and reenactment of the pathogenesis of type I diabetes. Trans Assoc Am Physicians 97:80–87.

Sutherland DER, Kendall DM, Moudry KC, Navarro X, Kennedy WR, Ramsay RC, Steffes MW, Mauer SM, Goetz FC, Dunn DL, Najarian JS (1988): Pancreas transplantation in nonuremic, type I diabetic recipients. Surgery 104:453–464.

Sutherland DER, Dunn DL, Goetz FC, Kennedy WR, Ramsay RC, Steffes MW, Mauer SM, Gruessner, RWG, Moudry-Munns KC, Morel P, Viste AB, Robertson RP, Najarian JS (1989a): A 10-year experience with 290 pancreas transplants at a single institution. Ann Surg 210:274–285.

Sutherland DER, Goetz FC, Sibley RK (1989b): Recurrence of disease in pancreas transplants. Diabetes 38:85–87.

Sutherland DER, Gruessner RWG, Gillingham KJ, Moudry-Munns KC, Dunn DL, Brayman KL, Morel P, Najarian JS (1992): A single institution's experience with solitary pancreas transplantation. In Terasaki PI (ed): "Clinical Transplants—1991." Los Angeles: UCLA Tissue Typing Lab, pp 141–152.

Sutherland DER, Gores PF, Farney AC, Wahoff DC, Matas AJ, Dunn DL, Gruessner RWG, Najarian JS (1993a): Evolution of kidney, pancreas, and islet transplantation for patients with diabetes at the University of Minnesota. Am J Surg 166:456–491.

Sutherland DER, Gruessner A, Moudry-Munns KC, Cecka M (1993b): Tabulation of cases from the International Pancreas Transplant Registry and analysis of United Network for Organ Sharing United States Transplant Registry data according to multiple variables. Transplant Proc 25:1707–1709.

Sutherland DER, Moudry-Munns KC, Gruessner A (1994): Pancreas Transplant Registry, United Network for Organ Sharing and International Data Report. In Terasaki PI (ed): "Clinical Transplants—1993." Los Angeles: UCLA Tissue Typing Laboratory, 47–69.

Ulrichs K, Muller-Ruchholtz W (1990): Mixed lymphocyte islet culture (MLIC) and its use in manipulation of human islet alloimmunogenicity. Horm Metab Res 25:123(abstract).

United States Renal Disease System (1992): Simultaneous kidney-pancreas transplantation versus kidney transplantation alone: Patient survival, kidney graft survival, and posttransplant hospitalization. Am J Kidney Dis 20(5):61–67.

Walter PK, Dickneite G, Schorlemmer HU (1987): Prolongation of graft survival in allogeneic islet transplantation by 15-deoxyspergualin in the rat. Diabetologia 30:38(abstract).

Wang TL, Stevens RB, Fioretto P, Lokeh A, Kunjummen D, Gruessner A, Schmidt W, Moudry-Munns KC, Mauer SM, Steffes MW, Sutherland DER (1993): Correlation of preoperative renal function and identification of risk factors for eventual native renal failure in cyclosporine-treated nonuremic diabetic recipient of pancreas transplants alone. Transplant Proc 25:1291–1292.

Xenos ES, Casanova D, Sutherland DER, Farney AC, Lloveras JJ, Gores PF (1993): The in vivo and in vitro effect of 15-deoxyspergualin on pancreatic islet function. Transplantation 56:144–147.

Zehrer CL, Gross CR (1991): Quality of life of pancreas transplant recipients. Diabetologia 34:S145–S140.

Zeng Y, Ricordi C, Lendoire J (1993): The effect of prednisone on pancreatic islet autografts in dogs. Surgery 113:98–102.

Chapter 9
Allogeneic Bone Marrow Transplantation

Richard J. O'Reilly, Esperanza Papadopoulos, and Farid Boulad

INTRODUCTION

In 1968, HLA-compatible marrow grafts derived from siblings were used to correct the lethal immunologic deficiencies of two children, one with severe combined immune deficiency (SCID) and the other with Wiskott–Aldrich syndrome (Bach et al., 1968; Gatti et al., 1968). These patients remain healthy chimeras to this day with lymphoid systems derived from their compatible siblings. Since that time, marrow transplantation has emerged as a treatment of choice for patients with acute leukemia who fail to sustain initial remission (Brochstein et al., 1987), chronic myelogenous leukemia (CML) (Goldman et al., 1988; Thomas et al., 1986) and the myelodysplastic syndromes (Appelbaum et al., 1990; O'Donnell et al., 1987). Marrow grafts are a treatment of choice for patients with aplastic anemia (Camitta et al., 1983; Storb et al., 1976) and several lethal congenital disorders of hematopoiesis and immunity, including Fanconi's anemia, Wiskott–Aldrich syndrome, and SCID (O'Reilly et al., 1984). Such transplants are also being applied with remarkable success to the treatment of patients with thalassemia (Lucarelli et al., 1990) and sickle cell anemia (Johnson et al., 1984; Milpied et al., 1988; Vermylen et al., 1988). Marrow transplants can also be used to provide a continuing source of enzymatically normal macrophages for the correction of several errors of metabolism, such as Gaucher's disease and certain mucopolysaccharidoses and mucolipidoses (Krivit et al., 1990b). They are also now being considered as a potential treatment for certain forms of autoimmune disease (Liu Yin and Jowitt, 1992), based on the striking reversals of autoimmune nephritis observed in genetically susceptible NZB/NZW mice transplanted with marrow from genetically resistant strains (Ikehara et al., 1985).

Marrow transplants differ radically from organ transplants in three critical respects. First, allogeneic marrow grafts are markedly more sensitive to rejection by residual host T cells than are organ grafts. As a consequence, patients undergoing marrow grafts must be immunoablated so that the host T cell immune system is completely replaced by the donor's own T cells or their precursors if the marrow graft is to achieve durable chimerism. Second, the requirements for histocompatibility between donor and recipient are considerably more stringent. Transplants from donors other than HLA-matched siblings are associated with a markedly increased incidence of graft rejection despite immunoablative cytoreduction (Anasetti et al., 1989). A third feature unique to marrow grafts is the fact that the marrow transplanted contains blood-derived T-lymphocytes that, upon engraftment, are capable of reacting against histoincompatibilities unique to the host and inciting an immune assault against host tissues, a disorder termed graft-versus-host disease (GvHD) (Streilein and Billingham, 1970). This complication is observed in 50–70% of individuals transplanted with marrow from HLA-matched siblings; its incidence and severity are higher when transplants from HLA-partially matched related or HLA-matched unrelated donors are used (Beatty et al., 1985, 1990; Gingrich et al., 1988; Gluckman, 1990; Hows et al., 1986).

Transplantation Immunology, pages 161–198
© 1995 Wiley-Liss, Inc.

Over the past 10 years, the results of HLA-matched sibling marrow grafts have markedly improved. The better results currently achieved reflect a clearer understanding of the biology of marrow transplantation, the development of new approaches for effective control of the cellular interactions contributing to graft rejection and GvHD, and radical improvements in supportive care, particularly our capacity to prevent and treat transplant-associated infections and the recognition that earlier application of marrow transplants can achieve dramatically better long-term results. These developments have also spawned approaches permitting the use of marrow transplants from donors other than HLA-matched siblings including donors from pools of unrelated volunteers.

In this chapter, we will review current knowledge of the biology of marrow transplantation, the therapeutic principles that govern its application to the treatment of lethal genetic and acquired disorders of hematopoiesis, and the new advances that have extended the application of marrow grafts to an increasing proportion of those individuals who do not have an HLA-matched sibling donor.

GENETIC AND CELLULAR INTERACTION AFFECTING THE BIOLOGY OF A MARROW ALLOGRAFT

Selection of Donor

The marrow constitutes the most immunogenic of the transplantable organs. It was recognized early that engraftment of hematopoietic cells could not be consistently achieved unless the host was immunoablated or genetically incapable of recognizing allodisparities unique to the donor, and conversely that donor T cells, if engrafted in a host expressing unshared major histocompatibility antigens, would react against tissues bearing those determinants resulting in a lethal GvH reaction. Subsequently, recognition of this need for compatibility between donor and host for major histocompatibility complex (MHC) antigens provided an immunogenetic basis for selection of donors, which led to the initial successful applications of HLA compatible marrow grafts in man (Bach et al., 1968; Gatti et al., 1968; see Chapter 1). HLA-identical siblings have been identified for 35–40% of patients. Non-sibling-related donors who are matched for all but one or two determinants encoded by one haplotype as well as "matched" unrelated donors may also be identified for an additional 5–10% and 20–30% of patients, respectively.

PREPARATION OF THE HOST FOR ALLOGENEIC MARROW TRANSPLANTS

Engraftment of allogeneic marrow, that is marrow from a donor other than an identical twin, in a relatively immunocompetent patient necessitates prior ablation of the host's capacity to reject the graft or resist its development. Only patients with SCID who lack functional T cells will regularly achieve engraftment following a transplant of unmanipulated HLA-matched marrow. Transplants for other conditions require immunoablative treatment in the immediate pretransplant period. Total body irradiation at doses of at least 9.0–10.0 Gy induces a degree of immunosuppression and myeloablation that is adequate to permit durable engraftment of an allogeneic marrow transplant (Thomas et al., 1971). Of the chemotherapeutic agents currently available, only cyclophosphamide and nitrogen mustard, administered in high doses, have been demonstrated to be sufficiently immunosuppressive to permit engraftment of foreign hematopoietic cells (Santos, 1974; Sullivan et al., 1982). While cyclophosphamide is the most immunosuppressive alkylating agent currently available, it provides effective preparation only for unsensitized patients with aplastic anemia (Storb et al., 1983). For diseases that do not compromise the overall cellularity of the patient's marrow, a myeloablative agent must be used in addition to cyclophosphamide to create sufficient space for the establishment of donor hematopoietic cells (Kapoor et al., 1981; Parkman, 1978). The myeloablative agents that have been used for this purpose include busulfan, dimethylmyleran, thiotepa, and melphalan (Kapoor et al., 1981).

MARROW TRANSPLANTATION TECHNIQUES AND PROCEDURES

The immunosuppressive and myeloablative regimens used to prepare a patient for an allogeneic marrow transplant, as summarized in Figure 1, entail intensive treatment with radiation and chemotherapy over 4–10 days prior to the marrow transplant procedure. The marrow harvest is usually performed under general anesthesia. Marrow is harvested by multiple needle aspirations from the anterior and posterior iliac crests bilaterally. The total volume of marrow harvested should be gauged so as to provide the recipient with a dose of nucleated cells in excess of 2.0×10^8 cells/kg body weight. Usually, 600–1100 mL of marrow provide a dose of cells adequate for the transplant. The heparinized marrow aspirates are pooled and thereafter filtered through micron steel mesh filters to remove bone chips. They can then be collected into transfusion bags and administered to the patient by the intravenous route.

Major red cell ABO incompatibilities (e.g., A into O) do not constitute a significant barrier to marrow transplantation. If there is a red cell incompatibility between donor and recipient such that the recipient has significant titers of antibodies against ABO or Rh determinants expressed on donor red cells, the red cells may be removed from the pool of marrow by differential centrifugation or sedimentation (Dinsmore et al., 1983b).

In order to prevent GvHD, the marrow may also be fractionated by any of several techniques to remove alloreactive donor T cells or subsets thereof.

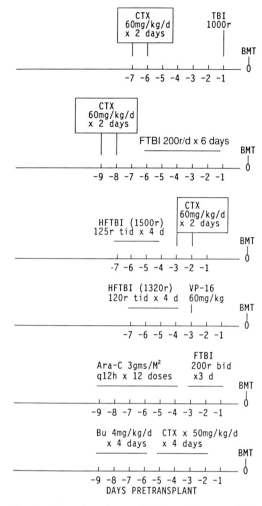

Fig. 1. Examples of cytoreduction regimens used for preparation of patients transplanted for leukemia. CTX = Cyclophosphamide; Bu = Busulfan; VP-16 = etoposide; HFTBI, FTBI and TBI = hyperfractionated, daily fractionated and single dose total body irradiation, respectively.

CLINICAL AND BIOLOGICAL DETERMINANTS OF ENGRAFTMENT OR GRAFT FAILURE

Following infusion of the marrow allograft, the hematopoietic progenitor cells migrate to sites in the marrow and spleen. Early engraftment is signaled by the development of myeloid and erythroid progenitors of donor origin in the marrow and the emergence of neutrophils in the blood 14–21 days posttransplant. By day 28–35, the cellularity of the marrow may be normal and peripheral blood, neutrophil, and platelet counts may be stable at levels > 1000/μl and 20,000/μl, respectively. In a proportion of cases, full recovery of peripheral blood counts may be impaired (Bolger et al., 1986) and require boost infusions of donor marrow. Persistent thrombocytopenia and leukopenia are also common in patients developing intercurrent

Table I. Disorders Correctable by Allogeneic BMT

Immunodeficiency Disorders
- Severe combined immunodeficiencies (SCID)
  - Autosomal recessive (ADA+ or ADA−)
  - X-linked recessive
  - Omenn's syndrome
  - Reticular dysgenesis
- Other immunodeficiency disorders
  - Bare lymphocyte syndrome
  - Nezeloff syndrome and other combined immunodeficiencies
  - Nucleoside phosphorylase deficiency
  - Wiskott Aldrich syndrome (WAS)
  - X-linked EBV lymphoproliferative disease

Erythroid Disorders
- Thalassemia major
- Sickle cell disease
- Diamond–Blackfan anemia

White Cell Disorders
- Kostmann agranulocytosis
- Chronic granulomatous disease (CGD)
- Leukocyte adhesion deficiency (LAD)
- Chediak–Higashi syndrome
- Familial erythrophagocytic lymphohistiocytosis (FEL)

Platelet Disorders
- Congenital amegakaryocytosis
- TAR syndrome
- Glanzmann's thrombasthenia

Constitutional Bone Marrow Failure Syndromes (AA)
- Fanconi's anemia
- Dyskeratosis congenita
- Osteopetrosis
- Schwachman–Diamond syndrome

Inborn Errors of Metabolism
- MPS: Hurler (MPS I-H), Hunter (MPS II),
             San Filippo syndrome (MPS III), Maroteaux–Lamy syndrome (MPS VI)
- Lipidoses: Gaucher disease, Metachromatic leukodystrophy

Acquired Aplastic Anemia (AA)

Malignant Disorders
- Acute lymphoblastic leukemia (ALL)
- Acute non-lymphoblastic leukemia (ANLL)
- Myelodysplastic syndromes (MDS)
- Chronic myelogenous leukemia (CML)
- Non-Hodgkin's lymphoma (NHL)
- Chronic lymphocytic leukemia (CLL)
- Multiple myeloma (MM)

infections with viruses such as cytomegalovirus (CMV) as well as GvHD (Baughan et al., 1984). However, proof of engraftment can be ascertained by demonstration of donor cells in T-lymphocyte and hematopoietic lineages by cytogenetics (Sparks, 1981), detection of donor-specific restriction fragment length polymorphisms (RFLP) (Blazar et al., 1985), or minisatellite allelic polymorphisms or, in sex-mismatched cases, detection of X and Y probes using fluorescence *in situ* hybridization techniques (Hutchinson et al., 1989).

Graft failure is empirically defined either as a failure to recover marrow function after transplantation or a reversion to marrow aplasia after initial hematopoietic reconstitution. Graft failure is also documented by the loss of donor type lymphoid and hematopoietic cells in the marrow and blood. Most instances of graft failure occur within the first 50 days posttransplant but have been documented as late as 4–5 months posttransplant.

The type of cytoreduction used to prepare the patient, the type of transplant administered, and the degree of HLA disparity existing between donor and recipient each contributes to the incidence of graft failure in the posttransplant period. For example, the incidence of graft failure ranges from 10 to 30% for patients with aplastic anemia prepared with cyclophosphamide alone depending on the patient's prior transfusion history (Champlin et al., 1989; Storb et al., 1977a,b). While unmodified, HLA-matched marrow grafts induce consistent engraftment in leukemic patients prepared with TBI and cyclophosphamide (Dinsmore et al., 1983a, & 1984; Thomas et al., 1971), unmodified grafts from HLA-nonidentical donors remain at increased risk of this complication, with the probability of graft failure ranging from 6 to 28% depending on the number and type of HLA allodisparities unique to the donor (Anasetti et al., 1989). In addition, depletion of T cells from a marrow allograft renders the transplant more susceptible to graft failure and rejection even when the graft is HLA matched with the recipient (Hale et al., 1988; Martin et al., 1988; O'Reilly et al., 1988). The incidence of graft failure ranges from 10 to 30% in leukemic recipients of T cell-depleted HLA-matched marrow (Hale et al., 1988; Kernan et al., 1989; Martin et al., 1985) and has been recorded to be as high as 40–50% in recipients of HLA-disparate grafts (O'Reilly et al., 1985).

Graft failures complicating allogeneic marrow transplants usually reflect active rejection of the donor cells by host resistance systems. In murine models, two types of marrow graft resistance have been identified: the resistance to parental marrow grafts exhibited by irradiated nonsensitized F_1 hybrids of specific genetic backgrounds, which has been ascribed to the activity of NK cells (Keissling et al., 1977), and the resistance of hosts presensitized to donor cells by transfusion, which is mediated by alloreactive cytotoxic host T cells (Dennert et al., 1985).

The fact that animals sensitized by transfusion are more susceptible to marrow graft rejection provided early evidence suggesting an immunologic basis for the failures observed (Storb et al., 1970). Recently, evidence directly implicating host T cells has been developed, through a series of studies documenting the emergence of host type $CD3^+$, $CD8^+$, $CD56^-$ T cells exhibiting specific reactivity against donor marrow cells at the time of rejection of an unmodified (Voogt et al., 1988) or a T cell-depleted marrow graft (Bordignon et al., 1989; Kernan et al., 1987). Following HLA-disparate T cell-depleted marrow grafts, cytotoxic, $CD3^+$, $CD8^+$ host T cells exhibiting specificity for single class I HLA alleles unique to the donor have been detected. In addition, in a smaller proportion of cases, $CD3^+$, $CD4^+$ cytolytic T cells of host origin exhibiting specific reactivity against donor unique HLA-DR and -DQ disparities have been identified. T cells detected in the circulation of patients rejecting HLA-matched marrow grafts are $CD3^+$, $CD8^+$, and $Leu7^+$ and have been shown to specifically inhibit donor colony-forming hematopoietic cells *in vitro* (Bordignon et al., 1989). While these cells have been found to be HLA restricted, the nature of the minor alloantigens targeted by these cells is still unclear. Two recently isolated antigens, the HY antigen expressed on male cells (Goulmy et al., 1977; Voogt et al., 1988) and the HA3 antigen, an autosomal antigen expressed on hematopoietic cells, have been implicated (Goulmy, 1988).

As the factors contributing to rejection or graft failure have been identified, strategies for the reversal or prevention of this complication have been developed and applied in preclinical and clinical trials. The strategies have principally explored intensifications of preparative immunosuppressive regimens, additional treatment with T cell-specific monoclonal and heteroantibodies (Atkinson et al., 1979; Bozdech et al., 1985; Camitta et al., 1983; Kernan et al., 1989), and the use of cytokines such as granulocyte–

macrophage colony-stimulating factor (GM-CSF) and G-CSF to induce early recovery of hematopoiesis posttransplantation (DeWitte et al., 1991; Masaoka et al., 1989; Nemunaitis et al., 1992). Early detection of infections with CMV and HHV-6 and treatment of these infections with ganciclovir or foscarnet coupled with hyperimmune globulin have also reversed graft failures in a proportion of cases (Emanuel et al., 1989).

GRAFT-VERSUS-HOST DISEASE

Graft-versus-host disease is a pathologic process initiated by the response of engrafted immunocompetent donor T-lymphocytes against alloantigens expressed on host cells. The principal targets thought to stimulate this reaction are cells derived from the host's lymphohematopoietic system (Streilein and Billingham, 1970). Of the many cells in this system, the most potent stimulants appear to be dendritic cells (Young et al., 1993). T-lymphocytes, in response to alloantigens, proliferate and mature to form both cytotoxic T cells and helper cells that can either directly injure targeted host tissues or recruit other cells, particularly natural killer (NK) cells and macrophages to destroy host cell targets (Ferrara et al., 1989; Xun et al., 1993). These T cells may also generate cytokines such as tumor necrosis factor (TNF), which may further contribute to the pathology observed (Piguet et al., 1987).

The principal clinical manifestations of acute GvHD are a maculopapular skin rash that may be focal or generalized, hepatitis, and enteritis, particularly affecting the colon and distal small bowel, and a delayed reconstitution of hematopoietic and lymphoid function (Glucksberg et al., 1974; Vogelsang et al., 1988; Witherspoon et al., 1984). Pathologic changes in the skin are distinctive but not pathognomonic and include infiltration of the perivascular spaces in the dermis and of the dermoepidermal junction with CD8$^+$ cytotoxic T-lymphocytes and NK cells and piecemeal necrosis of the overlying epidermis (Fig. 2A and B) (Slavin and Woodruff, 1974). This mononuclear cell infiltration is also seen in the epithelium of the oropharynx, at the bases of the intestinal crypts of the small and large bowel, and in the periportal areas of the liver (Slavin and Woodruff, 1974). In liver and bowel, the pathologic features are difficult to discriminate from those of an acute viral infection.

Acute GvHD is graded from I to IV (Glucksberg et al., 1974). Patients who have received an HLA-matched sibling marrow graft and have been treated with low dose methotrexate as prophylaxis against GvHD have experienced a 50–70% risk of developing this complication. Approximately 30% will develop grade II–IV acute GvHD, requiring immunosuppressive treatment.

The incidence and severity of acute GvHD are principally determined by the type and degree of allodisparity existing between donor and recipient. It is also strongly influenced by other host factors such as the patient's age, gender, the intensity of the cytoreductive regimen used to prepare the patient for transplantation, the presence or absence of intercurrent infection, and the type of resident microflora as well as donor features such as gender, prior sensitization to host minor alloantigens by pregnancy, and the number of T cells inoculated in the marrow allograft (Flowers et al., 1990; Gale et al., 1987; Storb et al., 1977b).

Chronic GvHD is a complex disorder that is pathologically distinct from acute GvHD. While it usually develops in patients with antecedent acute GvHD, it may evolve spontaneously late after transplantation in association with an intercurrent infection. Clinically, chronic GvHD presents with localized or widespread sclerodermic changes of the skin (Fig. 2c, 2d), xerostomia, xerophthalmia, biliary cirrhosis, malabsorption, failure to thrive, and debilitating skin and joint contractures (Sullivan et al., 1981). The pathologic features of chronic GvHD are strikingly different from those of acute GvHD: infiltration with mononuclear cells is sparse, if seen. Rather, there is marked sclerosis observed in the dermis, laminapropria of the intestinal tract, and biliary triads, as well as around the ducts of the salivary and lacrimal glands.

Detailed studies of the immunopathological

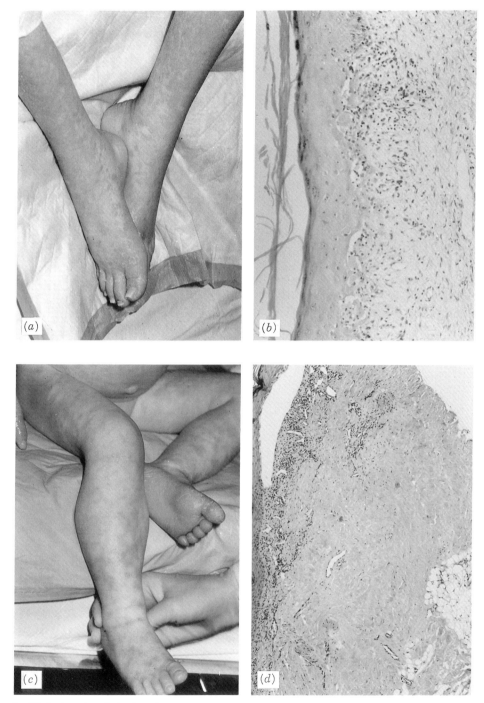

Fig. 2. Clinical and pathological features of acute and chronic GvHD. *a*: Maculopapular rash of acute GvHD involving leg and both dorsal and plantar aspects of feet. *b*: Pathological features of acute GvHD, including infiltration of mononuclear cells at dermoepidermal junction and in perivascular areas, with pyknotic necrosing cells in all layers of epidermis. *c*: Sclerosis, superficial ulceration of chronic GvHD. *d*: Marked deposition of collagen and fibrosis in the dermis, atrophic changes of epidermis with continuing infiltration with mononuclear cells at dermoepidermal junction in patient with chronic GvHD manifested by severe sclerosis and superficial ulcerations.

events precipitated by acute and chronic forms of GvHD have demonstrated distinctive features of each process. In murine models (Parkman, 1986), acute GvHD is usually marked by the development of donor-derived T cells that are specifically cytotoxic against host targets. In contrast, T cells cloned from animals with chronic GvHD express a helper phenotype, and, in response to either donor or host class II+ cells, proliferate and generate factors that stimulate collagen synthesis, the hallmark of chronic GvHD pathology. In humans with chronic GvHD, T-lymphocytes and monocytes capable of nonspecific suppression of antigen specific T cell immunity and B cell immunoglobulin production are regularly observed (Lum, 1987; Tsoi et al., 1979). As in the murine model, these T cells also generate cytokines that stimulate fibroblast proliferation and collagen secretion. In normal individuals, such broadly reactive potentially autocytotoxic cells can be detected at significant frequency in the blood by limiting dilution analyses (Rosenkrantz et al., 1987). However, such cells are usually limited in their activity by specific suppressor cells also detected in the circulation. In patients with chronic GvHD, such specific suppressor cells are either absent or markedly reduced in number (Rosenkrantz et al., 1987). Taken together, these findings suggest that chronic GvHD may reflect ineffectively controlled immunosuppressive and potentially autoreactive clones of cells, possibly generated in response to populations of host reactive donor T cells participating in acute GvHD reactions.

Chronic GvHD is reversible in a significant proportion of patients, but responses to treatment must be measured over months to years. Without systemic immunosuppressive treatment, only 18–23% of patients have survived over 18 months (Sullivan et al., 1986).

PREVENTION OF GRAFT-VERSUS-HOST DISEASE

The high mortality associated with severe forms of acute and chronic GvHD observed, particularly in older adult recipients of HLA-matched sibling marrow grafts and patients receiving transplants from matched unrelated donors, has continuously underscored the need for development of more effective methods for preventing this complication or abrogating its clinical expression. Recognition of the essential role of donor T cells in the initiation of GvHD (Streilein and Billingham, 1970) has focused attention on two principal approaches: (1) administration of combinations of immunosuppressive agents in the immediate posttransplant period to prevent or inhibit the proliferation and function of host-reactive donor T cells following engraftment of unmodified marrow, or (2) treatment of the marrow graft to remove alloreactive T cells capable of inducing GvHD.

Early studies in canine models lead to the recognition that low-dose methotrexate could significantly reduce both the incidence and severity of acute GvHD following DLA-identical marrow grafts. This standard approach was adopted in clinical trials in the 1970s. However, despite methotrexate prophylaxis, 50–70% of individuals receiving HLA-matched marrow grafts developed acute GvHD and 30% ultimately developed chronic GvHD. An alternative approach, the administration of a combination of ATG and prednisone, has been reported to reduce the severity of GvHD but has also been associated with a higher incidence of infectious mortality (Ramsay et al., 1982). As a result, long-term disease-free survival is not affected. In randomized trials, cyclosporine has been found to be equivalent to methotrexate in the prevention of GvHD (Storb et al., 1985). The combination of these two agents is significantly more effective than either alone in preventing the development of severe acute GvHD. Furthermore, this combination significantly improves survival in prospective trials (Storb et al., 1986). However, this combination has had little effect on either the incidence or the severity of chronic GvHD and has not been effective in preventing severe GvH reaction in 70–80% of recipients of HLA-disparate related or HLA-matched unrelated marrow grafts. A recent report suggests that the combination of prednisone, cyclosporine, and short-course methotrexate can reduce the incidence of Grade II–IV acute GvHD in good risk patients transplanted with HLA-matched sibling marrow to as low as 9% (Chao et al., 1993). However, this regimen is also associated with an increased incidence of chronic GvH (65%). Nevertheless, preliminary results with this regimen have been highly promising.

While no combination of agents administered to recipients of an unmodified marrow graft has prevented the development of GvHD in HLA-nonidentical recipients, GvHD can be prevented in both HLA-matched and HLA-disparate recipients through use of marrow grafts suitably depleted of T-lymphocytes prior to administration. Currently used techniques may differ by 1–2 $\log_{10}$-fold in the level of T cell depletion achieved (Frame et al., 1989). The incidence of moderate to severe acute and chronic GvHD recorded in results from large series tends to reflect the efficiency of the T cell depletion techniques used.

While several series have demonstrated that T cell-depleted marrow grafts may reduce the incidence and severity of acute GvHD and, with certain techniques, chronic GvHD, a clear advantage of such transplants of unmodified marrow grafts translating into a significant improvement in long-term disease-free survival has thus far been clearly documented only in patients with lethal congenital immune deficiencies transplanted from HLA and HLA-nonidentical donors (O'Reilly et al., 1989). In such cases, T cell-depleted transplants from HLA-A,B,DR haplotype parental donors may achieve rates of long-term disease-free survival with immunologic reconstitution that are comparable to those achieved with unmodified HLA-matched marrow grafts. However, among patients transplanted for leukemia and aplastic anemia, reductions in GvHD and GvH-associated mortality accrued by the use of T cell-depleted grafts have been largely counterbalanced by the sensitivity of such transplants to graft failure or rejection and by increased risk of leukemic relapse, particularly observed among patients who have received HLA-matched T cell-depleted grafts as treatment for chronic myelogenous leukemia (Goldman et al., 1988; Marmont et al., 1989; Gratwohl et al., 1993). This situation is now changing rapidly. With the introduction of tolerable, more effectively immunosuppressive pre-

paratory regimens, the risk of graft failure following T cell-depleted marrow transplants has been dramatically reduced (Aversa et al., 1993; Papadopoulos et al., 1992), resulting in a significant improvement in survival and 1 to 2 years disease-free survival rates, particularly among older recipients of matched sibling grafts and patients transplanted with marrow from unrelated donors (Papadopoulos et al., 1992). As regimens ensuring consistent engraftment and durable hematopoietic reconstitution have been introduced, a clearer estimate of the patient groups at increased risk for leukemic relapse following T cell-depleted transplants has also emerged.

That enhanced resistance to leukemia occurred as a result of an allogeneic marrow transplant was first suggested by comparisons of the actuarial risks of leukemic relapse following HLA-matched allogeneic as compared to syngeneic unmodified marrow grafts applied to the treatment of AML in first remission (Gale and Champlin, 1984). Subsequently, Weiden et al. (1979) presented evidence indirectly that risk of relapse was lower among patients developing grade II–IV acute GvHD and/or chronic GvHD. These data spawned the hypothesis that the antileukemic effect of a marrow allograft is largely or exclusively based on the activity of alloreactive T cells participating in GvHD. It is unclear, however, whether the T cells that induce clearance of leukemic population are limited to T cells recognizing donor alloantigens (Slavin et al., 1990). Indeed, recent evidence suggests that T cells exhibiting selective reactivity against donor leukemic cells may also arise postgrafting (Faber et al., 1992). In addition, NK cells that emerge early posttransplantation have also been shown to exhibit cytocidal activity against fresh host CML cells (Hauch et al., 1990; Mackinnon et al., 1990). Indeed, this leukemocidal activity has been correlated with low risk of leukemic relapse in one series (Hauch et al., 1990). Among patients transplanted for acute leukemias in early remission, the risk of relapse following a T cell-depleted marrow grafts has not been increased in several series suggesting that the enhanced leukemia resistance conferred by a marrow allograft may, in this circumstance, not depend upon alloreactive T cells for its expression (Antin et al., 1991; Hale and Waldmann, 1988; Young et al., 1992). Preliminary experience with unrelated marrow transplants applied to the treatment of leukemias also suggests a disease-free survival advantage for patients transplanted with T cell-depleted marrow and that among patients transplanted for CML, the incidence of relapse has been equally low following either an unmodified or a T cell-depleted marrow graft (McGlave et al., 1990). Taken together, these data strongly suggest that effector cells other than alloreactive T cells may also play an important role in the establishment of leukemic resistance following a marrow allograft.

OTHER EARLY COMPLICATIONS OF MARROW TRANSPLANTS

Prior to engraftment, patients are at highest risk for infections complicating neutropenia, particularly sepsis caused by gram negative and positive bacteria in the bowel flora, and fungi such as *Candida* species. Infections with HSV are also common during the first month posttransplant. Acute organ toxicities secondary to the cytoreductive regimen can also be seen during this early posttransplant period. These include varying degrees of oral, enteric, and vaginal mucositis, cyclophosphamide and radiation induced cardiomyopathy (Gottdiener et al., 1981), cyclophosphamide induced hemorrhagic cystitis and veno-occlusive disease of the liver (Gluckman et al., 1990).

Following engraftment and for the first 6–7 months posttransplant, patients are still markedly immunodeficient, and are particularly susceptible to interstitial pneumonias caused by viruses or *P. carinii*, sino-pulmonary infections caused by *Aspergillus* and encapsulated pyogenic bacteria, hepatic and enteric CMV and adenovirus infections, disseminated infections due to varicella zoster and other pathogens of severely immunocompromised hosts such as toxoplasma gondii, and mycobacteria.

Of these complications, interstitial pneumonia constitutes the most common cause of death in the first 3 months following a marrow

allograft. Overall, 10–25% of patients transplanted for leukemia will develop this process. CMV is detected and implicated as a pathogen in over 50% of cases; an additional 10% can be ascribed to infection by *Pneumocystis carinii* and other pathogens such as herpes simplex, adenovirus, fungi, mycobacteria, or other agents (Meyers et al., 1982; Neiman et al., 1977; Wingard et al., 1988a). At least 40% of cases cannot be ascribed to a pathogen and may represent the result of pathologic alterations in endothelial integrity and aberrant inflammatory responses induced by the combined effects of radiation and chemotherapy-induced injury, infection, and/or GvHD. CMV infections observed posttransplantation are usually due to reactivations of virus latent in the host or the donor graft (Winston et al., 1985). Such reactivations appear to be stimulated by allointeractions between donor and host, since the incidence of CMV infections is particularly high among patients with moderate–severe GvHD (Meyers et al., 1982; Neiman et al., 1977; Weiner et al., 1986). In contrast, recipients of syngeneic autologous marrow grafts are at low risk for CMV pneumonias (Wingard et al., 1988b).

The use of seronegative blood products for support of seronegative transplant recipients has reduced the risk of this complication. In addition, seroprophylaxis with CMV hyperimmune globulin also appears to be effective in reducing the incidence of CMV pneumonia (Sullivan et al., 1990) in seropositive older patients. In addition, gancyclovir with immune globulin has been shown to be able to reverse CMV interstitial pneumonia in 50–70% of cases (Emanuel et al., 1988; Reed et al., 1988; Schmidt et al., 1988).

LATE COMPLICATIONS OF MARROW TRANSPLANTS

There are several late complications of marrow transplantation that occur at significant frequency. These can be divided into those resulting from delays in immune reconstitution, particularly those induced by GvHD and its treatment, and those attributable to the toxic and oncogenic sequelae of the drugs and radiation used to prepare patients for transplant.

Redevelopment of a competent donor-derived immune system following a marrow allograft is a protracted process. T cell populations begin to redevelop within the first 2 months, but responses to mitogens and antigens may be severely depressed for at least 2–4 months posttransplant (Witherspoon et al., 1984; Keever et al., 1989). The risk of infections with HSV, CMV, and *Candida* falls off rapidly after the first 3–6 months posttransplant. The risk of *Aspergillus* infections extends further into the posttransplant period, particularly for patients receiving steroids for prevention or treatment of GvHD. The risk of reactivation and dissemination of varicella zoster virus infections also persists through the first 1 to 2 years (Locksley et al., 1985). Treatment with intravenous acyclovir effectively eradicates varicella zoster infections with low mortality (Shepp et al., 1986). Long-term prophylaxis with acyclovir may also prevent this complication (Perren et al., 1988).

Recovery of B cell function is more protracted, with antibody deficiency states persisting for 12–18 months (Keever et al., 1989; Lum, 1987; Witherspoon et al., 1984). In patients with chronic GvHD, severe humoral immune deficiencies may persist for 3–5 years. As a result, patients with chronic GvHD are particularly susceptible to infections, such as recurrent sinusitis, otitis media, pneumonia, and sepsis, caused by the same spectrum of pyogenic bacteria that affect children with agammaglobulinemia, such as pneumococci, streptococci, and *Hemophilus influenzae* (Atkinson et al., 1982; Winston et al., 1979).

The late sequelae of radiation and other alkylating agents used to prepare patients for transplant may be mild or severe, depending upon the type of agents used and their dose intensity, the treatment received by the patient prior to referral for transplantation, and the age of the patient at the time of transplant. In general, patients prepared with cyclophosphamide alone sustain limited and generally transient damage, while injury induced by total body irradiation tends to be more profound and enduring. Similarly, radiation administered in a single large dose tends to be more damaging than if this dose is administered in multiple fractions (Deeg et al., 1984a; Sanders et al., 1986).

The most devastating of late complications resulting from damage induced by total body irradiation and chemotherapy is leukoencephalopathy (Thompson et al., 1986). This complication occurs rarely and almost exclusively in patients transplanted for leukemia who have received cranial radiation and/or extended courses of intrathecal methotrexate as treatment or prophylaxis for CNS leukemia prior to referral for transplantation. In such patients, the risk of leukoencephalopathy has been reported to be 7% (Thompson et al., 1986).

Deficiencies of thyroid, pituitary, and gonadal hormones are potential sequelae of the cytoreductive regimens used for allogeneic marrow transplants. The linear growth of children prepared for transplantation with total body irradiation is also often limited. In part, this reflects injury to the hypothalamus, resulting in decreased production of growth hormone-releasing factor (GHRF) and consequently abnormal growth hormone secretion (Sanders et al., 1986; Leiper et al., 1987). However, total body irradiation also affects growing bone, reducing, to a variable degree, the ultimate growth potential of transplanted children. Whether and to what degree treatment with growth hormone or GHRF can partially correct short stature in these cases are now under study.

Radiation may also induce cataract formation in the lens late in the posttransplant period. In patients treated with single high doses of total body irradiation, the incidence of cataracts is 50%. This incidence is lower in patients treated with fractionated total body irradiation (10–20%) (Deeg et al., 1984a).

Treatment with alkylating agents also predispose to secondary malignancies. To date, such neoplasms have been recorded in only a relatively small proportion of marrow transplant recipients, and predominantly among patients transplanted for leukemia or aplastic anemia (Deeg et al., 1984b; Witherspoon et al., 1989). The most common neoplasms detected are

polyclonal or oligoclonal B cell lymphoproliferative disorders and monoclonal lymphomas
bearing Epstein–Barr virus (EBV)-associated
antigens with or without EBV DNA integrated
into the cell's DNA (Witherspoon et al., 1989).
Such lymphomas are uncommon following HLA-
matched conventional or marrow grafts depleted
of T- and B-lymphocytes by lectin agglutination
or Campath-1 (< 2%) (Witherspoon et al., 1989;
O'Reilly et al., 1989; Hale et al., 1988). On the
other hand, an estimated risk of 6.4% has been
observed following HLA-matched transplants
depleted with T cell-specific mouse monoclo-
nals (Zutter et al., 1988). Furthermore, the risk
has been reported to be as high as 8 to 24% in
patients treated with HLA-nonidentical grafts
depleted of T cells with T cell-specific monoclonal antibodies (Fischer, 1989), and in patients
receiving infusions of certain T cell monoclonal
antibodies for treatment of GvHD (Martin et al.,
1984). Usually, the lymphomas have been of donor rather than host origin (Martin et al., 1984).
The basis for susceptibility to such B cell transformations is unclear, but may, in part, reflect an
inability of such patients to generate T cells capable of regulating donor B cell expansions early
in the posttransplant periods.

Until recently, treatment of EBV-induced
lymphoproliferative disorders (LPD) in marrow
transplant recipients was discouraging since
these processes are refractory to classical chemotherapy and radiation. Polyclonal EBV LPD
have been reversed in some cases with interferon
or following infusions of B cell-specific monoclonal antibodies (Fischer et al., 1991; Shapiro
et al., 1988). However, monoclonal disease has
failed to respond. Recently, our group has shown
that infusions of small doses (10^6 CD3$^+$ T
cells/kg) of donor T-lymphocytes will induce
complete and durable remissions of EBV LPD in
a high proportion of cases (Papadopoulos et al.,
1993). The efficacy of this therapeutic approach
likely reflects the high frequency of EBV-
specific cytotoxic T cell precursors in the circulation of normal seropositive marrow donors
(Bourgault et al., 1991).

Solid tumors, including basal cell carcinomas, squamous cell carcinomas of the skin, ade-
nocarcinomas of the stomach, osteosarcomas,

and glioblastomas have also developed in a small
proportion (1–2%) of cases followed for 1–10
years posttransplant (Witherspoon et al., 1989).
Again, the incidence of these cancers appears to
be lower than that recorded in patients given
comparable or lower localized doses of radiation
and chemotherapy for other neoplasms such as
Hodgkin's disease. More prolonged follow-up is
still needed, however, before full assessments
can be made of the incidence of such tumors in
transplant recipients.

APPLICATIONS OF TRANSPLANTS OF MARROW DERIVED FROM HLA-MATCHED SIBLINGS

Lethal Immune Deficiencies

Over the past 20 years, marrow transplantation has become recognized as the treatment of
choice for several lethal immune deficiencies,
particularly the different variants of SCID
(O'Reilly et al., 1989). In a recent European
survey of patients transplanted with HLA-
matched marrow for SCID, 68% were surviving
with reconstitution of immunity through 1986
(Fischer et al., 1986b). For patients with SCID
diagnosed early in life who are referred for transplantation before they have acquired serious infections, the probability of a successful transplant is in excess of 90% (Fischer, 1989).

Patients with SCID usually do not require any
pretransplant cytoreduction in preparation for an
HLA-matched unmodified marrow transplant,
because they have little capacity to resist engraftment of HLA-matched marrow. However, in
over 50% of cases, the only cells engrafted following such transplants are donor T cells and
their precursors (O'Reilly et al., 1989). Despite
this limited chimerism, HLA-matched grafts
usually result in a full reconstitution of both T
and B cell function.

A series of lethal combined immunodeficiency (CID) states can be distinguished from SCID
by the fact that the response of T cells to allogeneic cells is at least partially preserved, even
though humoral and cell-mediated responses to
microbial antigens may not be detected. In most
of these disorders the etiology of the immune
deficiency observed is still unknown. However,

in recent years the pathogenetic bases for several syndromes have been described. These include a congenital deficiency of the interleukin 1 (IL-1) receptor (Chu et al., 1984), congenital deficiencies of T cell activation and IL-2 production (DiSanto et al., 1990; Pahwa et al., 1989; Weinberg and Parkman, 1990), defects of the T cell receptor (Alarcon et al., 1988), and the Bare Lymphocyte Syndromes, a series of genetic disorders resulting in defective transcription and ultimate expression of class I and/or class II HLA determinants on the surface of lymphoid and hematopoietic cells (Hadam et al., 1984; Touraine et al., 1978). In other diseases, distinctive functional abnormalities, such as aberrant antigen or mitogen-induced membrane capping (Gehrz et al., 1980) and cell membrane depolarization, have been described (Gelfand et al., 1979).

For patients with these lethal CID syndromes where T cells retain some capacity to respond to allogeneic cells, preparatory immunosuppression with high dose cyclophosphamide is likely required to secure engraftment. Thus, HLA-matched transplants administered to patients with CID syndromes without preparatory cytoreduction have often failed to achieve engraftment. In contrast, patients who have been pretreated with high doses of cyclophosphamide and either cytosine arabinoside or myleran have regularly engrafted and achieved long-term immunologic reconstitution (Fischer and Griscelli, 1983).

Several lethal congenital disorders of immunity also involve other hematopoietic lineages. Correction of these disorders requires replacement of both lymphoid and other hematopoietic cells with progenitor cells derived from the normal donor. To achieve this, patients must undergo both intensive immunosuppression with cyclophosphamide and myeloablation with an agent such as myleran, dimethylmyleran, or total body irradiation. The most frequently transplanted immune deficiency of this type is Wiskott–Aldrich syndrome, a sex-linked disorder characterized by deficiencies of both the T and B cell systems and thrombocytopenia (Cooper et al., 1968). Transplants administered to such patients prepared with cyclophosphamide alone have led to engraftment of donor lymphoid

cells with corrections of immune deficiencies but persistence of thrombocytopenia (Bach et al., 1968). In contrast, over 90% of patients prepared with cyclophosphamide in combination with myleran, dimethylmyleran, or total body irradiation have achieved engraftment of both lymphoid and hematopoietic progenitors from the donor, full corrections of both lymphoid and platelet abnormalities, and long-term disease-free survival (Brochstein et al., 1991; O'Reilly et al., 1984). Other rare disorders of immunity that have been successfully corrected by this approach include reticular dysgenesis, a disorder characterized by severe combined immunodeficiency coupled with profound leukopenia and anemia (Levinsky and Tiedman, 1983), Cartilage-Hair hypoplasia (Sorell et al., 1979), and the Bare Lymphocyte Syndromes (Touraine et al., 1980).

Congenital Aplasias and Disorders of Red Cell Formation and Function

Fanconi's anemia (FA) is an autosomal recessive disorder characterized by a variety of congenital malformations, and anemia progressing to marrow aplasia or leukemia (Fanconi, 1967). Bone marrow transplantation offers the potential for permanent correction of the stem cell defect of FA (Gluckman, et al., 1983; Gluckman et al., 1980).

Congenital erythroid hypoplasia (Diamond–Blackfan syndrome) is a genetic disorder of uncertain inheritance characterized by a selective failure of erythroid progenitor development that results in a profound anemia from early infancy. In 1976, August et al. reported a patient with this disease whose red cell production had been restored to normal following successful engraftment of an HLA-matched marrow transplant. Although this patient ultimately died of interstitial pneumonia, five subsequent patients transplanted for this disorder reported by Iriondo et al. (1984) and Lenarsky et al. (1988) have each achieved engraftment of donor hematopoietic cells, durable corrections of anemia, and long-term disease-free survival.

Thalassemia major currently represents the genetic disorder for which HLA-matched al-

logeneic marrow grafts are most frequently performed with over 222 patients transplanted by
Lucarelli et al. (1990), in Pesaro, and at least 90
patients reported so far from other centers in Europe and the United States (Lucarelli et al.,
1990; Gorin et al., 1989; Gottdiener et al.,
1981). For patients transplanted before the age of
16 years, at least 6 centers have reported incidences of long-term survival and disease-free
survival of 62–91 and 56–88%, respectively
(Barrett et al., 1988; Brochstein et al., 1986;
DiBartolomeo et al., 1987; Frappaz et al., 1988;
Hugh-Jones et al., 1988; Lucarelli et al., 1992;
Thomas et al., 1982) with the best results observed when transplants have been invoked before onset of pathologically detectable hemo-
siderosis or liver fibrosis (Lucarelli et al., 1990).
Recently, allogeneic marrow transplants have
also been applied as a curative approach to the
treatment of sickle cell anemia (Johnson et al.,
1984; Milpied et al., 1988; Vermylen et al.,
1988). Although experience with transplants for
this disease is limited, such grafts have been consistently successful.

Genetic Disorders of Platelet Production and Function

Marrow transplants have been used successfully to treat congenital amegakaryocytosis,
a lethal disorder producing severe sustained
thrombocytopenia from birth (Saunders and
Freedman, 1978). A separate disorder, the TAR
syndrome, is characterized by severe thrombocytopenia, absence of the radii, and other malformations. Our group has recently administered
an HLA-matched marrow graft to a 2-year-old
patient with TAR syndrome who had persistent
amegakaryocytosis resulting in repeated intracranial hemorrhages. The transplant, administered after preparation of the patient with busulfan and cyclophosphamide, has led to full
engraftment and durable correction of platelet
production (Brochstein et al., 1986b).

The autosomal recessive disorders, Glanzmann's thrombasthenia types I and II, constitute
another series of life-threatening disorders of
platelets. Recently, Belucci et al. (1985) corrected this disorder in a 4-year-old child through
a series of two HLA-matched transplants admin-

istered after myeloablation with CCNU and procarbazine and immunosuppression with cyclophosphamide.

Disorders of Myelopoiesis and Phagocyte Function

Allogeneic marrow grafts have been applied
as a corrective treatment for a series of lethal
disorders of phagocyte production or function
with variable results. The lethal disorder of neutrophil production of congenital agranulocytosis
(Kostmann's syndrome) (Kostmann, 1975) has
been corrected by allogeneic marrow grafts administered after suitable myeloablation and immunosuppression (Rappeport et al., 1980). Recently, however, an alternative approach has
been developed for the treatment of these disorders. Studies by Bonilla et al. (1989) and Welte
et al. (1990) indicate that production of normal
numbers of functional neutrophils can be induced in the vast majority of patients with severe
forms of Kostmann's agranulocytosis by the
daily administration of recombinant G-CSF.
Similarly, while treatment with G-CSF does not
prevent the periodic flux in neutrophil production associated with cyclic neutropenia, it can
increase neutrophil counts at the nadir of each
cycle (Hammond et al., 1989).

Disorders of phagocyte function such as the
different variants of chronic granulomatous disease (CGD) (Curnutte and Babior, 1987; DiBartolomeo et al., 1987; Dinauer et al., 1987), congenital deficiency of LFA-1, the adhesion
molecule on the surface of neutrophils critical to
their capacity to move from the bloodstream to
sites of infection (Fischer et al., 1988), and congenital actin deficiency (Camitta et al., 1977)
can also be corrected by eliminating the marrow
of the diseased host and replacing it with marrow
from a normal allogeneic donor. This approach
has led to long-term disease-free survival for
most patients transplanted for LFA-1 deficiency
(Fischer et al., 1988). However, in the experience accrued to date (Curnutte and Babior, 1987;
DiBartolomeo et al., 1987; Fischer et al., 1986b;
O'Reilly et al., 1984), all but one of the patients
transplanted for CGD (DiBartolomeo et al.,
1988) or congenital actin deficiency have suc-
cumbed to preexisting or intercurrent infections

early or late in the posttransplant period. Improved results would likely be achieved if such patients were transplanted when free of active infection.

Chediak–Higachi syndrome, an autosomal recessive disorder characterized by pigmentary dilution of the hair and skin, deficiencies of natural killer cells, and abnormalities of microtubular assembly in the phagocytes leading to the development of characteristic giant cytoplasmic granules and impairments of bactericidal activity (Chediak, 1952), has been repeatedly corrected by allogeneic marrow transplants (Vierlizier et al., 1982; Fischer et al., 1994).

An alternative preparative regimen has been required to successfully prepare patients with familial erythrophagocytic lymphohistiocytosis (FEL). This unique congenital myeloproliferative disorder produces pancytopenia and immunodeficiency with prominent infiltration of the spleen, liver, lymph nodes, bone marrow, and meninges with histiocytes exhibiting prominent erythrophagocytosis (Macmahon et al., 1963). Because the disorder is partially responsive to VP-16, a preparative cytoreductive regimen has been developed that incorporates this agent in combination with cyclophosphamide, myleran, and cytosine arabinoside. At least 7 of 9 patients transplanted with this approach have achieved full and durable reversals of the disease with correction of associated lymphoid and hematopoietic abnormalities (Fischer et al., 1994; O'Reilly, MSKCC Experience).

The juvenile, autosomal recessive form of osteopetrosis is a disorder characterized by functional deficiencies of osteoclasts that lead to an inability to resorb and reform bone (Brown and Dent, 1971). Encroachment of bone on the cranial cavity and its foramina produces cranial nerve palsies, blindness, deafness, and increased intracranial pressure early in life. The growth of long bones is also severely compromised. In addition, marrow spaces are gradually obliterated ultimately eliminating intramedullary sites of hematopoiesis and inducing aplastic anemia. Allogeneic marrow transplants can correct this disorder by replacing defective host osteoclasts with normal osteoclasts derived from monocyte/macrophage pools produced by the donor

marrow (Coccia et al., 1980; Sorell et al., 1981). Of the initial 10 patients transplanted for this disease (Gerritsen et al., 1990), 7 have achieved long-term survival with correction of hematopoietic function. Engraftment of donor-derived osteoclasts has led to extensive resorption of sclerotic bone with subsequent normalization of bone structure and growth. A recent report of the European transplant experience with this disease has confirmed these encouraging results (Fischer, 1989).

Marrow Transplantation for Genetic Disorders of Metabolism

Following engraftment of allogeneic marrow in a myeloablated, immunosuppressed host, donor-derived cells of the monocyte/macrophage lineage expand and migrate from the circulation, ultimately replacing populations of host-type macrophages fixed in the tissues. Cytogenetic analyses of cells in tissues biopsied from animals or from humans 2–3 months posttransplant have demonstrated that Langerhans' cells in the skin (Stingl et al., 1980), Kupffer cells in the liver (Gale et al., 1978), alveolar macrophages in the lung (Thomas et al., 1976), osteoclasts in bone (Coccia et al., 1980; Sorell et al., 1981), and microglial cells in the brain (Hoogerbrugge et al., 1988) are of donor origin. These findings, coupled with the results of *in vitro* experiments demonstrating that the pathologic features of fibroblasts or glial cells derived from patients with certain mucolipidoses and mucopolysaccharidoses could be corrected by coculture with fibroblasts, lymphocytes, or macrophages from enzymatically normal individuals (Abraham et al., 1985; Brooks et al., 1981; Conzelman and Sandhoff, 1984; Gruber et al., 1985; Kihara et al., Neufeld, 1973; Olsen et al., 1983; Weismann et al., 1971), have stimulated exploration of marrow transplants as a method for introducing into affected individuals a normal, constantly renewable source of progenitor cells capable of continuously supplying tissues with enzymatically intact macrophages for correction of these diseases.

Slavin and Yatziv (1980) were the first to demonstrate that a transplant of marrow could lead to normalization of levels of a lysosomal enzyme in leukocytes, liver, and plasma, when they used such grafts to correct β-glucuronidase deficiency in mice. Subsequent experiments demonstrated that marrow grafts from normal donors could reverse or prevent the visceral pathology of several storage diseases, including arylsulfatase B deficiency in cats (Gasper et al., 1984), type I mucopolysaccharidosis (Shull et al., 1987, 1988), and fucosidosis in dogs (Taylor et al., 1986), and Neimann–Pick disease in mice (Sakiyama et al., 1983). However, in the latter two models, while enzyme levels increased in the central nervous system of transplanted animals, symptoms of central nervous system degeneration progressed, and lethality was neither averted nor delayed. Recently, however, it has been found that transplants administered early in life to twitcher mice (a model of galactosyl ceramidase deficiency, or Krabbes disease in man) or to dogs afflicted with mucopolysaccharidosis type I (a model of Hurler syndrome), can not only increase levels of the deficient enzyme in the central nervous system but also retard the development of central nervous system pathology (Hoogerbrugge et al., 1988). In successfully transplanted twitcher mice, significant reversals of peripheral neuropathies, with remyelinization of affected nerves, are also observed (Yeager et al., 1984).

Experience with transplants for the treatment of metabolic diseases in man is still limited, but reiterates several of these issues. The transplantation programs at Westminster Hospital (Hobbs et al., 1986) and at the University of Minnesota (Krivit et al., 1990), which have most extensively studied this approach, have each recorded sustained increments in tissue and body fluid levels of deficient enzymes following engraftment and functional development of HLA-matched marrow transplants from normal donors in patients with types I, II, III, IV, and VI mucopolysaccharidosis (Desai et al., 1983; Hobbs et al., 1981, 1986; Hugh-Jones, 1982, 1986; Krivit et al., 1984, 1990b; Warkentin et al., 1986; Whitley et al., 1986) and mannosidosis (Will et al., 1987). Increments in the enzyme levels have led to reductions in tissue levels of abnormal storage products, with impressive improvements in the histological features and functions of affected organs such as the liver, spleen, corneas, heart, and skeletal system. The pathologic features of Gaucher's disease in the marrow, liver, and spleen have also been reduced following allogeneic marrow transplants (Rappeport et al., 1984). However, the improvements recorded have been incomplete and achieved over a much longer period of time (Ringden et al., 1988). At the other end of the spectrum, little, if any improvement in the histology, concentrations of storage products, or function of affected muscles has been recorded in patients transplanted for type II glycogen storage disease (Pompe's) (Harris et al., 1986), suggesting either that normal enzyme cannot be effectively transferred to these tissues or that abnormal stores of muscle glycogen cannot be mobilized or transported from the muscle cells for degradation by donor-derived macrophages.

For patients with metabolic disorders affecting the central nervous system, the effects of marrow transplants on the progression of degenerative changes induced by accumulations of storage products cannot yet be accurately assessed. However, at least two patients transplanted for metachromatic leukodystrophy have exhibited a stabilization of neurological symptoms and some improvement and developmental parameters (Bayever et al., 1985; Krivit et al., 1990a) associated with increases in arylsulfatase A activity in the cerebrospinal fluid (Krivit et al., 1990a). Similar stabilizations have also been recorded in patients transplanted for Krabbe's disease, Niemann–Pick disease (Krivit et al., 1990b), and adrenoleukodystrophy (Hobbs et al., 1981), as well as for Hurler's syndrome (MPS-I) (Hugh-Jones, 1986), and Sanfilippo's disease, type B (MPS-III) (Krivit et al., 1990b). In contrast, patients transplanted for Hunter's disease (MPS-II) to date have experienced progression of neurological symptoms despite a successful graft. Similarly, case reports of patients transplanted for Sanfilippo's disease type A (Hugh-Jones et al., 1982; O'Donnell et al., 1987) and Lesch–Nyhan disease (Nyhan et al., 1986) have failed to record any arrest in the progression of neurological symptoms. The progressive degenerative changes in the CNS associated with the latter disorders may not be altered by a marrow transplant; alternatively, different results might be achieved if a transplant were invoked earlier in the disease, before degenerative changes in CNS have become advanced.

HLA-MATCHED MARROW TRANSPLANTS FOR APLASTIC ANEMIA

Aplastic anemia in its severe form (marked hypocellularity of the marrow with lymphocyte constituting $> 65\%$ of marrow elements, an absolute neutrophil count $< 500/mm^3$, a platelet count $< 20,000/mm^3$, corrected reticulocyte count $< 1\%$) has been demonstrated to be lethal for over 75% of affected patients, over half of whom will die within 6 months of diagnosis (Lynch et al., 1975; Camitta et al., 1979). Treatment with androgens or steroids does not significantly improve their prognosis (Camitta et al., 1979). In 1978, HLA-matched allogeneic marrow grafts administered after high dose cyclophosphamide were demonstrated to be a treatment of choice for this disease, securing hematopoietic reconstitution and long-term survival for 57% of treated patients versus 23% for patients treated with autologous and supportive care alone (Camitta et al., 1979).

HLA-MATCHED MARROW TRANSPLANTS FOR LEUKEMIA

Between 1968 and 1978, marrow transplants were almost exclusively applied to the treatment of patients with leukemia who were already refractory to chemotherapy. Overall, 13–18% of such patients achieved durable disease-free survival (Thomas et al., 1977). However, for patients transplanted when in good physical condition, the probability of extended disease-free survival was 25%. Based on these results, transplants were then applied to patients in good clinical condition, at a stage in the disease when the leukemia cells burden was low and the residual leukemic cells were likely to be still sensitive to the cytoreduction employed (Thomas et al., 1979). In 1979, the Seattle group reported a series of patients with acute myelogenous leukemia transplanted in first remission of whom 63%

achieved long-term disease-free survival. In this series, the risk of relapse was only 12%. This study was quickly confirmed by several transplant centers, and led to the widespread exploration of HLA-matched marrow grafts in the treatment of acute leukemias in first or second remission and CML in first chronic phase. Approximately 10 years of this experience can now be evaluated. Results can also be compared with those achieved with current chemotherapy and with autologous marrow grafts at different stages in the disease course.

MARROW TRANSPLANTATION FOR ACUTE MYELOGENOUS LEUKEMIA (AML)

Transplants after First Relapse of AML

For patients with AML in second or later remission or relapse, an allogeneic HLA-matched marrow graft is generally regarded as the treatment of choice.

Transplants in First Remission of AML

The role of allogeneic marrow transplants in the treatment of patients with AML in first remission is considerably more controversial. Prospective clinical trials derived from six single institutions and two cooperative groups have compared HLA-matched marrow grafts and chemotherapy in the treatment of AML in first remission in young adults (< 40 years of age) (Appelbaum et al., 1984; Champlin et al., 1985; Clarkson et al., 1990; Conde et al., 1988; Powles et al., 1980; Zander et al., 1988). In each of these trials (Table II), the incidence of posttreatment relapse was significantly lower among transplant patients (9 to 40%) than among patients treated with chemotherapy alone (71 to 90%). In each of these studies, 3–5 year disease-free survival rates for patients transplanted were also superior to those achieved with chemotherapy alone. However, these differences were statistically significant in only three of the six single institution or multicenter trials. Other trials are in progress. However, continuing improvements in chemotherapy regimens and in transplantation approaches may make these studies obsolete before they are completed.

The role of marrow transplants in the treat-

Table II. Results of Prospective Trials Comparing Transplantation and Chemotherapy for the Treatment of AML in First Remission

Center	Bone marrow transplant			Chemotherapy			Reference
	DFS[a] (%)	N	Rate of relapse (%)	DFS (%)	N	Rate of relapse (%)	
Adults and children							
Fred Hutchinson	49*	33	15	20	46	74	Appelbaum et al. (1984)
UCLA, 1985	40	23	40*	27	44	71	Champlin et al. (1985)
UCLA, 1992	45	28	32*	38	54	60	Schiller (1992)
France	66*	20	18*	16	20	83	Reiffers (1989)
ECOG	42	54	13	30	29	NS	Cassileth (1992)
Royal Marsden	64*	22	22*	29	28	68	Powles et al. (1980)
University of Cantabria	70*	14	10*	17	13	88	Conde et al. (1988)
Memorial Sloan-Kettering Cancer Center	33	28	15	17	69	80	Clarkson et al. (1990)
M.D. Anderson	36	11	9*	18	27	85	Zander et al. (1988)
Children only							
St. Jude/Seattle	43	19	30*	31	42	62	Dahl et al. (1990)
Sweden	100	11	0*	7	15	93	Ringden et al. (1989)

[a]DFS, disease-free survival.
*Statistically significant difference.

ment of children with AML is particularly controversial since new chemotherapeutic regimens have significantly increased the proportion of children who achieve and remain in first remission. Currently, 40 to 50% of children treated with such regimens who achieve a first remission are alive and in sustained remission 5 years later (Creutzig et al., 1985; Weinstein et al., 1983). However, HLA-matched marrow grafts administered to children with AML in first remission have also achieved impressive results: 43 to 100% of such patients are alive and disease-free 3–5 years posttransplant (Brochstein et al., 1987; Dahl et al., 1990; Ringden et al., 1989). In a recent prospective trial conducted by the CCSG, 49% of children transplanted for AML in first remission were alive and in sustained remission 3 years posttreatment compared to 40% for patients treated with chemotherapy alone ($p <$ 0.05) (Feig et al., 1987). Thus, for children with AML in first remission, HLA-matched marrow grafts appear to be superior to chemotherapy alone.

The relative efficacy of autologous marrow grafts when compared with allogeneic marrow

grafts in the treatment of patients with AML in first remission is not yet established.

MARROW TRANSPLANTATION FOR ACUTE LYMPHOBLASTIC LEUKEMIA (ALL)

Transplants for ALL in First Remission

Current multidrug chemotherapeutic regimens combining systemic treatment and CNS prophylaxis chemotherapeutic regimens are able to induce sustained remissions or cures in 70 to 80% of children with ALL presenting with standard risk features (Tubergen et al., 1990). Furthermore, more intensive regimens applied to children at high risk for relapse have increased their probability of sustained disease-free survival to 60 to 70% (Clavell et al., 1986; Steinherz et al., 1986). Because of these results, it has been difficult to identify pediatric patients with ALL in first remission for whom an allogeneic transplant clearly affords an improved probability of cure. Indeed, allogeneic marrow grafts in children and adolescents with high risk features have been associated with long-term disease-free survival rates of 56 to 84%, which are not superior to those that can now be achieved with chemotherapy alone (Barrett et al., 1986, 1989; Bordigoni et al., 1989).

The place of allogeneic marrow grafts in the treatment of adults with ALL who have achieved an initial remission is only somewhat less controversial (Champlin and Gale, 1989). However, some results suggest that allogeneic marrow grafts may offer a significant advantage to the adult with ALL who presents with high risk features. Prospective trials are needed, however, to ascertain this point and also to evaluate transplantation as a general approach to the treatment of adults with both average and high risk forms of ALL who achieve a first remission.

Transplants for ALL in Second or Greater Remission or Relapse

Results reported for series of children who have received HLA-matched marrow grafts for acute lymphoblastic leukemia when in second remission vary considerably both in the incidence of relapse posttransplant and in the proportion of patients achieving long-term disease-free survival. Transplants administered after cytoreduction with variations of the Seattle regimen of single dose TBI and cyclophosphamide have been associated with relapse rates ranging from 30 to 57% at 2 years, and disease-free survival rates of 33 to 50% (Sanders et al., 1987; Woods et al., 1983). In contrast, newer approaches incorporating higher doses of hyperfractionated total body irradiation followed by cyclophosphamide (Brochstein et al., 1987)(Fig. 3a), or fractionated total body irradiation administered with high dose cytosine arabinoside (Coccia et al., 1988), etoposide (Blume et al., 1987), or altered doses of cyclophosphamide (Wingard et al., 1990), have reduced the incidence of relapse posttransplant to 5 to 16%, and concurrently improved long-term disease-free survival to 59 to 64% at 5 years. (Fig. 3a) Our own results strongly suggest that an allogeneic marrow graft is superior to chemotherapy for patients with ALL who relapse within 1 year of achieving their first remission. In our series, transplants may also be superior to chemotherapy when applied to patients with ALL who relapse late in their first remission (Fig. 3b). However, prospective trials comparing these

two approaches are still needed to ascertain this issue.

MARROW TRANSPLANTS FOR CHRONIC MYELOGENOUS LEUKEMIA (CML)

Allogeneic bone marrow transplantation is clearly the treatment of choice in patients with CML who are under the age of 55 and have an HLA-compatible donor. Single-agent chemotherapy applied to the treatment of CML has been only palliative, and has not been shown to significantly prolong survival (Sokal et al., 1988).

MARROW TRANSPLANTS FOR MYELODYSPLASTIC SYNDROMES

The myelodysplastic syndromes are a heterogeneous series of disorders marked by peripheral cytopenias associated with normal to increased marrow cellularity and abnormal maturation of the myeloid series. Intensive chemotherapeutic regimens have yielded only short-term remissions and have been associated with significant morbidity and mortality (Kantarjian et al., 1986). In contrast to these results, allogeneic marrow grafts administered to patients prepared with TBI or busulfan and cyclophosphamide have led to sustained remissions of disease in 40 to 50% of cases (Anderson et al., 1993; Appelbaum et al., 1990; Arnold and Heimpel, 1989; DeWitte et al., 1990; Guinan et al., 1989; O'Donnell et al., 1987).

MARROW TRANSPLANTS FOR LYMPHOMA

Current regimens employing multiple chemotherapeutic agents in dose-intensive protocols will induce durable curative remissions in approximately 50% of adults and over 70% of children with intermediate and high-grade lymphomas. Similarly, primary treatment of Hodgkin's disease is now curative for over 70% of cases. As a result, transplant of either allogeneic or autologous marrow, administered after myeloablative doses of total body radiation or alkylating agents and cyclophosphamide, has largely been applied

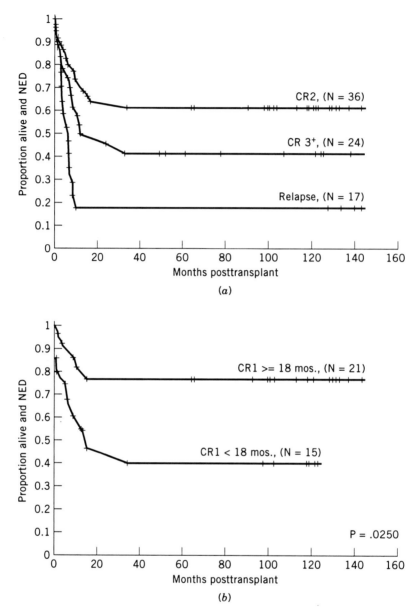

Fig. 3. Kaplan Meier plots comparing rates of disease-free survival for patients < 21 years of age transplanted for acute lymphoblastic leukemia after hyperfractionated total body irradiation and cyclophosphamide (The MSKCC experience). *a*: Results for patients in second or third degree remissions or relapse. *b*: Results for patients with acute lymphoblastic leukemia in second remission, dependent on duration of first remission (Memorial Sloan-Kettering Cancer Center).

to patients who fail to attain or sustain a primary remission of disease. Experience with allogeneic marrow transplants applied to the treatment of non-Hodgkin's lymphoma (NHL) while still limited, indicates that for patients with chemotherapy refractory NHL, prospects for extended disease-free survival (DFS) range from 0 to 23% (Copelan et al., 1990; Ernst et al., 1986; Phillips et al., 1986), compared to 25 to 44% of patients grafted in a second remission and up to 88% for patients reported who received transplants in first remission (Ernst et al., 1986; Troussard et al., 1990). It should also be noted that in large series, results of allogeneic marrow grafts have not differed in incidence of DFS or relapse post-transplant from those achieved with autologous marrow grafts if the autologous marrow was obtained during remission (Appelbaum et al., 1987; Gribben et al., 1987).

MARROW TRANSPLANTATION FOR PATIENTS LACKING AN HLA-IDENTICAL SIBLING

As recognition of the curative potential of al-logeneic marrow transplants has grown, the need to develop approaches that would permit transplants of normal marrow in the 60 to 70% of patients who lack an HLA-matched sibling has increased markedly. Several approaches to such patients are actively being explored, particularly the use of unmodified marrow grafts from partially matched related or HLA-compatible unrelated donors and the use of HLA nonidentical marrow grafts sufficiently depleted of T-lymphocytes so that they can be administered without the risk of lethal GvHD. Each of these approaches has shown considerable promise, but each is also associated with increased risks of either graft rejection or severe GvHD.

The genes within the HLA complex exhibit an extraordinary degree of polymorphism (see Chapter 1) (Bodmer et al., 1989). Molecular analyses further indicate that the allelic polymorphism detectable by serology is incomplete because several molecular variants of certain class I and class II alleles can be distinguished by isoelectric focusing, restriction fragment length polymorphism, or hybridization with sequence-specific oligonucleotide probes (Choo et al., 1986; Thomsen et al., 1989). Given the large number of different alleles that exist for each of the class I and class II genes of the HLA system and the assumption that the genes within the HLA region have been recombined at random over the course of evolution, it could be expected that the identification of a suitably compatible relative other than an HLA-matched sibling would be a rare event. In fact, however, HLA-phenotypically matched or partially matched related donors have been identified for up to 5 to 10% of patients. This is due, in part, to the high

frequency of several HLA class I and class II alleles and, in some cases, to the coassociation of certain HLA-A,-B, and -DR alleles to form specific haplotypes in certain ethnogeographic groups—a phenomenon termed genetic linkage disequilibrium (see Chapter 1) (Bauer et al., 1984).

For patients with certain lethal genetic disorders of hematopoiesis known to be common in specified ethnogeographic groups, such as Fanconi's anemia, Kostmann's agranulocytosis, and certain forms of severe combined immunodeficiencies, parents unrelated to one another often share one or more HLA alleles that are inherited on one of the patient's HLA haplotypes. In such circumstances a parent may be identified who is HLA compatible with a given patient. This situation may also be observed for patients with acquired blood diseases when both parents originate from a relatively restricted ethnogeographic background. Related donors may also be identified at significant frequency for patients who inherit an HLA-A,-B,-DR haplotype known to be in genetic linkage disequilibrium. Examples of common haplotypes detected among caucasians are summarized in Table III. In such cases, a search is made among the offspring of relatives sharing with the patient the uncommon or nonlinked haplotype. Through searches of this kind, a cousin can often be found who derives the common haplotype from a totally different pedigree together with the uncommon haplotype shared by the patient.

For a proportion of patients, particularly patients inheriting two HLA haplotypes containing alleles in genetic disequilibrium, unrelated donors may also be identified. For patients with two HLA haplotypes in linkage disequilibrium, the probability of identifying a suitably compatible donor from a relatively small pool of 10,000 individuals is high. In contrast, for patients inheriting haplotypes containing rare HLA alleles that are not linked to the other determinants in the haplotype, the probability of identifying a donor, even within the pool of a million donors, is remote (Sonnenberg et al., 1989). Based on the frequency of individual HLA-A,-B,-DR alleles and haplotypes in linkage disequilibrium, it has been estimated that a donor registry containing one million individuals would be sufficient to

Table III. Three-Locus Haplotype Frequencies (per 10,000) in Caucasians[a]

HLA-A, B, DR ($n = 1889$)

Haplotype HLA-			Haplotype frequency	Delta Value
A	B	DR		
2	w62	4	86	25
2	13	7	55	2
30	13	7	83	59
2	44	7	57	−37
29	44	7	111	76
1	w57	7	101	59
2	18	w11	84	33
24	35	w11	53	23
24	35	w11	53	23
2	44	w11	61	19
3	35	1	133	72
11	35	1	79	43
2	7	2	127	−9
3	7	2	260	115
24	7	2	69	3
25	18	2	69	44
2	44	2	62	9
1	8	3	477	280
2	8	3	74	−98
3	7	4	50	−12
2	51	w11	78	18
2	w62	w11	53	10

[a]From Bauer et al. (1984).

provide an HLA-A,-B,-Dr matched donor for at least an additional 35% of individuals who lack an HLA-matched sibling (Beatty et al., 1988).

To establish a donor pool of this size, the National Bone Marrow Donor Program has, over the past 6 years, conducted an intensive recruiting effort. At present this registry maintains a computerized bank of over 1.3 million typed donors. Furthermore, this registry is now connected to several other donor registries in Europe. Principal among these is the Anthony Nolan Foundation, a registry of over 200,000 donors based in London. Additional, smaller registries have been established in France, Holland, Italy, the Scandinavian countries, and Russia. Currently, these registries are identifying serologically matched, MLC compatible donors for up to 20 to 30% of patients who are of European caucasian background and particularly for patients inheriting two common HLA-A,-B,

-DR haplotypes. However, the proportion of successful searches for patients who are black, oriental, hispanic, or native american is very low, due to the limited number of donors from these minority groups in the donor registries.

UNMODIFIED MARROW GRAFTS FROM PARTIALLY MATCHED RELATED DONORS

Since the early 1970s, several groups have conducted limited explorations of the use of HLA-partially matched related donors in an attempt to identify tolerable histoincompatibilities within the HLA region. These early studies concentrated on the use of HLA haplotype-identical but MLC-compatible related donors because of results in murine transplantation models indicated that marrow grafts from MHC class II disparate donors were most likely to induce lethal GvHD (Klein and Park, 1973). Initial studies, which were conducted in patients with SCID, tended to support this approach to donor selection, since disparities for HLA-A and/or -B on one haplotype were tolerated without lethal GvHD.

Experience with partially matched related donor marrow grafts in the treatment of aplastic anemia underscores the incremental risk of marrow graft rejection when HLA-disparate grafts are used. In 1985, Beatty et al. (1985) reported that transplants administered to leukemic patients differing from their donors at a single HLA allele developed grade II–IV GvHD in over 75% of cases. However, long-term disease-free survival was comparable to that observed following HLA-matched sibling marrow transplants. In this series, no one allelic disparity (i.e., HLA-A, or -B, or -D) could be identified that placed the patient at greater risk for severe GvHD. Graft rejections were observed in 9% of such cases, an incidence increased over that following HLA-matched sibling grafts.

TRANSPLANTS OF UNMODIFIED MARROW FROM UNRELATED DONORS

In 1977, our group reported a successful reconstitution of immunologic function in a child with SCID engrafted with marrow from an HLA-compatible unrelated donor (O'Reilly et al.,

1977). Subsequent case reports demonstrated that unrelated marrow grafts could also reconstitute hematopoiesis in patients transplanted for leukemia or aplastic anemia. In 1988, a series of 40 patients was reported with refractory forms of leukemia and aplastic anemia who had received marrow grafts from unrelated, HLA-matched or partially mismatched donors obtained from a statewide registry developed in Iowa (Gingrich et al., 1988). Of these patients, 15% survived disease free for periods of more than a year. Acute severe GvHD was observed in 67%, and all but one of the surviving patients also had chronic GvHD.

Recently, the cumulative results of the first 462 transplants performed using donors identified by the National Marrow Donor Program have been summarized (Kernan et al., 1993). Of these patients, 352 received transplants for leukemia, 38 for myelodysplastic or lymphoid malignancies, and 72 for aplasias and congenital disorders of immunity or metabolism. In this series, early or late graft failures were observed in 14% of cases. Acute GvHD of grade II or greater severity was observed in 64% of cases; in 47%, grade III–IV acute GvHD was observed. Severe grade III–IV acute GvHD was significantly increased among recipients of unmodified marrow grafts (60%) when compared to the group transplanted with T cell-depleted marrow (30%). Limited or extensive chronic GvHD was observed in 55% of cases, again particularly among recipients of unmodified marrow grafts.

The basis for the marked increase in the incidence of severe acute GvHD in recipients of HLA-phenotypically matched unrelated marrow when compared with that observed in recipients of HLA-genotypically matched sibling marrow is still poorly understood. It may reflect alloreactions generated against molecular differences in class I and II alleles that can be detected only by more discriminatory molecular approaches such as isoelectric focusing or hybridization with HLA-microvariant sequence-specific oligonucleotides. In recent studies, up to 30% of HLA-serologically matched MLC compatible unrelated individuals selected as potential donors were found to differ from their intended recipient by 1 or 2 alleles distinguishable by isoelectric focusing (Kernan et al., 1990), and over 60% by

sequence analyses of HLA class I determinants (Santamaria et al., 1994). Preliminary evidence suggests that microvariant disparities for class II determinants also occur at significant frequency among HLA- and MLC-matched unrelated donor recipient pairs (Al-Daccak et al., 1990; Howard et al., 1992). These molecular differences in HLA class I and II alleles likely also explain the increased frequency of allocytotoxic T cells that can be generated in mixed lymphocyte cultures between HLA-phenotypically matched unrelated donor recipient pairs in comparison with the low frequency of such cells generated in mixed lymphocyte cultures between HLA-matched siblings (Beatty et al., 1990).

T CELL-DEPLETED HLA-NONIDENTICAL RELATED AND HLA-COMPATIBLE UNRELATED MARROW GRAFTS

A central limitation to the use of single HLA-disparate related donors and suitably matched unrelated donors is that such donors are realistically available only for 20 to 30% of individuals lacking an HLA-matched sibling. Furthermore, it is already clear that restricted donor availability will persist even when registries in excess of one million unrelated donors have been recruited (Sonnenberg et al., 1989). Development of more sensitive techniques for the selection of donors matched for HLA class I and class II microvariants, while important to our understanding of incompatibilities contributing to graft rejection, GvHD, and impaired immunologic reconstitution posttransplantation, will nevertheless serve only to further restrict the proportion of patients for whom an adequately compatible donor will be identified. Thus, there is a continuing need for the development of transplantation approaches whereby consistent engraftment and functional reconstitution can be achieved in HLA-disparate recipients without severe or lethal GvHD.

The development of techniques for depleting T-lymphocytes from a marrow allograft has provided one such approach to this dilemma. In 1981, our group showed that transplants of HLA-A,-B or HLA haplotype disparate parental marrow depleted of T cells by agglutination with a soybean lectin followed by E-rosette depletion could reconstitute hematopoietic and lymphoid function in children with leukemia or SCID (Reisner et al., 1981) without GvHD. In our series of 60 patients with SCID who have been transplanted with T cell-depleted HLA-haplotype disparate parental marrow over the last 12 years, 47 currently survive with reconstitution of immunity and stable donor lymphoid chimerism. In this series, only three patients have developed grade I acute GvH reactions. The actuarial disease-free survival at 6 years for this group (74%) is not different from that achieved following unmodified HLA-matched grafts in severe combined immunodeficiency. Other centers incorporating this and other approaches to T cell depletion have reported similar results (O'Reilly et al., 1989). These studies of T cell-depleted HLA disparate marrow grafts applied to children with SCID demonstrate the potential of this approach and illustrate the feasibility of broad application of marrow grafts to patients lacking a matched sibling donor. Unfortunately, when T cell-depleted HLA-nonidentical marrow grafts have been used for the treatment of other genetic and acquired diseases of hematopoiesis or leukemia, they have been considerably less effective because of their enhanced susceptibility to rejection. Recently, however, new techniques employing more intensive cytoreductive measures, coupled with less stringent or more selective T cell depletion methods and the administration of T cell-specific immunotoxins or antithymocyte globulin in the early posttransplant period, have reduced the incidence of rejection without unduly increasing the risk of severe GvHD. For example, in a series of patients transplanted with T cell-depleted marrow from unrelated donors for hematologic malignancies (Ash et al., 1990), patients transplanted for acute leukemia in early remission or chronic phase CML achieved a 48% extended disease-free survival. In this series, HLA-matched unrelated marrow grafts were associated with a 20% incidence of grade II–IV GvHD, a result that is markedly lower than that observed among unmodified marrow transplants. As a result, the T cell-depleted grafts were also associated with significant improvement in disease-free survival (60 vs 29% at 3

months), a difference that was not observed among recipients of HLA-matched sibling marrow grafts. Similarly, in the review of results of marrow grafts from donors identified by the National Marrow Donor Program applied to patients with CML, McGlave et al. (1993) found the incidence of durable engraftment following T cell-depleted grafts (94%) did not differ from that following unmodified grafts (88%) reflecting improvements in the cytoreductive regimen used for these transplants. As expected, the incidences of severe (grade II–IV) acute GvHD and chronic GvHD were significantly reduced in recipients of T cell-depleted grafts. Strikingly, the incidence of relapse following a T cell-depleted unrelated graft (16% at 2 years) did not differ significantly from that observed following an unmodified graft (10% at 2 years). As a result, T cell-depleted grafts were again shown to be associated with a significant improvement in long-term disease-free survival.

The results of T cell-depleted partially matched related and HLA-phenotypically compatible unrelated marrow transplants in children have yielded particularly promising results. In a series of 10 children, with aplastic anemia, 5 have achieved long-term reconstitution (Camitta et al., 1989). Similarly, in a report of 31 children transplanted with HLA-nonidentical T cell-depleted marrow for leukemia, 54% were able to secure extended disease-free survival (Trigg et al., 1989).

While the results of trials incorporating techniques that permit more consistent engraftment together with a low incidence of severe GvHD are encouraging, HLA-partially matched related or HLA-matched unrelated marrow grafts have still not attained rates of extended disease-free survival comparable to those achieved following HLA-matched sibling grafts. In most of these series, the difference is due to a disturbingly high frequency of infectious complications following HLA-partially matched related or unrelated marrow grafts, complications that may reflect the relatively profound and protracted state of immunodeficiency observed following these marrow transplants (Marks et al., 1993). The basis for these immunodeficiencies is not clear, but may indicate limitations to the redevelopment or reeducation of donor cells in a partially HLA-disparate environment. Research in this critical area is urgently needed to identify and potentially circumvent such limitations to immune reconstitution. On the positive side, however, the incidence of relapse following such transplants, when applied to the treatment of patients with acute and chronic leukemias, has been strikingly low, possibly reflecting advantages of increased genetic disparity between donor and host for the expression of the antileukemic effects of a marrow allograft.

REFERENCES

Abraham LD, Muir H, Olsen I, Winchester B (1985): Direct enzyme transfer from lymphocytes corrects a lysosomal storage. Biochem Biophys Res Commun 129:415–417.

Alarcon B, Regueiro JR, Arnaiz-Villena A, Terhorst C (1988): Familial defect in the surface expression of the T-cell receptor-CD3 complex. N Engl J Med 319:1203–1208.

Al-Daccak R, Loiseau P, Rabian C, Devergie A, Bourdeau H, Raffoux C, Gluckman E, and Colombani J (1990): HLA-DR, DQ, and/or genotypic mismatches between recipient-donor pairs in unrelated bone marrow transplantation and transplant clinical outcome. Transplantation 50:960–964.

Anasetti C, Amos D, Beatty PG, Appelbaum FR, Bensinger W, Buckner CD, Clift R, Doney K, Martin PJ, Mickelson E, Nisperios B, O'Quigley J, Ramberg R, Sanders JE, Stewart P, Storb R, Sullivan KM, Witherspoon RP, Thomas ED, Hansen JA (1989): Effect of HLA compatibility of engraftment of bone marrow transplants in patients with leukemia or lymphoma. N Engl J Med 320:197–204.

Anderson JE, Appelbaum FR, Fisher LD, Schoch G, Shulman H, Anasetti C, Bensinger WI, Bryant E, Buckner CD, Doney K, Martin PJ, Sanders JE, Sullivan KM, Thomas ED, Witherspoon RP, Hansen JA, Storb R (1993): Allogeneic bone marrow transplantation for 93 patients with myelodysplastic syndrome. Blood 82:677–681.

Antin JH, Bierer BE, Smith BR, Ferrara J, Guinan EC, Sieff C, Golan DE, Macklis RM, Tarbell NJ, Lynch E, Reichert TA, Blythman H, Bouloux C, Rappeport JM, Burakoff SJ, Weinstein HJ (1991): Selective depletion of bone marrow T-lymphocytes with anti-CD5 monoclonal antibodies: Effective prophylaxis for graft-versus-host disease in patients with hematologic malignancies. Blood 78:2139–2149.

Appelbaum FR, Dahlberg S, Thomas Ed, Buchner CD, Cheever MA, Clift RA, Crowley J, Deeg HJ, Fefer A, Greenberg PD, Kadin M, Smith W, Smith W, Stewart P, Sullivan K, Storb R, Weiden P (1984): Bone marrow transplantation for chemotherapy after remission induction for adults with acute nonlymphoblastic leukemia: A prospective comparison. Ann Intern Med 101:581–588.

Appelbaum FR, Sullivan KM, Buckner CD, Clift RA, Deeg HJ, Fefer A, Hill R, Mortimer J, Neiman PA, Sanders JE, Singer J, Stewart P, Storb R, Thomas ED (1987): Treatment of malignant lymphoma in 100 patients with chemotherapy, total body irradiation, and marrow transplantation. J Clin Oncol 5(9):1340.

Appelbaum FR, Barrall J, Storb R, Fisher LD, Schoch G, Ramberg RE, Shulman H, Anasetti C, Bearman SI, Beatty P, Bensinger WI, Buckner CD, Clift RA, Hansen JA, Martin P, Petersen FB, Sanders JE, Singer J, Stewart P, Sullivan KM, Witherspoon RP, Thomas ED (1990): Bone marrow transplantation for patients with myelodysplasia: Pretreatment variables and outcome. Ann Intern Med 112(8):590–597.

Arnold R, Heimpel H (1989): Allogeneic bone marrow transplantation for myelodysplastic syndromes (MDS). Bone Marrow Transplant 4(suppl 4):101.

Ash RC, Casper JT, Chitambar CR, Hansen R, Burnin N, Truitt RL, Lawton C, Murray K, Hunter J, Baxter-Lowe LA (1990): Successful allogeneic transplantation on T-cell depleted bone marrow from closely HLA-matched unrelated donors. N Engl J Med 322:485–494.

Atkinson K, Storb R, Prentice RL, Weiden PL, Witherspoon RP, Sullivan K, Noel D, Thomas ED (1979): Analysis of late infections in 89 long-term survivors of bone marrow transplantation. Blood 53(4):720–731.

Atkinson K, Farewell V, Strob R, Tsoi MS, Sullivan KM, Witherspoon RP, Fefer A, Clift R, Goodell B, Thomas ED (1982): Analysis of late infections after human bone marrow transplantation: Role of non-specific suppressor cells in patients with chronic graft-versus-host disease and genotypic non-identity between marrow donor and recipient. Blood 60:714–719.

August CS, King E, Githens JH, McIntosh K, Humbert JR, Greensheer A, Johnson FB (1976): Establishment of erythropoiesis following bone marrow transplantation in a patient with congenital hypoplastic anemia (Diamond-Blackfan syndrome). Blood 48:491–498.

Aversa F, Terenzi A, Carrotti A, Martelli MP, Latini P, Gambelunghe C, Martelli MF (1993): Addition of thiotepa improves results in T-cell depleted bone marrow transplant for advanced leukemia. Blood 82:81a.

Bach FH, Albertini RJ, Joo P, Anderson JL, Bortin MM (1968): Bone marrow transplantation in a patient with the Wiskott-Aldrich syndrome. Lancet 2:1364–1366.

Barrett AJ, Joshi R, Kendra JR, Phillips RH, Ashford R, Shaw PJ, Hugh-Jones K, Hobbs JR (1986): Prediction and prevention of relapse of acute lymphoblastic leukaemia after bone marrow transplantation. Br J Haematol 64:179.

Barrett AJ, Lucarelli G, Gale RP, Sobocinski A, Horowitz M, Bortin MM (1988): Bone marrow transplantation for thalassemia-A preliminary report from the International Bone Marrow Transplant Registry. In Buckner CD, Gale RP, Lucarelli G (eds): "Advances and Controversies in Thalassemia Therapy." New York: Alan R. Liss, pp 173–185.

Barrett AJ, Horowitz MM, Gale RP, Biggs JC, Camitta BM, Dicke KA, Gluckman E, Good RA, Herzig RH, Lee MB, Marmont AM, Masaoka T, Ramsay NKC, Rimm AA, Speck B, Zwaan FE, Bortin MM (1989): Marrow transplantation for acute lymphoblastic leukemia: Factors affecting relapse and survival. Blood 74(2):862–871.

Bauer MP, Neugebauer M, Albert ED (1984): Reference tables of three-locus haplotype frequencies and delta values. In Albert ED (ed): "Caucasians, Orientals, and Negroids in Histocompatibility Testing 1984." Berlin/Heidelberg: Springer-Verlag, pp 767–760.

Baughan AS, Worsley AM, McCarthy DM, Hows JM, Catovsky D, Gordon-Smith ED, Galton DAG, Goldman JM (1984): Haematological reconstitution and severity of graft-versus-host disease after bone marrow transplantation for chronic granulocytic leukaemia: The influence of previous splenectomy. Br J Haematol 56:445–454.

Bayever E, Philippart M, Nuwer M, Ladisch S, Brill N, Sparkes RS, Feig SA (1985): Bone marrow transplantation for metachromatic leukodystrophy. Lancet 2:471–473.

Beatty PG, Clift RA, Michelson EM, Nisperos BB, Flournoy N, Martin PJ, Sanders JE, Stewart P, Buckner CD, Storb R, Thomas ED, Hansen JA (1985): Marrow transplantation from related donors other than HLA-identical siblings. N Engl J Med 313:765–771.

Beatty PG, Dahlberg S, Mickelson EM, Nisperos B, Opelz G, Martin PJ, Hansen JA (1988): Probability of finding HLA-matched unrelated marrow donors. Transplantation 45:714–718.

Beatty PG, Hansen JA, Anasetti C, Sander J, Martin PJ, Buckner CD, Storb R, Thomas ED (1990): Significance of different levels of histocompatibility in patients receiving marrow grafts from unrelated donors. Exp Hematol 15:509a.

Bellucci S, DeVergie A, Gluckman E, Tobelem G, Lethielleux P, Benbunan M, Schaison G, Boiron M (1985): Complete correction of Glanzmann's thrombasthenia by allogeneic bone marrow transplantation. Br J Haematol 56:635–641.

Blazar, BR, Orr HT, Arthur DC, Kersey JH, Filipovich AH (1985): Restriction fragment length polymorphisms as markers of engraftment in allogeneic marrow transplantation. Blood 66:1436–1444.

Blume KG, Forman SJ, O'Donnell MR, Doroshow JH, Krance RA, Nademanee AP, Snyder DS, Schmidt GM, Fahey JL, Metter GE, Hill LR, Findley DO, Sniecinski IJ (1987): Total body irradiation and high-dose etoposide: A new preparatory regimen for bone marrow transplantation in patients with advanced hematologic malignancies. Blood 69(4):1015–1020.

Bodmer WF, Albert E, Bodmer JG, Dupont B, Mach B, Mayr WR, Sasazuki T, Schreuder GM, Svejgaard A, Terasaki PI (1989): Nomenclature for factors of the HLA system, 1987. In Dupont B (ed): "Immunobiology of HLA, Histocompatibility Testing 1987," Vol 1. New York: Springer-Verlag, pp 72–79.

Bolger GB, Sullivan KM, Storb R, Witherspoon RP, Weiden PL, Stewart P, Sanders J, Meyers JD, Martin PJ, Doney KC, Deeg HJ, Clift RA, Buchner CD, Appelbaum FR, Thomas ED (1986): Second marrow infusion for poor graft function after allogeneic marrow transplantation. Bone Marrow Transplant 1:21–30.

Bonilla MA, Gillio AP, Ruggiero M, Kernan NA, Brochstein JA, Abboud M, Fumagalli L, Vincent M, Gabrilove JL, Welte K, Souza LM, O'Reilly RJ (1989): Effects of recombinant human granulocyte colony-stimulating factor on neutropenia in patients with congenital agranulocytosis. N Engl J Med 320:1574–1580.

Bordignon C, Keever CA, Small TN, Flomenberg N, Dupont B, O'Reilly RJ (1989): Graft failure after T-cell-depleted human leukocyte antigen identical marrow transplants for leukemia: In vitro analyses of host effector mechanisms. Blood 74(6):2227–2236.

Bordigoni P, Vernant JP, Souillet G, Gluckman E, Marininchi D, Milpied N, Fischer A, Lemoine EB, Jouet JP, Reiffers J (1989): Allogeneic bone marrow transplantation for children with acute lymphoblastic leukemia in first remission: A Cooperative Study of the Groupe d'Etude de la Greffe de Moelle Osseuse. J Clin Oncol 7:747–753.

Bourgault I, Gomez A, Gomard E, Levy JP (1991): Limiting-dilution analysis of the HLA restriction of anti-Epstein-Barr virus-specific cytolytic T lymphocytes. Clin Exp Immunol 84:501–507.

Bozdech MJ, Sondel PM, Trigg ME, Longo W, Kohler PC, Flynn B, Billing R, Anderson SA, Hank JA, Hong R (1985): Transplantation of HLA-haploidentical T-cell depleted marrow for leukemia: Addition of cytosine arabinoside to the pretransplant conditioning prevents rejection. Exp Hematol 13:1201–1210.

Brochstein JA, Kirkpatrick D, Giardina P, Weinberg RS, Alter BP, Driscoll C, Wolfe L, Shank B, O'Reilly RJ (1986a): Bone marrow transplantation in two multiply-transfused patients with thalassemia major. Br J Haematol 63:445–456.

Brochstein JA, Kernan NA, Laver J, Emanuel D, Rabellino E, O'Reilly RJ (1986b): Bone marrow transplantation for thrombocytopenia-absent radii (TAR) syndrome. Proc XXI Congr Int Soc Haematol, Sydney, Australia.

Brochstein JA, Kernan NA, Groshen S, Cirrincione C, Shank B, Emanuel D, Laver J, O'Reilly RJ (1987): Allogeneic bone marrow transplantation after hyperfractionated total-body irradiation and cyclophosphamide in children with acute leukemia. N Engl J Med 317(26):1618–1624.

Brochstein JA, Gillio A, Ruggiero M, Kernan NA, Emanuel D, Laver J, Small TN, O'Reilly RJ (1991): Bone marrow transplantation (BMT) from HLA-identical or haploidentical donors for correction of Wiskott-Aldrich syndrome. J Pediat 119(6):907–912.

Brooks SE, Adachi M, Hoffman LM, Amsterdam D, Schneek L (1981): Enzymatic biochemical and morphological correction of Tay-Sachs disease glial cells in vitro. In Calahan W, Lowden JL (eds): "Lysosomes and Lysosomal Storage Diseases." New York: Raven Press, pp 195–203.

Brown DM, Dent PB: Pathogenesis of osteopetrosis (1971): A comparison of human and animal spectra. Pediat Res 5:181–191.

Camitta BM, Quesenberry PS, Parkman R et al. (1977): Bone marrow transplantation for an infant with neutrophil dysfunction. Exp Haematol 5:109–116.

Camitta BM, Thomas ED, Nathan DG, Gale RP, Ko-pecky J, Rappeport JM, Santos G, Gordon-Smith EC, Storb R (1979): A prospective study of androgens and bone marrow transplantation for treatment of severe aplastic anemia. Blood 53:504–514.

Camitta B, O'Reilly RJ, Sensenbrenner L, Rappeport J, Champlin R, Doney K, August C, Hoffmann RG, Kirkpatrick D, Stuart R, Santos G, Parkman R, Gale RP, Storb R, Nathan D (1983): Antithoracic duct lymphocyte globulin therapy of severe aplastic anemia. Blood 62:883–888.

Camitta B, Ash R, Menitove J, Murray K, Lawton C, Hunter J, Casper J (1989): Bone marrow transplantation for children with severe aplastic anemia: Use of donors other than HLA-identical siblings. Blood 74(5):1852–1857.

Champlin RE, Gale RP (1989): Acute lymphoblastic leukemia: Recent advances in biology and therapy. Blood 73(8):205.

Champlin RE, Ho WG, Gale RP, Winston D, Selch M, Mitsuyasu R, Lenarsky C, Elashoff R, Zieghelboim J, Feig SA (1985): Treatment of acute myelogenous leukemia: A prospective controlled trial of bone marrow transplantation versus consolidation chemotherapy. Ann Intern Med 102:285–291.

Champlin RE, Horowitz MM, van Bekkum DW, Camitta BM, Elfenbein GE, Gale RP, Gluckman E, Good RA, Rimm AA, Rozman C, Speck B, Bortin MM (1989): Graft failure following bone marrow transplantation for severe aplastic anemia: Risk factors and treatment results. Blood 73(2): 606–613.

Chao NJ, Schmidt GM, Niland JC, Amylon MD, Dagis AC, Long GD, Nademanee AP, Negrin RS, O'Donnell MR, Parker PM, Smith EP, Snyder DS, Stein AS, Wong RW, Blume K, Forman SJ (1993): Cyclosporine, methotrexate and prednisone compared with cyclosporine and prednisone for prophylaxis of acute graft-versus-host disease. N Engl J Med 329:1225–1230.

Chediak M (1952): Novvelle anomalie leucocytaire de caractere contitutional et familial. Rev Hematol 7:362.

Choo SY, Antonelli P, Nisperos B, Nepom GT, Hansen JA (1986): Six variants of HLA-B27 identified by isoelectric focusing. Immunogenetics:23: 24–29.

Chu E, Rosenwasser LJ, Dinarello CA, Rosen FS, Geha RS (1984): Immunodeficiency with defective T-cell response to interleukin-1. Proc Natl Acad Sci USA 81:4945–4949.

Clarkson B, Berman E, Little C, Andreeff M, Kempin S, Kolitz J, Gabrilove J, Arlin Z, Mertelsmann R, Cunningham I, Castro-Malaspina H, Gulati S,

O'Reilly RJ, Gee T (1990): Update on clinical trials of chemotherapy and bone marrow transplantation in acute myelogenous leukemia in adults at Memorial Sloan-Kettering Cancer Center 1966 to 1989. In "Acute Meylogenous Leukemia: Progress and Controversies." New York: Wiley-Liss, pp 239–272.

Clavell LA, Gelber RD, Cohen JH, Hitchcock-Bryan S, Cassady JR, Tarbell NJ, Blattner SR, Tantravahi R, Leavitt P, Sallan SE (1986): Four-agent induction and intensive asparaginase therapy for treatment of childhood acute lymphoblastic leukemia. N Engl J Med 315:657.

Coccia PE, Krivit W, Cervenka J, Clawson C, Kersey JH, Kim T, Nesbit M, Ramsay NKC, Warkentin PI, Teitelbaum SL, Kahn AJ, Brown DM (1980): Successful bone-marrow transplantation for infantile malignant osteopetrosis. N Engl J Med 302:701–708.

Coccia PF, Strandjord SE, Warkentin PI, Cheung NK, Gordon EM, Novak LJ, Shina DC, Herzig RH (1988): High-dose cytosine arabinoside and fractionated total-body irradiation: An improved preparative regimen for bone marrow transplantation of children with acute lymphoblastic leukemia in remission. Blood 71(4):888–893.

Conde E, Iriondo A, Rayon C, Fanjul E, Garigo J, Hermos V, Coma A, Bello C, Carrera D, Baro J, Zubizarreta A (1988): Allogeneic bone marrow transplantation versus intensification chemotherapy for acute myelogenous leukaemia in first remission: A prospective controlled trial. Br J Haematol 68:219–226.

Conzelmann E, Sandhoff K (1984): Partial enzyme deficiencies; residual activities and the development of neurological disorders. Dev Neurosci 6:58–71.

Cooper MD, Chae HP, Lowman JT, et al. (1968): Immunologic defects in patients with Wiskott-Aldrich syndrome. Birth Defects 4:378.

Copelan EA, Kapoor N, Gibbons B, Tutschka PJ (1990): Allogeneic marrow transplantation in non-Hodgkin's lymphoma. Bone Marrow Transpl 5:47.

Creutzig V, Ritter J, Riehm H, Langermann HJ, Henze G, Kabisch H, Niethammer D, Jurgens H, Stollmann B, Lasson U, Kaufmann U, Loffler H, Schellong G (1985): Improved treatment results in childhood acute myelogenous leukemia: A Report of the German Cooperative Study AML-BFM 78. Blood 65:298–304.

Curnutte JT, Babior BM (1987): Chronic granulomatous disease. Adv Hum Genet 16:229–297.

Dahl GV, Kalwinsky DK, Mirro J, Look AT, Pui C-H, Murphy SB, Mason C, Ruggiero M, Schell M, Johnson FL, Thomas ED (1990): Allogeneic bone marrow transplantation in a program of intensive sequential chemotherapy for children and young adults with acute nonlymphocytic leukemia in first remission. J Clin Oncol 8:295–303.

Deeg HJ, Flournoy N, Sullivan KM, Sheehan K, Buckner CD, Sanders J, Storb R, Witherspoon RP, Thomas Ed (1984a): Cataracts after total body irradiation and marrow transplantation: A sparing effect of dose fractionation. Int J Radiat Oncol Biol Phys 10:957–964.

Deeg HJ, Sanders JE, Martin P, Fefer A, Neiman P, Singer J, Strob R, Thomas ED (1984b): Secondary malignancies after marrow transplantation. Exp Hematol 12:660–666.

Dennert G, Anderson CG, Warner J (1985): T killer cells play a role in allogeneic bone marrow graft rejection but not in hybrid resistance. J Immunol 135:3729–3734.

Desai S, Hobbs JR, Hugh-Jones K, Williamson S, Barnes I, Kendra J, White S (1983): Morquio's disease (mucopolysaccharidosis IV) treated by bone marrow transplant. Exp Hematol 11:Suppl: 98–100.

DeWitte T, Zwaan F, Hermans J, Vernant J, Kolb H, Vossen J, Lonnqvist B, Beelen D, Ferrant A, Gmur J, Yin JL, Troussard X, Cahn J, Van Lint M, Gratwohl A (1990): Allogeneic bone marrow transplantation for secondary leukaemia and myelodysplastic syndrome: A survey by the leukaemia working party of the European Bone Marrow Transplantation Group (EMBTG). Br J Haematol 74:151–155.

DeWitte T, Gratwohl A, Van der Lely N, Bacigalupo A, Stern AC, Speck B, Schattenberg A, Nissen C (1991): Recombinant human granulocyte-macrophage colony-stimulating factor (rhGM-CSF) reduces infection-related mortality after allogeneic T-depleted bone marrow transplantation. Bone Marrow Transplant 7 (Suppl 2):83.

DiBartolomeo P, DiGirolamo G, Angrilli F, Schettini F, DeMattia D, Ciancarelli M, Catinella V, Betti S, Dragani A, Iacone A, Torlontano G (1987): Successful allogeneic bone marrow transplantation (BMT) in a patient with chronic granulomatous disease (CGD). Bone Marrow Transplant 2 (Suppl 1):131.

DiBartolomeo P, DiGirolamo G, Angrilli F (1988): Bone marrow transplantation for thalassemia in Pescaro. In: Buckner CD, Gale RP, Lucarelli G (eds): "Advances and Controversies in Thalassemia Therapy." New York: Alan R. Liss, pp 193–200.

Dinauer MC, Orkin SH, Brown R, Jesaitis AJ, Parkos CA (1987): The glycoprotein encoded by the X-linked chronic granulomatous disease locus is a component of the neutrophil cytochrome b complex. Nature (London) 327:717–720.

Dinsmore R, Kirkpatrick D, Flomenberg N, Gulati S, Kapoor N, Shank B, Reid A, Groshen S, O'Reilly RJ (1983a): Allogeneic bone marrow transplantation for patients with acute lymphoblastic leukemia. Blood 62(2): 381–388.

Dinsmore R, Reich L, Kapoor N, Kirkpatrick D, O'Reilly RJ (1983b): ABO incompatible bone marrow transplantation: Removal of erythrocytes by starch sedimentation. Br J Haematol 54:441–449.

Dinsmore R, Kirkpatrick D, Flomenberg N, Gulati S, Kapoor N, Brochstein J, Shank B, Reid A, Groshen S, O'Reilly RJ (1984): Allogeneic bone marrow transplantation for patients with acute nonlymphocytic leukemia. Blood 63(3):649–656.

DiSanto J, Keever CA, Small TN, Nichols G, O'Reilly RJ, Flomenberg N (1990): Absence of IL-2 production in a severe combined immunodeficiency disease syndrome with T-cells. J Exp Med 171:1697–1704.

Emanuel D, Cunningham I, Jules-Elysee K, Brochstein J, Kernan NA, Laver J, Stover D, White D, Fels A, Polsky B, Castro-Malaspina H, Peppard J, Bartus P, Hammerling U, O'Reilly RJ (1988): Cytomegalovirus pneumonia after bone marrow transplantation successfully treated with the combination of ganciclovir and high-dose intravenous immune globulin. Ann Intern Med 109(12):777–782.

Emanuel D, Kernan NH, Castro-Malaspina H, Cunningham I, Taylor J, Small T, Keever C, Flomenberg N, Young J, O'Reilly RJ (1989): Cytomegalovirus-associated bone marrow failure after allogeneic bone marrow transplantation successfully treated with the combination of ganciclovir and high dose CMV immune globulin. Blood 74 (Suppl. 1):905a.

Ernst P, Maraninchi D, Jacobsen N, Kolb HJ, Bordigoni P, Ljungman P, Bandini G, Parker AC, Volin L, Powles R, Gorin NG, Rio B (1986): Marrow transplantation for non-Hodgkin's lymphoma: A multi-centre study from the European co-operative bone marrow transplant group. Bone Marrow Transpl 1:81.

Faber LM, Luxemburg-Heijs SAP, Willemze R, Falkenburg JHF (1992): Generation of leukemia-reactive cytotoxic T lymphocyte clones from the HLA-identical bone marrow donor of a patient with leukemia. J Exp Med 176:1283–1289.

Fanconi G (1967): Familial constitutional panmyelocytopathy Fanconi's anaemia. Clinical aspects. Sem Hematol 4:233–240.

Feig S, Nesbit M, Buckley J, Lampkin B, Bernstein I, Kim T, Piomelli S, Kersey J, Coccia P, O'Reilly RJ, Thomas ED, August C, Hammond C (1987): Superiority of allogeneic bone marrow transplantation over conventional maintenance chemotherapy in children with acute non-lymphocytic leukemia. Exp Hematol 15:373a.

Ferrara JL, Guillen FJ, Dijken PJ, Marion A, Murphy GF, Burakoff SJ (1989): Evidence that large granular lymphocytes of donor origin mediate acute graft-versus-host disease. Transplantation 47:50–54.

Fischer A (1989): Bone marrow transplantation in immunodeficiency and osteopetrosis. Bone Marrow Transplant 4(Suppl 14):12–14.

Fischer A, Griscelli C (1983): Which conditioning regimen should be used for bone marrow transplantation in children with inherited diseases? Exp Hematol 11 (Suppl 1):84–95.

Fischer A, Cerf-Bensussan N, Blanche S, Le Deist F, Bremard-Oury C, Leverger G, Schaison G, Duranay A, Griscelli C (1986a): Allogeneic bone marrow transplantation for erythrophagocytic lymphohistiocytosis. J Pediat 108:267–270.

Fischer A, Griscelli C, Friedrich W, Kubanek B, Levinsky R, Morgan G, Vossen J, Wagemaker G, Landais P (1986b): Bone marrow transplantation for immunodeficiencies and osteopetrosis: Eur Survey 1968–1985. Lancet 2:1080–1084.

Fischer A, Lisowska-Grospierre B, Anderson DC, Springer TA (1988): Leukocyte adhesion deficiency: Molecular basis and functional consequences. Immunodefic Rev 1:39–54.

Fischer A, Blanche S, LeBidois J, Bordignon C, Garnier JL, Niaudet P, Morinet F, LeDeist F, Fischer AM, Griscelli C, Hirn M (1991): Anti-B-cell monoclonal antibodies in the treatment of severe B-cell lymphoproliferative syndrome following bone marrow and organ transplantation. N Engl J Med 324:1451–1456.

Fischer A, Landais P, Friedrich W, Gerritsen B, Fasth A, Porta F, Vellodi A, Benkerrou M, Jais JP, Cavazzana-Calvo M, Souillet G, Bordigoni P, Morgan G, Van Dijken P, Vossen J, Locatelli F, deBartolomeo P (1994): Bone marrow transplantation in Europe for primary immunodeficiencies other than severe combined immunodeficiency: A report from the European Group For BMT and the European Group For Immunodeficiency. Blood 83:1149–1154.

Flowers MED, Pepe MS, Longton G, Doney KC, Monroe D, Witherspoon RP, Sullivan KM, Storb R (1990): Previous donor pregnancy as a risk factor for acute graft-versus-host disease in patients with aplastic anaemia treated by allogeneic marrow transplantation. Br J Haematol 74:492–496.

Frame J, Collins NH, Cartagena T, Waldmann H, O'Reilly RJ, Kernan NA (1989): T-cell depletion of human bone marrow: Comparison of Campath-1 plus complement, anti-t-cell ricin A chain immunotoxin and soybean agglutinin alone or in combination with sheep erythrocytes or immunomagnetic beads. Transplantation 47:984–988.

Frappaz D, Gluckman E, Souillet G, Maraninchi D, Demeocq F, Fischer A, Lutz P, Bergerat P, Herve P, Freycon F (1988): Bone marrow transplantation (BMT) for thalassemia major (TM). The French experience. In Buckner CD, Gale RP, Lucarelli G (eds): "Advances and Controversies in Thalassemia Therapy." New York: Alan R. Liss, pp 207–216.

Gale R, Champlin R (1984): How does bone marrow transplantation cure leukaemia? Lancet 2:28–30.

Gale RP, Sparkes RS, Golde DW (1978): Bone marrow origin of hepatic macrophages (Kupffer cells) in humans. Science 201:937–938.

Gale RP, Bortin MM, van Bekkum DW, Biggs JC, Dicke KA, Gluckman E, Good RA, Hoffman RG, Kay HEM, Kersey JH, Marmont A, Masaoka T, Rimm AA, van Rood JJ, Zwaan FE (1987): Risk factors for acute graft-versus-host disease. Br J Haematol 67:397–406.

Gasper PW, Thrall MA, Wenger DA, Macy DW, Ham L, Dornsife RE, McBiles K, Quackenbush SL, Kesei ML, Gillette EL, Hoover EA (1984): Correction of feline arysulfatase B deficiency (mucopoly-saccharidosis VI) by bone marrow transplantation. Nature (London) 312:467–469.

Gatti RA, Meuwiissen HJ, Allen HD, Hong R, Good RA (1968): Immunological reconstitution of sex-linked lymphopenic immunological deficiency. Lancet 2:1366–1369.

Gehrz RC, McAuliffe JJ, Linner KM, Kersey JH (1980): Defective membrane function in a patient with severe combined immunodeficiency disease. Clin Exp Immunol 39:344–348.

Gelfand EW, Oliver JM, Schuurman RK, Matheson DS, Dosch HM (1979): Abnormal lymphocyte capping in a patient with severe combined immu-

nodeficiency disease. N Engl J Med 301:1245–1249.

Gerritsen EJA, Van Loo IHG, Fischer A (1990): European results of allogeneic bone marrow transplantation in juvenile osteopetrosis. Bone Marrow Transplant 5 (Suppl 2):12.

Gingrich RD, Ginder GD, Goeken D, Howe CWS, Wen BC, Hussey DH, Fyfe MA (1988): Allogeneic marrow grafting with partially mismatched, unrelated donors. Blood 71:1375–1381.

Gluckman E (1990): Bone marrow transplantation for Fanconi anemia. In Shahidi NT (ed): "Aplastic Anemia and Other Bone Marrow Failure Syndromes." New York: Springer-Verlag, pp 134–144.

Gluckman E, Devergie A, Schaison G, Bussel A, Berger R, Sohier J, Bernard J (1980): Bone marrow transplantation in Fanconi Anemia. Br J Haematol 45:557–564.

Gluckman E, Devergie A, Dutreix J (1983): Radiosensitivity in Fanconi Anemia: Application to the conditioning regimen for bone marrow transplantation. Br J Haematol 54:431–440.

Gluckman E, Jolivet I, Scrobohaci ML, Devergie A, Traineau R, Bourdeau-Esperon H, Lehn P, Foure P, Drouet L (1990): Use of prostaglandin E_1 for prevention of liver veno-occlusive disease in leukaemic patients treated by allogeneic bone marrow transplantation. Br J Haematol 74:277–281.

Glucksberg H, Storb R, Fefer A, Buckner CD, Neiman PE, Clift RA, Lerner KG, Thomas ED (1974): Clinical manifestations of GvHD in human recipients of marrow from HLA-matched sibling donors. Transplantation 18:295–304.

Goldman JM, Gale RP, Horowitz MM, Biggs JC, Champlin RE, Gluckman E, Hoffmann RG, Jacobsen SJ, Marmont AM, McGlave PB, Messner HA, Rimm AA, Rozman C, Speck B, Tura S, Weiner RS, Bortin MM (1988): Bone marrow transplantation for chronic myelogenous leukemia in chronic phase: Increased risk for relapse associated with T-cell depletion. Ann Intern Med 108(6):806–814.

Gorin NC, Aegerter P, Auvert B (1989): Autologous bone marrow transplantation (ABMT) for acute leukemia in remission: Fifth European Survey. Evidence in favour of marrow purging. Bone Marrow Transplant 4(Suppl 1):206.

Gottdiener JS, Appelbaum FR, Ferrans VJ, Deisseroth A, Ziegler J (1981): Cardiotoxicity associated with high-dose cyclophosphamide therapy. Arch Inter Med 141:758–763.

Goulmy E (1988): Minor histocompatibility antigens

in man and their role in transplantation. In Morris J, Tilney NL (eds): "Transplant Reviews." New York: W. B. Saunders.

Goulmy E, Termijtzlen A, Bradley BA, van Rood JJ (1977): Y-antigen killing by T-cells of woman is restricted by HLA. Nature (London) 226:544–545.

Gratwohl A, Hermans J, Niederwieser D, Frassoni F, Arcese W, Gahrton G, Bandini G, Carreras E, Vernant JP, Bosi A, de Witte T, Fibbe WE, Zwaan F, Michallet M, Ruutu T, Devergie A, Iriondo A, Apperley J, Reiffers J, Speck B, Goldman J (1993): Bone marrow transplantation for chronic myeloid leukemia: Long-term results. Bone Marrow Transplant 12:509–516.

Gribben J, Goldstone AH, Ernst P, Philip T, Maraninchi D, Gorin NC, Ricci P, Singer P (1987): Bone marrow transplantation for non-hodgkin's lymphoma in remission—allogeneic versus autologous. Bone Marrow Transplant 2(Suppl 1):204.

Gruber HE, Koenker R, Luchtman LA, Willis RC, Seegmiller JE (1985): Glial cells metabolically cooperate: Potential requirements for gene replacement therapy. Proc Natl Acad Sci USA 82:6662–6666.

Guinan EC, Tarbell NJ, Tantravahi R, Weinstein HJ (1989): Bone marrow transplantation for children with myelodysplastic syndromes. Blood 73(2): 619–622.

Hadam MR, Dopfer R, Peter HH, Niethammer D (1984): Congenital agammablobulinemia associated with lack of expression of HLA-D region antigens. In Griscelli C, Vossen J (eds): "Progress in Immunodeficiency Research and Therapy." Amsterdam: Excerpta Medica, pp 43–50.

Hale G, Waldmann H (1988): Campath-1 for prevention of graft-versus-host disease and graft rejection. Summary of results from a multi-centre study. Bone Marrow Transplant 3:11–14.

Hale G, Cobbold S and Waldmann H (1988): T-cell depletion with Campath-1 in allogeneic bone marrow transplantation. Transplantation 45:753–759.

Hammond WP, Price TH, Souza LM, Dale DC (1989): Treatment of cyclic neutropenia with granulocyte colony stimulating factor. N Engl J Med 320:1306–1311.

Harris RE, Hannon D, Vogler C, Hug G (1986): Bone marrow transplantation in type IIa glycogen storage disease. Birth Defects 22:119–132.

Hauch M, Gazzola MV, Small T, Bordignon C, Barnett L, Cunningham I, Castro-Malaspina H, O'Reilly RJ, Keever CA (1990): Anti-leukemia potential of interleukin-2 activated natural killer cells after bone marrow transplantation for chronic myelogenous leukemia. Blood 75:2250–2262.

Hobbs JR, Hugh-Jones K, Barrett AJ, Byrom N, Chambers D, Hehry K, James DC, Lucas CF, Rogers TR, Benson PF, Tansley LR, Patrick AD, Mossman J, Young EP (1981): Reversal of clinical features of Hurler's Disease and biochemical improvement after treatment by bone marrow transplantation. Lancet 2:709–712.

Hobbs JR, Hugh-Jones K, Chambers JD, et al. (1986): Lysosomal enzyme replacement therapy by displacement bone marrow transplantation with immunoprophylaxis. Adv Clin Enzymol 3:184–201.

Hoogerbrugge PM, Suzuki K, Suzuki K, Poorthuis BJ, Kobayashi T, Wagemaker G, van Bekkum DW (1988): Donor-derived cells in the central nervous system of twitcher mice after bone marrow transplantation. Science 239:1035–1038.

Howard MR, Brookes P, Bidwell JL, Bidwell EA, Clay TM, Evans JLM, Hows JM, Bradley BA (1992): HLA-DR and DQ matching by DNA restriction fragment length polymorphism methods and the outcome of mixed lymphocyte reaction tests in unrelated bone marrow donor searches. Bone Marrow Transplant 9:161–166.

Hows JM, Yin JL, Marsh D, Swirsky D, Jones L, Apperley JF, James DCO, Smithers S, Batchelor JR, Goldman JM, Gordon-Smith EC (1986): Histocompatible unrelated volunteer donors compared with HLA-non-identical family donors in marrow transplantation for aplastic anemia and leukemia. Blood 68:1322–1328.

Hugh-Jones K (1986): Psychomotor development of children with mucopolysaccidosis type I-H following bone marrow transplantation. Birth Defects 22:25–29.

Hugh-Jones K, Kendra J, James DCQ, et al. (1982): Treatment of San Filippo B disease (MPS III B) by bone marrow transplant. Exp Hematol 10 (Suppl 1):50–51.

Hugh-Jones K, Vellodi A, Jones ST, Hobbs JR, Rogers JRF, Abdul-Ahad A (1988): Bone marrow transplantation for thalassemia: Westminster Children's Hospital and United Kingdom Experience. In Buckner CD, Gale RP, Lucarelli G (eds): "Advances and Controversies in Thalassemia Therapy." New York: Alan R. Liss, pp 201–205.

Hutchinson RM, Pringle JH, Potter L, Patel I, Jeffreys AJ (1989): Rapid identification of donor and recipient cells after allogeneic bone marrow transplantation using specific genetic markers. Br J Haematol 72:133–140.

Ikehara S, Good RA, Nakamura T, Sekita K, Inoyes S, Oo M, Muso E, Ogawa K, Hamashima Y (1985): Rationale for bone marrow transplantation in the treatment of autoimmune diseases. Proc Natl Acad Sci USA 82:2483–2487.

Iriondo A, Garijo J, Baro J, Conde E, Pastor JM, Sabanes A, Hermosa V, Sainz MC, Perez de la Lastra L, Zubizarreta A (1984): Complete recovery of hemopoiesis following bone marrow transplant in a patient with unresponsive congenital hypoplastic anemia (Blackfan-Diamond syndrome). Blood 64:348–351.

Johnson FL, Look AT, Gockerman J, Ruggiero MR, Dall-Pozza L, Billings FT (1984): Bone marrow transplantation in a patient with sickle cell anemia. N Engl J Med 311:780–783.

Kantarjian HM, Keating MJ, Walters RS, Smith TL, Cork A, McCredie KB, Freireich EJ (1986): Therapy related leukemia and myelodysplastic syndrome: Clinical, cytogenetic and prognostic features. J Clin Oncol 4:1748.

Kapoor N, Kirkpatrick D, Blaese RM, Oleske J, Hilgartner MH, Chaganti RSK, Good RA, O'Reilly RJ (1981): Reconstitution of normal megakaryocytopoiesis and immunologic functions in Wiscott-Aldrich syndrome by marrow transplantation following myeloablation and immunosuppression with busulfan and cyclophosphamide. Blood 57:692–696.

Keever CA, Small TN, Flomenberg N, Heller G, Pekle K, Black P, Kernan NA, O'Reilly RJ (1989): Immune reconstitution following bone marrow transplantation: Comparison of recipients of T-cell depleted marrow with recipients of conventional marrow grafts. Blood 73:1340–1350.

Keissling R, Hochman PS, Haller O, Shearer GM, Wigzell H, Cudkowicz G (1977): Evidence for a similar or common mechanism for natural killer activity and resistance to hemopoietic grafts. Eur J Immunol 7:655.

Kernan NA, Flomenberg N, Dupont B, O'Reilly RJ (1987): Graft rejection in recipients of T-cell depleted HLA-non-identical marrow transplants for leukemia. Transplantation 43:842–847.

Kernan NA, Bordignon C, Heller G, Cunningham I, Castro-Malaspina H, Shank B, Flomenberg N, Burns J, Dupont B, Collins NH, O'Reilly RJ (1989): Graft failure after T-cell-depleted human leukocyte antigen identical marrow transplants for leukemia: I. Analysis of risk factors and results of secondary transplants. Blood 74(6):2227–2236.

Kernan NA, Khan R, Landrey C, O'Reilly RJ, Dupont B, Yang SY (1990): Identification of unrelated bone marrow donors based on matching for class I IEF subtypes. Blood 76:548a.

Kernan NA, Bartsch G, Ash RC, Beatty PG, Champlin R, Filipovich A, Gajewski J, Hansen JA, Henslee-Downey J, McCullough J, McGlave P, Perkins HA, Phillips GL, Sanders J, Stroncek D, Thomas ED, Blume KG (1993): Analysis of 462 transplantations from unrelated donors facilitated by the national marrow donor program. N Engl J Med 328:593–602.

Kihara H, Porter MT, Fluharty AL: Enzyme replacement in cultured fibroblasts from metachromatic leukodystrophy. N Engl J Med 328:19–26.

Klein J, Park JM (1973): Graft-versus-host reaction across different regions of the H-2 complex of the mouse. J Exp Med 137:1213–1225.

Kostmann R (1975): Infantile genetic agranulocytosis. ACTA Paediatr Scand 64:362–368.

Krivit W, Pierpont ME, Ayaz K, Tsai M, Ramsay NKC, Kersey JH, Weisdorf S, Sibley R, Snover D, McGovern MM, Schwartz MF, Desnick RJ (1984): Bone marrow transplantation in the Maroteaux-Lamy syndrome (mucopolysaccharidosis type VI). N Engl J Med 311:1606–1611.

Krivit W, Shapiro E, Kennedy W, Lipton M, Lockman LK, Smith S, Summers GC, Wenger DA, Tsai MM, Ramsay NKC, Kersey JH, Yao JK, Kay E (1990a): Treatment of late infantile metachromatic leukodystrophy by bone marrow transplantation. N Engl J Med 322:28–32.

Krivit W, Whitley CB, Chang PN (1990b): Lysosomal storage diseases related by bone marrow transplantation: Review of 21 patients: Bone marrow transplantation in children. In Johnson L, Pochedly C (eds): New York: Alan R. Liss, pp 261–287.

Leiper AD, Stanhope R, Lau T, Grant DB, Blacklock H, Chesselis JM, Plowman PN (1987): The effect of total body irradiation and bone marrow transplantation during childhood and adolescence on growth and endocrine function. Br J Haematol 67:419–426.

Lenarsky C, Weinberg K, Guinan E, Dukes PP, Barak Y, Ortega J, Siegel S, Williams K, Lazerson J, Weinstein H, Parkman r (1988): Bone marrow transplantation for constitutional pure red cell aplasia. Blood 71:226–229.

Levinsky RJ, Tiedman K (1983): Successful bone marrow transplantation for reticular dysgenesis. Lancet 1:671–673.

Liu Yin JA, Jowitt SN (1992): Resolution of immune-mediated diseases following allogeneic bone marrow transplantation for leukaemia. Bone Marrow Transplant 9:31–33.

Locksley RM, Flournoy N, Sullivan KM, Meyers JD (1985): Infection with varicella-zoster virus after marrow transplantation. J Infect Dis 152:1172–1178.

Lucarelli G, Galimberti M, Polchi P, Angelucci E, Baronciani D, Giardini C, Politi P, Durazzi SMT, Muretto P, Albertini F (1990): Bone marrow transplantation in patients with thalassemia. N Engl J Med 322:417–421.

Lucarelli G, Galimberti M, Polchi P, Angelucci E, Baronciani D, Durazzi SMT, Giardini C, Albertini F, Clift RA (1992): Bone marrow transplantation in adult thalassemia. Blood 80:1603–1607.

Lum LG (1987): The kinetics of immune reconstitution after human marrow transplantation. Blood 69:369–380.

Lynch RE, Williams DM, Reading JC, Cartwright GE (1975): The prognosis of aplastic anemia. Blood 45:517–528.

Mackinnon S, Hows JM, Goldman JM (1990): Induction of in vitro graft-versus-leukemia activity following bone marrow transplantation for chronic myeloid leukemia. Blood 76:2037–2045.

Macmahon HE, Bedizel M, Ellis CA (1963): Familial erythrophagocytic lymphohistiocytosis. Pediatrics 32:868–879.

Marks DI, Cullis JO, Ward KN, Lacey S, Szydlo R, Hughes TP, Schwarer AP, Lutz E, Barrett AJ, Hows JM, Batchelor JR, and Goldman JM (1993): Allogeneic bone marrow transplantation for chronic myeloid leukemia using sibling and volunteer unrelated donors: A comparison of complications in the first 2 years. Ann Intern Med 119:207–214.

Marmont AM, Gale RP, Butturini A, Goldman JM, Martelli MF, Prentice HG, Slavin S, Storb R, Truitt RL, Van Bekkum DW (1989): T-cell depletion in allogeneic bone marrow transplantation: Progress and problems. Haematologica 74:235–248.

Martin PJ, Shulman HM, Schubach WH, Hansen JA, Fefer A, Miller G, Thomas ED (1984): Fatal Epstein-Barr-virus-associated proliferation of donor B-cells after treatment of acute graft-versus-host disease with a murine anti-T-cell antibody. Ann Intern Med 101:310–315.

Martin PJ, Hansen JA, Buckner CD, Sanders JE, Deeg HJ, Stewart P, Appelbaum FR, Clift R, Fefer A, Witherspoon RP, Kennedy MS, Sullivan KM, Flournoy N, Storb R, Thomas ED (1985): Effects of in vitro depletion of T-cells in HLA-identical allogeneic marrow grafts. Blood 66:664–672.

Martin PJ, Hansen JA, Torok-Storb B, Durnam D, Pzrepiorka D, O'Quigley J, Sanders J, Sullivan KM, Witherspoon RP, Deeg HJ, Appelbaum FR, Stewart P, Weiden P, Doney K, Buckner CD, Clift R, Storb R, Thomas ED (1988): Graft failure in patients receiving T-cell depleted HLA-identical allogeneic marrow transplants. Bone Marrow Transplant 3:345–356.

Masaoka T, Takaku F, Kato S, Moriyama Y, Kodera Y, Kanamaru A, Shimosaka A, Shibata H, Nakamura H (1989): Recombinant human granulocyte colony-stimulating factor in allogeneic bone marrow transplantation. Exp Hematol 17:1047–1050.

McGlave PB, Beatty PG, Ash R, Hows JM (1990): Therapy for chronic myelogenous leukemia with unrelated donor bone marrow transplantation: Results in 102 cases. Blood 75:1728–1732.

McGlave P, Bartsch G, Anasetti C, Ash R, Beatty P, Gajewski J, Kernan NA (1993): Unrelated donor marrow transplantation therapy for chronic myelogenous leukemia: Initial experience of the national marrow donor program. Blood 81:543–550.

Meyers JD, Fluornoy N, Thomas ED (1982): Nonbacterial pneumonia after allogeneic marrow transplantation: A review of ten year's experience. Rev Infect Dis 4:1119–1132.

Meyes JD, Fluornoy N, Thomas ED (1986): Risk factors for cytomegalovirus infection after human marrow transplantation. J Infect Dis 153:478–488.

Milpied N, Harousseau JL, Garand R, David A (1988): Bone marrow transplantation for sickle cell anaemia. Letters to the Editor. Lancet II:328–329.

Neiman PE, Reeves W, Ray G, Fluornoy N, Lerner KG, Sale GE, Thomas ED (1977): A prospective analysis of interstitial pneumonia and opportunistic viral infection among recipients of allogeneic bone marrow grafts. J Infect Dis 136(6):754–767.

Nemunaitis J, Anasetti C, Storb R, Bianco JA, Buckner CD, Onetto N, Martin P, Sanders J, Sullivan K, Mori M, Shannon-Dorcy K, Bowden R, Appelbaum FR, Hansen J, Singer JW (1992): Phase II trial of recombinant human granulocyte-macrophage colony stimulating factor (rhGM-CSF) in patients undergoing allogeneic bone marrow transplantation from unrelated donors. Blood 79:2572–2577.

Neufeld EF (1973): Replacement of genotype specific proteins in mucopolysaccharidosis enzyme therapy in genetic disease. In Desnick RJ, Bernlohr LRW, Krivit W (eds): Birth Defects March of Dimes Original Series, Vol IX, No. 2. New York: Alan R. Liss, pp 27–30.

Nyhan WL, Page T, Gruber HE, Parkman R (1986): Bone marrow transplantation in Lesch-Nyham disease. Birth Defects 22:113–117.

O'Donnell MR, Nademanee AP, Snyder DS, Schmidt GM, Parker PM, Bierman PJ, Fahey JL, Stein AS, Krance RA, Stock AD, Forman SJ, Blume KG (1987): Bone marrow transplantation for myelodysplastic and myeloproliferative syndromes. J Clin Oncol 5(11):1822–1826.

Olsen I, Muir H, Smith R, Fensome A, Watt DJ (1983): Direct enzyme transfer from lymphocytes is specific. Nature (London) 306:75–77.

O'Reilly RJ: Experience of the Memorial Sloan-Kettering Cancer Center Transplantation Service.

O'Reilly RJ, Dupont B, Pahwa S, Grimes E, Smithwick EM, Pahwa R, Schwartz S, Hansen JA, Siegel FP, Sorell M, Svejgaard A, Jersild C, Thomsen M, Platz PI, L'Esperance P, Good RA (1977): Reconstitution in severe combined immunodeficiency by transplantation of marrow from an unrelated donor. N Engl J Med 297:1311–1318.

O'Reilly RJ, Brochstein J, Dinsmore R, Kirkpatrick D (1984): Marrow transplantation for congenital disorders. Semin Hematol 21:188–221.

O'Reilly RJ, Collins NH, Kernan NA, Brochstein J, Dinsmore R, Kirkpatrick D, Siena S, Keever C, Jordon B, Shank B, Wolf L, Dupont B, Reisner Y (1985): Transplantation of marrow depleted of T-cells by soybean lectin agglutination and E-rosette depletion: Major histocompatibility complex-related graft resistance in leukemia transplant patients. Transplant Proc 17:455–459.

O'Reilly RJ, Kernan NA, Cunningham I, Brochstein J, Castro-Malaspina H, Laver J, Flomenberg N, Emanuel D, Gulati S, Keever C, Small T, Collins NH, Bordignon C (1988): Allogeneic transplants depleted of T-cells by soybean lectin agglutination and E-rosette depletion. Bone Marrow Transplant 3:3–6.

O'Reilly RJ, Keever CA, Small T, Brochstein JA (1989): The use of HLA-non-identical T-cell-depleted marrow transplants for correction of severe combined immunodeficiency disease. Immunodef Rev 1:273–309.

Pahwa R, Chatila T, Pahwa S, Paradise C, Day NK, Geha R, Schwartz SA, Slade H, Oyaizu N, Good RA (1989): Recombinant IL-2 therapy in severe combined immunodeficiency disease. Proc Natl Acad Sci USA 86:5069–5073.

Papadopoulos E, Carabasi M, Young JW, Castro-Malaspina H, Childs B, Mackinnon S, Taylor J, Collins NH, Lindsley K, Black P, Kernan NA, O'Reilly (1992): Results of T-cell depleted (TCD) allogeneic BMT after TBI, thiotepa and cyclo-

phosphamide in patients with leukemia. Blood 80:170a.

Papadopoulos E, Ladanyi M, Emanuel D, Mackinnon S, Rosenfield N, Boulad F, Carabasi MH, Castro-Malaspina H, Childs B, Gillio AP, Small TN, Young JW, Kernan NA, O'Reilly RJ (1994): Infusions of donor leukocytes as treatment of Epstein-Barr virus associated lymphoproliferative disorders complicating allogeneic marrow transplantation. N Engl J Med 330:1185–1191.

Parkman R (1986): Clonal analysis of murine graft-versus-host-disease. I. Phenotypic and functional analysis of T-lymphocyte clones. J Immunol 136:3543–3548.

Parkman R, Rappeport J, Geha R, Belli J, Cassady R, Levey R, Nathan DG, Rosen FS (1978): Complete correction of the Wiskott-Aldrich syndrome by allogeneic bone marrow transplantation. N Engl J Med 298:921–927.

Perren TJ, Powles RL, Easton D, Stolle K, Selby PJ (1988): Prevention of herpes zoster in patients by long-term oral acyclovir after allogeneic bone marrow transplantation. Am J Med 85(Suppl 2A):99.

Phillips GL, Herzig RH, Lazarus HM, Fay JW, Griffith R, Herzig GP (1986): High-dose chemotherapy, fractionated total-body irradiation, and allogeneic marrow transplantation for malignant lymphoma. J Clin Oncol 4(4):480.

Piguet PF, Grau GE, Allet B, Vassali P (1987): Tumor necrosis factor/cachectin is an effector of skin and gut lesions of the acute phase of graft-versus-host disease. J Exp Med 166:1280–1289.

Powles RL, Morgenstern G, Clink HM, Hedley D, Bandini G, Lumley H, Watson JG, Lawson D, Spence D, Barrett A, Jameson B, Lawler S, Kay HEM, McElwain TJ (1980): The place of bone marrow transplantation in acute myelogenous leukemia. Lancet 1:1047–1050.

Ramsay NKC, Kersey JH, Robinson LL, McGlave PB, Woods WG, Krivit W, Kim TH, Goldman AI, Nesbit ME (1982): A randomized study of the prevention of acute graft-versus-host disease. N Engl J Med 306:392–397.

Rappeport J, Ginns EI (1984): Bone marrow transplantation in severe Gaucher's Disease. N Engl J Med 311:84–92.

Rappeport J, Parkman R, Newburger P, Camitta BM, Chusid MJ (1980): Correction of infantile agranulocytosis (Kostmann's syndrome) by allogeneic bone marrow transplantation. Am J Med 68:605–609.

Reed EC, Bowden RA, Dandliker PS, Lilleby KE, Meyers JD (1988): Treatment of cytomegalovirus pneumonia with ganciclovir and intravenous cytomegalovirus immunoglobulin in patients with bone marrow transplants. Ann Intern Med 109(12):783–788.

Reisner Y, Kapoor N, Kirkpatrick D, Pollack MS, Dupont B, Chaganti RSK, Good RA, O'Reilly RJ (1981): Transplantation for acute leukemia with HLA-A and B non-identical parental marrow cells fractionated with soybean agglutinin and sheep blood cells. Lancet 2:327–331.

Ringden O, Groth, C-G, Erikson A, Backman L, Granqvist S, Mansson JE, Svennerholm L (1988): Longterm follow up of the first successful bone marrow transplantation in Gaucher's disease. Transplantation 46:66–70.

Ringden O, Bolme P, Lonnqvist B, Gustafsson G, Kreuger A (1989): Allogeneic bone marrow transplantation versus chemotherapy in children with acute leukemia in Sweden. Pediat Hematol Oncol 6:137–144.

Rosenkrantz K, Keever C, Kirsch J, Horvath A, Bhimani K, O'Reilly RJ, Dupont B, Flomenberg N (1987): In vitro correlates of graft-host tolerance after HLA-matched and mismatched marrow transplants: Suggestions from limiting dilution analysis. Transplant Proc XIX (6):98–103.

Sakiyama T, Tsuda M, Owada M, Joh K, Miyawaki S, Kitagawa T (1983): Bone marrow transplantation for Niemann-Pick mice. Biochem Biophys Res Commun 113:605–610.

Sanders JE, Pritchard S, Mahoney P, Amos D, Buchner CD, Witherspoon RP, Deeg HJ, Doney KC, Sullivan KM, Appelbaum FR, Storb R, Thomas ED (1986): Growth and development following marrow transplantation for leukemia. Blood 68:1129–1135.

Sanders JE, Thomas ED, Buckner CD, Doney K (1987): Marrow transplantation for children with acute lymphoblastic leukemia in second remission. Blood 70:324.

Santamaria P, Reinsmoen NL, Lindstrom AL, Boyce-Jacino MT, Barbosa JJ, Faras AJ, McGlave PB, and Rich SS (1994): Frequent HLA class I and DP sequence mismatches in serologically (HLA-A, HLA-B, HLA-DR) and molecularly (HLA-DRB1, HLA-DQA1, HLA-DQB1) HLA-identical unrelated bone marrow transplant pains. Blood 83:280–287.

Santos GW (1974): Immunosuppression for clinical marrow transplantation. Semin Hematol 11:341–351.

Saunders LEF, Freedman MH (1978): Constitutional aplastic anemia: Defective haematopoietic stem cell growth in vitro. Br J Haematol 40:277–287.

Schmidt GM, Kovacs A, Zaia JA, Horak DA, Blume

KG, Nademanee AP, O'Donnell MR, Snyder DS, Forman SJ (1988): Gancyclovir/immunoglobulin combination therapy for the treatment of human cytomegalovirus-associated interstitial pneumonia in bone marrow allograft recipients. Transplantation 46:905–907.

Shapiro R, Chauvenet A, McGuire W, Pearson A, Craft AW, McGlave P, Filipovich A (1988): Treatment of B-cell lymphoproliferative disorders with interferon alfa and intravenous gammaglobulin. N Engl J Med 318:1334.

Shepp DH, Dandiliker PS, Meyers JD (1986): Treatment of varicella-zoster virus infection in severely immunocompromised patients—A randomized comparison of acyclovir and cidarabine. N Engl J Med 314:208–212.

Shull RM, Hastings HE, Selcer RR, Jones JB, Smith JR, Cullen WC, Constantopoulos G (1987): Bone marrow transplantation in canine mucopolysaccharidosis I. J Clin Invest 79:435–443.

Shull RM, Breider MA, Constantopoulos GG (1988): Longterm neurological effects of bone marrow transplantation in a canine lysosomal storage disease. Pediat Res 24:347–352.

Slavin RE, Woodruff JM (1974): The pathology of bone marrow transplantation. Pathol Ann 91:291–344.

Slavin S, Yatziv S (1980): Correction of enzyme deficiency in mice by allogeneic bone marrow transplantation with total lymphoid irradiation. Science 210:1150–1152.

Slavin S, Ackerstein A, Naparstek E, Or R, Weiss L (1990): The graft-versus-leukemia (GVL) phenomenon: Is GVL separable from GVHD? Bone Marrow Transplant 6:155–161.

Sokal JE, Baccarani M, Russo D, Tura S (1988): Staging and prognosis in chronic myelogenous leukemia. Semin Hematol 25(1):49–61.

Sonnenberg FA, Eckman MH, Pauker SG (1989): Bone marrow donor registries: The relation between registry size and probability of finding complete and partial matches. Blood 74:2569–2578.

Sorell M, Kirkpatrick D, Kapoor N, et al (1979): Bone marrow transplant for combined immune deficiency (CID) and agranulocytosis associated with cartilage-hair hypoplasia (CHH). Pediatr Res 13:455.

Sorell M, Kapoor N, Kirkpatrick D, Rosen JF, Chaganti RSK, Lopez C, Dupont B, Pollack MS, Terrin BN, Harris MB, Vine D, Rose, JS, Goossen C, Lane J, Good RA, O'Reilly RJ (1981): Marrow transplantation for juvenile osteopetrosis. Am J Med 70:1280–1287.

Sparks RS (1981): Cytogenetic analysis in human

bone marrow transplantation. Cancer Genet Cytogenet 4:345–352.

Steinherz PG, Gaynon P, Miller DR, Reaman G, Bleyer A, Finklestein J, Evans RG, Meyers P, Steinherz L, Sather H, Hammond D (1986): Improved disease free survival of children with acute lymphoblastic leukemia at high risk for early relapse with the New York Regimen—A new intensive therapy protocol: A report from the Children's Cancer Study Group. J Clin Oncol 4:744.

Stingl S, Tamaki K, Katz SI, Katz S (1980): Origin and function of epidermal langerhans cells. Immunol Rev 53:149–174.

Storb R, Epstein RB, Rudolph RH, Thomas ED (1970): The effect of prior transfusion on marrow grafts between histocompatible canine siblings. J Immunol 107:409–413.

Storb R, Thomas ED, Weiden PL, Buckner CD, Clift RA, Fefer A, Fernando LP, Giblett ER, Goodell BW, Johnson FL, Lerner K, Neiman P, Sanders JE (1976): Aplastic anemia treated by allogeneic bone marrow transplantation: A report of 49 new cases from Seattle. Blood 48 817–841.

Storb R, Prentice RL, Thomas ED (1977a): Marrow transplantation for treatment of aplastic anemia: An analysis of factors associated with graft rejection. N Engl J Med 296(2):61–66.

Storb R, Prentice RL and Thomas ED (1977b): Treatment of aplastic anemia by marrow transplantation from HLA identical siblings. J Clin Invest 59:625–632.

Storb R, Prentice RL, Thomas ED, Applebaum FR, Deeg HJ, Doney K, Fefer A, Goodell BW, Mickelson E, Stewart P, Sullivan KM, Witherspoon RP (1983): Factors associated with graft rejection after HLA-identical marrow transplantation for aplastic anaemia. Br J Haematol 55:573–585.

Storb R, Deeg HJ, Thomas ED, Appelbaum FR, Buckner CD, Cheever MA, Clift RA, Doney KC, Flournoy N, Kennedy MS, Loughran TP, McGuffin RW, Sale GE, Sanders JE, Singer JW, Stewart PS, Sullivan KM, Witherspoon RP (1985): Marrow transplantation for chronic myelocytic leukemia: A controlled trial of cyclosporine versus methotrexate for prophylaxis of graft-versus-host disease. Blood 66:698–702.

Storb R, Deeg HJ, Farewell V, Doney K, Appelbaum F, Beatty P, Bensinger W, Buckner CD, Clift R, Hansen J, Hill R, Longton G, Lum L, Martin P, McGuffin R, Sanders J, Singer J, Stewart P, Sullivan K, Witherspoon R, Thomas ED (1986): Marrow transplantation for severe aplastic anemia: Methotrexate alone compared with a combination of methotrexate and cyclosporine for prevention of acute graft-versus-host disease. Blood 68(1):119–125.

Streilein WJ and Billingham RE (1970): An analysis of graft-versus-host disease in syrian hamsters. J Exp Med 132:163–180.

Sullivan KM, Shulman HM, Storb R, Weiden PL, Witherspoon RP, McDonald GB, Schubert MM, Atkinson K, Thomas ED (1981): Chronic graft-versus-host disease in 52 patients: Adverse natural course and successful treatment with combination immunosuppression. Blood 57:267–276.

Sullivan KM, Storb R, Shulman HR, Shaw CM, Spence A, Beckman C, Clift RA, Buckner CD, Stewart P, Thomas ED (1982): Immediate and delayed neurotoxicity after mechlorethamine preparation for bone marrow transplantation. Ann Intern Med 97:182–189.

Sullivan KM, Deeg HJ, Sanders J, Klosterman A, Amos D, Shulman H, Sale G, Martin P, Witherspoon R, Appelbaum F, Doney K, Stewart P, Meyers J, McDonald GB, Weiden P, Fefer A, Buckner CD, Storb R, Thomas ED (1986): Hyperacute graft-v-host disease in patients not given immunosuppression after allogeneic marrow transplantation. Blood 67(4):1172–1175.

Sullivan KM, Kopecky KJ, Jocom J, Fisher L, Buckner CD, Meyers JD, Counts GW, Bowden RA, Petersen FB, Witherspoon RP, Budinger MD, Schwartz RS, Appelbaum FR, Clift RA, Hansen JA, Sanders JE, Thomas ED, Storb R (1990): Immunomodulatory and antimicrobial efficacy of intravenous immunoglobulin in bone marrow transplantation. N Engl J Med 323(11):705–712.

Taylor RM, Farrow BRH, Stewart GJ, Healy PJ (1986): Enzyme replacement in nervous tissue after allogeneic bone marrow transplantation for fucosidosis in dogs. Lancet 2:722–724.

Thomas ED, Buckner CD, Rudolph RH, Fefer A, Storb R, Neiman PE, Bryant JI, Chard RL, Clift RA, Epstein RB, Fialkow PJ, Funk DD, Giblett E, Lerner KG, Reynolds FA, Slichter S (1971): Allogeneic marrow grafting for hematologic malignancy using HLA matched donor recipient sibling pairs. Blood 38:267–287.

Thomas ED, Ramberg RE, Sale GE (1976): Direct evidence for a bone marrow origin of the alveolar macrophages in man. Science 192:1016–1018.

Thomas ED, Buckner CD, Banaji M, Clift RA, Fefer A, Flournoy N, Goodell, BW, Hickman RO, Lerner KG, Neiman PE, Sale GE, Sanders JE, Singer J, Stevens M, Storb R, Weiden PL (1977): One hundred patients with acute leukemia treated by chemotherapy, total body irradiation and allogeneic marrow transplantation. Blood 49:511–533.

Thomas ED, Buckner CD, Clift RA, Fefer A, Johnson FL, Neiman PE, Sale GE, Sanders JE, Singer JW, Shulman H, Storb R, Weiden PL (1979): Marrow transplantation for acute nonlymphoblastic leukemia in first remission. N Engl J Med 301:597–599.

Thomas ED, Buckner CD, Sanders J (1982): Marrow transplantation for leukemia. Lancet 2:279.

Thomas ED, Clift RA, Fefer A, Applebaum FR, Beatty P, Bensinger WI, Buckner CD, Cheever MA, Deeg HJ, Doney K, Flournoy N, Greenberg P, Hansen JA, Martin P, McGuffin R, Ramberg R, Sanders JE, Singer J, Stewart P, Storb R, Sullivan K, Weiden PL, Witherspoon R (1986): Marrow transplantation for the treatment of chronic myelogenous leukemia. Ann Intern Med 104(2):155–163.

Thomsen M, Alvarez C, Carpenter CB (1989): Analysis of HLA recombinant families by Southern blots. In Dupont B (ed): "Immunobiology of HLA, Histocompatibility Testing," Vol 1. New York: Springer-Verlag, pp 900–908.

Thompson CB, Sanders JE, Flournoy N, Buchner CD, Thomas ED (1986): The risks of central nervous system relapse and leukoencephalopathy in patients receiving marrow transplants for acute leukemia. Blood 67:195–199.

Touraine JL, Betuel H, Souillet G, Jeune M (1978): Combined immunodeficiency disease associated with absence of cell surface HLA-A and B antigens. J Pediatr 93:47–51.

Touraine JL, Betuel H, Phillipe N (1980): The bare lymphocyte syndrome. I. Immunological studies before and after bone marrow transplantation. BLUT 41:198–202.

Trigg ME, Gingrich R, Goeken N, deAlarcon P, Klugman M, Padley D, Rumelhart S, Giller R, Wen BC, Strauss R (1989): Low rejection rate when using unrelated or haploidentical donors for children with leukemia undergoing marrow transplantation. Bone Marrow Transplant 4:431–437.

Troussard X, Leblond V, Kuentz M, Milpied N, Jouet JP, Cordonnier C, Leporrier M, Vernant JP (1990): Allogeneic bone marrow transplantation in adults with Burkitt's lymphoma or acute lymphoblastic leukemia in first complete remission. J Clin Oncol 8(5):809.

Tsoi MS, Storb R, Dobbs S, Kopecky KJ, Santos E, Weiden PL, Thomas ED (1979): Non-specific suppressor cells in patients with chronic graft-versus-host disease after marrow grafting. J Immunol 123:1970.

Tubergen D, Gilchest G, Coccia P, Nouak L, O'Brien R, Waskerwitz M, Sather H, Bleyer A, Hammond D (1990): The role of intensified chemotherapy in intermediate risk acute lymphoblastic leukemia (ALL) of childhood. Proc Am Soc Clin Oncol 9:216.

Vermylen C, Fernandez-Robles E, Ninane J, Cornu G (1988): Bone marrow transplantation in five children with sickle cell anaemia. Lancet 1:1427–1428.

Vierlizier JL, Lagrue A, Durandy A, Arenzana F, Oury C, Griscelli C (1982): Reversal of natural killer defect in a patient with Chediak-Higashi syndrome after bone marrow transplantation. N Engl J Med 306:1055–1056.

Vogelsang GB, Hess AD and Santos GW (1988): Acute graft-versus-host disease: Clinical characteristics in the cyclosporine era. Medicine 67:163–174.

Vogelsang GB, Farmer EB, Hess AD, Altamonti V, Beschorner WE, Jabs DA, Cario RL, Levin LS, Colvin OM, Wingard JR, Santos GW (1992): Thalidomide for the treatment of chronic graft versus host disease. N Engl J Med 326:1055–1058.

Voogt PJ, Goulmy WE, Fibbe WE, Veenhof WFJ, Brand A, Falkenberg JHF (1988): Minor histocompatibility antigen H-Y is expressed on human hematopoietic progenitor cells. J Clin Invest 82:906–912.

Warkentin PI, Dixon MS, Schafer I, Strandjord SE, Coccia PF (1986): Bone marrow transplantation in Hurler syndrome: A preliminary report. Birth Defects 22:31–39.

Weiden PL, Flournoy N, Thomas ED, Prentice R, Fefer A, Buchner D, Storb R (1979): Antileukemic effects of graft versus host disease in human recipients of allogeneic marrow grafts. N Engl J Med 300:1068–1073.

Weinberg K, Parkman R (1990): Severe combined immunodeficiency due to a specific defect in the production of interleukin-2. N Engl J Med 322:1718–1723.

Weinberg K, Moser A, Watkins P, Lenarsky C, Winter S, Moser H, Parkman R (1988): Bone marrow transplantation (BMT) for adrenoleukodystrophy (ALD). Pediatr Res 23:334a.

Weiner RS, Bortin MB, Gale RP, Gluckman E, Kay HEM, Kolb HJ, Hartz AJ, Rimm AA (1986): Interstitial Pneumonitis after bone marrow transplantation: Assessment of risk factors. Ann Intern Med 104(2):168–175.

Weinstein HJ, Mayer RL, Rosenthal DS, Coral FS, Camitta BM, Gelber RD (1983): Chemotherapy for acute myelogenous leukemia in children and adults: VAPA update. Blood 62:315–319.

Weismann VN, Rossi EE, Hirschowitz NN (1971): Treatment of metachromatic leukodystrophy fibroblasts by enzyme replacement. N Engl J Med 204:672–673.

Welte K, Zeidler C, Reiter A, et al (1990): Differential effects of granulocyte-macrophage colony-stimulating factor and granulocyte colony-stimulating factor in children with severe congenital neutropenia. Blood 75:1056–1063.

Whitley CB, Ramsay NKC, Kersey JH, Krivit W (1986): Bone marrow transplantation for Hurler syndrome: Assessment of metabolic correction. Birth Defects 22:7–24.

Will A, Cooper A, Hatton C, Sardharwalla IB, Evans DI, Stevens RF (1987): Bone marrow transplantation in the treatment of alpha-mannosidosis. Arch Dis Child 62:1044–1049.

Wingard JR, Mellits ED, Sostrin MB, Chen YH, Burns WH, Santos GW, Vriesendorp HM, Beschorner WE, Saral R (1988a): Interstitial pneumonitis after allogeneic bone marrow transplantation. Nine year experience at a single institution. Medicine 67:175–186.

Wingard JR, Chen DY, Burns WH, Fuller DJ, Braine HG, Yeager AM, Kaiser H, Burke PJ, Graham ML, Santos GW, Saral R (1988b): Cytomegalovirus infection after autologous bone marrow transplantation with comparison to infection after allogeneic bone marrow transplantation. Blood 71(5):1432–1437.

Wingard JR, Piantadosi S, Santos GW, Saral R, Vriesendorp HM, Yeager AM, Burns WH, Ambinder RF, Braine HG, Elfenbein G, Jones RJ, Kaizer H, May WS, Rowley, SD, Sensenbrenner LL, Stuart RK, Tutschka PJ, Vogelsang GB, Wagner JE, Beschorner WE, Brookmeyer R, Farmer, ER (1990): Allogeneic bone marrow transplantation for patients with high-risk acute lymphoblastic leukemia. J Clin Oncol 8(5):820–830.

Winston DJ, Schiffman G, Wang DC, Feig SA, Lin CH, Marso EL, Ho, WG, Young LS, Gale RP (1979): Pneumococcal infections after human bone marrow transplantation. Ann Intern Med 91:835–841.

Winston DJ, Huang E, Miller MJ, Lin CH, Ho WG, Gale RP Champlin RE (1985): Molecular epidemiology of cytomegalovirus infections associated with bone marrow transplantation. Ann Intern Med 102(1):16–20.

Witherspoon RP, Lum LG, Storb R (1984): Immu-nologic reconstitution after human marrow grafting. Semin Hematol 21:2–10.

Witherspoon RP, Fisher LD, Schoch G, Martin P, Sullivan KM, Sanders J, Deeg HJ, Doney K, Thomas D, Storb R, Thomas ED (1989): Secondary cancers after bone marrow transplantation for leukemia or aplastic anemia. N Engl J Med 321:784–789.

Woods WG, Nesbit ME, Ramsay NKC, Krivit W, Kim TH, Goldman A, McGlave PB, Kersey JH (1983): Intensive therapy followed by bone marrow transplantation for patients with acute lymphocytic leukemia in second or subsequent remission: Determination of prognostic factors (a report from the University of Minnesota Bone Marrow Transplantation Team). Blood 61(6):1182–1189.

Xun C, Brown SA, Jennings CD, Henslee-Downey PJ, Thompson JS (1993): Acute graft-versus-host-like disease induced by transplantation of human activated natural killer cells into SCID mice. Transplantation 56:409–417.

Yeager AM, Brennan S, Tiffany C, Moser NW, Santos GW (1984): Prolonged survival and remyelination after hematopoietic cell transplantation in the twitcher mouse. Science 225:1052–1054.

Young JW, Papadopoulos E, Cunningham I, Castro-Malaspina H, Flomenberg N, Carabasi MH, Gulati SC, Brochstein JA, Heller G, Black P, Collins NH, Shank B, Kernan NA, O'Reilly RJ (1992): T-cell depleted allogeneic bone marrow transplantation in adults with acute nonlymphocutic leukemia in first remission. 79:3380–3387.

Young JW, Baggers J and Soergel SA (1993): High-dose UV-B radiation alters human dendritic cell costimulatory activity but does not allow dendritic cells to tolerize T-lymphocytes to alloantigen in vitro. Blood 81:2987–2997.

Zander AR, Keating M, Dicke K, Dixon D, Pierce S, Jagannath S, Peters L. Horwitz L, Cockerill K, Spitzer G, Vellekoop L, Kantarjian H, Walters R, McCredie K, Freireich EJ (1988): A comparison of marrow transplantation with chemotherapy for adults with acute leukemia of poor prognosis in first complete remission. J Clin Oncol 6:1548–1557.

Zutter MM, Martin PJ, Sale GE, Shulman HM, Fisher L, Thomas ED, Durnam DM (1988): Epstein-Barr virus lymphoproliferation after bone marrow transplantation. Blood 72:520–529.

Chapter 10
New Small Molecule Immunosuppressants for Transplantation: Review of Essential Concepts

Randall E. Morris

INTRODUCTION

Until recently, there was ample time to become familiar with a new immunosuppressant before the next one came along. This is no longer true. As can be seen from Figure 1, many new drugs have appeared in just the last few years (Morris, 1993). Since none of these agents has been approved for use by the FDA, their widespread use cannot not be assured. In addition, many controlled clinical trials will be needed to prove that these new drugs offer clear advantages over conventional immunosuppression. Nevertheless, these drugs have demonstrated sufficient efficacy and safety in preclinical studies to merit the substantial investment required for their entry into serious clinical trials. This is a rare accomplishment. These new drugs are not perfect, but they have progressed much further than the thousands of other molecules that have failed in preclinical development. Many of these failures have been biologicals that were developed to exploit the newest fashions in molecular immunology and promised to achieve exquisitely antigen-specific suppression of graft rejection. In the uncompromising world of immunosuppressive drug development, the decision to move a new drug to the clinic is based on its raw performance not its theoretical elegance.

The new drugs now in clinical testing are generating so much information that their fundamental aspects are becoming increasingly obscured. Rather than recite endless details about each drug, this review will attempt to distill the information on the agents into essential concepts necessary to understand how these drugs work, how they differ, and how they might be used in patients. This core knowledge is the best weapon against the misconceptions, rumors, and innuendo that contribute to the chaos in this rapidly developing field.

Before discussing each drug separately, it is worth noting that their development represents the continuation of a clear trend toward more specific immunosuppression (Fig. 2). None of the new small molecule drugs depends on a reduction in the number of lymphocytes for its efficacy. The actions of these drugs are directed primarily to T and B cells rather than to all white cells. In contrast, T cell depleting antibodies, steroids, and azathioprine are crude: they need to eliminate lymphocytes to be effective, they inhibit the function of granulocytes and macrophages, or they are myelotoxic. These older drugs are responsible for most of the morbidity and mortality in transplant patients. They need to be replaced.

CYCLOSPORINE ANALOGUES

There are two analogues that have been recently evaluated in clinical trials: cyclosporin G (CsG) and IMM125 (Hiestand et al., 1992; Henry et al., 1993a,b). Both analogues effectively suppress immune responses in preclinical mod-

Transplantation Immunology, pages 199–210
© 1995 Wiley-Liss, Inc.

```
                              – MIZORIBINE
                                   – DEOXYSPERGUALIN
                                   – FK506
                                     – MYCOPHENOLIC
                                       ACID
                                     – RAPAMYCIN
                                       – BREQUINAR
                                         SODIUM
        AZATHIOPRINE                     – LEFLUNOMIDE
        STEROIDS              CYCLOSPORINE & ANALOGUES
        XRT    ANTI-T CELL Abs        OKT3 & OTHER MAbs
```

Fig. 1. Shown are the approximate periods when different immunosuppressive therapies were initially used in transplantation.

els *in vitro* and *in vivo*. There is insufficient published clinical data to predict the potential utility of IMM125, but a small number of studies with CsG in patients has shown that it has immunosuppressive efficacy similar to cyclosporine (CsA) and might be less nephrotoxic. The hepatotoxic effects of CsG are controversial, and hepatotoxicity caused by IMM125 may cause clinical work to be placed on hold. It is unlikely that either CsG or IMM 125 will offer a substantial increase in the therapeutic index compared to

CsA, since the molecular mechanisms of action of all three drugs are identical. Rather, the differences in structure of CsG and IMM125 compared to their parent may produce a widening of the therapeutic window by favorably altering these analogues' pharmacokinetics or tissue distribution.

Ultimately, it may be a question of cost that determines whether a new analogue or new CsA formulation will replace CsA. Since CsA is ending its patent life, less expensive generic forms

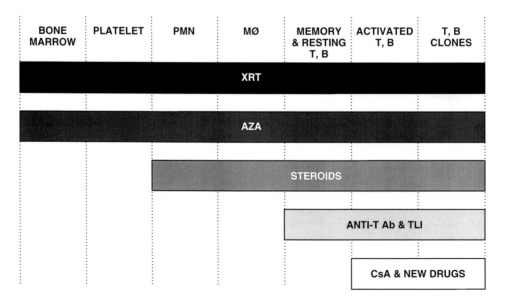

Fig. 2. Schematic of effects of different immunosuppressive therapies on cells of the hematopoietic system including polymorphonuclear (PMN) cells and macrophages (MØ).

may be available. The use of an expensive alternative to CsA would then have to be justified based on the presumption that the costs associated with the toxicity of CsA are significantly more than the expense of purchasing an improved version of CsA. Without knowing how much less toxic or how much more expensive the analogues will be compared to CsA, it is impossible to predict how important an advance they will represent.

FK506

For all intents, FK506 can be regarded as a more potent and, for some applications, a more effective alternative to CsA (or its analogues). Both CsA and FK506 are prodrugs, since they must form a complex with cellular proteins known as immunophilins (cyclophilin or CyP binds CsA, and FK506 binding protein or FKPB binds FK506.) (Figs. 3 and 4). Once bound to its immunophilin, the surface of the drug–immunophilin complex associates with a complex of other proteins containing calcineurin. Unimpeded, calcineurin is a phosphatase, but when associated with the drug–immunophilin

complex, calcineurin's enzymatic activity is inhibited. Although the precise steps are not known, it appears that the enzymatic activity of calcineurin is part of the biochemical cascade that transduces activation signals from the surface of a T cell to its nucleus causing genes for cytokines to be transcribed. By inhibiting the activity of calcineurin, the production of interleukin 2 (IL-2) and other cytokines is reduced, though calcineurin may not be the only target of these drugs (Thomson and Woo, 1989; Thomson, 1990; Sigal and Dumont, 1992).

Since FK506 inhibits T cell activation, it inhibits primary humoral responses that are T cell dependent but not secondary, T-cell independent B cell responses. The cytokines produced after T cell activation amplify the immune response by stimulating the proliferation of immune cells and activating nonimmune cells at the site of an immune response. These cytokine actions are not blocked by FK506. Similarly, T cells stimulated through the CD28 pathway are resistant to suppression by FK506 (Fig. 3).

Both *in vitro* and *in vivo,* FK506 is a far more potent immune suppressant than CsA. The high potency of FK506 may be related to the fact that

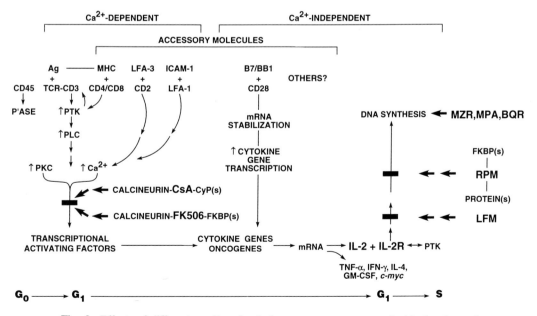

Fig. 3. Effects of different small molecule immunosuppressants on the biochemistry of T cell activation.

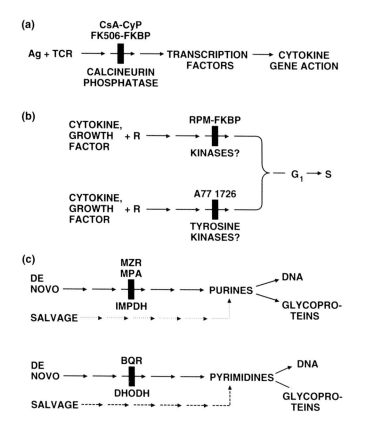

Fig. 4. (a) Possible mechanisms of action of inhibition of cytokine synthesis by cyclosporine (CsA) and FK506 after binding to cyclophilin (CyP) and FK binding protein (FKPB). (b) Possible mechanism of action of rapamycin (RPM) and A77 1726, the active metabolite of leflunomide. Both agents appear to use different mechanisms to interrupt the signals transduced by cytokines and growth factors that cause cells to progress into DNA synthesis after binding to their receptors. (c) Possible mechanisms of action of mizoribine (MZR), mycophenolic acid (MPA), and brequinar sodium (BQR) in T and B cells. Inosine monophosphate dehydrogenase (IMPDH) is inhibited by MZR and MPA; dihydroorotate dehydrogenase (DHODH) is inhibited by BQR.

FK506 binds with much greater affinity to FKBP than CsA binds to CyP, thus more efficiently blocking T cell activation signals that cause cytokine synthesis. It is also possible that FK506 partitions more efficiently from plasma into cells than does CsA. These differences between FK506 and CsA may account for the ability of FK506 to reverse rejections that have been refractory to treatment with CsA, steroids, and anti-T cell antibodies. In this application, the efficacy of FK506 is probably due to its ability to turn off the synthesis of cytokines by T cells that have infiltrated the graft. The use of FK506 to control ongoing rejection is an indication that clearly differentiates this drug from CsA.

Data from controlled trials in liver transplant recipients have shown that FK506 plus low dose steroids prevents rejection as effectively as CsA combined with steroids, azathioprine, and anti-T cell antibodies. There was more nephrotoxicity in patients treated with FK506, however (Fig. 5). This complication might have been less with lower blood levels of FK506, but since FK506 was being relied on as the primary immunosuppressant, lower doses of FK506 would probably have resulted in more rejection. In an uncontrolled trial in pediatric heart transplantation, FK506 was suggested to have many advantages over conventional immunosuppression including suppression of rejection, less need for ste-

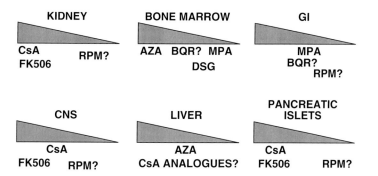

Fig. 5. Known and potential toxicities of different immunosuppressants in transplant patients. For each system that is the target of toxicity, drugs are listed in order of known or suspected toxicity with the level of toxicity decreasing from left to right. Drugs are abbreviated as follows: cyclosporine (CsA), rapamycin (RPM), azathioprine (AZA), brequinar sodium (BQR), deoxyspergualin (DSG), and mycophenolic acid (MPA). Some drugs are shown with a question mark to indicate that while these toxicities may have occurred in animals (RPM) or in nontransplant patients (BQR), it is not yet known whether immunosuppressive doses of these drugs produce these toxic effects in transplant patients.

roids, and less hypertension (Armitage et al., 1993). FK506 is diabetogenic and causes central nervous system toxicity, but does not cause gingival hypertrophy or hirsutism. Frequent blood level monitoring of FK506 levels is required for this drug to be used effectively and safely, since the therapeutic index is low.

Several pharmaceutical companies have mounted major efforts to identify FK506 analogues with a greater therapeutic indexes. While some improvement may be possible, there is little room to maneuver. Changes in the structure of FK506 that decrease toxicity decrease its immunosuppressive efficacy equally, thus implying that the same or very similar mechanisms are responsible for both efficacy and toxicity. If the same or similar FK506-sensitive biochemical pathways are as critical to the function of certain non-T cells as they are for T cells, toxicity is the inevitable result (Parsons et al., 1993).

FK506 is approved for use in transplantation in Japan and should receive FDA approval in 1994 (Fig. 6). Perhaps when this drug is used more commonly, the accumulated experience can be used to maximize its therapeutic index and to define indications in transplantation where it is clearly superior to other immunosuppressants. FK506 might find its widest application in combination with other new drugs (Fig. 7). In this role, blood levels might be able to be

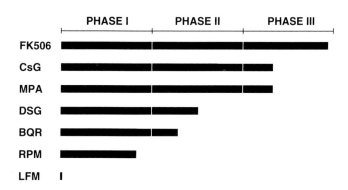

Fig. 6. Approximate current clinical trial status of new immunosuppressive drugs.

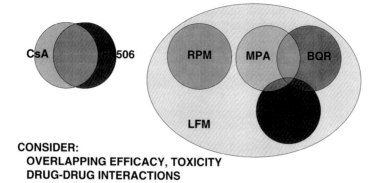

CONSIDER:
OVERLAPPING EFFICACY, TOXICITY
DRUG-DRUG INTERACTIONS

Fig. 7. Schematic diagram to show approximate overlapping mechanisms of immunosuppressive action and toxicities of different immunosuppressive drugs. Drugs are abbreviated as follows: cyclosporine (CsA), rapamycin (RPM), azathioprine (AZA), brequinar sodium (BQR), deoxyspergualin (DSG), mycophenolic acid (MPA), and leflunomide (LFM).

lowered enough to avoid nephrotoxicity but high enough to contribute to suppression of T cell activation. This strategy may bring us closer to eliminating the need for steroids, azathioprine, and T cell-depleting antibody therapy. It is unlikely that CsA and FK506 will be used in combination, since they potentiate each other's nephrotoxicity.

RAPAMYCIN

Part of this molecule has the same structure as the segment of FK506 that binds to FKBP, so it is not surprising that rapamycin (RPM) also binds to FKPB. The structural similarity between FK506 and RPM prompted the first studies of RPM in transplantation (Calne et al., 1989; Morris and Meiser, 1989). In fact, RPM, like CsA and FK506, is a prodrug that must first complex with its immunophilin before it can block immune cell activation. The part of the RPM molecule that faces away from FKBP is structurally very different from FK506. This structural difference explains why the RPM–FKBP complex neither inhibits calcineurin phosphatase activity nor the synthesis of T cell cytokines. Instead, RPM blocks cell proliferation caused by growth factors by preventing cells from progressing from the G_1 to the S phase of the cell cycle by affecting the proteins that are required for cell cycle progression (Figs. 3 and 4). The precise molecular

targets for the RPM–FKBP complex are unknown, but may involve kinases; RPM affects T and B cells directly by preventing cytokines from activating these cells; CsA and FK506 cannot interrupt cytokine-mediated activation pathways (Kahan et al., 1991; Morris, 1992; Sigal and Dumont, 1993).

Since RPM appears to be capable of blocking only cell proliferation stimulated by growth factors, the actions of RPM are more restricted than many antiproliferative drugs that halt the division of all cells. The full spectrum of activity of RPM is not yet known, but it is already clear that its effects are not restricted to lymphoid cells. RPM can inhibit the mitogenic response of fibroblasts, hepatocytes, endothelial cells, and smooth muscle cells to growth factors. Other growth factor-dependent cells must be resistant to inhibition by RPM, otherwise it would be toxic to cells in the marrow and other tissues. Without knowing more about the specific cellular targets of RPM, it is not possible to understand how RPM can inhibit the mitogenic effects of some, but not all, growth factors.

Since RPM has not entered Phase II trials in transplant patients and Phase I trials have yet to be completed (Fig. 6), the therapeutic profile and therapeutic index can be assessed only from animal studies. In summary, RPM has been shown to prevent and reverse acute rejection, suppress primary and secondary antibody synthesis, and prevent graft vascular disease. It has been especially effective when combined with CsA or FK506. Dogs are unusually sensitive to the toxicity of RPM, but in other animals that may more accurately predict toxicity in humans, RPM's toxicity has been limited to weight loss, testicular atrophy, and lethargy (Fig. 5); it causes diabetes in rodents but not in large animals. No nephrotoxicity has been seen when the drug is used at immunosuppressive doses.

Single dose Phase I pharmacokinetic studies have been completed and 2 week safety trials are ongoing; despite attaining higher trough levels than are maximally tolerated for FK506, dose-limiting toxicity has not been reached. Phase II trials in organ transplant recipients and patients with psoriasis are being designed.

Assuming that RPM is reasonably safe in humans and that human immune cells are as sensitive to RPM's actions as the cells of experimental animals, RPM might be a valuable adjunct to treatment with CsA or FK506 to prevent acute rejection (Fig. 7). Since RPM is believed to inhibit cytokine action, it should complement the effects of CsA and FK506, since these drugs suppress cytokine synthesis. Cytokines and growth factors are believed to play important roles in ongoing rejection and in all forms of chronic rejection (Gregory et al., 1993); RPM may be an effective therapy for the treatment of these conditions.

LEFLUNOMIDE

Leflunomide (LFM) has been used in hundreds of patients in Europe for the treatment of rheumatoid arthritis and only recently has been considered for use in transplantation (Bartlett et al., 1991; Kuchle et al., 1991; Chong et al., 1993; Williams et al., 1993). After oral absorption, LFM is converted in the blood into its active form, A77 1726. LFM was developed as a prodrug to reduce the gastrointestinal irritation caused by ingesting A77 1726. Very little is known about how LFM suppresses the actions of immune cells other than recent data that suggest that tyrosine kinases associated with growth factor receptors are inhibited by this drug (Figs. 3 and 4). At the cellular level, LFM has been shown to inhibit immune cell proliferation. Like RPM, LFM blocks the action of IL-2 and other immune cytokines as well as the mitogenic effects of growth factors on nonimmune cells.

In vivo, LFM has prevented and reversed allo- and xenograft rejection in rodents. LFM also very effectively inhibits both primary and secondary antibody synthesis. We have recently found that it can reduce graft vascular disease in vessel allografts in rats. Dr J. Williams' group at Rush Medical School in Chicago has used LFM to prevent kidney allograft rejection in dogs. Since LFM is converted into a toxic aniline in dogs, the efficacy of LFM monotherapy was limited in this species. When low dose CsA was combined with low dose LFM, long-term dog renal allograft survival was achieved. We have recently found in preliminary studies that LFM effectively suppresses graft rejection in cynomolgus recipients of heterotopic heart allografts. Blood levels of A77 1726 in these animals were similar to blood levels that were well tolerated in patients with rheumatoid arthritis. One of our recipients was treated with LFM for 100 days posttransplantation and with a subtherapeutic dose of CsA for 55 days. The graft in this animal rejected on day 130.

Studies of this drug in transplant patients have been restricted to a study at Rush Medical Center of its pharmacokinetics and interaction with other standard immunosuppressants (Fig. 6). Because its manufacturer is focusing on its use in autoimmune diseases, its future in transplantation is unclear.

Although much more preclinical work needs to be done to understand the potential roles of LFM as a suppressant of graft rejection, there are several reasons to continue to evaluate its potential: (1) it has been well tolerated in patients at blood levels required to treat rheumatoid arthritis, (2) its ability to inhibit cytokine and growth factor action defines an unusual mechanism of action similar to RPM, (3) its actions are not limited to T cells, since it very effectively blocks antibody synthesis, (4) it effectively prolongs allograft survival in small and large animal models, and (5) since it produces neither myelo- nor nephrotoxicity, it should be able to be used in combination with other drugs to minimize their toxicities without sacrificing overall immuno-suppressive efficacy (Fig. 7).

MIZORIBINE AND MYCOPHENOLATE MOFETIL

Both of these drugs have an identical mechanism of action (Fig. 4), but only mycophenolate mofetil (MM, previously known as RS-61443) is being developed for widespread clinical use (Turka et al., 1991; Dayton et al., 1992; Allison et al., 1993). Mizoribine (MZR, also known as bredinin) was used in Japan well before preclinical work on MM began, but there has been little clinical development of MZR outside Japan. Both MZR and MM are prodrugs: MZR needs to be phosphorylated to be active, and MM needs to be converted in the blood to its active drug, mycophenolic acid (MPA). By inhibiting the enzyme inosine monophosphate dehydrogenase either competitively (MZR) or noncompetitively (MPA), these drugs block the *de novo* synthesis of the purine, guanosine that is required for DNA synthesis. The proliferation of T and B cells is especially sensitive to inhibition by MZR and MM, since these cells are highly dependent on a functioning *de novo* pathway for guanosine synthesis. These drugs do not impair the synthesis of IL-2 by T cells, since they do not inhibit early events after cell activation. Since most other cell types can meet their requirement for guanosine using enzymes in the salvage pathway that are not inhibited by MZR or MPA, these cells are more resistant to the antiproliferative effects of these drugs. This accounts for the lack of myelotoxicity seen with the use of MZR and MPA at doses that suppress immune cells.

It has recently been found *in vitro* that T cells stimulated in the presence of MPA do not process glycoprotein adhesion molecules normally. This may be caused by a depletion of guanosine, which is a biosynthetic intermediate required for the assembly of cell surface glycoproteins.

MZR was first used clinically more than a decade ago in Japan and was found to be a non-myelotoxic, nonhepatotoxic, and a steroid sparing alternative to azathioprine. Since these studies were not controlled, the advantages of MZR over azathioprine have been difficult to prove convincingly.

MM has been more extensively studied than MZR in preclinical animal models. Since early work had shown that MPA only very weakly suppressed skin graft rejection in mice, MM was developed at Syntex by Dr. A. Allison and his team as therapy for rheumatoid arthritis. Since I felt the true potential of MM in transplantation had been overlooked, and since Syntex was not pursuing this application, I requested samples of MM for evaluation in transplant models in my laboratory in 1987 (Morris et al., 1989). Our finding that MM effectively prevented acute and chronic rejection and reversed ongoing rejection in rat allograft models was the initial stimulus for its development as an immunosuppressant for transplantation. MM has now been used to suppress rejection in large animal and in human organ allograft recipients (Morris et al., 1991; Platz et al., 1991a,b; Sollinger et al., 1992a,b; Ensley et al., 1993). Rejection episodes have been reversed by MM in dog renal allograft recipients and in patients whose rejections were refractory to conventional immunosuppressants. To compensate for poor gastrointestinal absorption in some patients, an intravenous form is being developed. As expected, treatment of human graft recipients with MM has been remarkably free from myelotoxicity.

The known mechanisms of action of MPA *in vitro* can be related to its immunosuppressive effects *in vivo*. It is likely that MM prevents acute rejection by inhibiting alloantigen- and cytokine-driven proliferation of T cells, B cell proliferation, and antibody synthesis as well as the function of certain cell-surface adhesion molecules. The same effects may be responsible for the ability of MM to reverse ongoing rejection. In addition to its immunosuppressive actions, high concentrations of MPA have been shown to inhibit growth factor-stimulated proliferation of smooth muscle cells *in vitro* (Allison et al., 1993). Each of these actions could contribute to the ability of MM to suppress graft vascular disease in rodent models.

Even though MM is highly bioavailable, large doses (2–4 g/person/day) are required to suppress the alloimmune response. The low potency of MM may be due to its effective conversion into an inactive metabolite, its low binding affinity to inosine monophosphate dehydrogenase, or perhaps because plasma proteins compete with inosine monophosphate dehydrogenase for binding to MPA. Whatever the reason, the large doses required may reduce patient compliance. It will be important for patients to maintain immunosuppressive blood levels of MPA, because T and B cell proliferation can begin as soon as there is insufficient MPA to block inosine monophosphate dehydrogenase. Also, since MPA blocks lymphocyte proliferation at a late stage of activation, the biochemical machinery in lymphocytes is engaged and ready to proceed once inhibition by MPA has ceased. HPLC can be used to monitor blood levels of MPA to ensure adequate levels are maintained.

All the information to date suggests that MM is an effective and well-tolerated immunosuppressant in transplant patients. There should be enough data from clinical trials for this drug to be approved by the FDA in the next few years (Fig. 6). For MM to be adopted as a replacement of azathioprine, however, clinical trials will have to show that MM is less toxic than azathioprine at doses that are as effective as azathioprine. No studies have been done to prove that the efficacy and therapeutic index of MM are superior to azathioprine in large animal models. If additional clinical studies can conclusively show that MM reduces the need for steroids and CsA or FK506, is preferable to other drugs for reversing ongoing rejection, and reduces the incidence of chronic rejection, MM will be an important advance in immunosuppression.

BREQUINAR SODIUM

In many ways brequinar sodium (BQR) has much in common with MM and MZR. All three drugs inhibit T and B cell proliferation by interfering with nucleotide biosynthesis (Fig. 4). BQR inhibits the action of dihydroorotate dehydrogenase in the *de novo* biosynthetic pathway leading to the synthesis of pyrimidines needed for DNA and RNA synthesis (Simon et al., 1993). Evidently, the salvage pathway in T and B cells cannot compensate for the reduction in pyrimidine synthesis caused by the inhibition of the *de novo* pathway by BQR. Inhibition of the *de novo* synthesis of uridine by BQR could reduce plasma levels of uridine, which is a sub-

strate for the salvage pathway in lymphocytes. Like MM, BQR decreases the function of adhesion molecules on lymphocytes *in vitro,* because glycosylation of adhesion molecules requires pyrimidine– as well as purine–sugar intermediates (Allison and Eugui, 1993).

Even though the actions of MM and BQR are restricted to the inhibition single enzymes in the *de novo* pathways of purine or pyrimidine biosynthesis, BQR is a less specific inhibitor of lymphocyte proliferation than MM. At immunosuppressive and slightly higher doses, BQR is more myelotoxic and toxic to the epithelium in the gastrointestinal tract than MM. Therefore, the proliferation of marrow and epithelial cells must depend more on the *de novo* pathway for pyrimidine biosynthesis than on the *de novo* pathway for purine synthesis. Since the therapeutic window of BQR may be narrow in transplant recipients, BQR blood levels will have to be carefully monitored by HPLC.

The efficacy of BQR as an immunosuppressant has been primarily determined from work in rodents (Murphy and Morris, 1991, 1992; Cramer et al., 1992). These experiments have shown that BQR effectively prolongs the survival of organ allografts when the dose and schedule are modified to minimize toxicity and maximize efficacy. BQR has also been shown to reverse ongoing rejection. BQR very effectively controls antibody synthesis by its direct action on B cells, and it is one of the most effective drugs available for treatment of two forms of antibody-mediated rejection: accelerated allograft rejection and rejection of hamster grafts by rats (Cramer et al., 1992b). Since BQR is a less specific antiproliferative than MM, its inability to prevent intimal thickening in a rat aortic allograft model is surprising; these results need to be confirmed. Used as monotherapy, BQR produced moderate prolongation of survival of heterotopic cardiac allografts in nonhuman primates (Makowka et al., 1993). In several rodent models, BQR potentiated the effects of CsA treatment (Cramer et al., 1992a; Murphy and Morris, 1992).

There is no question that BQR very effectively inhibits the actions of T and B cells that cause different forms of graft rejection. Since its mechanism of action does not allow it to be completely lymphocyte specific, its utility in clinical transplantation will depend on how much more sensitive lymphocytes are to its antiproliferative effects than cells in the marrow and GI tract. Based on what we now know, it is unlikely that BQR can replace CsA as a primary immunosuppressant. Used with CsA, however, BQR could play an important role as an inhibitor of antigraft antibody, and as a means of reversing intractable rejection. If an effective dose can be found that is not myelotoxic, BQR might be preferable to azathioprine as part of a regimen designed to prevent acute rejection.

DEOXYSPERGUALIN

Deoxyspergualin (DSG) has little in common with the other new immunosuppressive drugs (Morris, 1991). It can be administered only parenterally, and typical treatment schedules last from 5 to 10 days. It does not inhibit the synthesis of IL-2 but does reduce IL-1 synthesis. By blocking the maturation of T and B cells, DSG halts the development of cytotoxic T cells and development of B cells into antibody-secreting cells. DSG can be added several days after stimulation of immune cells *in vitro* without loss of efficacy (Takahara et al., 1992). How DSG causes these effects is unknown, but it has recently been found that it binds to a cytoplasmic heat shock protein and this interaction may ultimately give a clue about this drug's mechanism of action.

DSG has been used extensively in preclinical animal models (Yuh and Morris, 1993). This work has shown DSG to suppress acute allograft rejection when DSG is used alone or with CsA. It has been used successfully to reverse allograft rejection. Because DSG is an effective inhibitor of antibody synthesis, it has been used to prolong survival of xenografts (Marchman et al., 1992). One of its most successful applications has been as treatment to suppress islet graft rejection (Stephanian et al., 1992).

Despite numerous clinical studies of DSG in transplant patients in Japan (Okubo et al., 1993), the ultimate role of DSG in transplantation remains to be seen. For now, its predicted uses might include treatment of ongoing rejection and prevention or suppression of unwanted primary or secondary antibody responses.

SUMMARY

There has always been a seemingly unending stream of "new and improved" ways to suppress graft rejection, but the vast majority of these ideas have been disregarded, since they have not been clinically useful. Now, however, there are more new drugs that are progressing toward FDA approval. Even if only some of the new drugs are finally approved, they will affect the way the immune system is managed in transplant patients. In view of the time it takes from initial concept to completion of all clinical trials, it is likely that the small molecule immunosuppressants reviewed here will be the only drugs of this type approved for general use before the end of the century. Therefore, it is important to understand these new drugs so that when they are approved for clinical use, they will be used intelligently.

Although this review summarized the current views of the mechanisms of action of the new drugs, it should be emphasized that our understanding of how these drugs affect immune cells is based primarily on *in vitro* experiments. There is very little information on the precise molecular actions of these drugs on immune cells *in vivo*. Furthermore, our concepts of how these drugs work is limited by our present understanding of normal immune cell function. As more is learned about the immune system, the greater the possibility that additional effects of these drugs will be appreciated.

Regardless of exactly how these drugs suppress lymphocyte function, they will be of value only if they enable pharmacologic suppression of graft rejection to be less toxic and more effective than it is with conventional immunosuppressants. From what we know now, no one drug has such superior efficacy and margin of safety that it can be used as monotherapy. Fortunately, many of the drugs have different mechanisms of action and nonoverlapping toxicities. These drugs will have fulfilled some of their promise if they allow the dose of CsA to be reduced so that it is nonnephrotoxic. Another high priority will be to determine whether steroid use can be substantially reduced or completely eliminated. FK506 is rarely used with azathioprine or anti-T cell-depleting antibodies, and perhaps the use of other drugs will perpetuate this trend. In addition it will be important to know whether these new drugs, many with mechanisms of action that differ from conventional immunosuppressants, will control acute cellular and humoral rejection and chronic rejection more effectively than the drugs in current use.

Based on their mechanisms of action and their preclinical and clinical performance, there is certainly reason to be optimistic about the potential of these new molecules. Many complex, rigorous, and lengthy clinical trials will be required, however, before the true benefits and limitations of these drugs are known.

REFERENCES

Allison AC, Eugui EM (1993): Inhibitors of de novo purine and pyrimidine synthesis as immunosuppressive drugs. Transplant Proc 25(3, suppl 2):8–18.

Allison AC, Kowalski CJ, Muller CJ, Waters RV, Eugui EM (1993): Mycophenolic acid and brequinar, inhibitors of purine and pyrimidine synthesis, block the glycosylation of adhesion molecules. Transplant Proc 25(3, suppl 2):76–70.

Armitage JM, Fricker FJ, del Nido P, Starzl TE, Hardesty RL, Griffith BP (1993): A decade (1982 to 1992) of pediatric cardiac transplantation and impact of FK 506 immunosuppression. J Thorac Cardiovasc Surg 105(3):464–473.

Bartlett PR, Dimitrijevic M, et al. (1991): Leflunomide (HWA 486), a novel immunomodulating compound for the treatment of autoimmune disorders and reactions leading to transplantation rejection. Agents Actions 32(1/2):10–21.

Calne RY, Collier DS et al. (1989): Rapamycin for immunosuppression in organ allografting. Lancet 2:227.

Chong AS-F, Finnegan A, Jiang X, Gebel H, Sankary HN, Foster P, Williams JW (1993): Leflunomide, a novel immunosuppressive agent. Transplantation 55(6):1361–1366.

Cramer DV, Chapman FA, Jaffee BD, Jones EA, Knoop M, Hreha-Eiras G, Makowka L (1992a): The effect of a new immunosuppressive drug, brequinar sodium, on heart, liver, and kidney allograft rejection in the rat. Transplantation 53:303–308.

Cramer DV, Chapman FA, Jaffee BD, Zajac I, Hreha-Eiras G, Yasunaga C, Wu G-D, Makwka L (1992b): The prolongation of concordant hamster-

to-rat cardiac xenografts by brequinar sodium. Transplantation 54(3):403–408.

Dayton JS, Turka LA, Thompson CB, Mitchell BS (1992): Comparison of the effects of mizoribine with those of azathioprine, 6-mercaptopurine, and mycophenolic acid on T lymphocyte proliferation and purine ribonucleotide metabolism. Mol Pharmacol 41:671–676.

Ensley DR, Bristow MR, Olsen SL, Taylor DO, Hammond EH, O'Connell JB, Dunn D, Osburn L, Jones KW, Kauffman RS, Gay WA, Renlund DG (1993): The use of mycophenolate mofetil (RS-61443) in human heart transplant recipients. Transplantation 56(1):75–82.

Gregory CR, Huie P, Billingham ME, Morris RE (1993): Rapamycin inhibits arterial intimal thickening caused by both alloimmune and mechanical injury: Its effect on cellular, growth factor and cytokine responses in injured vessels. Transplantation 55(6):1409–1418.

Henry ML, Tesi RJ, Elkhammas, EA, Ferguson RM (1993a): A randomized, prospective, double-blinded trial of cyclosporine vs. OG37-325 in cadaveric renal transplantation—a preliminary report. Transplantation 55(4):748–752.

Henry ML, Tesi RJ, Elkhammas EA, Ferguson RM (1993b): Trial of cyclosporine vs OG37-325 in cadaveric renal transplantation: A preliminary report. Transplant Proc 25(1):689–690.

Hiestand PC, Graber M, Hurtenbach U, Hermann P, Cammisuli S, Richardson BP, Eberle MK (1992): The new cyclosporine derivative, SDZ IMM 125: In vitro and in vivo pharmacological effects. Transplant Proc 24(2):31–38.

Kahan BD, Chang JY, et al. (1991): Preclinical evaluation of a new potent immunosuppressive agent, rapamycin. Transplantation 52(2):185–91.

Kuchle CCA, Thoenes GH, Langer KH, Schorlemmer HU, Bartlett RR, Schleyerbach R (1991): Prevention of kidney and skin allograft rejection in rats by leflunomide, a new immunomodulating agent. Transplant Proc 23(1):1083–1086.

Makowka L, Tixier A, Chaux A, Hill D, O'Neill P, Eiras-Hreha G, Wu GD, Cuneen S, Cajulis E, Zajac I, Jaffee BD, Chapman FA, Cramer DV (1993): Use of brequinar sodium for preventing cardiac allograft rejection in primates. Transplant Proc 25(3 suppl 2):48–53.

Marchman W, Araneda D, DeMasi R, Taylor D, Larkin E, Alqaisi M, Thomas F (1992): Prolongation of xenograft survival after combination therapy with 15-deoxyspergualin and total-lymphoid irradiation in the hamster-to-rat cardiac xenograft model. Transplantation 53(1):30–34.

Morris RE (1991): ± 15 deoxyspergualin: A mystery wrapped within an enigma. Clin Transplant 5(2): 530–533.

Morris RE (1992): Rapamycins: Antifungal, antitumor, antiproliferative and immunosuppressive macrolides. Transplant Rev 6:39–87.

Morris RE (1993): Commentary on new xenobiotic immunosuppressants for transplantation: Where are we, how did we get here and where are we going? Clin Transplant 7(1, Part 2):138–145.

Morris RE, Meiser BM (1989): Identification of a new pharmacologic action for an old compound. Med Sci Res 17:609–10.

Murphy MP, Morris RE (1991): Brequinar sodium (Dup 785) is a highly potent antimetabolite immunosuppressant that suppresses heart allograft rejection. Med Sci Res 19:835–836.

Murphy MM, Morris RE (1992): Brequinar sodium (Dup 785) selectively, effectively and potently suppresses allograft rejection in a heterotopic mouse heart transplant model. Transplant Proc 25(3, Suppl 2):75–76.

Morris RE, Hoyt EG et al. (1989): Prolongation of rat heart allograft survival by RS-61443. Surg Forum 40:337–338.

Morris RE, Wang J, et al. (1991): Immunosuppressive effects of the morpholinoethyl ester of mycophenolic acid (RS-61443) in rat and nonhuman primate recipients of heart allografts. Transplant Proc 23(2, Suppl 2):19–25.

Okubo M, Tamura K, Kamata K, Tsukamoto Y, Nakayama Y, Osakabe T, Sato K, Go Mikitoshi G, Kumano K, Endo T (1993): 15-Deoxyspergualin "rescue therapy" for methylprednisolone-resistant rejection of renal transplants as compared with anti-T cell monoclonal antibody. Transplantation 55(3):505–508.

Parsons WH, Sigal NH, Wyvratt MJ (1993): FK-506—a novel immunosuppressant. Ann NY Acad Sci 685:22–36.

Platz KP, Bechstein WO, et al. (1991a): RS-61443 reverses acute allograft rejection in dogs. Surgery 110(4):736–741.

Platz KP, Eckhoff DE, et al. (1991b): Prolongation of dog renal allograft survival by RS-61443, a new, potent immunosuppressive agent. Transplant Proc 23(1):497–498.

Sigal SN, Dumont FJ (1993): Rapamycin: In vitro profile of a new immunosuppressive macrolide. Ann NY Acad Sci 685:58–67.

Sigal NL, Dumont FJ (1992): Cyclosporin A, FK-506, and rapamycin: Pharmacologic probes of lymphocyte signal transduction. Annu Rev Immunol 10: 519–560.

Simon P, Townsend RR, Harris EA, Jones EA, Jaffee BD (1993): Brequinar sodium: Inhibition of dihydroorotic acid dehydrogenase, depletion of pyrimidine pools, and consequent inhibition of immune functions in vitro. Transplant Proc 25(3 suppl 2):77–80.

Sollinger HW, Belzer FO, Deierhoi MH, Diethelm AG, Gonwa TA, Kauffman RS, Klintmalm GB, McDiarmid SV, Roberts J, Rosenthal JT, Tomlanovich SJ (1992a): RS-61443 (mycophenolate mofetil. A multicenter study for refractory kidney transplant rejection. Ann Surg 216(4):513–519.

Sollinger HW, Seierhoi MH, Belzer FO, Diethelm A, Kauffman RS (1992b): RS-61443—a phase I clinical trial and pilot rescue study. Transplantation 53:428–432.

Stephanian E, Lloveras JJ, Sutherland DER, Farney AC, Field MJ, Kaufman DB, Matteson BD, Gores PF (1992): Prolongation of canine islet allograft survival by 15-deoxyspergualin. J Surg Res 52: 621–624.

Takahara S, Jiang H, Takano Y, Kokado Y, Ishibashi M, Okuyama A, Sonada T (1992): The in vitro immunosuppressive effect of deoxymethylspergualin in man as compared with FK506 and cyclosporine. Transplantation 53(4):914–918.

Thomson AW (1990): FK-506: Profile of an important new immunosuppressant. Transplant Rev 4(1): 1–13.

Thomson AW, Woo J (1989): Immunosuppressive properties of FK-506 and rapamycin [letter]. Lancet 2(8660):443–444.

Turka LA, Dayton J, et al. (1991): Guanine ribonucleotide depletion inhibits T cell activation. J Clin Invest 87:940–948.

Williams JW, Xiao F, Foster PF, Chong A, Sharma S, Bartlett R, Sankary HN (1993): Immunosuppressive effects of leflunomide in a cardiac allograft model. Transplant Proc 25(1):745–746.

Yuh DD Morris RE (1993): The immunopharmacology of immunosuppression by 15-deoxyspergualin. Transplantation 55(3):578–591.

Chapter 11
Strategies to Induce Tolerance

Hugh Auchincloss, Jr.

INTRODUCTION

Tolerance is the long-lasting nonreactivity of the immune system to a specific set of antigens, maintained without on-going immunosuppression. Tolerance to self-antigens is, of course, a fundamental feature of the immune system. The induction of tolerance to a set of donor antigens is, in turn, the fundamental goal of transplantation immunology. Many different strategies have been developed to achieve transplantation tolerance, some of which have led to indefinite graft survival in rodents. Nonetheless, none of these strategies has yet been applied to human patients in a way that allows reliable withdrawal of exogenous immunosuppression.

In this section several authors describe the features of the strategies that they have developed or studied. Here, we provide an organizational framework for considering these strategies and suggest some of the open issues that still need to be resolved by further research. The underlying question throughout this chapter is why has it proven so difficult to achieve tolerance in human patients when it can apparently be achieved so easily in smaller animals.

MECHANISMS OF TOLERANCE INDUCTION

The older literature on tolerance induction frequently made use of the terms *central* and *peripheral* tolerance and sometimes used the term *thymic* tolerance interchangeably with *central*. As immunologists learned more about tolerance-inducing mechanisms, the term "central" was

sometimes used synonymously with *deletional*, while the term *peripheral* was loosely associated with *suppressor* mechanisms. Now, however, we have enough understanding of these mechanisms that it is no longer appropriate to confuse references to place with those to mechanism. Studies of self-tolerance induction have revealed that both deletional and nondeletional mechanisms can occur in the thymus and, similarly, that more than one mechanism for tolerance induction is available in the periphery. Thus it is time for us to try to characterize strategies for transplantation tolerance induction according to the mechanisms that seem to be involved, specifying in addition the place when that is useful.

Table I shows one possible outline of the mechanisms of tolerance induction. Overall, immune tolerance can be maintained in one of three basic ways. First, reactive lymphocytes can fail to respond to a set of antigens if they never encounter them. This has been described as *ignorance* and it probably accounts for some of self-tolerance. The mechanism is not generally important in clinical transplantation, however, and will not be considered further in this chapter. Second, reactive lymphocytes can be *deleted* from the mature repertoire. This is probably the most important mechanism of self-tolerance and is the mechanism underlying several strategies to achieve transplantation tolerance. While most deletion occurs in the thymus, there is evidence that mature lymphocytes can also be deleted in the periphery. Third, antigen-specific lymphocytes can remain in the mature repertoire, can encounter their particular antigens, but tolerance can still be maintained if something suppresses

Transplantation Immunology, pages 211–218
© 1995 Wiley-Liss, Inc.

Table I. Mechanisms of Tolerance Induction

Ignorance
Deletion
    Thymic
    Peripheral
Suppression
    External
        Antigen-specific
            Th1 vs. Th2
            T suppressor cells
        Receptor-specific
            Veto and natural suppressors
            Antiidiotype
    Internal = anergy

the function of these lymphocytes. Such suppressor mechanisms can be divided into two types: those external to the lymphocyte and those internal. All suppressor mechanisms that induce tolerance must have specificity since the term tolerance means antigen-specific nonreactivity. There are two ways that external suppressors could achieve such specificity: (1) by themselves recognizing the relevant antigens and then causing down-regulation of other lymphocytes (these are *antigen-specific suppressors*), or (2) by recognizing the particular receptors of the responding lymphocytes, either by having receptors that recognize those receptors or by expressing the antigens recognized by the receptors (these are *receptor-specific suppressors*). Internal suppression refers to changes inside a lymphocyte that cause engagement of its receptor to fail to activate an immune response. The term *anergy* describes this state, although anergy may result from more than one cellular mechanism.

STRATEGIES TO ACHIEVE TRANSPLANTATION TOLERANCE

Although it is relatively easy to generate an organizational outline for the mechanisms of tolerance induction (such as shown in Table I), it is much harder to determine which mechanism is involved for each of the numerous strategies that have been developed in rodents. In some cases we know too little about the mechanisms involved and in others there is ongoing controversy. Some strategies may use more than one

mechanism. In later chapters in this volume individual authors describe their particular strategies in some detail, providing, in some cases, interpretations that differ from those suggested here.

Deletional Strategies

The first demonstration of induced transplantation tolerance was *neonatal tolerance* induction in mice and was achieved by Medawar and his colleague in the late 1940s (Billingham et al., 1953). According to his memoirs, Medawar initiated these studies as a result of an off-hand comment made at a cocktail party to the veterinarian Hugh Douglas in 1946. Douglas was involved in studies of heredity versus the environment using twin cattle and needed a reliable way to determine whether the twins were fraternal or genetically identical. Medawar apparently told him that this could be accomplished easily by exchanging skin grafts between the animals. If the grafts were rejected, the twins were fraternal, if they were accepted, they were genetically identical. He even offered to help perform the experiments. Perhaps to Medawar's distress, Douglas accepted the offer, thus leading to dozens of trips across back roads of rural England by Medawar and his team to perform skin grafts on cows. As it turned out, Medawar's prediction was proven wrong. The skin grafts were accepted, whether or not the twins were genetically identical. Searching for an explanation for these findings, Medawar realized that Owen had already published studies that might explain the outcome (Owen, 1945). Owen had shown that twin cows of different blood groups failed to produce antibodies to the blood group antigens of their siblings and that this probably resulted from the unusual shared placental circulation of fraternal twin cattle. By exchanging antigens early in ontogeny, the twins had become tolerant to the foreign antigens.

Medawar and his colleagues set out to recapitulate this phenomenon in mice by injecting allogeneic cells into murine fetuses *in utero*. Mature animals that developed after these injections were able to accept skin grafts from the original allogeneic donor. This was characterized as *actively acquired tolerance* in the landmark article describing these experiments (Billingham et al., 1953). Medawar received the Novel prize for his work on tolerance.

Medawar's strategy to induce tolerance almost certainly involves a deletional mechanism. We now believe (1) that bone marrow-derived cells in the allogeneic inoculum populate the recipient's thymus before the development of mature, functional T cells, (2) that such bone marrow-derived cells from both the donor and recipient are responsible for eliminating maturing thymocytes that are reactive with their antigens, and (3) that the mature T cells that leave the thymus are therefore tolerant to both donor and self antigens.

In mice it turns out that tolerance can be induced by injection of allogeneic cells even after birth if they are given within the first few days of life. Careful analysis by Streilein (1979) of the relevant mechanisms under these circumstances, however, suggests that more than one process may be involved, perhaps because some elements of the immune system have fully matured by this time.

Studies more exactly recapitulating Medawar's original experiments have recently been reported in larger animals, with the idea that the strategy might be applied when severe congenital abnormalities are diagnosed *in utero* (Flake et al., 1986). Fetus's rendered tolerant to a particular donor could then receive transplants after birth without requiring immunosuppression.

Most transplant candidates, of course, already have mature immune systems. Therefore, all strategies that seek to apply Medawar's deletional approach to adult animals must include treatment to eliminate that mature system. Then, in common with Medawar's strategy, they all introduce bone marrow-derived cells designed to enter the thymus where they can delete newly maturing lymphocytes that repopulate the immune system.

Table II lists the more widely recognized strategies that attempt to create tolerance by deletion in adult animals. The earliest such strategy was the creation of *allogeneic bone marrow chimeras* following lethal, whole body irradiation. Although quite successful in rodents, this strategy has the disadvantages of requiring a lethal condi-

Table II. Deletion Strategies for Tolerance Induction

Bone marrow chimeras
Mixed bone marrow chimeras
Mixed chimeras (nonmyeloablative)
Total lymphoid irradiation with bone marrow
Transduced autologous marrow
Intrathymic injection
Neonatal tolerance induction

Not: Bone marrow ± ATG
     Organ Tx + immunosuppression

tioning regimen, of allowing the potential for graft-versus-host (GvH) disease, and of generating immunocompromised recipients even after reconstitution. This last feature occurs because the hematopoietic elements of donor B that repopulate an A animal will mature and undergo positive selection in a thymus with epithelium of type A. However, mature T cells, selected by the A epithelium for their ability to recognize pathogens presented in the context of A MHC antigens, will have only antigen-presenting cells (derived from the bone marrow) of type B with which to work (Zinkernagel et al., 1980).

To overcome these problems several modifications of the allogeneic bone marrow chimera strategy have been developed. Mixed bone marrow chimeras and mixed chimeras created with nonlethal, nonmyeloablative regimens will be described by Sachs (Chapter 12). The approach avoids GvH and the problem of immunoincompetence and is designed to be less toxic in the manner of recipient conditioning. It has been very successful in rodent experiments.

Total lymphoid irradiation is another nonlethal conditioning program that has been used in conjunction with bone marrow transplantation to induce tolerance. In this form it is probably a deletional strategy, although without the addition of bone marrow (as it is generally used clinically) it probably helps promote the induction of anergy as discussed below.

The strategy of transducing autologous marrow with genes encoding donor antigens has the same advantages as the mixed chimera approach, plus the feature that less recipient conditioning appears to be required to introduce autologous cells expressing a limited set of foreign antigens (Sykes et al., 1993). The approach has the corresponding disadvantage that the range of tolerance that can be achieved is limited. Most recently, as described by Naji et al. (Chapter 13), the technique of *intrathymic injection* of donor cells has taken advantage of the "privileged site" offered by the thymus such that engraftment in the thymus is more easily achieved than elsewhere (Posselt et al., 1993). In addition, of course, injection directly into the thymus places the donor cells where they are needed to accomplish thymic deletional tolerance. Several recent studies of intrathymic injection have indicated that it does work through a deletional mechanism. Therefore, application of this strategy also requires treatment to eliminate the mature immune system at the time of thymic injection.

Two common features of the deletional strategies are the use of bone marrow and the long-term achievement of hematopoietic chimerism. This is because bone marrow-derived cells must populate the thymus to cause deletion and because the successful engraftment of these bone marrow elements leads to chimerism. It does not necessarily follow, however, that all strategies that use bone marrow or that are associated with chimerism necessarily use a deletional mechanism. Specifically, the use of donor marrow in association with antilymphocyte antibodies and the microchimerism found after successful clinical organ transplantation are considered later in this mechanism as reflecting different mechanisms.

External Suppressor Strategies

Table III lists the strategies for tolerance induction that appear to use external suppressor mechanisms. Only one of the listed strategies (the use of nondepleting anti-CD4 antibodies (described by Waldmann in Chapter 14) appears to involve antigen-specific suppressor cells (Qin et al., 1990). In this case, the lymphocytes induced by anti-CD4 treatment at the time of organ transplantation appear to remain responsive to donor antigens, but to produce an altered profile of cytokines. The change may represent a shift

Table III. External Suppression Strategies for Tolerance Induction

Antigen-specific
  Nondepleting anti-CD4
Receptor-specific
  Bone marrow plus ATG
  Bone marrow
  Blood transfusions

from Th1 to Th2 types of helper lymphocytes, although this feature has not been clearly defined. Whatever the precise mechanism, elimination of the "suppressor" CD4 cells allows graft rejection by CD8 cells to proceed. The conditions under which nondepleting anti-CD4 treatment induces tolerance by suppression are relatively limited and not yet sufficiently understood to allow clinical application of this strategy. Other types of suppressor T cells have been characterized over the years, primarily in systems involving DTH responses to protein antigens. Although these systems have provided fascinating information on suppressor networks, they have not produced strategies that seem relevant to organ transplantation. The one exception may be the finding that oral and intravenous administration of peptides of donor antigens, especially MHC class II antigens, seems to suppress more general immune responses to a donor graft. Studies of these findings are too preliminary to have yet defined another strategy for tolerance induction.

The strategy of using donor bone marrow with or without antithymocyte globulin (ATG) treatment is listed here as an external suppressor strategy, using a receptor-specific mechanism, because the evidence at this point suggests that veto cells and perhaps natural suppressor cells in the donor bone marrow are the critical elements in the donor-specific immunosuppression seen with this approach (Thomas et al., 1991; Hartner et al., 1991). This evidence is discussed by Monaco et al. (Chapter 15). Some of the strategies using donor-specific blood transfusions, as discussed later by Morris (Dallman et al., 1991), may also rely on the function of veto cells for their effect.

Veto cells are cells that destroy lymphocytes that would otherwise destroy them while natural suppressor cells, plentiful especially in bone marrow, are less specific in their function, suppressing reactive lymphocytes in their environment. Veto cells are discussed in more detail by Miller (Chapter 16). Strategies relying on veto cells might alternatively be listed as peripheral deletional mechanisms since veto cells seems to induce apoptosis in mature T cells.

Antiidiotypic suppressors would also represent a receptor-specific technique for inducing tolerance. Although there was great interest in this approach for several years, there have been few reports of successful control of graft rejection using antiidiotypic reagents and none that appears clinically relevant.

Internal Suppressor Strategies—
Anergy Induction

The finding that T cells can sometimes encounter antigen in ways that down-regulate rather than activate the immune responses demonstrated the existence of internal suppressor mechanisms. Jenkins describes this process of anergy induction in Chapter 18 (Jenkins et al., 1987). The fundamental requirement for the mechanism seems to be the engagement of a T cell's receptor without simultaneously providing "the second signal." There are probably several elements to this second signal. Without their coactivating stimulus, T cells not only fail to respond normally to the antigen triggering them, but in addition their internal gears are disengaged, such that they fail to respond to receptor stimulation in the future, even when the appropriate costimulatory signals are provided.

It now seems likely that anergy induction is the mechanism underlying several strategies for tolerance induction (see Table IV) some of which were described before the mechanism of T cell anergy was identified. The successful engraftment of some endocrine tissues with subsequent tolerance induction after depletion of antigen-presenting cells (APC), for example, probably reflects the engagement of T cell receptors without costimulation provided by APCs. Some strategies using pretransplant donor-specific

Table IV. Anergy-Inducing Strategies for Tolerance Induction

APC depletion or modification
Donor-specific blood transfusions
Blocking the "second signal"
Organ transplantation

blood transfusions may also be anergy inducing when they depend primarily on APC depletion rather than enrichment for veto or natural suppressor cells. Similarly, techniques that modify the function of APCs, such as UV irradiation, are probably anergy-inducing strategies. A number of strategies have also been developed that are designed to block the action of the second signal, including CTLA4-Ig (which interferes with the interaction between CTLA4 on T cells and its costimulatory ligand, B7, on APCs) (Lenshow et al., 1992), a combination of anti-LFA-1 and anti-ICAM-1 (to block the adherence of T cells to APCs) (Isobe et al., 1992), and anti-CD4 depleting antibodies (to prevent IL-2 delivery to CD8 cells at the time of antigen exposure).

Unfortunately, experimental strategies using reagents to block the delivery of second signals have generally been performed in rodents and almost always with a simultaneous primarily vascularized organ or pancreatic islet transplants. It is rarely pointed out that these types of transplants in rodents are themselves highly tolerogenic, especially after they have survived for several weeks. Some of the reagents reported to be tolerance inducing are more likely simply immunosuppressive, and the tolerance seen following their use reflects instead the presence of the organ transplant.

The phenomenon that some organs are tolerogenic in rodents (and sometimes even in larger animals such as the pig) has been recognized since the early 1970s (Russell et al., 1979). The evidence now suggests that the liver is especially powerful in this regard, followed by the kidney, the heart, and pancreatic islets. Skin grafts never seem to induce tolerance merely by their own survival. It now seems likely that some degree of tolerance induction by persistent organ transplant survival occurs even in larger animals, including in human patients. For example, pig kidney transplants with limited MHC antigen disparities, kept in place initially with a short course of high-dose cyclosporine, can go on to survive indefinitely and to induce tolerance in their recipients (Rosengard et al., 1992). In addition, human patients almost always require less immunosuppression late after a transplant than in the early stages. A few patients can even stop their immunosuppression entirely without losing their organs.

The phenomenon that organ transplantation itself is tolerogenic is listed here as an anergy-inducing strategy—based on the supposition that anergy induction by the vast presentation of donor antigens on parenchymal cells (without APC function) can dominate the smaller (and diminishing) effect of donor APCs under some circumstances. However, many investigators would disagree with this characterization. Sachs' group, for example, has suggested that a suppressor mechanism is involved when their pig kidneys survive for a prolonged time and induce tolerance. Alternatively, Starzl has noted the persistent microchimerism that accompanies long-term successful organ transplantation and postulated that these chimeric cells are responsible for tolerance induction, presumably though a deletional mechanism. We lack the information at this point, however, to determine whether microchimerism is responsible for or simply reflects the fact of prolonged graft survival.

THE DIFFICULTIES IN APPLYING TOLERANCE-INDUCING STRATEGIES TO CLINICAL TRANSPLANTATION

With so many strategies to induce tolerance in rodents, it is frustrating that clinical transplantation is still practiced today without application of these approaches. here more than anywhere, the persistent separation between the science of transplantation immunology and the practice of clinical medicine is apparent. It is worth asking, therefore, what is keeping us from applying the research strategies to our patients, not with the purpose of diminishing the importance of the experimental work, but with the idea of identifying the problems that still need to be solved.

In the first place, clinical transplantation has become the victim of its own success. With the majority of patients maintaining successful transplants and leading productive lives by taking nonspecific immunosuppressive drugs, it is difficult to identify the circumstances where unproven protocols to induce tolerance can be tested ethically in human patients. Perhaps the use of xenografts, which are likely to fare less well than corresponding allogeneic organs unless tolerance accompanies their use, will provide the opportunity for trials of new tolerance-inducing strategies.

Beyond this practical issue, however, the tolerance-inducing strategies that have worked so well in rodents have been less successful even when tested in nonhuman primates and other large animals. Large animal trials of these strategies, using vascularized organs, have generally produced results more similar to those using rodent skin grafts than to those using the corresponding organ. As a practical consequence, it seems reasonable to focus especially on those strategies that have proven effective even for rodent skin grafts—essentially only the deletional, bone marrow chimera strategies. One biologic difference between rodent solid organs and those of larger animals is that rodents do not express class II antigens on their vascular endothelium. Whether this is the reason for the greater ease of tolerance induction in these animals is not clear, however.

There are other important issues that limit the simple application of the many tolerance-inducing strategies to human patients.

Deletional Strategies

1. All thymic deletional strategies require that the recipient's mature immune system be eliminated so that newly maturing lymphocytes, without donor-reactive cells, will represent the complete mature repertoire. Treatments that accomplish immune ablation and that are well-tolerated in rodents (such as whole body irradia-

tion) would not be appropriate for clinical transplantation. Although monoclonal antibody therapy has also proven effective for this purpose in rodents, similarly effective antibodies for humans have not been identified.

2. Reconstitution of the mature immune system requires that the thymus be capable of repopulating mature T cells. Most experimental studies have been performed with relatively young animals, whereas the adult human thymus is a scant remnant of the original organ. It is not yet clear how completely, and under what circumstances, the adult human thymus can function adequately.

3. Tolerance induced to bone marrow-derived cells cannot be expected to provide tolerance to tissue-specific antigens. Although such antigens can be the target of rejection in some experimental systems, it is not yet clear whether such responses are clinically relevant.

External Suppressor Strategies

1. The best source of veto and suppressor cells is in the bone marrow compartment. However, to achieve the most benefit from these cells, with the least risk, requires learning to select more precisely for these populations by phenotypic markers, while eliminating those cells that may cause GvH disease.

Anergy-Inducing Strategies

1. Experimental studies of T cell anergy have indicated that the condition can be reversed under some circumstances. Exactly what conditions and how to prevent them remain to be determined.

2. The process of graft rejection can involve responses initiated by donor APCs and also responses initiated by recipient APCs presenting donor antigens. Anergy-inducing strategies can be applied permanently only to the donor APC pathway, since recipient APCs must eventually be left competent to allow responses to new environmental pathogens. The long-term stimulus to graft rejection provided by recipient APC function can presumably never be controlled entirely by an anergy-inducing strategy alone.

All Tolerance-Inducing Strategies

All of the tolerance-inducing strategies discussed here attempt to eliminate the recipient's response to donor antigens and none of them makes provision for adding cells back to the mature T cell repertoire that have receptors specific for viral peptides presented by donor antigens. Experimental evidence suggests that tolerance induced without a positive selection process will leave the recipient immunologically compromised for responses to pathogens in the donor tissue. While the defect is not likely to be worse than that suffered by transplant patients today (who are taking exogenous immunosuppression), it is likely to remain a significant issue even if the problem of rejection could be eliminated completely from clinical transplantation.

CONCLUSION

This brief review of tolerance-inducing strategies has been designed to provide an organizational framework for considering and comparing the multitude of approaches that researchers are exploring. It is also designed to highlight some of the issues that should be considered and the questions that should be asked when evaluating these different strategies. The potential that transplantation tolerance can be achieved clinically has now been apparent for more than 40 years and thus enthusiastic predictions accompanying the introduction of each new strategy have begun to seem stale. Although more than a dozen different techniques to induce tolerance in rodents are now available, the fact remains that none of them has been used successfully in the clinic. Inducing transplantation tolerance in humans must, therefore, be very hard to do. Readers of this chapter should, therefore, be wary of simple solutions to this complex problem. They should also realize that fresh approaches (perhaps new ones, perhaps combinations of elements from old techniques) may be needed to solve this most important problem in transplantation immunology.

REFERENCES

Billingham RE, Brent L, Medawar PB (1953): "Actively acquired tolerance" of foreign cells. Nature (London) 172:603–606.

Dallman MJ, Shiho D, Page TM, Wood KJ, Morris PJ (1991): Peripheral tolerance to alloantigen results from altered regulation of the interleukin 2 pathway. J Exp Med 173:79–87.

Flake AW, Harrison MR, Adzick NS et al. (1986): Transplantation of fetal hematopoietic stem cells in utero: The creation of hematopoietic chimeras. Science 233:776–778.

Hartner WC, Markees TG, De Fazio SR, Khouri W, Maki T, Monaco AP, Gozzo JJ (1991): The effect of antilymphocyte serum, fractionated donor bone marrow, and cyclosporine on renal allograft survival in mongrel dogs. Transplantation 52:784–789.

Isobe M, Yagita H, Okumura K, Ihara A (1992): Specific acceptance of cardiac allograft after treatment with antibodies to ICAM-1 and LFA-1. Science 255:1125–1127.

Jenkins MK, Pardoll DM, Mizuguchi J, Chused TM, Schwartz RH (1987): Molecular events in the induction of a nonresponsive state in interleukin 2-producing helper T-lymphocyte clones. Proc Natl Acad Sci USA 84:5409–5413.

Lenshow DJ, Zeng Y, Thistlewaite JR, Montag A, Brady W, Gibson MG, Linsley PS, Bluestone JA (1992): Long-term survival of xenogeneic pancreatic islet grafts induced by CTLA-4 Ig. Science 257:789–792.

Owen RD (1945): Immunogenetic consequences of vascular anastomoses between bovine twins. Science 102:400.

Posselt AM, Campos L, Mayo GL, O'Connor TP, Odorico JS, Markmann JF, Barker CF, Naji A (1993): Selective modulation of T-cell immunity by intrathymic cellular transplantation. Transplant Rev 7:200–213.

Qin SX, Wise M, Cobbold SP, Leong L, Kong YC, Parnes JR, Waldmann H (1990): Induction of tolerance in peripheral T cells with monoclonal antibodies. Eur J Immunol 20:2737–2745.

Rosengard BR, Ojikutu CA, Guzetta PC, Smith CV, Sundt TM III, Nakajima K, Boorstein SM, Hill GS, Fishbein JM, Sachs DH (1992): Induction of specific tolerance to class I-disparate renal allografts in miniature swine with cyclosporine. Transplantation 54:490–497.

Russell P, Chase C, Colvin R, Plate J (1979): Kidney transplants in mice: An analysis of the immune status of mice bearing long-term H-2 incompatible transplants. J Exp Med 147:1449–1468.

Streilein JW (1979): Neonatal tolerance: Toward an immunogenetic definition of self. Immunol Rev 46:125.

Sykes M, Sachs DH, Nienhuis AW, Pearson DA, Moulton AD, Bodine DM (1993): Specific prolongation of skin graft survival following retroviral transduction of bone marrow with an allogeneic MHC gene. Transplantation 55:197–202.

Thomas JM, Carver FM, Cunningham PR, Olson LC, Thomas FT (1991): Kidney allograft tolerance in primates without chronic immunosuppression—the role of veto cells. Transplantation 51:198–207.

Zinkernagel RM, Althage A, Callahan G, Welsh RM Jr. (1980): On the immunocompetence of H-2 incompatible irradiation bone marrow chimeras. J Immunol 124:2356–2365.

Chapter 12
Mixed Chimerism as an Approach to Transplantation Tolerance

David H. Sachs

It has been known for many years that production of fully allogeneic chimeras through bone marrow transplantation carries with it the induction of transplantation tolerance to other tissues and organs from the donor of the allogeneic marrow (Rapaport et al., 1978; Rayfield and Brent, 1983; Ildstad and Sachs, 1984). However, there are two major problems with this procedure as a means of inducing tolerance: (1) if mature T cells are not removed from the allogeneic bone marrow, then graft-versus-host disease may result; and (2) if mature T cells are removed from the allogeneic bone marrow inoculum, then the chimeras that result are relatively immunoincompetent.

The probable reason for this immunocompetence was first suggested by Zinkernagel and colleagues (Zinkernagel et al., 1980a,b),and is illustrated in Figure 1. As seen in Figure 1A, fully allogeneic chimeras result from lethal irradiation of a recipient and reconstitution with T cell-depleted allogeneic bone marrow. New T cells that subsequently arise in such recipients are of the allogeneic MHC type (B), but are educated in a thymus of host MHC type (A). These new T cells therefore acquire restriction specificities for A + X, in which X is the peptide of a nominal antigen presented by MHC molecules of type A. However, the antigen-presenting cells that are responsible for presenting environmental antigens to mature T cells in the periphery are also replaced by the bone marrow transplant, and are, therefore, of MHC type B. The mature T cells thus encounter B + X rather than the A + X to which they are restricted. Some sharing of specificities is undoubtedly responsible for the weak immune responses that occur in such fully allogeneic chimeras, but the majority of MHC-restricted responses are disabled, leading to relative immunoincompetence.

This concept was later validated by Singer and colleagues (Singer et al., 1981) who demonstrated that mature T cells from fully allogeneic chimeras are capable of responding if appropriate antigen-presenting cells of MHC type A are provided. As illustrated in Figure 1B, reconstitution of irradiated strain A recipients with a mixture of T cell-depleted bone marrow cells from strain A plus strain B leads to production of new mature T cells of both MHC haplotypes. In this case, both mature T cell populations are restricted through positive selection in the thymus to the recognition of A + X. However, now antigen-presenting cells are present in the periphery of the appropriate strain A type, and immunocompetent interactions can occur.

We have referred to animals reconstituted with both allogeneic and self-lymphohematopoietic elements as mixed chimeras (Ildstad et al., 1985b; Sykes and Sachs, 1988). As will be described further below, the allogeneic bone marrow-derived elements in such animals are responsible for conferring transplantation tolerance, while the host type elements confer immunocompetence. Thus, unlike the situation in which bone marrow transplants are used to treat leukemia, full ablation of host lymphoid elements is neither necessary nor desirable when the transplant is used as a means of inducing mixed chimerism for the purpose of achieving transplantation tolerance.

Transplantation Immunology, pages 219–225
© 1995 Wiley-Liss, Inc.

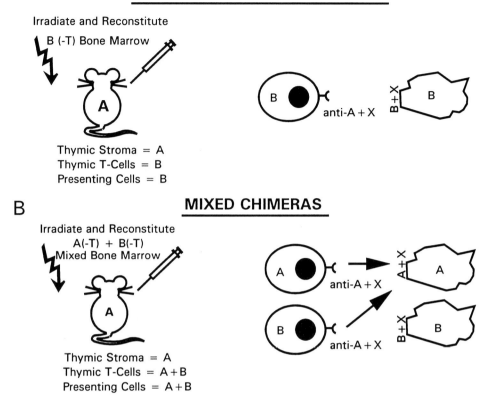

A FULLY ALLOGENEIC CHIMERAS

Irradiate and Reconstitute
B (-T) Bone Marrow

Thymic Stroma = A
Thymic T-Cells = B
Presenting Cells = B

B MIXED CHIMERAS

Irradiate and Reconstitute
A(-T) + B(-T)
Mixed Bone Marrow

Thymic Stroma = A
Thymic T-Cells = A + B
Presenting Cells = A + B

Fig. 1. Schematic representation of the cellular interactions required for immunocompetence in allogeneic chimeras. (**A**) Fully allogeneic chimeras develop mature T cells with restriction specificities for host MHC type, but encounter donor MHC type presenting cells in the periphery and are consequently immunoincompetent. (**B**) Mixed allogeneic chimeras develop mature T cells with the same host MHC-restricting specificities, but now have appropriate host MHC type presenting cells in the periphery and are consequently immunocompetent.

MIXED ALLOGENEIC CHIMERAS FOLLOWING LETHAL IRRADIATION

Our early attempts to produce mixed chimerism involved lethal irradiation of C57BL/10 (B10) recipient mice followed by reconstitution with mixtures of syngeneic B10 and fully allogeneic B10.D2 bone marrow, both of which were depleted of mature T cells by antibodies and complement prior to reconstitution (Ildstad and Sachs, 1984; Ildstad et al., 1985b, 1986). By titrating relative proportions of bone marrow cells, it was determined that a 1:3 ratio of host to donor bone marrow achieved the best results in terms of producing mixed chimeras. An example

of the peripheral blood lymphocyte typing of animals in one such experiment is shown in Table I. These animals were reconstituted with B10 + B10.D2 bone marrow 60–120 days prior to the assay. As seen in Table I, all animals demonstrated mixed chimerism among their peripheral blood lymphocytes (PBL), with the percent donor (B10.D2) cells ranging from 5 to 92%. Repeat assays on the same animals over a period of months showed fluctuations, but the animals always demonstrated PBL of both host and donor type.

Mixed chimeras and controls (syngeneic and fully allogeneic reconstituted animals) were subsequently tested for immune responsiveness to a

Table I. Characterization of Mice Reconstituted with Mixed Allogeneic Bone Marrow (B10 + B10.D2 → B10)

Animal number	Percent B10.D2 cells by complement-mediated cytotoxicity (PBL)
1	92
2	23
3	79
4	87
5	74
6	19
7	82
8	33
9	49
10	64
11	42
12	70
13	48
14	32
15	49
16	64
17	5
Normal B10	0
Normal B10.D2	100

single dose of sheep red blood cells (Ildstad et al., 1985b). Assessment of plaque-forming cells in the spleens of these animals demonstrated equal numbers of plaques for mixed chimeras and syngeneically reconstituted animals, but severely reduced plaques among spleen cells from fully allogeneic chimeras. This result was consistent with the prediction of improved immunocompetence, which might be expected for mixed chimeras in comparison to fully allogeneic chimeras.

In addition, these mixed chimeras were found to be specifically tolerant to skin grafts from the allogeneic donor strain (Ildstad and Sachs, 1984; Ildstad et al., 1985b). Thus, as illustrated in Figure 2, the vast majority of mixed chimeras retained skin grafts from B10.D2 animals permanently, while they were capable of rejecting third party skin grafts (C3H) just as promptly as did normal B10 animals. Thus, induction of mixed chimerism by this procedure resulted in animals that were both immunocompetent and specifically tolerant.

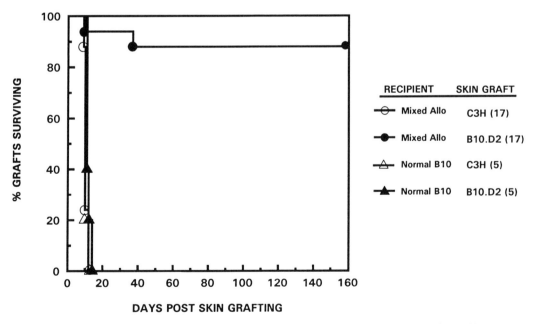

RECIPIENT	SKIN GRAFT
Mixed Allo	C3H (17)
Mixed Allo	B10.D2 (17)
Normal B10	C3H (5)
Normal B10	B10.D2 (5)

DAYS POST SKIN GRAFTING

Fig. 2. Survival of skin grafts on mixed chimeras. Mixed chimeras [B10+B10.D2→B10] retained skin grafts from B10.D2 animals permanently, while they were capable of rejecting third party skin grafts (C3H) just as promptly as did normal B10 animals.

MIXED CHIMERISM BY A NONLETHAL PREPARATIVE REGIMEN

The major problem with the protocol so far described for inducing tolerance through mixed chimerism is that it requires lethal irradiation as a preparative regimen for bone marrow engraftment. Despite the advantages that induction of tolerance would have over long-term conventional immunosuppression with drugs, most clinicians would agree that lethal irradiation is too toxic and dangerous a procedure to be considered for clinical application in organ transplantation. Therefore, over the past several years we have investigated methods for producing mixed chimerism without the need for lethal irradiation. One such regimen that will be described in detail here involves the use of monoclonal antibodies to remove the mature T cells, which are the main impediment to allogeneic engraftment.

This work was inspired by reports from Cobbald et al. (1986) indicating that treatment of mice with antibodies to mature T cell subsets (CD4 and CD8) was capable of permitting transient engraftment of MHC mismatched bone marrow or skin grafts. However, despite the fact that this antibody treatment was shown to deplete all peripheral mature T cells, and despite the fact that these authors used a low dose of whole-body irradiation (3–6 Gy) to make "room," bone marrow engraftment was only transient and disappeared within a few weeks. As an extension of this work, we attempted to determine why the engraftment was only transient. When lymphoid compartments of treated animals were examined, depletion of all mature CD4 and CD8 T cells was observed in peripheral blood, lymph nodes, and spleen (Sharabi and Sachs, 1989). However, T cells were found in the thymus that were coated with antibody but not depleted. It was concluded that the mechanism by which antibody treatment leads to depletion of mature T cells does not function efficiently within the thymus. A boost of irradiation to the thymus was therefore added to the preparative regimen. Utilizing a protocol consisting of 3 Gy whole-body irradiation, 7 Gy thymic irradiation and treatment with monoclonal antibodies to CD4 and CD8, mixed allogeneic chimerism could be induced in the majority of recipient animals (Sharabi and Sachs, 1989). The pattern of reconstitution of animals prepared by this non-myeloablative regimen was indistinguishable by FACS analysis from that of animals prepared by lethal irradiation and reconstitution with T cell-depleted host plus donor bone marrow. By 2 weeks after treatment and administration of allogeneic bone marrow, cells of both host and donor type were observed in both the T cell and non-T cell compartments in this analysis. Levels of T cells in both host and donor compartments increased over the next month, and subpopulations in all four compartments remained for the rest of the life of the animals. Like their counterparts prepared by the lethal preparative regimen, these mixed chimeras showed specific tolerance to subsequent skin grafts, retaining B10.B2 skin permanently and rejecting third party skin promptly. In addition, these animals were far more healthy than those produced by the lethal preparative regimen, and showed none of the toxic effects of lethal irradiation. Premature graying, for example, was observed only in the small area of the neck where thymic irradiation had been carried out, and the animals gained weight equivalent to untreated cohorts. Lastly, if no bone marrow was administered, these animals all survived and reconstituted their hematopoietic systems, indicating that the preparative regimen was indeed nonlethal.

Because this regimen is far less toxic than the lethal preparative regimen, we have considered it for potential clinical applicability. We have, therefore, recently begun a trial of a similar protocol in cynomolgus monkeys as a preclinical large animal model (Kawai et al., 1995). The test organ for transplantation tolerance in these studies has been a kidney transplant between fully mismatched monkeys. The preliminary data so far are very encouraging, with one monkey already achieving greater than 500 days of normal kidney function without any immunosuppressive treatment beyond 30 days.

MIXED XENOGENEIC CHIMERISM

Shortly after determining that mixed bone marrow reconstitution of lethally irradiated recipients could produce long-term mixed chimerism and transplantation tolerance in an allogeneic model, we turned our attention to a xenogeneic application of the same protocol (Ildstad and Sachs, 1984; Ildstad et al., 1984). We utilized the very close, or concordant, species combination of rat→mouse, and administered 4×10^7 T cell-depleted F344 rat bone marrow cells plus 5×10^6 syngeneic T cell-depleted B10 bone marrow cells to lethally irradiated B10 recipients. In this case, unlike the situation for allogeneic reconstitution, the mixed chimerism achieved was only transient, and disappeared over a few weeks. Nevertheless, skin grafts from F344 rats showed markedly prolonged survival, with a median survival time of approximately 80 days, as compared to less than 10 days for third party allogeneic (C3H) or xenogeneic (WF rat) skin grafts. We believe that the loss of the skin grafts was not necessarily due to a loss of tolerance, but rather to skin-specific antigens toward which bone marrow was unable to induce tolerance. Skin is indeed the hardest tissue to prolong by most immunosuppressive regimens, and some of these same animals that eventually rejected F344 skin grafts were capable of permanently accepting an F344 vascularized heart transplant placed intraabdominally (Ildstad et al., 1985a). Tolerance was also confirmed by the absence of antidonor MLR and CML. We hypothesize that sufficient rat–mouse mixed chimerism persists in the necessary location (possibly the thymus) to maintain tolerance to a vascularized graft in this situation.

We have subsequently extended our nonmyeloablative protocol to concordant xenogeneic transplants as well (Sharabi et al., 1990). In this case, it was found necessary to deplete not only mature T cells, but also natural killer (NK) cells from the recipients to achieve mixed chimerism and prolonged skin graft survival. The best specific survival of F344 skin grafts was achieved utilizing antibodies to CD4, CD8, Thy1, and NK1.1 antigens.

MIXED CHIMERISM FOR DISCORDANT XENOGRAFTS

Because donor organ availability has become a major limitation to the field of transplantation, there has been a resurgence of interest in xenografting over the past few years. Although nonhuman primates would provide the closest potential donors for man phylogenetically, there are a variety of reasons, including availability and ethical considerations, that mitigate against widescale use of primates as xenograft donors. We and others have therefore turned our attention to more discordant species as a potential xenograft donor source. The miniature swine that we have inbred over the past 20 years as a large animal model for transplantation (Sachs et al., 1976; Sachs, 1992) have a variety of advantages over other potential xenograft donors as indicated in Table II. The chief advantage of pigs is their breeding characteristics, which make it possible to manipulate the genetics of these animals in a relatively short time. These characteristics include large litter size (3–10 piglets), short gestation time (15 weeks), frequent estrus cycles (every 3 weeks), and sexual maturity at the early age of 4–6 months. Thus, the generation time of these animals is approximately 1 year, with the potential for selection of breeders at every generation. These characteristics have enabled us to establish three herds of MHC homozygous pigs as well as several intra-MHC recombinant strains. Another advantage of these animals is their size, which is very similar to that of human beings, with maximal weights of approximately 250 pounds. Thus, one might choose an appropriate donor for any potential human recipient.

We have recently begun studies attempting to extend the nonmyeloablative regimen for production of mixed chimerism to this discordant

Table II. Advantages of Inbred Miniature Swine as Xenograft Donors

Size
Immunologic characterization
Breeding characteristics
Reproducibility of genetics
    For absorption of natural antibodies
    For cellular plus organ transplants
Genetic therapy
    One set of genes for all donors
    For breeding of transgenics

pig→primate combination (Latinne et al., 1993). We have utilized intraoperative *ex vivo* perfusion of a pig liver as a means of absorbing natural antibodies from cynomolgus monkeys. Otherwise, the protocol we have developed is very similar to that used for the rat→mouse concordant procedure. The steps of this protocol are illustrated in Figure 3. Preliminary results utilizing this model have recently been reported (Latinne et al., 1993; Tanaka et al., 1994), using a pig kidney xenograft as the test organ for induction of tolerance. Our results so far have demonstrated elimination of hyperacute rejection by the absorption technique, and we have obtained kidney graft survival times of up to 13 days. During this period the pig xenograft kidneys have functioned essentially normally, maintaining a normal creatinine and acid–base balance in the recipient monkey. However, we have not yet achieved persistent mixed chimerism in these animals, nor has long-term tolerance been accomplished. Among the approaches being tested to further extend these results are (1) the use of specific immunoabsorbent columns rather than whole liver to remove natural antibodies, (2) production and use of new specific monoclonal antibodies rather than antithymocyte globulin (ATG) to eliminate host T cells and NK cells, and (3) production and use of pig-specific cytokines and growth factors that may be needed to sustain xenogeneic bone marrow engraftment. Nevertheless, we are encouraged by the survivals achieved already without additional immunosuppressive agents. We hope that further extensions of this model will eventually provide a clinically applicable protocol for discordant xenografting.

ACKNOWLEDGMENTS

This work was supported in part by NIH Grant CA55553 and by a Sponsored Research Agreement between the M.G.H. and BioTransplant, Inc. We thank Ms. Rachael Supple for expert secretarial assistance and Drs. Megan Sykes and Pierre Gianello for review of the manuscript and helpful comments.

REFERENCES

Cobbold SP, Martin G, Qin S, Waldmann H (1986): Monoclonal antibodies to promote marrow engraftment and tissue graft tolerance. Nature (London) 323 6084):164–166.

Ildstad ST, Sachs DH (1984): Reconstitution with syngeneic plus allogeneic or xenogeneic bone marrow leads to specific acceptance of allografts or xenografts. Nature (London) 307(5947):168–170.

Ildstad ST, Wren SM, Sharrow SO, Stephany D, Sachs DH (1984): In vivo and in vitro characterization of specific hyporeactivity to skin xenografts in mixed xenogeneically reconstituted mice (B10 + F344 rat→B10). J Exp Med 160:1820–1835.

Ildstad ST, Russell PS, Chase CM, Sachs DH (1985a): Long-term survival of primarily vascularized cardiac xenografts in mice repopulated with syngeneic plus xenogeneic bone marrow (C57BL/

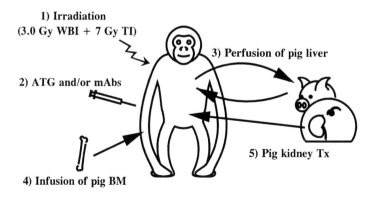

Fig. 3. Proposed nonmyeloablative protocol for induction of mixed xenogeneic chimerism and tolerance in the discordant system, pig to cynomolgus monkey.

10Sn + F344 rat→C57BL/10Sn). Transplant Proc 17:535–538.

Ildstad ST, Wren SM, Bluestone JA, Barbieri SA, Sachs DH (1985b): Characterization of mixed allogeneic chimeras. Immunocompetence, in vitro reactivity, and genetic specificity of tolerance. J Exp Med 162:231–244.

Ildstad ST, Wren SM, Bluestone JA, Barbieri SA, Stephany D, Sachs DH (1986): Effect of selective T cell depletion of host and/or donor bone marrow on lymphopoietic repopulation, tolerance, and graft-vs-host disease in mixed allogeneic chimeras (B10 + B10.D2→B10). J Immunol 136:28–33.

Kawai T, Cosimi AB, Colvin RB, Powelson J, Eason J, Kozlowski T, Sykes M, Monroy R, Tanaka M, Sachs DH (1995): Mixed allogeneic chimerism and renal allograft tolerance in cynomolgus monkeys. Transplantation (in press).

Latinne D, Gianello P, Smith CV, Nickeleit V, Kawai T, Beadle M, Haug C, Sykes M, Lebowitz E, Bazin H, Colvin R, Cosimi AB, Sachs DH (1993): Xenotransplantation from pig to cynomolgus monkey: Approach toward tolerance induction. Transplant Proc 25:336–338.

Rapaport FT, Bachvaroff RJ, Watanabe K, Hirasawa H, Mollen N, Ferrebee JW, Amos DB, Cannon FD, Blumenstock DA (1978): Induction of allogeneic unresponsiveness in adult dogs: Role of non-DLA histocompatibility variables in conditioning the outcome of bone marrow, kidney, and skin transplantation in radiation chimeras. J Clin Invest 61:790–800.

Rayfield LS, Brent L (1983): Tolerance, immunocompetence, and secondary disease in fully allogeneic radiation chimeras. Transplantation 36:183–189.

Sachs DH (1992): MHC homozygous miniature swine. In Swindle MM, Moody DC, Phillips LD (eds): "Swine as Models in Biomedical Research." Ames: Iowa State University Press, pp 3–15.

Sachs DH, Leight G, Cone J, Schwarz S, Stuart L, Rosenberg S (1976): Transplantation in miniature swine. I. Fixation of the major histocompatibility complex. Transplantation 22:559–567.

Sharabi Y, Sachs DH (1989): Mixed chimerism and permanent specific transplantation tolerance induced by a nonlethal preparative regimen. J Exp Med 169:493–502.

Sharabi Y, Aksentijevich I, Sundt III TM, Sachs DH, Sykes M (1990): Specific tolerance induction across a xenogeneic barrier: Production of mixed rat/mouse lymphohematopoietic chimeras using a nonlethal preparative regimen. J Exp Med 172: 195–202.

Singer A, Hathcock KS, Hodes RJ (1981): Self recognition in allogeneic radiation bone marrow chimeras. J Exp Med 153:1286–1301.

Sykes M, Sachs DH (1988): Mixed allogeneic chimerism as an approach to transplantation tolerance. Immunol Today 9:23–27.

Tanaka M, Latinne D, Gianello P, Sablinski T, Lorf T, Bailin M, Nickeleit V, Colvin R, Lebowitz E, Sykes M, Cosimi AB, Sachs DH (1994): Xenotransplantation from pig to cynomolgus monkey: The potential for overcoming xenograft rejection through induction of chimerism. Transplant Proc 26:1326–1327.

Zinkernagel RM, Althage A, Callahan G, Welsh RM (1980a): On the immunocompetence of H-2 incompatible irradiation bone marrow chimeras. J Immunol 124:2356.

Zinkernagel RM, Althage A, Waterfield E, Kindred B, Welsh RM, Callahan G, Pincetl P (1980b): Restriction specificities, alloreactivity, and allotolerance expressed by T cells from nude mice reconstituted with H-2-compatible or -incompatible thymus grafts. J Exp Med 151:376–399.

Chapter 13
Induction of Tolerance by Intrathymic Cellular Transplantation

Luis Campos, Andrew M. Posselt, George L. Mayo, Jon S. Odorico, James F. Markmann, Clyde F. Barker, and Ali Naji

INTRODUCTION

The inevitability of allograft rejection and the sustained threat to recipients of deleterious effects of immunosuppression continue to be important limitations to treatment of human disease by transplantation. The cellular and humoral networks that orchestrate the interaction of multiple graft and host-determined factors are extremely complex and still incompletely understood. Of central importance to both the initiation of the immune response and the effector phase that later destroys the alien target organ is the recognition by recipient T cells of MHC antigens expressed on the foreign tissue. The identification of allogeneic antigens by recipient T cells is mediated by clonally restricted T cell receptors that provide specificity to the response by interacting with the polymorphic regions of the MHC antigens (Krensky et al., 1990).

It seems unlikely that the evolution of this complex process by even the most primitive species took place in anticipation of man's eventual ambition to replace diseased organs and for the seemingly perverse purpose of preventing successful transplantation. Thus implicit in the concept that allogeneic rejection represents a specific immune response to foreign histocompatibility antigens is the ability of the immune system of the recipient to recognize and destroy harmful foreign antigens while granting amnesty to its own tissues. In the case of B cells, acquisition of the capacity to distinguish self from nonself begins during their maturation in the bone marrow and continues after their residence in secondary lymphoid organs (Goodnow et al., 1989). The acquisition of T cell tolerance, on the other hand, appears to be achieved primarily within the thymus (Kappler et al., 1987).

Three mechanisms have been proposed as possible explanations of the induction and maintenance of immunologic tolerance to self-antigens: (1) clonal deletion, (2) clonal anergy, and (3) specific suppression. These mechanisms are not mutually exclusive. In fact, there is considerable evidence that they all may coexist in certain circumstances. The acquisition of T cell tolerance in the thymus is probably achieved primarily by selective deletion of self-reactive T cells, whereby the interaction between self-antigen and the T cell receptor at an immature stage in T cell differentiation aborts further development of the cell (Kappler et al., 1987). In experimental models other forms of tolerance have been observed that are not dependent on deletional mechanisms. In some of these systems the tolerant state is the result of functional inactivation (anergy) of mature antigen-reactive lymphocytes (Ramsdell and Fowlkes, 1990). This effect appears to result from the interaction of T cells with specific antigens in the absence of requisite costimulatory signals necessary for T cell activation. Finally, suppression represents another means by which tolerance within the mature T cell repertoire can be achieved. This process in which T cells are generated capable of down-regulating immunity was originally invoked to explain the empiric observation that in

Transplantation Immunology, pages 227–238
© 1995 Wiley-Liss, Inc.

certain models of allograft acceptance, unresponsiveness could be transferred to naive hosts by lymphoid cells from tolerant donors (Hall et al., 1990).

Induction of tolerance to a specific donor would be the ideal method of protecting a transplant from rejection and sparing the recipient from deleterious effects of long-term immunosuppression while leaving the immune system fully capable of responding to all other non-self-antigens. The feasibility of promoting tolerance of grafted foreign tissue was first demonstrated in 1953 by the ingenious experiment of Billingham, Brent, and Medawar, who obtained donor-specific tolerance in mice by inoculating them *in utero* with lymphohematopoietic cells (Billingham et al., 1953). This strategy is highly effective in that it establishes a state of life long tolerance permitting the recipients to accept donor strain grafts of any tissue. The tolerant state achieved in this model is likely the result of several mechanisms; however, the prevailing view is that intrathymic deletion–inactivation of high avidity donor-reactive T cells is most important (Streilein, 1991).

Other strategies devised to induce a similar state of transplantation tolerance in adult recipients have all proved inferior to neonatal tolerance. Most of these have relied on pretreatment of hosts with radiation or immunosuppressive agents to ablate the lymphoid system followed by reconstitution with donor lymphohematopoietic cells. The immunosuppressive step promotes engraftment of the donor cells by disabling the host's mature T cells and, in effect, simulates the immunologic naivete of the neonates used in the Billingham model of tolerance. However, the risks associated with the intense conditioning regimen renders such protocols impractical for clinical utility. Therefore induction of transplantation tolerance in humans will require development of strategies in which safer preparative protocols can be used.

Such an objective could potentially be accomplished by manipulating T cell development at either the thymic or postthymic level. Within the thymus as noted above, tolerance induction can be profoundly influenced by the repertoire of antigens expressed on nonlymphoid cellular components of the thymus. In the studies reviewed here we have taken advantage of the knowledge that exposure of immature prothymocytes to donor alloantigens at a stage when the developing T cell is most sensitive to tolerance induction can influence the functional state of the peripheral immune repertoire. The following sections will summarize our attempts to manipulate intrathymic maturation of T cells for therapeutic purposes by employing a novel strategy that involves inoculation of foreign antigens directly into the thymus. Specifically, studies that characterize the influence of intrathymic cellular inoculation on allogeneic, xenogeneic, as well as autoimmune T cell-mediated responses will be reviewed.

Our rational for induction of transplantation tolerance by intrathymic inoculation of donor cells was a reconsideration of the findings of Billingham and colleagues that whereas donor cells of lymphohematopoietic origin were highly effective in inducing tolerance in neonatal rodents, parenchymal cells of organs such as liver, testicle, and kidney lacked this capacity. We reasoned that the consistent efficiency of lymphohematopoietic cells to promote transplantation tolerance was due not to a unique expression of alloantigens that they share with most cell types but to their ability to migrate to and populate the thymic microenvironment where they would be able to influence T cell maturation. If the failure of parenchymal cells to induce tolerance was due to their inability to home to the thymic microenvironment, the direct introduction of cellular grafts into the thymus may obviate the necessity to use cells with the capability to migrate to the thymus and permit assessment of nonlymphoid populations to promote specific tolerance. There was in fact considerable support for this hypothesis. Shimonkevitz and Bevan (1988) had reported that intrathymic injection of allogeneic $CD4^-/CD8^-$ prothymocytes into lethally irradiated, bone marrow-reconstituted mice induced a marked reduction in the frequency of donor reactive cytotoxic T-lymphocyte precursors, suggesting that deletion or inactivation of allo-reactive cells had occurred. Earlier studies examining the effect of intrathymic inoculation of soluble (Staples et al., 1966) and cellular antigens (Vojtiskova and Lengerova, 1968) had indicated a subsequent reduction of the immune responsiveness of the host to those antigens. In these studies, inoculation of bovine γ-globulin into the thymus of sublethally irradiated rats resulted in decreased anti-γ-globulin antibody synthesis and DTH responses to this antigen.

INTRATHYMIC TRANSPLANTATION OF PANCREATIC ISLET ALLOGRAFTS

In our initial studies we investigated whether the thymus as a transplant site could support the engraftment and physiologic function of isolated endocrine cells (pancreatic islets) in recipients rendered diabetic with the β cell toxin, streptozotocin (Posselt et al., 1990). Islets were isolated from Lewis (RT1^l) or DA (RT1^a) donors and transplanted to histoincompatible WF (RT1^u) recipients (Table I). Isolated islets were inoculated into conventional islet transplant sites (the renal subcapsule or into the liver via portal vein), into a known immunologically privileged site (the testicle) or into the thymus. Intraportal and renal subcapsule Lewis islet allografts were uniformly rejected promptly by nonimmunosuppressed WF recipients. Survival of intrathymic Lewis allografts was usually about doubled and in one recipient permanent allograft survival was achieved. In an attempt to further extend transplant survival we immunosuppressed the recipients of islet allografts with a single intraperitoneal dose of antilymphocyte serum (ALS) at the time of islet transplantation, again comparing the outcome of intrathymic and extrathymic islet allografts. ALS resulted in moderate pro-

longation of extrathymic islet allografts but a much more striking impact was observed in recipients of intrathymic islets. Virtually all intrathymic islet allografts survived permanently.

Given the unique function of the thymus in the induction of T cell tolerance, we next explored whether persistence of the allogeneic islets in the thymus might induce specific unresponsiveness to extrathymic alloantigens of the same donor strain. Therefore, WF rats that had harbored long-term intrathymic Lewis islets for >100 days were challenged with extrathymic Lewis islet allografts transplanted to extrathymic sites (renal subcapsule) in which prompt rejection was the expected outcome. No immunosuppression was administered at the time of the extrathymic islet transplantation or at any time thereafter. Nevertheless, the extrathymic donor-strain Lewis islets enjoyed permanent survival in WF rats harboring long-term intrathymic Lewis islets. In other rats harboring long-term intrathymic Lewis islets, "third-party" DA renal subcapsular islet transplants were not accepted, indicating that the induction of the unresponsiveness was specific for the donor strain (Fig. 1).

To evaluate the possibility that if the prolonged survival of islet allografts in transplant sites other than the thymus (if it could be achieved) would similarly weaken the host response to donor antigens, we evaluated the fate of secondary extrathymic donor-strain islets in recipients of islet allografts transplanted to the testicle—a known immunologically privileged site. In WF rats that had retained the intratesticular islet allografts for 200 days, second Lewis islet allografts transplanted under the kidney

Table I. Survival of Fresh Lewis Islet Allografts in WF Recipients

Site of islet transplantation	Days of islet allograft survival	
	Without ALS	With ALS
Liver (intraportal)	5, 8, 8, 9, (8)[a]	6, 22, 29, 35, 36, (29)
Renal subcapsule	9, 9, 10, 13, (9.5)	27, 33, 38, 47, 61, >200 × 2, (47)
Testicle	—	50, 50, 76, 110, >200 × 2, (76)
Thymus	13, 13, 16, 17, 17, 18, >200, (17)	28, 33, 57, >200 × 10, (>200)

[a] Numbers in parentheses denote median survival time (MST).

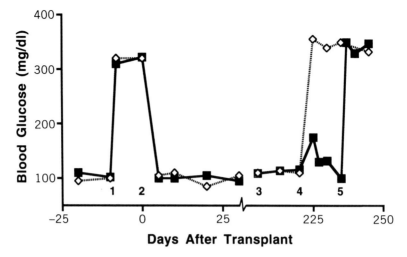

Fig. 1. Representative blood glucose profiles of WF rats transplanted with freshly isolated pancreatic islets. (1) Streptozotocin administration. (2) Intrathymic transplantation of fresh Lewis islets with con- comitant intraperitoneal administration of ALS. (3) Second renal subcapsular transplants of either Lewis (■) or DA (◇) islets. (4) Islet-bearing thymectomy. (5) Removal of islet-bearing kidneys.

capsule were rejected within 2 weeks, indicating that the established extrathymic islet allografts did not share the unique capacity of intrathymic islets for induction of unresponsiveness.

Pancreatic islets are complex structures comprised of endocrine and nonendocrine bone marrow-derived cells of dendritic/macrophage lineage, which are endowed with antigen-presenting capability. To study which cell population was responsible for inducing the tolerant state observed after intrathymic islet transplantation, we examined the capacity of intrathymic inocula of islets depleted of antigen-presenting cells (APCs) by *in vitro* culture to promote survival of secondary donor-strain grafts transplanted beneath the renal capsule (Campos et al., 1994). WF rats in which long-term (>120 days) normoglycemia had been achieved by intrathymic transplantation of cultured Lewis islets in conjunction with a single intraperitoneal dose of ALS received freshly isolated Lewis islets beneath the renal capsule 120 days after thymic inoculation. All animals promptly developed hyperglycemia, demonstrating that retransplantation had provoked the rejection of both the primary intrathymic and subsequent extrathymic test grafts. Thus it appears that tolerance induction in this model requires the presence of intraislet APCs.

The above findings demonstrate that the thymus constitutes a hospitable environment for islet engraftment and physiologic endocrine activity. Even more interesting was the concomitant observation that the thymus is an immunologically privileged site. Islet allografts transplanted intrathymically to nonimmunosuppressed rats enjoyed substantially prolonged survival and, if the hosts were briefly immunosuppressed with a single dose of ALS, permanent allograft survival was observed. Although the precise mechanisms responsible for these findings remain to be elucidated, a partial explanation is suggested by several known morphologic and physiologic characteristics of the organ. Ultrastructural as well as kinetic studies have demonstrated the presence of a blood–thymus barrier surrounding the capillaries in the thymic cortex that prevents extravasation of low-molecular-weight proteins and radiolabeled cells (Raviola and Karnovsky, 1972). This situation is in some ways analogous to that in the central nervous system where the blood–brain barrier may be in part responsible for the immunologically privileged status of this organ (Barker and Billingham, 1977). In addition, although the thymus possesses efferent lymphatics, it lacks an afferent lymphatic supply (Weiss, 1977). These details of vascular anatomy and the markedly reduced capacity of mature T lymphocytes to recirculate through the thymic parenchyma may in part account for the immune privileged environment of the thymic milieu (Michie et al., 1988).

Though these anatomic and physiological features might account for the survival of allografts implanted into the thymus, they do not explain why intrathymic islet recipients will accept subsequent donor-strain grafts transplanted extrathymically. Several mechanisms could be responsible for promoting the unresponsive state exhibited by long-term recipients of intrathymic allogeneic islets to subsequent extrathymic transplants. These include (1) nonspecific immunosuppression resulting from disruption of thymic function, (2) deletion or inactivation within the thymus of donor-reactive T cell populations that could otherwise be expected to destroy extrathymic grafts, and (3) generation of suppressor/regulatory T cells. Immunofluorescent analysis showed no differences in the phenotypic composition of lymphocyte subpopulations between thymic allograft recipients and naive controls, demonstrating that the trauma and disruption of the thymic parenchyma caused by the inoculation had not led to global T cell immunodeficiency. To assess the second possibility, mixed lymphocyte cultures (MLC) and limiting dilution analyses (LDA) of donor-specific cytotoxic T lymphocyte precursors (pCTL) were performed using lymphoid cells from long-term recipients of intrathymic islets. The proliferative responses of lymph node cells from islet allograft acceptors to donor-strain and third party stimulator cells were no different than the responses of naive animals. However, LDA analysis of lymph node cells from these animals showed significantly reduced (40 to 60%) pCTL frequencies to donor-strain alloantigens (Lewis) as compared with those from untransplanted controls. In the same recipients, the pCTL frequencies for DA alloantigens were unchanged (Fig. 2).

To assess active suppression by a population of regulatory T cells as a possible cause of the tolerant state, we performed adoptive transfer studies in which $250–300 \times 10^6$ spleen cells from either nontransplanted WF controls or WF rats harboring established (>200 days) intrathymic Lewis islet allografts were transferred to sublethally irradiated WF hosts. Twenty-four hours later, these animals received islets from Lewis donors beneath the renal capsule. Islet survival in rats given splenocytes from intrathymic recipients was not significantly different from that of the control group and thus provided no evidence for the presence of suppressor cells in tolerant animals. Together, these results support the conclusion that the unresponsive state induced by long-term residence of the intra

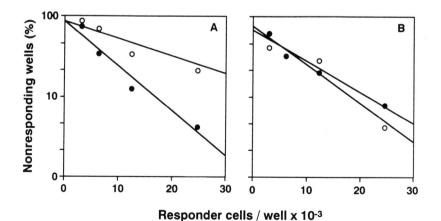

Fig. 2. Effect of intrathymic islet transplantation on pCTL frequencies. (**A**) Anti-Lewis pCTL of lymph node cells from control WF (●, $1/f = 6,240$) and WF recipients of intrathymic Lewis islets (○, $1/f = 16,000$). (**B**) Anti-DA pCTL of lymph node cells from control WF (●, $1/f = 6,930$) and WF recipients of intrathymic Lewis islets (○, $1/f = 6,500$).

thymic allograft is the result of intrathymic deletion or inactivation of T cell precursors recognizing alloantigens expressed on the graft. The inability to induce unresponsiveness in rats bearing *in vitro* cultured intrathymic islets indicates that islet endocrine cells per se are ineffective as tolerogens and demonstrates the importance of intraislet APC populations in intrathymic tolerance induction.

Intrathymic Islet Transplantation in Spontaneously Diabetic BB Rats

The spontaneously diabetic BB rat is a model with many similarities to human type I diabetes mellitus. As in the human disease damage to pancreatic β cells in BB rat appears to be mediated by diabetogenic T cells responding to a putative islet β cell autoantigen(s). This contention is supported by experiments in which pancreatic islets from donors of a variety of other rat strains were found to be destroyed promptly if transplanted to acutely diabetic BB rats (Naji et al., 1981). This destruction occurred just as rapidly in BB recipients that had been rendered tolerant to islet donor alloantigens by neonatal inoculation or ones in which pretransplant *in vitro* culture of the islet grafts prevented rejection (Woehrle et al., 1986). These findings proved that recurrent anti-β cell autoimmunity could in itself damage the graft, just as was later shown to be the case for human pancreatic isografts to diabetic patients (Sutherland et al., 1989).

To determine whether the favorable influence of the thymus on allograft survival could also protect islets from damage by recurrent anti-β cell autoimmunity, we examined survival of MHC-incompatible (Lewis) islets in acutely diabetic BB rats (RTl^u) (Posselt et al., 1991). Pancreatic islets isolated from Lewis donors and transplanted by portal vein inoculation into spontaneously diabetic BB rats were rejected promptly in every instance (MST, 9 days) (Table II). In contrast to the results in extrathymic sites, none of the BB rats that received intrathymic Lewis islets rejected their grafts.

To determine whether intrathymic islets transplanted to diabetic BB rats would induce an unresponsive state that could protect subsequent extrathymic islets from either rejection or autoimmunity, BB rats that had harbored an intrathymic Lewis islet transplant for >120 days received secondary Lewis islets intraportally. All animals remained normoglycemic, and remained so after primary islet bearing thymectomy confirming the functional survival of the extrathymic islet transplants.

Intrathymic Islet Xenografts (Rat → Mouse)

The unique advantage of the thymus as a transplant site for pancreatic islet allografts has prompted evaluation of the capability of this organ to promote survival of xenogeneic islets (Mayo et al., 1994; Zeng et al., 1993). In these experiments, WF (RTl^u) rat islets were transplanted to the thymus of diabetic C57BL/6 mice (Table III). In the absence of immunosuppression, intrathymic islet xenografts did not fair significantly better than those transplanted to a control transplant site, the renal subcapsule. However if a single dose of rabbit anti-mouse thymocyte serum (ATS) was given to the recipients, intrathymic islet xenograft survival was significantly increased and one-half of the animals remained normoglycemic for >100 days. Similar to the situation brought about by intrathymic allografts, recipients harboring longterm intrathymic islet xenografts were found unresponsive to subsequent donor-strain rat islets transplanted to an extrathymic site with no requirement for immunosuppression at the time

Table II. Survival of MHC-Compatible and Incompatible Islet Allografts in Spontaneously Diabetic BB Rats

Site of islet transplantation	Donor strain	Days of islet allograft survival
Liver (intraportal)	Lewis	8, 9, 9, 19, 24, (9)
Thymus	Lewis	>120 × 11, (>120)
	WF	>120 × 5, (>120)

Table III. Effect of Intrathymic Transplantation on Islet Xenograft Survival

	Days of islet xenograft survival	
Site of islet transplantation	Without ATS	With ATS
Renal subcapsule	12 × 3, 14, 20, 21 × 2, 26, (17.3)	31, 39, 43, 43, 53, (41.8)
Thymus	11, 12 × 3, 13, 22 × 2, 39, (17.9)	39, 40, 57, 59, 68, 70, 90, >100 × 7, (>94.5)

of the second transplant. In contrast, rat islet xenografts from a different strain (Lewis) were promptly rejected. Thus, the thymus of briefly immunosuppressed mice provides sanctuary to concordant islet xenografts from rat donors and renders the recipients unresponsive to extrathymic xenogeneic islets if they are from the same rat strain donors.

INDUCTION OF TOLERANCE BY INTRATHYMIC INOCULATION OF LYMPHOHEMATOPOIETIC CELLS

In several experimental models of transplantation tolerance, such as neonatal tolerance and radiation chimeras, the use of bone marrow as the tolerance-inducing inoculum has been found to be particularly effective. Therefore we examined the capacity of intrathymic inocula of donor lymphohematopoietic cells in promoting the survival of cellular or vascularized organ allografts in allogeneic hosts. In addition, as our results using *in vitro* cultured islets demonstrated, the component of the islets that appears to be crucial for tolerance induction is antigen-presenting cells within the islets rather than endocrine cells (Campos et al., 1994). Bone marrow, which can differentiate into cells with antigen-presenting capability, might therefore be predicted to be especially efficient in promoting tolerance after intrathymic inoculation (Bowers and Berkowitz, 1986).

Induction of Tolerance to Islets by Intrathymic Inoculation of Donor Strain Bone Marrow

The protocol employed in these experiments involved treatment of prospective recipients with donor strain lymphohematopoietic cells and concomitant administration of a single dose of ALS. Unlike the previous experiments in which the intrathymic inoculum was followed only months later by the extrathymic test graft, the recipients received the test allografts (islets, vascularized heart, or liver) within 10–14 days after the intrathymic inoculum (Posselt et al., 1992).

Normal WF recipients not pretreated with intrathymic Lewis bone marrow cells (BMC) or ALS rapidly rejected Lewis islet grafts transplanted 14 days after inoculation (Table IV). In a second control group, WF recipients that received intrathymic injections of saline in conjunction with ALS 2 weeks prior to islet transplantation also promptly rejected Lewis islet allografts in virtually all instances. In another control group intravenous injection of Lewis BMC in conjunction with ALS 2 weeks prior to islet grafting led to modest prolongation of Lewis islet allograft survival; however, all allografts eventually underwent rejection within 32 days. In contrast, in the experimental group in which Lewis BMC were administered intrathymically, 5 of 7 WF recipients of Lewis islet allografts remained permanently normoglycemic. Histologic examination of surviving grafts at the conclusion of the experimental period revealed numerous clusters of well-granulated islets with no cellular infiltration or other evidence of rejection. The specificity of the tolerant state induced by inoculation of Lewis BMC was assessed by grafting WF rats that had received intrathymic Lewis BMC with islets from DA (RTl[a]) donors. These third party grafts were all rejected within 10 days.

Prolonged residence of allogeneic tissue in other immunologically privileged sites has sometimes been found to weaken the host's immune responsiveness to subsequent donor-strain

Table IV. Survival of Lewis Islet Allografts in WF Recipients

Site of Lewis bone marrow cell inoculation	ALS treatment	Days of islet allograft survival
None	None	9, 9, 10, 13, (9.5)
None	+	8, 9, 14, 15, 18, >173,[a] (14.5)
Intravenous	+	13, 16, 21, 23, 32, 32, (22)
Thymus	+	12, 28, >130 × 2, >148, >159, >183, (>130)
Testicle	+	7, 8, 8, 10, (8)

[a] Animal reverted to hyperglycemia after removal of islet-bearing kidney.

allografts transplanted to conventional sites (Barker and Billingham, 1977). Since the thymic parenchyma is relatively inaccessible to the peripheral immune system, it was conceivable that the unresponsiveness observed in intrathymically treated rats was solely due to the presence of the conditioning BMC inoculum and that the special immunologic functions of the thymus were not relevant (i.e., its role in T lymphocyte maturation and induction of self-tolerance). To evaluate this possibility, we inoculated allogeneic Lewis BMC into another immunologically privileged site, the testicle, of WF recipients given a single injection of ALS. Two weeks following intratesticular BMC inoculation, these recipients were rendered diabetic and transplanted with Lewis islet allografts. All animals rapidly rejected the islets, indicating that the protective influence of the intrathymic bone marrow inoculum on subsequent allografts was unlikely to be explained entirely by the thymus' capability as a privileged site.

Tolerance to Cardiac and Liver Allografts Induced by Intrathymic Inoculation of Bone Marrow

In studies using a "high-responder" combination (DA to LEW) we found that the usual vigorous response of LEW rats to orthotopic DA liver allografts could be overcome without chronic immunosuppression by intrathymic inoculation of recipients with donor strain BMC and a single dose of ALS (Table V) (Campos et al., 1993). This effect occurred only if the cellular inoculum was introduced into the thymus, as demonstrated by the inability of donor-strain cells adminis-

tered intravenously to promote survival of liver allografts. The donor specificity of the unresponsive state was confirmed by the failure of intrathymic inocula from WF donors to prolong survival of DA liver allografts.

Similar results were obtained when cardiac allografts rather than liver allografts were used as the test graft (Table VI)(Odorico et al., 1992). WF recipients not pretreated with ALS or BMC rapidly rejected heterotopically placed Lewis cardiac allografts (MST: 14 days); pretreatment with 1 ml ALS and an intrathymic inoculation of saline 14 days prior to grafting modestly prolonged survival (MST: 24 days), but all recipients eventually rejected their grafts. Similarly, administration of Lewis BMC intravenously in conjunction with ALS was not protective and five of six cardiac grafts were rejected (MST: 10 days). The results in recipients pretreated with intrathymic Lewis bone marrow were quite different and eight of nine animals in this group retained functional grafts for more than 200 days.

Other attempts to induce tolerance with intrathymic inocula have demonstrated the feasibility of promoting prolonged survival of cardiac allografts in adult rodents by the intrathymic inoculation of donor spleen cells or thymocytes (Goss et al., 1992; Odorico et al., 1993a,b; Oluwole et al., 1993; Krokos et al., 1993). The induction of the unresponsive state required brief immunosuppression of the host with ALS or sublethal doses of irradiation to induce a transient state of T cell depletion. Since antigen-presenting cells have been demonstrated to play a critical role in the development of T cell tolerance in the thymus, the unresponsiveness ob-

Table V. Survival of Bone Marrow Cell-Pretreated LEW Recipients of DA Orthotopic Liver Allografts

Pretreatment of recipients		
Inoculum	ALS[a]	Survival of LEW recipients
None	None	11, 12 × 2, 13 × 4, 14, 15, 20, (13)
IT saline	+	8, 23, 24 × 2, 28, 29, 39, 41, 44 × 2, 86, >150, (29)
IT DA BMC	+	24, 31, 33, 41, 53, 54, >150 × 8, (>150)
IT WF BMC	+	25, 27, 29, 31, 33, 60, >150, (31)
IV DA BMC	+	28, 29, 39, 44, 46, 52, 54, (44)

[a] Fourteen days before orthotopic liver transplantation.

served after intrathymic inoculation of spleen cells may be attributable to the presence of these populations in the conditioning inoculum. Remuzzi et al. (1991) have also reported prolonged survival of renal allografts in rats pretreated with intrathymic inocula of glomerular cells and a short course of cyclosporine and corticosteroids. However, Odorico et al. (1993) found that substitution of a short course of cyclosporine for ALS failed to promote cardiac allograft survival, suggesting that a T cell-depleting regimen is crucial to tolerance induction by intrathymic protocol. The efficacy of intrathymic inocula of spleen cells to promote survival of skin allografts have been examined in a murine model (Ohzato and Monaco, 1992). Prolonged survival of skin allografts was achieved in ALS-treated mice inoculated intrathymically with donor spleen cells.

Mechanisms of Unresponsiveness Induced by Intrathymic Bone Marrow

In accordance with the *in vivo* findings, intrathymic inoculation of allogeneic Lewis BMC

was found to have a marked influence on T cell-mediated responses to donor alloantigens *in vitro*. In mixed lymphocyte culture the lymph node cells from recipients in which long-term Lewis islet allograft survival was achieved by intrathymic BMC inoculation responded normally to third-party DA stimulators; however proliferation of these cells to Lewis stimulators was consistently decreased as compared with responses of unmanipulated controls (Fig. 3).

Analysis of pCTL frequencies in recipients bearing established islet allografts as a result of pretreatment with intrathymic bone marrow yielded somewhat variable results. Although the majority of recipients demonstrated significant reductions in pCTL frequencies toward donor (Lewis) alloantigens, some animals had frequencies similar to those of unmanipulated animals. All animals had similar pCTL frequencies to third-party DA alloantigens.

In several models of unresponsiveness induced by conditioning with allogeneic BMC, tolerance has been shown to be characterized by the presence of microchimerism in the thymus

Table VI. Survival of Lewis or DA Cardiac Allografts in WF Recipients

Site of Lewis BMC inoculation	ALS	Donor	Days of allograft survival
None	None	Lewis	14, 14, 14, 17, 17, (14)
None	+	Lewis	10, 14, 17, 23, 25, 38, 50, 62, (24)
Intravenous	+	Lewis	3, 5, 9, 11, 16, >150, (10)
Thymus	+	Lewis	14, >200 × 4, >220 × 4, (>200)
Thymus	+	DA	6, 7, 9, 10, 11, (9)

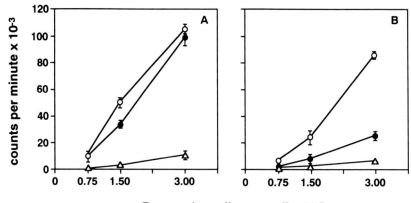

Fig. 3. Mixed lymphocyte culture proliferative responses of lymph node cells from (A) WF controls and (B) WF recipients in which long-term Lewis islet allograft survival was achieved by intrathymic inoculation of Lewis BMC. Graded numbers of responder cells were cultured alone ($\triangle$) or with irradiated Lewis ($\bullet$) or DA ($\bigcirc$) lymph node stimulators for 3 days, and pulsed with tritiated thymidine for an additional 24 hr prior to harvesting. Values are depicted as the arithmetic mean $\pm$ SD of triplicate cultures.

and peripheral lymphoid organs of the recipients (Sharabi and Sachs, 1989). To determine whether a similar chimeric state was present in our model, the lymphoid organs of WF rats that had received intrathymic Lewis BMC (without subsequent islet grafts) were examined at various intervals after inoculation by immunofluorescence (FACS) and immunohistochemistry utilizing a murine monoclonal antibody specific for Lewis class I alloantigens (Posselt et al., 1992). Using the FACS analysis, chimerism could be detected in the thymus for only 4–5 days after intrathymic inoculation and was never demonstrated in the lymph nodes. However, by the immunohistochemical method we routinely demonstrated the presence of donor strain cells scattered throughout the thymus in animals inoculated with Lewis BMC 2 to 45 days earlier. Similarly, in animals that had accepted Lewis islet grafts after conditioning with intrathymic Lewis BMC, donor-strain cells were found in the thymus when it was examined 140–170 days after inoculation, although the number of allogeneic cells appeared to decrease progressively with time. In contrast, donor-strain cells were not detected in the thymus or lymph node of animals given intravenous or intratesticular BMC. Thus, it appears that the thymic microenvironment can support the long-term survival of

implanted allogeneic hematopoietic cells and is capable of protecting them (or their descendants) from elimination by immune mechanisms.

It is now well established that the thymus is responsible for generating mature functional T cells with a diverse set of T cell receptors that recognizes foreign antigens. During development in the thymus, T cells are rendered tolerant to self-antigens. Increasing experimental evidence has been provided to demonstrate that thymocytes bearing self-reactive T cell receptors are physically eliminated (clonal deletion) or functionally inactivated (clonal anergy) and that intrathymic tolerance induction can be profoundly influenced by the repertoire of antigens expressed on nonlymphoid epithelial components of the thymus. In the studies reviewed here, we attempted to exploit these mechanisms for induction of unresponsiveness to histocompatibility antigens by employing the strategy of direct inoculation of foreign alloantigens into the thymus. These studies suggest that the successful induction of tolerance by the method of intrathymic inoculation depends on the persistence of chimerism within the thymic microenvironment.

Although the immunologically privileged environment of the thymus facilitates the survival of the foreign cells in the thymus, their persistent survival requires a transient reduction of the pool of mature peripheral T cells, which we achieved with one dose of ALS. The reduction of the pool of T cells in the peripheral tissues probably prevents the alloimmune destruction of the intrathymic inoculum by impeding the migration of a small population of mature T cells that would otherwise gain entry into the chimeric thymus. Additionally, the reduction of mature peripheral T cells encourages migration of immature T cell precursors to the thymus, inviting their interaction with the intrathymic allogeneic cells prior to their exit from the thymus to repopulate the peripheral immune repertoire with tolerant cells.

The demonstration that intrathymic inoculation of donor cells into the thymus is efficient in promoting the induction of specific tolerance to allogeneic and xenogeneic histocompatibility antigens provides encouragement that intrathymic cellular implantation may be useful in inducing unresponsiveness in adults possibly allowing successful transplantation without chronic immunosuppression.

REFERENCES

Barker CF, Billingham RE (1977): Immunologically privileged sites. In Kunkel HG, Dixon FJ (eds): "Advances in Immunology." New York: Academic Press, 1–54.

Billingham RE, Brent L, Medawar PB (1953): "Actively acquired tolerance" of foreign cells. Nature (London) 172:603–606.

Bowers WE, Berkowitz MR (1986): Differentiation of dendritic cells in cultures of rat bone marrow cells. J Exp Med 163:872–883.

Campos L, Alfrey EJ, Posselt AM, Odorico JS, Barker CF, Naji A (1993): Prolonged survival of rat orthotopic liver allografts after intrathymic inoculation of donor-strain cells. Transplantation 55: 866–870.

Campos L, Posselt AM, Mayo GL, Pete K, Deli BC, Barker CF, Naji A (1994): The failure of intrathymic transplantation of non-immunogenic islet allografts to promote induction of donor-specific unresponsiveness. Transplantation 57:950–953.

Goodnow CC, Crosbie J, Jorgensen H, Brink RA, Basten A (1989): Induction of self-tolerance in mature peripheral B cells. Nature (London) 342:385–391.

Goss J, Nakafusa Y, Flye W (1992): Intrathymic injection of donor alloantigens induces donor-specific

vascularized allograft tolerance without immunosuppression. Ann Surg 216:409–416.

Hall BM, Pearce NW, Gurley KE, Dorsch SE (1990): Specific unresponsiveness in rats with prolonged cardiac allograft survival after treatment with cyclosporine. III further characterization of the CD4+ suppressor cell and its mechanisms of action. J Exp Med 171:141–157.

Kappler JW, Roehm N, Marrack P (1987): T cell tolerance by clonal elimination in the thymus. Cell 49:273–280.

Krensky A, Weiss A, Crabtree G, Davis M, Parham P (1990): T-lymphocyte-antigen interactions in transplant rejection. N Engl J Med 322:510.

Krokos NV, Brons IGM, Sriwatanawongsa V, Makisalo H, Katami M, Davies HS, Calne RY (1993): Intrathymic injection of donor antigen-presenting cells prolongs heart graft survival. Transplant Proc 25:303–304.

Mayo GL, Posselt AM, Campos L, Barker CF, Naji A (1994): Intrathymic transplantation promotes survival of islet xenografts (rat to mouse). Transplant Proc 26(2):758.

Michie SA, Kirkpatrick EA, Rouse RV (1988): Rare peripheral T cells migrate to and persist in normal mouse thymus. J Exp Med 168:1929–1934.

Naji A, Silvers WK, Bellgrau D, Barker CF (1981): Spontaneous diabetes in rats: Destruction of islets is prevented by immunological tolerance. Science 213:1390–1392.

Odorico JS, Barker CF, Posselt AM, Naji A (1992): Induction of donor-specific tolerance to rat cardiac allografts by intrathymic inoculation of bone marrow. Surgery 112:370–377.

Odorico JS, Barker CF, Markmann JF, Posselt AM, Naji A (1993a): Prolonged survival of rat cardiac allografts after intrathymic inoculation of donor thymocytes. Transplant Proc 25:295–296.

Odorico JS, Posselt AM, Naji A, Markmann JF, Barker, CF (1993b): Promotion of rat cardiac allograft survival by intrathymic inoculation of donor splenocytes. Transplantation 55:1104–1107.

Ohzato H, Monaco AP (1992): Induction of specific unresponsiveness (tolerance) to skin allografts by intrathymic donor-specific splenocyte injection in antilymphocyte serum treated mice. Transplantation 54:1090–95.

Oluwole SF, Chowdhury NC, Fawwaz R, James T, Hardy MA (1993): Induction of specific unresponsiveness to rat cardiac allografts by pretreatment with intrathymic donor major histocompatibility complex class I antigens. Transplant Proc 25:299–300.

Posselt AM, Barker CF, Tomaszewski JE, Markmann JF, Choti MA, Naji A (1990): Induction of donor-specific unresponsiveness by intrathymic islet transplantation. Science 249:1293–1295.

Posselt AM, Naji A, Roark JH, Markmann JF, Barker CF (1991): Intrathymic islet transplantation in the spontaneously diabetic rat. Ann Surg 214:363–373.

Posselt AM, Odorico JS, Barker CF, Naji A (1992): Promotion of pancreatic islet allograft survival by intrathymic transplantation of bone marrow. Diabetes 41:771–775.

Ramsdell F, Fowlkes BJ (1990): Clonal deletion versus clonal anergy: The role of the thymus in inducing self tolerance. Science 248:1342–1348.

Raviola E, Karnovsky MJ (1972): Evidence for a blood-thymus barrier using electron-opaque tracers. J Exp Med 136:466–470.

Remuzzi G, Rammi M, Limberti O, Perico N (1991): Kidney graft survival in rats without immunosuppression after intrathymic glomerular transplantation. Lancet 337:750.

Sharabi Y, Sachs DH (1989): Mixed chimerism and permanent specific transplantation tolerance induced by a nonlethal preparative regimen. J Exp Med 169:493–502.

Shimonkevitz RP, Bevan MJ (1988): Split tolerance induced by the intrathymic adoptive transfer of thymocyte stem cells. J Exp Med 168:143–156.

Staples PJ, Gery I, Waksman BH (1966): Role of the thymus in tolerance. III. Tolerance to bovine gamma globulin after direct injection of antigen into the shielded thymus of irradiated rats. J Exp Med 124:127–139.

Streilein JW (1991): Neonatal tolerance of H-2 alloantigens. Procuring graft acceptance the "old-fashioned" way. Transplantation 52:1–10.

Sutherland DE, Goetz FC, Sibley RK (1989): Recurrence of disease in pancreas transplantation. Diabetes 38 (suppl 1):85–87.

Vojtiskova M, Lengerova A (1968): Thymus mediated tolerance to cellular alloantigens. Transplantation 6:13–16.

Weiss L (1977): "The Blood Cells and Hematopoietic Tissues." New York: McGraw-Hill, pp 503–522.

Woehrle M, Markmann JF, Silvers WK, Barker CF, Naji A (1986): Transplantation of cultured pancreatic islets to BB rats. Surgery 100:334–340.

Zeng JA, Bluestone ST, Ildstad MA, Torres AG, Montag RJ, Thistlethwaite Jr (1993): Long-term functional xenograft tolerance after intrathymic islet transplantation (Lewis rat → B6 mouse). Transplant Proc 25:438–439.

Chapter 14
Transplantation Tolerance with Monoclonal Antibodies

Herman Waldmann and Stephen Cobbold

INTRODUCTION

Despite the emergence of numerous immunosuppressive drugs over the past 20 years, there is still no comprehensive solution to the rejection problem. Most of the drugs need to be given long-term, if not indefinitely, and a balance has to be struck between prevention of rejection, and risking infection and other side effects. Even with best management, chronic rejection and increased malignancy still remain major problems. This will always be so with immunosuppression geared to penalize the whole immune system for misdemeanors of a minority of its lymphocytes. If one could selectively control just those lymphocytes that were involved in the rejection process, while sparing others, one would have the ideal solution.

In short, the ideal form of immunosuppression would induce immunological tolerance to the transplanted tissue.

THE CHALLENGE OF TOLERANCE

The goal of achieving tolerance in the mature immune system is far from simple, for the following reasons.

1. We know that self-tolerance is something that happens to lymphocytes that are immature. It has been hard to accept that one might could easily tolerize "mature" cells.

2. Even if only 1 in 10,000 lymphocytes recognized the graft as foreign, there would still be a huge number of lymphocytes to control. In humans that number might be somewhere between 10^7 and 10^9. Even if one could tolerize them at one point in time, what of the lymphocytes that would continue to develop? How could one ensure that these would become tolerized as well?

3. The diversity of histocompatibility (major and minor) antigens is great, and variable within each donor–recipient combination. One would not expect to isolate all the donor antigens for modification for use as tolerogens. This means that any therapeutic intervention to achieve tolerance must involve manipulation of the host immune system (rather than antigen) so as to alter "perception" of the donor tissue as "*something not to be rejected.*"

4. Even if animal experiments lead us to discover tolerance-inducing strategies, it might still be difficult to apply these clinically, as this would probably require withdrawal of the "currently acceptable" drugs.

5. Even then, if clinical research showed tolerance to be possible, would the pharmaceutical industry be prepared to provide drugs for short-term use? This is not a trivial issue, as commercial interests figure strongly in drug development programs.

Clearly there are many issues to be resolved for clinical transplantation tolerance to ever be achieved. From the immunological standpoint this applied goal is a driving force for a deeper understanding of *self–nonself recognition*. The field began with Medawar's demonstration that mice could become tolerized to foreign trans-

Transplantation Immunology, pages 239–246
© 1995 Wiley-Liss, Inc.

plantation antigens by the neonatal injection of donor bone marrow (Billingham et al., 1953). This simple demonstration has provided the impetus to discover how the same could be achieved in the adult. Tolerance research (with its far-reaching therapeutic implications) is now becoming one of the most exciting areas of immunology.

SELF-TOLERANCE

Clonal Deletion and Anergy

Research into self-tolerance has demonstrated that self-reactivity is largely avoided by deletion of any self-reactive lymphocytes within the primary lymphoid organs. This phenomenon has become known as *central tolerance*. For T cells *central tolerance by clonal deletion* provides the mechanism of tolerance to all ubiquitous self-antigens. Any immature T cell confronting antigen within the thymus will delete or die through a process called *apoptosis*. There must, however, be a diversity of tissue-specific peptides that are not represented within the thymus. What happens to T cells with receptors for these? There must be further downstream "peripheral" mechanisms to prevent self-reactivity to those particular tissues. These mechanisms described are responsible then for *peripheral tolerance*. It is still not clear which of the mechanisms are the most important. Part of the uncertainty comes from the very contrived model systems that have been used to study peripheral "self"-tolerance. These have mostly involved the use of mice transgenic for a surrogate self-antigen located on a variety of different tissues (islets, liver, skin, brain), and mice transgenic for T cell receptors (TCR) to those antigens (Arnold et al., 1993; Lo et al., 1989; Miller et al., 1990; Zinkernagel et al., 1991). The F_1 hybrid mice, that have both the transgenic antigen and the TCR, do not suffer from autoimmune disease, do not respond to challenge with the test antigen, and are therefore deemed tolerant. It is relatively simple to follow the fate of antigen-reactive T cells by using anti-clonotypic antibodies directed to the transgenic TCR, and using such reagents immunologists have documented mechanisms for peripheral tolerance ranging from deletion, receptor down-modulation, anergy (receptor there but cell refractory to stimulation), and sheer ignorance.

T Cell-Mediated Suppression

The limitation of the studies above is that they ignore the contribution of lymphocytes that do not have the transgenic TCR, and so the conclusions may be heavily biased. In some of the models, it has been noted that tolerance is hard to break by transfusion of naive lymphocytes into the tolerant animal. It is surprising that these data have been largely ignored or dismissed as unimportant by those who describe it. There can be no doubt that the phenomenon of "resistance" provides an important clue to the mechanism that must be followed up, if we are to properly understand peripheral self-tolerance.

Very recently, there have been a number of compelling reports showing that regulatory T cells with immunosuppressive properties play an important part in self-tolerance. In two different animal species (rat and mouse), it would seem that CD4 T cells that express the CD45RB isoform at high levels (CD45RB[hi]) are able to induce a severe autoimmune syndrome when injected into mice (Powrie and Mason, 1990; Fowell and Mason, 1993; Morrisey et al., 1993). This can be prevented by coinjecting CD4 T cells that are CD45RB[lo]. It is implicit that such regulation should go on within the normal animal, and that this would provide one of mechanisms by which tissue-specific autoimmunity would be prevented.

How Do Peripheral T Cells Know That They Should Become Tolerant Rather Than Respond?

Once T cells leave the thymus they may have the opportunity of confronting tissue-specific peptides in the context of self class I or class II. Of course, many tissues do not express MHC class II, and here the only presentation that would be possible would be through reprocessed peptides that have been acquired indirectly by other MHC class II-bearing cells (e.g., cells of hematopoietic origin). This might mean that T cells might be ignorant of those peptides that could not "make it" to MHC class I presentation, and tolerant of the others. How, though, could a

T cell distinguish between a self-peptide and a foreign one, so as to take the tolerance decision. We can consider three possible reasons.

1. The T cell may still remain immature and obligatorily tolerance sensitive even after it has left the thymus, at least long enough to experience the peripheral self-antigen before it commits suicide.

2. The T cell has the potential to mount an immune response, but in the absence of collaboration from other T cells it fails to do so, and as a result of *helplessness* it registers the antigen for tolerance. There are numerous examples in the literature to show that mature CD8 T cells might become tolerant in the absence of CD4 help (e.g., Guerder and Matzinger, 1992), and that B cells may do the same. Indeed, it is most likely that the immune system demands collaboration between rare antigen-specific T cells as part of its safeguard strategy for self-tolerance. If the first T cell is inactivated, then the second one

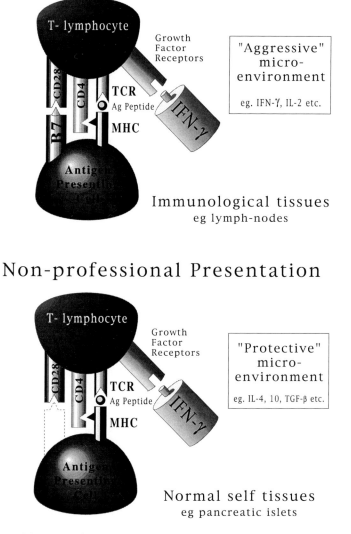

Fig. 1. Professional (**A**) and nonprofessional (**B**) presentation.

will also fail to find a collaborator, and itself become tolerant, and so on. This is unlike the situation of a mature immune system confronting a foreign graft where the frequency of alloreactive T cells is so high that T cell–T cell collaboration is almost inevitable.

3. The context in which the self-antigen is presented may favor tolerance, while that for the foreign antigen may favor an immune response. "Professional" presentation by dendritic cells may be the most influential form of foreign antigen, while "nonprofessional" presentation by cells such as small resting B cells, quiescent macrophages, and others may dominate "self-antigen" presentation (see Fig. 1). One popular view is that it is the absence of particular costimulator molecules (such as the ligand for CD28) from the antigen-presenting cells (APC) that determines the nonprofessional status of those cells (Schwartz, 1992). Another line of thinking suggests that it is the microenvironment within which the T cell and APC interact that determines the final outcome, where local cytokines, and other soluble mediators determine what line of the development the T cell should take (aggressive or protective). The contribution of the particular tissue to that microenvironment should not be underestimated. The poor immunogenicity of transplanted allogeneic kidney and vascularized heart grafts in mouse probably is part of the explanation in such a hypothetical tissue-specific influence on antigen presentation. The finding of a range of cytokines that can control aggressive reactions of T cells [interleukins 4, 10, and 13 (IL-4, IL-10, IL-13) and transforming growth factor β (TGF-β)] suggests that any or all of these could be important ingredients of a "nonaggressive" microenvironment. TGF-β seems a good example of one whose influence would vary from tissue to tissue, depending on the endogenous levels. This will surely be a growth area of tolerance research.

ANTIBODIES FOR TRANSPLANTATION TOLERANCE

Why Antibodies?

Therapy with monoclonal antibodies has elicited much interest in tolerance research. This comes from the opportunity to target so many molecules in the immune system, to establish which targets serve best for immunosuppression (Waldmann, 1989). Antibodies can be used to kill cells, to block the function of a cell surface molecule, to neutralize humoral factors, and to deliver signals to cells.

STRATEGIES

There have been two general conceptual approaches to tolerance induction using monoclonal antibodies.

The first aims to reprogram the immune system through *"central" tolerance,* by targeting a permanent source of antigen to the primary lymphoid tissues. This requires a two-stage strategy, where in the first stage, antibodies are simply used with the purpose of ablating or inactivating the peripheral T cell pool, so as to clear the old while the new are given the opportunity to develop in the presence of antigen. A foreign bone marrow given under the umbrella of the ablative umbrella would provide a source of stem cells that could seed the primary lymphoid organs and provide a continuous source of tolerogen. This is in essence the simulation of the classical Medawar approach applied to the adult (see Qin et al., 1989; Sykes and Sachs, 1990; Leong et al., 1992).

This first stage is not, however, as straightforward as one might imagine. For the stem cells to seed one has to ensure marrow acceptance and growth. This requires both immunosuppression and myeloablation to create "space" for the stem cells. The most extreme way of doing this is to lethally irradiate the host, thus simultaneously ablating immunity and creating new space. Although feasible in animal models, this is extremely impractical in the clinic. This is why much research has focused on so-called "nonablative" regimens for the purpose. Ablative monoclonal antibodies together with nonlethal myeloablation with drugs or limited irradiation have proven very effective for the purpose of establishing a robust state of mixed chimerism.

In the second stage, the desired donor tissue is then transplanted. From that time on it is very likely that both sources of the antigen act as reinforcing tolerogens operating to maintain the tolerant state.

Although, such procedures are eminently feasible in animal models, it is still doubtful whether they would be sufficiently reliable and safe to be extended to humans. Nor is it entirely clear that the tolerance achieved with nonlethal therapy is purely central as was hoped. Caution is certainly needed before taking such vigorous strategies to the clinic.

In an attempt to simplify the process, others have tried to introduce antigen into the thymus by direct injection (Posselt et al., 1990). Again antilymphocyte antibodies are used to provide the umbrella under which antigen is smuggled in. Whether this approach can ever be used clinically is still uncertain, but not impossible.

The second approach involves the use of antibodies in one stage therapy, so as to induce *peripheral tolerance* to the foreign tissue graft given under the antibody umbrella. For that tolerance to be sustained lifelong, there needs to be a mechanism by which any new T cells are also brought under control. As T cells are continuously generated in the thymus, then so must tolerance be continuously induced in them, even after the antibody therapy has stopped. As these new T cells would be confronting foreign grafts bearing numerous alloantigens, *they could become tolerant only if their perception of the graft were altered.*

In recent years, it has proven possible to use nonlytic antibodies to certain T cell surface molecules to block T cell function and guide the T cell system toward tolerance. By far the most powerful have been antibodies to CD4 and CD8 (Qin et al., 1989, 1990; Cobbold et al., 1990, 1993). Tolerance to relatively weak antigens has also been reported for antibodies to CD3 (Nicholls et al., 1993), CD25 (Wood et al., 1993), LFA-1 (Benjamin et al., 1988), and the combination of LFA-1 and I-CAM1 (Isobe et al., 1992). A chimeric protein of CTLA4 (a member of the CD28 family) fused to the heavy chain constant region of IgG has also proven capable of tolerance to xenografts of islets (Lenschow et al., 1992), and when combined with tolerogenic blood transfusion enabling tolerance to vascularized heart grafts (Lin et al., 1993). This chimeric protein blocks the interaction between CD28 and its ligands on APC, and was tried on the basis of *in vitro* studies that predicted anergy

as the outcome. To our knowledge, there has not yet been a formal demonstration of anergy after CTLA4-Ig therapy.

Because so many different antibodies can induce tolerance, it is our belief that the antibodies are simply "blindfolding" the T cells they would reject, buying time for "natural" peripheral tolerance mechanisms to take place. In other words the *therapeutic antibodies do not induce tolerance, they simply permit it to happen.*

Very little research has been performed on the mechanisms by which antibodies other than CD4 induce tolerance. We will, therefore, concentrate on tolerance induction with CD4 monoclonal antibody (MAb) therapy where tolerance has been demonstrated for grafts mismatched for both minor and major histocompatibility antigens (Qin et al., 1990; Cobbold et al., 1990).

MECHANISMS OF CD4 MAb TOLERANCE

Our own studies have revealed three mechanisms that contribute to peripheral tolerance induced with CD4 MAbs (see Qin et al., 1990, 1993; Cobbold et al., 1990, 1993). All have been defined in models where skin grafts differing in multiple minor antigens have been transplanted into recipients treated with non-lytic CD4 MAbs, or nonlytic CD4 and CD8 MAbs given together.

1. Naive animals given skin grafts under the umbrella of nonlytic CD4 antibodies alone did not reject their grafts. CD8 T cells from such animals became tolerant without the need for any CD8 antibodies (Leong, Cobbold, and Waldmann, in preparation). It was not possible to generate cytotoxic T cells *in vitro*, even when all conventional sources of "help" were provided. This can be considered an example of "helplessness" whereby the CD8 T cells are simply incapable of generating their own "helper" function, and consequently become inactivated when confronted with antigen.

2. In a model using bone marrow as the tolerogen, where donor and recipient differed for the self-superantigen M1s, CD4 T cells with receptors preoccupied with binding that self-superantigen (Vβ6) were shown to be present but anergic. In some animals the T cells expressing Vβ6 could not be triggered *in vitro* by either

the "antigen" or by ligation of their receptor with antibodies. In others there was selective anergy, in the sense that antibodies could trigger the T cells while "antigen" could not (Waldmann et al., 1989). This suggests that anergic T cells might set their triggering thresholds at variable levels, which can occasionally be overcome by a sufficiently strong stimulus.

3. Perhaps the most exciting yet surprising mechanism is one we have termed "infectious tolerance," a previously popularized phrase that once represented T cell-mediated suppression (Qin et al., 1993). We were able to observe that once tolerance had been induced, it is maintained by "infectiousness." By this we mean that the first cohort of tolerant T cells is able to guide naive T cells to the same sort of tolerance, so that they too influence further generations of T cells. The conclusion that an infectious form of T cell suppression determines long-term tolerance stems from the following findings:

a. It takes many weeks for T cells to become tolerant. This can be documented by adoptive transfer of T cells from antibody-treated animals into new hosts. It took some 4 weeks after the completion of 1 week of antibody therapy before the T cells became fully tolerant. Even if antibody therapy was continued for the full 5 weeks, T cells still became tolerant. One concludes that saturating CD4 antibody levels were sufficient to prevent T cells from recognizing the graft antigens for rejection, but not for tolerance induction (Cobbold et al., 1993).

b. Once animals are tolerant, it is not possible to break that tolerant state by lymphocyte transfusion (at least with naive lymphocytes). This "resistance" is mediated by T cells as their elimination with lytic antibodies eliminated "resistance" (Qin et al., 1993).

c. T cells from tolerant animals are capable of suppressing naive lymphocytes when transferred together into new hosts (Qin et al., 1993).

d. Using genetically marked T cells, one can demonstrate that naive cells parked with antigen in tolerant mice themselves became tolerant. Two weeks of coexistence of the naive cells with tolerant cells is sufficient, because prior ablation of the "tolerant-host" T cells prevents the "infectious" spread of tolerance (see Fig. 2). Nor can one break this *acquired* tolerance by transfusion

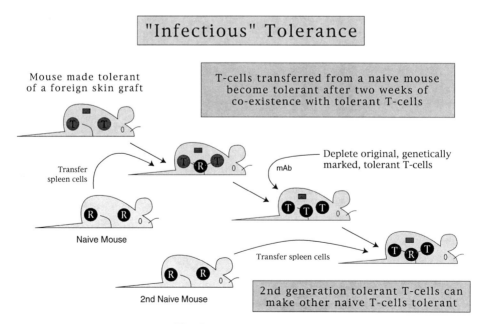

Fig. 2. Infectious tolerance.

of further populations of naive cells. This shows that the second generation of tolerant cells is also capable of suppression.

e. T cells transfused from mice tolerant to MHC-mismatched cardiac allografts were also able to prevent naive mice from rejecting a fresh cardiac allograft. This shows that suppression and infectious tolerance are also responsible for long-term tolerance over MHC-incompatible combinations (Chen et al., 1993).

AN HYPOTHESIS ON HOW ANTIBODY THERAPY LEADS TO "INFECTIOUS TOLERANCE"?

We have discussed the concept that antigen could be presented to the immune system in two types of microenvironment. One, considered as *permissive,* depends upon the *professional* presentation of antigen by specialized APC together with collaborative interactions from other T cells. The other, which is *nonpermissive* or *pro-tolerance,* would involve antigen presentation by nonspecialist APC, or *professional* APC that have been down regulated for *professional* function. This nonpermissive microenvironment (whether in the lymphoid or nonlymphoid tissue) might also be unsuitable for collaborative interactions between T cells.

At present, our favored hypothesis (which tries to accommodate all the experimental findings) is that a prolonged "blockade" of the immune system with antibodies favors "nonprofessional" presentation to T cells, and selectively promotes the emergence of regulatory T cells (Waldmann and Cobbold, 1993). This may be because the "professional" APC (unlike nonprofessional APC) have only a limited time frame in which they can behave as *professionals,* or because the regulatory T cells are refractory to antibody "blockade." Either way the result would be dominance of T cells with regulator function. Once dominant, such cells would be responsible for creation of further nonpermissive microenvironments, which would result in other T cells being guided into the same role. *This is how infectiousness of tolerance might arise.*

There are precedents for "infectious" behavior in T cells as, for example, in the competition between Th1 and Th2 subsets of CD4 T cells. Once the immune system gets set into Th2 function, the Th2-type cytokines influence naive T cells to follow the same Th2 life style.

CLINICAL IMPLICATIONS

Once we accept that there are a wealth of natural regulatory mechanisms within the immune system, we can equally accept that they could be exploited for therapeutic purposes. This line of immunosuppressive therapy will require a detailed knowledge of which drugs promote T cell suppression, and which are antagonistic. The mere fact that a drug is immunosuppressive will not predict its ability to promote T cell suppression. This concept clearly undermines all previous strategies for selection of immunosuppressive drugs. The knowledge that will come from the intensive analysis of studying basic mechanisms should eventually provide the clinician with new drugs and diagnostics by which tolerance can be promoted and monitored. This will be the future of immunosuppression in general, and the pharmaceutical industry will need to adjust itself to accept the concept of *short-term drug therapy for a long-term effect.*

REFERENCES

Arnold B, Schonrich G, Hammerling GJ (1993): Multiple levels of peripheral tolerance. Immunol Today 14:12–14.

Benjamin RJ, Qin S-X, Wise M, Cobbold SP, Waldmann H (1988): Mechanisms of monoclonal antibody facilitated tolerance induction. A possible role for CD4 and CD11a in self non-self discrimination. Eur J Immunol 18:1079–1088.

Billingham RE, Brent L, Medawar PB (1953): Actively acquired tolerance to foreign cells. Nature (London) 172:603–606.

Chen Z, Cobbold S, Waldmann H, Metcalfe S (1993): Stability of tolerance in mice generated by CD4 and CD8 monoclonal antibody treatment: Cell transfer experiments. Transplant Proc 25:790–791.

Cobbold SP, Martin G, Waldmann H (1990): The induction of skin graft tolerance in major histocompatibility complex-mismatched or primed recipients: Primed T cells can be tolerized in the periphery with anti-CD4 and anti-CD8 antibodies. Eur J Immunol 20:2747–2755.

Cobbold SP, Qin S, Leong LY, Martin G, Waldmann H (1993): Reprogramming the immune system for peripheral tolerance with CD4 and CD8 monoclonal antibodies. Immunol Rev 129:165–201.

Fowell D, Mason D (1993): Evidence that the T cell repertoire of normal rats contains cells with the potential to cause diabetes. Characterisation of the CD4+ T cell subset that inhibits this autoimmune potential. J Exp Med 771:627–636.

Guerder S, Matzinger P (1992): A fail-safe mechanism for maintaining self-tolerance in mature peripheral cytotoxic T-cells. J Exp Med 176:553.

Isobe M, Yagita H, Okamura K, Ihatra A (1992): Specific acceptance of cardiac allograft after treatment with antibodies to ICAM-1 and LFA-1. Science 2545:1125–112.

Lenschow DJ, Zheng Y, Thistlethwaite JR, Montag A, Brady W, Gibson MG, Linsley PS, Bluestone JA (1992): Long term survival of xenogeneic pancreatic islet grafts induced by CTLA4Ig. Science 357:789–792.

Leong LYW, Qin S-X, Cobbold SP, Waldmann H (1992): Classical transplantation tolerance in the adult: The interaction between myeloablation and immunosuppression. Eur J Immunol 22:2285–2830.

Lin H, Bolling SF, Linsley PS, Wei R-Q, Gordon D, Thompson CB, Turka LA (1993): Long term acceptance of major histocompatibility complex mismatched cardiac allografts induced by CTLA4-Ig plus donor specific transfusion. J Exp Med 178:1801–1906.

Lo D, Burkly LC, Flavell R, Palmiter RD, Brinster RL (1989): Tolerance in transgenic mice expressing class II major histocompatibility complex on pancreatic acinar cells. J Exp Med 170:87–95.

Miller JFAP, Morahan G, Allison (1990): Extrathymic acquisition of tolerance by T-lymphocytes. Cold Spring Harb Symp Quant Biol 54:807–812.

Morrisey PJ, Charrier K, Bradley S, Liggit D, Watson JD (1993): CD4+ T-cells that express high levels of CD45RB induce wasting disease when transferred into congenic severe combined immunodeficient mice. Disease development is prevented by cotransfer of purified CD4+ T-cells. J Exp med 178:237–244.

Nicolls MR, Aversa GG, Pearce NW, Spinelli A, Berger MF, Gurley KE, Hall BM (1993): Induction of long-term specific tolerance to allografts in rats by

therapy with an anti-CD3-like monoclonal antibody. Transplantation 55:459–468.

Posselt AM, Barker CF, Tomaszewski JE, Markman JF, Choti MA, Naji A (1990): Induction of donor-specific unresponsiveness by intrathymic islet transplantation. Science 249:293–1295.

Powrie F, Mason D (1990): Ox22high CD4 T-cells induce a wasting disease with multiple organ pathology: Prevention by the Ox22lo subset. J Exp Med 122:1701–1708.

Qin S, Cobbold SP, Benjamin R, Waldmann H (1989): Induction of classical transplantation tolerance in the adult. J Exp Med 169:779–794.

Qin S, Wise M, Cobbold SP, Leong L, Kong YC, Parnes JR, Waldmann HI (1990): Induction of tolerance in peripheral T cells with monoclonal antibodies. Eur J Immunol 20:2737–2745.

Qin S, Cobbold SP, Pope H, Elliott J, Kioussis D, Davies, Waldmann H (1993): Infectious transplantation tolerance. Science 259:974–977.

Schwartz RH (1992): The role of CD28, CTLA-4 and B7/BB1 in interleukin-2 production and immunotherapy. Cell 71:1065–1068.

Sykes M, Sachs D (1990): Bone marrow transplantation as a means of inducing tolerance. Semin Immunol 2:401–417.

Waldmann H (1989): Manipulation of T-cell responses with monoclonal antibodies. Annu Rev Immunol 7:407–444.

Waldmann H, Cobbold SP (1993): Monoclonal antibodies for the induction of transplantation tolerance. Curr Opin Immunol 5:753–758.

Waldmann H, Cobbold SP, Qin S, Benjamin RJ, Wise M (1989): Tolerance induction in the adult using monoclonal antibodies to CD4; CD8 and CD11a. 54th Symposium on Quantitative Biology: Immunological Recognition. Cold Spring Harbour Lab. Press LIV:885–889.

Wood-MJ, Sloan-DJ, Dallman-MJ, Charlton-HM (1993): Specific tolerance to neural allografts induced with an antibody to the interleukin 2 receptor. J-Exp Med 177:597–601.

Zinkernagel RM, Pircher HP, Ohashi H, Ochen S, Odermatt B, Mak T, Arnheiter H, Burki K, Hengartner H (1991): T and B cell tolerance and responses to viral antigens in transgenic mice: Implications for pathogenesis of autoimmune versus immunopathological disease. Immunol Rev 122:133–171.

Chapter 15
Induction of Immunological Tolerance to Allografts with Antilymphocyte Serum and Donor-Specific Bone Marrow

Anthony P. Monaco, Mary L. Wood, and Takashi Maki

CLINICAL CONCEPTS AND EFFECTS OF CHRONIC IMMUNOSUPPRESSION

Over the past two decades, clinical organ transplantation has become the most effective therapy for end organ failure. This progress has been due to extraordinary advances in the understanding of the allograft response and its modification with various types of immunosuppression. Modern concepts of clinical immunosuppression for organ transplantation utilize high levels of immunosuppressive drugs at the time of induction (the time of placement of the organ allograft) with progressive reduction of daily immunosuppressive drugs to maintenance levels over time. Furthermore, newer immunosuppressive treatments have utilized drugs and biological reagents with more and more restricted effects on the various steps in the allograft response to minimize the nonspecific immune suppression of the recipient's immune reactivity. Nevertheless, the requirement for use of chronic immunosuppression has been associated with significant morbidity and mortality due to opportunistic infection, spontaneous neoplasms, as well as direct drug toxicity and metabolic complications. Thus, the ability to transplant organ allografts without the necessity for chronic immunosuppression, i.e., the induction of specific immunological tolerance, remains an important goal.

NEONATAL ALLOGRAFT TOLERANCE

In an effort to explain the natural self-tolerance to self-tissues, Burnett (1959) postulated that exposure to antigen during fetal and neonatal development of an animal when it is still immunologically immature or incompetent would result in total and specific obliteration of the capacity to make an immune response to that antigen (so-called clonal deletion). Billingham, Brent, and Medawar (1953) were the first to induce tolerance to foreign tissues. They postulated that certain unexpected instances of tolerance to foreign tissues in certain pairs of nonidentical twins of several species might have been due to the exchange of foreign blood cells between the twin partners *in utero* due to vascular (placental) abnormalities. These authors reproduced these experiments of nature by injecting replicating allogeneic lymphoid cells from one adult mouse strain into fetal and (later) neonatal mice of another strain. The injected animals were specifically tolerant (i.e., did not reject) to donor tissues (skin) as adults. Medawar and colleagues noted that tolerant mice were chimeras (i.e., the inoculated cells persisted in the adult tolerant mice), the chimerism correlated with the tolerant state, and tolerance (and chimerism) could be abrogated by addition of syngeneic (recipient strain) normal adult lymphoid cells. Billingham, Brent, and Medawar

Transplantation Immunology, pages 247–265
© 1995 Wiley-Liss, Inc.

(1953) designated the allograft tolerance that they induced actively acquired immunological tolerance.

MODERN CONCEPTS OF NEONATAL ALLOGRAFT TOLERANCE

Although originally thought to be an all-or-none phenomenon in which the immune response was totally and specifically obliterated by neonatal antigen exposure (so-called clonal deletion), it is now clear that states of unresponsiveness (tolerance) induced in neonates and adults can involve multiple mechanisms that evolve sequentially during tolerance induction and maintenance. These mechanisms include clonal deletion (absence of specific alloreactive cells), clonal reduction (reduction of specific alloreactive cells), clonal anergy (presence of specific alloreactive cells that cannot appropriately function), and specific active suppression (presence of cells or factors that block the allograft response).

The elegant experiments of Streilein and colleagues (1991) have analyzed the activation mechanisms in a model of tolerance induced by neonatal injection of semiallogeneic hematopoietic cells (bone marrow and spleen cells). These authors demonstrated that all neonatal recipients become chimeric in the thymus and peripheral lymphoid organs. Subsequently, the recipients lose specific alloreactive cells in the thymus and lack peripheral T cells capable of responding to the tolerogen. They noted, however, that these usual consequences of neonatal allogeneic cell injection could not explain the skin graft acceptance (tolerance) demonstrated when the animals matured. They demonstrated that the type of tolerogen (class I and/or class II alloantigen differences) influences the eventual mechanism involved in tolerance. Thus, mice rendered tolerant as neonates with hematopoietic cells from donors with class I and/or class II alloantigen differences become chimeras in the thymus and peripheral lymphoid compartments. Tolerance in these animals was not transferred adoptively but was abrogated by transfusion of normal syngeneic lymphoid cells. These tolerant animals did not reject skin grafts, their lympho-

cytes failed to respond to tolerogens *in vitro* [in mixed lymphocyte reactions (MLR) and cell-mediated lymphocytotoxicity reactions (CML)] and suppressor cells could never be demonstrated at any time. Furthermore, evidence was accumulated that these tolerant animals had significantly reduced precursor cytotoxic T cells and the T cell receptor (TCR) repertoire of the remaining tolerogen-reactive cells was abnormal. Thus, clonal deletion (and/or reduction) is an important mechanism in tolerance in these animals. In contrast, in certain recipients (B10 strain background) rendered tolerant to class II alloantigen different donors, chimerism is present, tolerance cannot be abrogated by infusion of normal syngeneic cells, but tolerance can be transferred adoptively. Anergic, tolerogen-specific T cells are present and active suppressor mechanism(s) are also important in maintaining the tolerant state. In further contrast, in other class II differences (recipient with A strain background) tolerant animals are not chimeras, but tolerance can be transferred adoptively. Although these animals fail to reject skin grafts, their lymphocytes react vigorously *in vitro* when stimulated with class II tolerogen-bearing cells. These important studies clearly show that rather than being an all-or-none phenomenon as emphasized by Medawar and colleagues (1953), neonatal tolerance can involve a multiplicity of mechanisms.

INDUCTION OF IMMUNOLOGICAL TOLERANCE TO TISSUE ALLOGRAFTS IN IMMUNOCOMPETENT ADULT ANIMALS

To achieve a situation analogous to neonatal tolerance induction, the overwhelming number of experimental models to induce immunological tolerance in adult immunologically competent animals have utilized a transient period of induced nonspecific immunosuppression in association with or in close temporal relation to exposure to specific alloantigen (Monaco et al., 1989). The alloantigens utilized may be the graft itself but usually additional donor-specific antigen is required. Although varying degrees of tolerance have been induced with cell-free antigenic tissue extracts or nonreplicating parenchymal cells, the best tolerogenic alloantigens have been replicating cells, especially lymphoid cells, and particularly bone marrow cells (Monaco and Wood, 1970; Gozzo et al., 1970). Replicating cells may provide a continued source of antigen. Replicating lymphoid cells, especially bone marrow cells, may also be tolerogenic by virtue of their content of self-suppressive or veto cells (see below). All forms of nonspecific immunosuppression to prepare adult immunologically competent animals for tolerance induction have been utilized. These have included physical agents (total body irradiation, total lymphoid irradiation), biological reagents (polyclonal antilymphocyte sera, specific anti-CD4 and CD8 monoclonal antibodies, etc.), and chemical reagents, particularly cyclosporine A, rapamycin FK506, and 15-deoxyspergualin (DSG). A number of parameters facilitate or mitigate against tolerance induction. Histocompatibility facilitates tolerance induction, and presensitization is a profound barrier to tolerance induction. Depending upon the donor–recipient combination and species involved, the time, dose, and route of antigen administration for tolerance induction utilized will affect the degree and duration of tolerance induced. Also, the type of graft to be tolerized significantly affects tolerance induction. Highly immunogenic skin allografts are difficult to tolerize; islets and whole organ grafts (heart, liver) are frequently easy to tolerize.

hematopoietic cells and treatment with cyclophosphamide. In these studies, unresponsiveness involved three successive stages in which a separate cellular mechanism was responsible for tolerance. Immediately after induction, alloreactive T cells were absent in the periphery, but were still present in the thymus. At the time of application of skin grafts (2 weeks post-cyclophosphamide treatment and cell infusion), tolerogen-specific T cells were absent in the periphery but cells with tolerogen specific TCR were still present in the thymus. Graft acceptance resulted from peripheral but not central clonal deletion of antigen reactive T cells. After 4 weeks, recipients became chimeric both in the peripheral lymphoid organs and the thymus. At this time, thymocytes with TCR specific for the donor cells disappeared from the thymus. Coincidentally, T cells specific for the tolerogen appeared in the periphery but were anergic, i.e., they failed to respond to donor alloantigen *in vitro*. During this second stage, tolerance could not be transferred adoptively. Clonal reduction and anergy are responsible for tolerance. In the third stage (day 75–135), chimerism disappears in the lymphoid compartments, tolerogen-reactive cells are identifiable in the peripheral lymphoid organs by *in vitro* assays, and tolerance becomes transferable to syngeneic recipients with recipient lymphoid cells. Thus, suppressor cells are responsible for tolerance maintenance in the third stage.

THE CONCEPT OF MULTIPLE MECHANISMS IN ALLOGRAFT TOLERANCE IN ADULT ANIMALS

As demonstrated with neonatal allograft tolerance, evidence now emphasizes that multiple mechanisms of immune modification are involved in certain tolerance states induced in adult animals. An excellent series of experiments was reported by Mayumi and colleagues (1990) who demonstrated the sequential involvement of multiple mechanisms in transplantation tolerance in adult animals. These authors induced tolerance in adult mice across weak histocompatibility barriers using infusion of T cell-depleted allogeneic

THE USE OF POLYCLONAL ANTILYMPHOCYTE SERUM AND DONOR-SPECIFIC BONE MARROW TO INDUCE TOLERANCE TO TISSUE AND ORGAN ALLOGRAFTS

The author and his collaborators (Monaco and Wood, 1970; Gozzo et al., 1970) first described the use of polyclonal antilymphocyte serum and donor specific bone marrow to induce tolerance to tissue allografts. Although the original description was in mice to skin allografts, this model has been successfully applied to immediately vascularized whole organ renal allografts in dogs, primates, and in man.

Standard Protocol

A standard protocol was devised that could be used in all species and with application to human cadaveric organ tranplantation in mind (Fig. 1). Since antigen would not be available from cadaveric harvesting until the time of or after transplantation, protocols in which antigen was administered after grafting were studied. In initial studies, recipient strain mice were transiently immunosuppressed with antilymphocyte serum (ALS) before and after (day −1 and +2) skin grafting (on day 0) and were subsequently infused iv with donor type cells a week later (day +7). Using this protocol, nonreplicating cells (epidermal, renal, hepatic) did not induce tolerance. Replicating lymphoid cells were effective in inducing tolerance to varying degrees. Bone marrow cells were clearly superior to splenocytes, which in turn were much more efficacious than lymphocytes and thymocytes, which were not significantly tolerogenic. Tolerance was defined as specific survival of donor-specific skin grafts in ALS-treated, bone marrow (BM)-infused animals over that seen in recip-

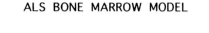

ALS BONE MARROW MODEL

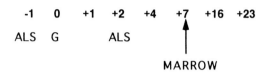

Fig. 1. Induction of specific unresponsiveness. Mice are treated with ALS on days −1 and +2 (0.5 ml, ip) relative to skin grafting on day 0. Donor strain bone marrow is given iv on day +7. Assays to determine mechanism of tolerance induced by this protocol are performed at various times.

ients given ALS alone. In these initial experiments, only 10–20% of ALS–BM recipients had significant tolerance greater than 100 days (Fig. 2). As with other forms of adult experimental tolerance induction, the dose and timing of tolerogen (BM) injection were critical for maximal effect. The optimal tolerance-inducing effect was achieved with 10^7 BM cells per recipient given iv on day +4 to +7. Lesser or larger doses of

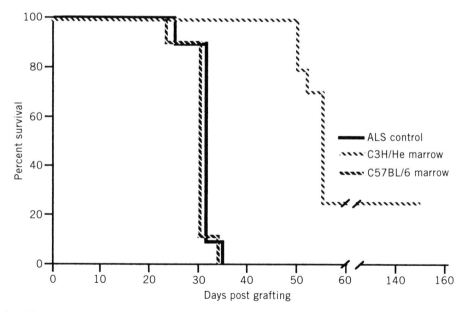

Fig. 2. Effect of ALS and bone marrow on skin allograft survival. B6AF$_1$ mice received ALS (0.5 ml ip) on days −1 and +2 and C3H/He skin allografts on day 0 (control group). Other groups received ALS and skin grafts as described, but also received either donor strain bone marrow (C3H/He) or third-party (C57BL/6) bone marrow iv on day +7.

BM induced less tolerance and in some instances even shortened graft survival (i.e., induced sensitization). BM given before grafting or after day +21 failed to induce tolerance (Wood et al., 1971). Unlike other experimental models of tolerance induction in adult animals, the intravenous route of BM cell administration was not obligatory, i.e., significant tolerance could be induced with BM cells administered intravenously, intraperitoneally, and even by direct intraorgan (into the liver or spleen) injection.

In Vitro and In Vivo Analysis of Alloreactivity of Mice Rendered Tolerant with ALS and Donor BM

Recipients given ALS only in the standard protocol exhibit nonspecific depression of the immune response for 3–4 weeks during which they fail to reject skin allografts. Thereafter, nonspecific immune responses recover and specific antidonor alloreactivity is evident and grafts are rejected (Fig. 3). In contrast, ALS-treated BM-infused mice recover nonspecific immune responses after the effect of ALS is dissipated, but exhibit specific nonreactivity against donor antigens during which time donor specific allografts are not rejected. Lymphocytes from tolerant ALS–BM recipients do not re-

spond in MLR to donor antigens and fail to exhibit direct lymphocyte mediated cytotoxicity to donor target antigens unless donor grafts have been rejected. However, lymphocytes from tolerant recipients can exhibit secondary cytotoxic reactivity after mixed lymphocyte culture and reexposure to donor target alloantigens (Maki et al., 1981) (Fig. 4).

Microchimerism

Mice rendered tolerant with ALS and BM are not gross chimeras. However, various studies have demonstrated that small numbers of donor bone marrow cells (or their descendants) persist at very low levels for varying periods of time in animals rendered tolerant with ALS and BM. This was postulated very early in the analysis and development of the model and confirmed by Liegeois et al. (1974) using a T6T6 chromosome marker technique. In these studies, it was evident that the degree of chimerism in recipients given ALS and BM but no donor skin graft was significantly less than recipients given ALS, BM, and a donor-specific graft. Thus, this suggests that the presence of the additional alloantigen in the graft provides a stimulus for proliferation of the donor-specific BM cells. Very recently, Thomas et al. (1994) used PCR meth-

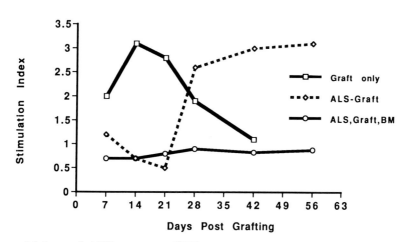

Fig. 3. Sequential changes in MLR response to C3H/He alloantigens. B6AF$_1$ mice received C3H/He skin allografts on day 0. Group 1 received no other treatment, group 2 received ALS on days −1 and +2, and group 3 received ALS on days −1 and +2, and C3H/He marrow on day +7. Spleen cells were harvested at various times and assayed in standard MLR coculture with C3H/He spleen cells.

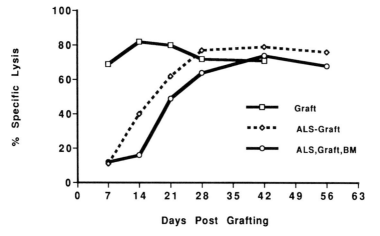

Fig. 4. Sequential changes of cytotoxic responses to C3H/He alloantigens. B6AF$_1$ spleen cells from mice from graft only, ALS and graft, or ALS, graft, and marrow groups were cocultured with C3H/He spleen cells in standard MLR for 6 days. Cytotoxicity was determined by assaying the effector cells against ^{51}Cr-labeled L929 cells.

ods to demonstrate BM chimerism in this model. Similarly, Barber et al. (1994) demonstrated donor BM microchimerism in human recipients given polyclonal antilymphocyte serum and donor BM following cadaveric renal allografts. The potential significance of microchimerism in this model of tolerance will be discussed below.

Suppressor Cell Analysis

As with a number of other adult tolerance models, the presence of various types of suppressor cells can be demonstrated at various times in the tolerant period. What is unique in the ALS–BM model is that the presence of different types of suppressor cells can be established depending on the time in the evolution of tolerance. Thus, using standard suppressor cell adoptive transfer assay techniques, tolerance could be transferred by spleen cells from tolerant animals injected into syngeneic nonspecifically immunosuppressed hosts indicating the presence of suppressor cell mechanisms. Furthermore, *in vitro* analysis of the ALS–BM model using coculture of mixed lymphocyte reaction assays demonstrates that ALS treatment alone initially induces nonspecific host-derived suppressor cells. If such ALS-treated recipients are also skin grafted, an antigen-specific host-derived sup-

pressor cell is associated with the prolonged graft survival produced by ALS alone. Most importantly, donor-specific BM infusion 7 days later after skin grafting subsequently leads to development of an antigen-specific donor-derived (from the BM) suppressor cell that suppresses anti-self-MHC alloreactivity (Maki et al., 1981). Since the cell suppresses anti-self alloreactivity, it has some of the characteristics of a veto cell.

Separation and Characterization of the Active Bone Marrow Cell Fraction(s) Capable of Tolerance Induction

An important area of research has been the nature of the BM cell that produces the specific tolerance induced in the ALS and BM model. As noted above, specific T suppressor cells of donor haplotype can be identified from the spleens of tolerant ALS–BM-treated mice bearing long surviving donor type skin allografts; it is highly likely that these mature antigen-specific cells are descendants of donor bone marrow precursor cells. Active BM fractions that induce tolerance in ALS-treated recipients as well or better than whole unfractionated BM can be prepared using Ficoll or Percoll gradients (Gosso et al., 1982; De Fazio et al., 1987). These fractions contain cells that are of relatively light density and of medium size and histologically have the appearance of immature lymphocytes. Investigations have been performed to characterize the surface markers of the active bone marrow cells. Marker positive populations were either depleted or enriched by panning techniques or killed with specific antibody and complement and then assayed for their ability to induce tolerance in the standard ALS-BM protocol (De Fazio et al., 1987b). These studies have shown that BM cells that induce tolerance in ALS-treated mice appear to be Ia⁻, Thy-1⁻, complement receptor negative, and Ig⁻ but are largely positive for Fcγ receptors. These phenotype characteristics suggest that the active BM tolerance-inducing cell is an early non-T, non-B cell consistent with a natural regulatory or natural suppressor cell of the type found in normal adult BM, neonatal spleens, and mice recovering after treatment with total lymphoid irradiation. It is important to note that the spleen cell(s) active in prolonging graft survival in ALS-treated mice is also a non-T cell non-B cell, as it also lacks Thy 1, Ia, surface markers. Both FcγR⁺ and FcγR⁻ cells are effective in prolonging grafts, but FcγR⁻ cells are the most effective. In contrast, the active cell in lymph node and thymus (both poor tolerogens) is Thy-1 positive, indicating that they are T lymphocytes.

Effect of Bone Marrow Growth Factors on Tolerance Induction

Since an early immature stem-like cell was identified as the active cell in BM capable of inducing allograft tolerance, it was logical to determine if certain bone marrow stem cell growth factors might facilitate tolerance in this model. Interleukin 3 (IL-3) and granulocyte-macrophage colony-stimulating factor (GM-CSF) stimulate the differentiation and proliferation of early multilineage precursor cells. In these studies (Monaco et al., 1991) C3H/He lymphoid cell donors were treated with GM-CSF prior to cell donation. Either normal or GM-CSF-treated cells were injected into ALS-treated B6AF₁ mice grafted with C3H/He skin in the otherwise standard protocol. GM-CSF treatment significantly augmented the effect of BM in prolonging graft survival at doses of 1 to 25 × 10⁶ cells (Fig. 5).

In contrast, GM-CSF had no effect on the graft-prolonging effect of spleen cells when 50 × 10⁶ were given. When the dose of spleen cells was reduced to 25 × 10⁶, graft survival in the group given GM-CSF-treated cells was prolonged compared with survival in the group given normal cells. Grafts in the group given GM-CSF-treated lymph node cells were rejected in sensitized fashion. When active whole BM or spleen cells are separated on a Percoll gradient, the active cell in promoting graft survival is recovered primarily in the 52.5% fraction. The graft-prolonging effect of the 52.5% fraction was not affected by GM-CSF treatment. In contrast, GM-CSF-treated marrow cells in the 60% fraction significantly prolonged graft survival, while normal marrow cells in this fraction had no effect on graft survival. GM-CSF-treated spleen cells in the 52.5 and 60% fractions significantly decreased graft survival compared with normal cells when given at a dose equal to the number of cells recovered from 50 × 10⁶ whole spleen cells. When the dose of fractionated spleen cells was reduced, GM-CSF-treated spleen cells were more effective than normal cells in prolonging graft survival. These results indicate that GM-CSF activates a cell in the marrow that promotes graft survival. This cell is recovered in the 60% Percoll fraction. In contrast, GM-CSF appears to affect two cell populations in spleen, one beneficial and one detrimental to graft survival. The predominant effect depends on the dose of GM-CSF-treated spleen cells given for tolerance induction.

These observations suggest that it might be possible to treat cadaveric organ donors from whom tolerance-inducing BM is also harvested with specific BM growth factors prior to donation to enhance the tolerogenicity of donor-specific marrow.

Cloning of Self-Major Histocompatibility Complex Antigen-Specific Suppressor Cells from Normal Adult Bone Marrow

Since the tolerance induced by ALS and BM treatment is associated with suppressor cells that suppress anti-self-alloimmune responses, it was logical to determine if suppressor cell clones

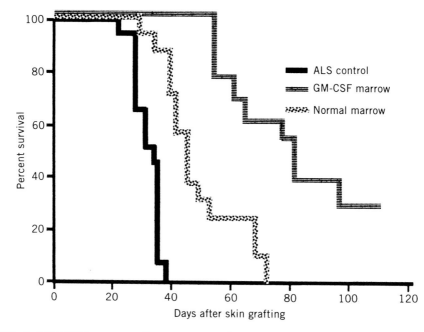

Fig. 5. Effect of GM-CSF treatment of bone marrow donors on skin allograft survival. C3H/He mice were treated with GM-CSF (20 μg/day, ip, 10–15 days). Various numbers of marrow cells (1, 5, or 10 × 10⁶ from treated or normal donors were then given iv into ALS-treated, C3H skin-grafted B6AF₁ mice. Most significant prolongation was seen in recipients of 10 × 10⁶ BMC from treated donors.

could be established from adult bone marrow that contain a population of cells capable of specifically down-regulating the immune response directed toward self-major histocompatibility complex (MHC) antigens (Takahashi and Maki, 1990). In these studies, freshly prepared adult C3H (H-2^k) marrow cells were cultured in medium containing IL-2, IL-3, or a mixture of IL-2 and IL-3. After 7–10 days in culture, cells grown in IL-3-containing medium were screened for their capacity to suppress cytotoxic T lymphocyte (CTL) generation against self-MHC antigen in allogeneic mixed lymphocyte culture. Cells capable of suppressing anti-C3H CTL generation were cloned by limiting dilution. Several suppressor clones were established that exhibited strong suppression of anti-H-2^k, anti-H-$2K^k/I^k$, and anti-H-$2D^k$ CTL generation but failed to suppress anti-H-2^d and anti-H-2^b responses (Fig. 6). When tested in a skin allograft model, intravenous injections of donor bone marrow-derived anti-self-suppressor cell clones together with IL-3 induced prolongation of C3H skin allografts in antilymphocyte serum-treated B6AF₁ mice. Injection of IL-3 alone had no effect on allograft survival. Moreover, these

Fig. 6. MHC antigen specificity suppression by IL-3-dependent clones 11.7 and 3.2. 5 × 10⁴ irradiated (2,000 rad) clone 11.7 cells (●---●), clone 3.2 cells (▲---▲), or C3H splenocytes (○—○) were added to each 16-mm well containing 5 × 10⁶ responder nylon wool–nonadherent splenocytes and 10⁵ irradiated stimulator splenic adherent cells. Responder cell–stimulator cell combinations are as indicated above. After a 5-d culture, surviving cells were assayed at various E/T ratios against ⁵¹Cr-labeled 3-d Con A-stimulated spleen cells. C3H blast targets were used for C57BL/6 anti-C3H, DBA/2 anti-A, and DBA/2 anti-C3H.OH, DBA/2 blasts for C57BL/6 anti-DBA/2 and C3H anti-DBA/2, C57BL/6 blasts for DBA/2 anti-C57BL/6, and B10.MBR blasts for DBA/2 anti-B10.MBR effector cells. Results are expressed as percent specific lysis. (A) One experiment and (B) two experiments in which suppression of DBA/2 anti-C3H and no suppression of DBA/2 anti-C57BL/6 were always confirmed (parts of data not shown). Spontaneous release was ~20–30% of maximal release in all experiments.

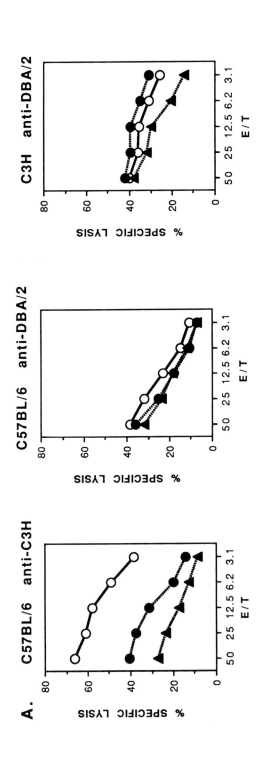

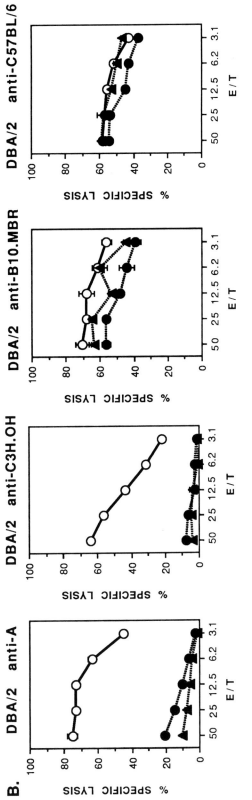

Fig. 6.

cells failed to prolong B10.AKM skin allografts on B6AF$_1$ recipients. Northern blot analysis showed that these cells expressed full-length transcripts of the T cell receptor (TCR) *a* gene, but not those of the TCR *B* or *b* genes. However, no rearrangement of the *a* gene was observed by Southern blot analysis. Flow cytometric analysis revealed that bone marrow-derived suppressor cells are strongly positive for Thy-1 antigen but negative for CD3, CD4, and CD8 surface markers and express only class I MHC antigens. It is possible that these cells may represent a unique population of immature lymphoid cells that remain in the extrathymic environment. Suppression of anti-self immunity by these cells could represent an alternative mechanism to intrathymic elimination of self-reactive T cells for induction of self-tolerance. These cells may remain dominant in the bone marrow except when suppression of anti-self-MHC reactivity is required during early development of T cell differentiation. Presumably, in the ALS–BM model, activation and proliferation of these cells in donor marrow occur as a result of increased production of IL-3 by the host T-lymphocytes after alloantigen stimulation.

Cellular Events in Tolerance Induction with ALS and Donor-Specific Bone Marrow

Immunosuppression with ALS alone causes severe peripheral T cell depletion and induces a state of nonspecific unresponsiveness to alloantigen; the MLR and CML responses are nonspecifically suppressed, and allograft survival is prolonged. Antidonor MLR and CML responses eventually recover and grafts are rejected. If ALS-treated grafted recipients receive donor bone marrow, the state of nonspecific unresponsiveness is converted to a state of specific nonreactivity to graft antigens and graft survival is significantly prolonged beyond the period of nonspecific immunosuppression. Spleen cell proliferation in MLR to C3H/He stimulation is significantly suppressed in the majority of tolerant B6AF$_1$ mice after ALS and marrow, although a small percentage of mice bearing long-term grafts exhibit a normal MLR. However, the CML responses to donor antigens after *in vitro* culture of spleen cells from ALS-treated, marrow-

injected mice returns to normal after recovery from the nonspecific immunosuppressive effects of ALS (approximately 21 days postgrafting) even in mice whose grafts remain intact for 60 days or more (Maki et al., 1981). Streilein and colleagues (1989) have noted a similar discrepancy between *in vivo* and *in vitro* reactivity in mice made tolerant as neonates to class II antigens that permanently accept skin grafts from the donor but can exhibit normal reactivity to the donor antigens in MLR and can produce IL-2 when stimulated with donor antigens. These results suggest that the MLR and CML assays do not necessarily reflect the true immune status of unresponsive mice. *In vitro* conditions may be permissive for responses that are abrogated by *in vivo* conditions. MLR and CML assays monitor the entire graft-reactive T-lymphocyte population in a qualitative rather than a quantitative manner, which makes it difficult to document the evolution of functional changes in the cell populations. The activity of cells specifically involved in graft prolongation may be masked by the delicate balance between cells with immune and suppressor function in unresponsive animals. Generation of CML might be possible *in vitro* in bulk cultures using a large number of responders and stimulators, when, *in vivo,* in the unresponsive recipient, the CTL population specific for the graft antigens could in fact be significantly suppressed.

A quantitative assay such as the limiting dilution assay (LDA) may be more accurate in demonstrating the immune status of unresponsive animals. This assay can determine the frequency of a defined population of cells and can be used to detect small numbers of CTL that are specific for a given set of alloantigens. Traditional LDA techniques identify the total number of antigen-reactive CTL, regardless of their stage of differentiation, i.e., precursor, naive, and memory, not all of which are necessarily activated *in vivo* by graft alloantigens. Alternatively, a modified LDA assay can be used in which the population of CTL activated *in vivo* by alloantigens [antigen-conditioned CTL (cCTL)] can be distinguished from the total CTL (tCTL) population (Wood et al., 1992). This modification is based on the fact that CTL that have been stimulated *in vivo* by appropriate antigen proliferate and maintain specific cytolytic activity *in vitro* for a period of time without further alloantigen restimulaion, if a source of mitogenic lymphokine is provided in the culture. In contrast, nonactivated CTL require *in vitro* alloantigenic stimulation, as well as lymphokine, to develop cytolytic activity in culture. To obtain the frequency of the total CTL population, responder cells are stimulated with the appropriate allogeneic cells plus exogenous growth factors. To obtain the frequency of the subpopulation of *in vivo* alloantigen-conditioned CLT, the responder cells are cultured with syngeneic feeder cells plus exogenous growth factors, so that only those cells previously stimulated *in vivo* by alloantigen can proliferate and develop cytolytic activity.

To identify the sequential cellular events associated with unresponsiveness induced by ALS and donor BMC, the precursor frequencies of donor-reactive CTL in the spleen and lymph nodes of ALS-treated, grafted mice given donor bone marrow were compared with CTL frequencies in ALS-treated, grafted controls used the modified LDA assay. Figure 7 shows that no C3H/He-reactive CTL could be detected on day +8 in either marrow-injected mice or controls (no BMC). By day +14, a small number of

donor-reactive CTL (9% of normal) were present in spleens of marrow injected mice and reached 55% by day +42 in BMC-injected mice that maintained their grafts. In mice that still maintained their grafts for 1 year, the number of +CTL in the spleen had only risen to 54% of normal. In control mice that did not receive marrow, the number of tCTL had recovered to 21% of normal by day +14 and to 67% of normal by day +21. All grafts in the control group were rejected by day +42, and the number of tCTL in the spleen was three times the normal number. This rebound phenomenon was seen in the control spleens after graft rejection in all the groups assayed.

The percentage of tCTL represented by cCTL in both groups is shown in Figure 8. In the BMC-injected group, the cCTL constituted a majority of the tCTL present at both days +14 and +21. At this peak level on day +14, 99% in the BMC-injected group were cCTL and 69% tCTL were cCTL on day +21. In the control group, the cCTL were only 51% of tCTL at their peak on day +14 and dropped to 21% on day +21. Of interest, the number of C3H/He-reactive CTL was 50% of normal in spleen of BMC-injected mice bearing perfect grafts on day +58 while it had returned to normal in similar mice that had

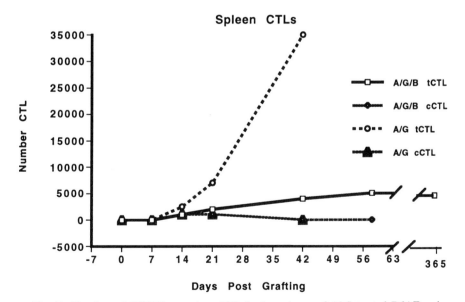

Fig. 7. Number of C3H/He-reactive cCTL in the spleens of ALS-treated B6AF$_1$ mice grafted with C3H/He skin and injected with C3H/He marrow (A/G/B) and of ALS-treated, grafted controls (A/G). Assays were performed at various days after grafting.

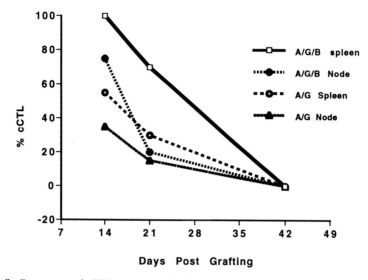

Fig. 8. Percentage of cCTL present in the tCTL in the spleens and lymph nodes of ALS-treated B6AF$_1$ mice grafted with C3H/He skin and injected with C3H/He marrow (A/G/B) and of ALS-treated grafted controls (A/G). The assays were performed on various days after grafting.

rejected grafts at this time. The CTL frequency to third party DBA/2 alloantigens was normal in both groups of mice. Figure 9 shows a similar analysis of cCTL and tCTL in regional nodes draining grafts sites of BMC-injected and noninjected controls. On day +8, no CTL were detected in either marrow or control mice. On day +14, a small number of tCTL were detectable in the nodes of BMC injected mice (7% of normal), which rose to 13% by day +21, and this number did not change essentially in the marrow-injected

mice with surviving grafts up to 1 year postgrafting when the number of tCTL was extremely low. Significantly, there was no overlap in the frequency range in normal mice and in the BMC-injected mice bearing grafts at 1 year. In control mice (no BMC), the frequency of donor-reactive CTL remained in the normal range at all times tested, but the number of tCTL/site remained below normal even on day +42 when all grafts of the group were rejected. Antigen conditioned cCTL were present in the nodes of marrow-

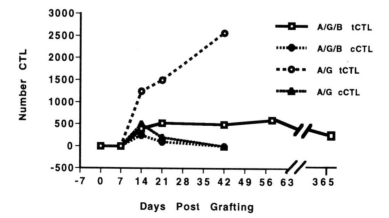

Fig. 9. Number of C3H/He-reactive tCTL and cCTL in the lymph nodes of ALS-treated B6AF$_1$ mice grafted with C3H/He skin and injected with C3H/He marrow (A/G/B) and of ALS-treated, grafted controls (A/G). The nodes were assayed at various times postgrafting.

injected and control mice between days +14 and +21 as observed with the spleen. The majority of tCTL in marrow-injected mice was cCTL (72%) at day +14 while only 33% of control tCTL were cCTL. By day +21, the number of cCTL had fallen to a low level in both groups. The number of tCTL in lymph nodes of mice bearing unrejected grafts on day +58 was significantly suppressed while the number and frequency had returned to normal in mice that had rejected their grafts. Third party reactivity to DBA/2 was normal in the nodes of mice bearing C3H/He grafts. In contrast to results with donor BMC injection, C3H/He graft survival in ALS-treated B6AF$_1$ recipients injected with C3H/He lymph node cells is not significantly prolonged compared with ALS-treated controls (Wood et al., 1992). The effect of injecting lymph node cells instead of BMC in ALS-treated, grafted recipients has been studied. tCTL was suppressed in both the spleen and lymph nodes on day +14 after lymph node cell injection, but by day +21 the tCTL frequency in the spleen had returned to normal. In contrast, the frequency and number of tCTL in the lymph nodes remained markedly suppressed. Also, no cCTL were detected in the lymph nodes or spleen in recipients injected with lymph node cells.

These data on the frequency of donor-reactive CTL in ALS-treated, grafted mice with and without marrow suggest that a primary effect of donor marrow is to suppress the regeneration of donor-reactive CTL after recovery from the immunosuppressive effects of ALS. Donor-reactive CTL frequency correlated well with graft survival, in contrast to our previous finding using the CML response as an assay for donor reactivity (Maki et al., 1981). In BMC mice the frequency and number of CTL reactive to C3H/He remained significantly suppressed in the spleen and lymph nodes as long as the recipients maintained their skin grafts. Even at 1 year postgrafting, the number of C3H/He-reactive CTL was only 55% of normal in the spleen and 6% of normal in the lymph nodes while the frequency of CTL to third-party antigens was normal. In contrast, in the mice given no marrow C3H/He-reactive CTL returned to normal as the recipients recovered from the effects of ALS. Furthermore, presentation of donor alloantigen in this model does not necessarily result in the inhibition of regeneration of donor-reactive cells, as shown by comparing the effect of injecting lymph node cells and marrow. In ALS-treated mice injected with donor lymph node cells, the frequency of donor-reactive CTL had returned to normal in the spleen by day +21 shortly before graft rejection occurred, although the frequency in the nodes was still suppressed. This correlates with the original finding that marrow is markedly superior to lymph node cells in prolonging graft survival in ALS-treated mice (Monaco and Wood, 1970; Gozzo et al., 1970).

When CTL began to regenerate in the spleen and lymph nodes 14 day postgrafting, a majority of CTL present initially in both ALS controls and marrow-injected mice were committed CTL, activated in vivo to donor antigens. The significance of these activated cells is unclear. Their appearance does not correlate with graft rejection, as grafts in the marrow-injected group did not begin to reject until day +50. Even in the control group, grafts remained in good condition until day +25. The characteristic that distinguished the groups that did not maintain long-term grafts, i.e., the ALS controls and the group injected with lymph node cells, from the marrow-injected group was a more rapid recovery of tCTL, particularly in the spleen and not a higher percentage of alloactivated cells. This suggests that after repopulation of the lymphoid tissues with CTL, the maturation and activation of CTL into committed CTL take place mainly in the graft, and rejection occurs. This would be consistent with the studies in normal mice by Ascher et al. (1983) that showed that precytotoxic cells recruited from the lymphoid tissues could mature into cytotoxic cells in the graft without any evidence of concomitant cytotoxicity in the spleen or nodes. Also, Bishop et al. (1990) compared tCTL and cCTL in spleen, lymph nodes, and sponge allografts in normal mice and found that the cCTL present in the spleen and nodes at the time of graft rejection represented only a small fraction of the tCTL, while almost all the CTL in the graft were cCTL. The failure of donor-reactive CTL to regenerate in the spleen and nodes after the injection of marrow would prolong graft survival by removing the source of precursor cytotoxic cells.

Suppression of CTL regeneration has been demonstrated in other models of unresponsiveness after the injection of lymphoid cells, and the underlying mechanism has been ascribed to veto cell activity. This could also be one of the mechanisms operating in our marrow model. The veto cell was first described by Muraoka and Miller (1980) as a Thy 1-negative cell in marrow that had the unique ability to suppress the cytotoxic response against its own H-2 antigens when assayed *in vitro* in MLR. The suppression occurred at the level of precursor CTL (pCTL) resulting in a reduction in the number of pCTL activated. The pCTL are most sensitive to veto activity within a few days after exposure to antigen while mature CTL cannot be inactivated. The marrow cell active in inducing unresponsiveness in our ALS marrow model has been characterized as a Thy 1-negative cell. If this cell in the donor marrow is acting as a veto cell in the ALS-treated, grafted recipients, precursor CTL would be particularly vulnerable to veto activity as they regenerate after ALS treatment and are exposed to graft antigens.

Thy 1-negative marrow cells that have veto activity can differentiate in culture into Thy 1-positive cells (Muraoka and Miller, 1980). Thy 1-positive cells that can specifically suppress the host response to donor antigens have been demonstrated in the spleens and lymph nodes, as well as at the graft site in ALS-treated, marrow-injected mice bearing long-term skin grafts (Wood and Monaco, 1980). These cells can transfer suppression to naive syngeneic recipients and are thought to be active in maintaining unresponsiveness. The cells capable of adoptively transferring suppression have not been analyzed for donor and host H-2 antigens, so it is not possible to say whether they are of donor or host origin. However, a donor-derived Thy 1-positive cell that can specifically suppress the MLC response to donor antigens in coculture *in vitro* has been identified in mice with long-term grafts after ALS and marrow treatment (Maki et al., 1981). It is possible that both the cells that suppress the regeneration of CTL after ALS and marrow and the cells that can transfer suppression from long-term survivors are derived from the donor marrow.

Effect of Additional Immunosuppression on Tolerance Induction with ALS and Donor BM

In a number of experimental models of adult allograft tolerance induction, the addition of additional finite courses of immunosuppression frequently augments the degree and duration of tolerance induced. As noted above, with tolerance induced by ALS and BM, only a small number (10–20%) of recipients had significant (>100 days) tolerance induced. For clinical application to be reasonably possible, a higher degree of efficacy would be required. Also, since current clinical immunosuppressive protocols are extremely efficacious, any tolerance-inducing regimen would have to be introduced as an adjunctive protocol to current immunosuppressive regimens, i.e., it would be ethically unacceptable to initially substitute an unproved questionably efficacious tolerance protocol for a highly efficacious although nonspecific immunosuppressive protocol. Thus, it was extremely important to see if the ALS–BM tolerance protocol could be incorporated and possibly be augmented by current immunosuppressive drug regimens.

A finite course of cyclosporine given for 1 week before marrow injection in the standard tolerance protocol does not significantly enhance the tolerance induced in ALS–BM-injected mice. However, a similar course of cyclosporine given after BM injection dramatically increases the degree of tolerance induced (Wood et al., 1988) so that up to 60–70% of ALS-treated, BM-injected, cyclosporine-treated recipients become tolerant over 100 days (Fig. 10). In a similar study (Bobbio et al., 1993), rapamycin was substituted for cyclosporine post-BM injection. Figure 11 shows that with a brief course of adjuvant rapamycin, 100% of the recipients become tolerant over 100 days (Fig. 11). These studies emphasize that in the clinical application of the ALS–BM tolerance model, immunosuppressive therapies such as cyclosporine already used in clinical transplantation can be used as adjuvant therapy to enhance specific tolerance.

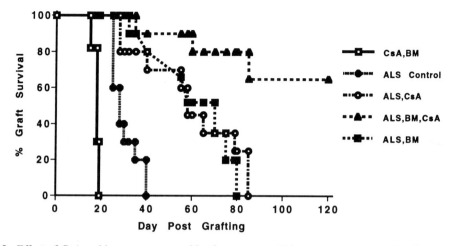

Fig. 10. Effect of CsA and bone marrow on skin allograft prolongation. The effect of CsA treatment started after marrow on the survival of C3H/He skin grafts on ALS-treated B6AF₁ mice given donor bone marrow. CsA treatment was started on day +9 relative to skin grafting on day 0 and marrow injection on day +7.

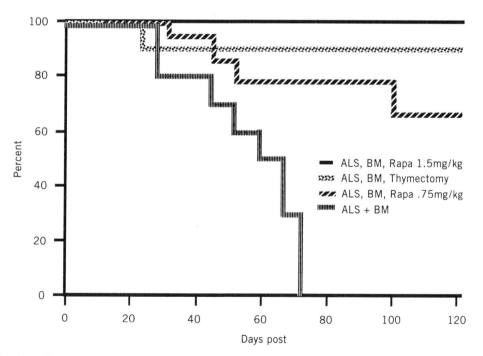

Fig. 11. Effect of ALS, bone marrow, and rapamycin on skin allograft prolongation. B6AF₁ mice were treated with ALS on days −1 and +2 relative to grafting with C3H/He skin on day 0 and donor marrow on day +7. Rapamycin was given from day +9 to +21; thymectomy was performed 1 month prior to grafting.

Induction of Specific Unresponsiveness to Renal Allografts in Antilymphocyte Serum-Treated Dogs Given Donor-Specific Bone Marrow

The use of donor-specific bone marrow infusion in ALS-treated recipients is one of the few adult rodent models of tolerance induction that can be translated to large outbred species using immediately vascularized organs (Caridis et al., 1973; hartner et al., 1986, 1991). The standard canine model involves treatment of a recipient with polyclonal ALS before and after (usually from day −7 through day +7) renal allografting on day 0 followed by infusion of donor specific BMC ($1 - 3 \times 10^8$ bone marrow cells per kilogram) on day +14. In the dog model, the easiest way to obtain adequate BMC is isolation from the ribs. Rib marrow has less blood contamination than from other marrow sources such as the

pelvic bones. This is an advantage since contamination with mature T cells present in the blood can reduce the tolerogenicity of donor BMC (De Fazio et al., 1987a).

In a typical canine renal allograft experiment, normal dogs reject renal allografts in 10–12 days. When only ALS treatment is given, renal allograft survival is increased to 18–40 days. For those recipients given donor-specific BMC after ALS treatment, donor renal allograft survival is significantly augmented beyond that achieved with ALS alone. Typically, 15–20% of grafts in ALS–BMC recipients survive over 150 days or longer with no other immunosuppressive therapy (Fig. 12). *In vitro* immunological studies of these animals strongly suggest that specific immunological tolerance has been induced in ALS–BMC recipients in which there is long-term graft survival. Nonspecific mitogen responses are suppressed for up to 50 days post-

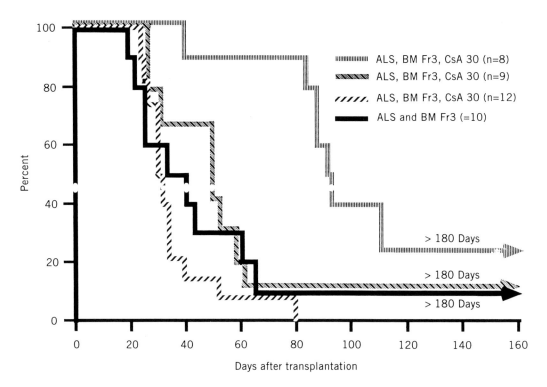

Fig. 12. Effect of CsA dose on renal allograft survival in ALS and BMC fraction 3 (Fr3)-treated outbred dogs. Outbred dogs received renal allografts, bone marrow (fraction 3), and various doses of cyclo-sporine following transplantation. Prolonged survival is observed in all groups compared to ALS control (MST = 27.1 days) with best results obtained when high (30 mg/kg) doses of CsA were used.

ALS treatment due to the nonspecific immunosuppressive effects of ALS. Thereafter, mitogenic responses recover as ALS nonspecific immunosuppressive effects are dissipated. In the case of the mixed lymphocyte responses, both specific donor and third-party MLC responses are suppressed for approximately 50 days after ALS treatment. Thereafter, third-party MLC responses return to normal, but donor-specific MLC responses are dramatically suppressed, emphasizing that donor-specific unresponsiveness has been induced. Furthermore, when ALS-treated, donor BMC recipients with longstanding well-tolerated renal allografts were transplanted with third-party renal allografts to the cervical region, third-party renal allografts were vigorously rejected while the original graft remained well-tolerated without rejection. As with the rodent model, whole bone marrow can be replaced with an active bone marrow fraction prepared by density gradient separation. Also, whole bone marrow or the active fraction can be frozen and stored prior to use, a property that is important for clinical application in human cadaveric transplantation. When protocols emphasizing preparation with polyclonal antilymphocyte serum followed by donor-specific BMC only are used, only 20% or less long-term recipients tolerant to renal allografts was achieved. Again, as with the mouse ALS–BMC protocol, finite courses of supplemental immunosuppression using cyclosporine can increase the percentage of long-term tolerant animals to up to 40% (Fig. 12). In a typical supplemental protocol, recipient dogs are prepared as above with ALS, renal allografting, and donor-specific bone marrow followed by cyclosporine A 5 to 10 mg/kg/day for 30 to 120 days. Although additional long-term tolerant animals can be obtained with such protocols, the number of tolerant animals rarely exceeds 40%. The duration of tolerance is variable, but some long-term tolerant dogs have maintained renal allografts after ALS and donor BMC (with or without temporary cyclosporine A) for up to 5 years. Such animals have maintained normal serum creatinine and persistent nonreactivity to specific donors in MLC for prolonged periods. These canine studies demon-

strated clearly that the ALS–BMC tolerance protocol could be applied with significant efficacy in larger outbred species using a vascularized whole organ, a finding supporting a trial of clinical application.

Induction of Specific Unresponsiveness to Renal Allografts in Antilymphocyte Serum-Treated Nonhuman Primates Given Donor-Specific Bone Marrow

Thomas and colleagues have performed an elegant series of experiments in which the ALS donor BMC protocol has been applied to induce tolerance to renal allografts in nonhuman primates (Rhesus monkey) (Thomas et al., 1991). In these studies, rabbit antihuman thymocyte serum is used for transient immunosuppression and whole bone marrow or bone marrow fractions have been used effectively. As with the rodent and dog experiments, the percentage of animals rendered tolerant can be augmented with supplemental immunosuppression in the form of total lymphoid irradiation or additional immunosuppression with azathioprine or cyclosporine. These authors have provided dramatic evidence for the role of veto cells from the bone marrow as a supplemental mechanism in this model. These investigators compared the ability of various donor bone marrow subpopulations to suppress MLR-induced CML responses of the recipient's peripheral blood cells to the marrow donor. These same marrow subpopulations that were well characterized for phenotypic markers were also compared for their ability to prolong the survival of a renal allograft from the marrow donor. There was an excellent correlation between the *in vivo* and *in vitro* results. The same fractions of whole marrow that induced long-term survival of kidney grafts *in vivo* also suppressed antidonor CML responses *in vitro*. They concluded that the cell in the marrow responsible for the suppressive effect was a veto cell. Since it has already been shown in rodents that long-term tolerance is also associated with suppressor cells (Maki et al., 1981), it is possible that the induction phase of unresponsiveness may be mediated by donor-derived veto cells while the maintenance of unresponsiveness may be regulated by host and donor-derived suppressor cells.

Induction of Unresponsiveness to Human Cadaveric Renal Allografts with Polyclonal Antilymphocyte Serum and Donor-Specific Bone Marrow

Barber and Diethelm and associates (1991) have pioneered the application of the antilymphocyte serum-donor bone marrow tolerance protocol to human renal allotransplantation. In their studies, both kidneys were harvested from standard cadaver donors who also contributed donor bone marrow. Bone marrow was allocated to one of the two recipients of the kidneys in a nonrandom fashion with the recipient of the contralateral kidney entered into the control (no bone marrow) group. These authors demonstrated that recipients given donor-specific bone marrow had improved 1-year graft survival and reduced numbers of rejection reactions. Also, a significant number of bone marrow recipients were able to have their prednisone immunosuppressive drug doses reduced or eliminated. Recently, this group has provided an elegant analysis of the presence and potential role of donor cell chimerism in these ALS–BM-treated recipients (McDaniel et al., 1994). Using polymerase chain reaction techniques to detect HLA antigenic or Y chromosome differences specific for the donor, these authors showed that immediately posttransplant and prior to bone marrow infusion, 26.4% of the marrow group and 18% of the untransfused controls showed allogeneic chimerism in the peripheral blood. In the marrow group chimerism was detected frequently 1–3 months after BM transfusion (65%) and then chimerism diminished to 50–56% of recipients during the interval 3–12 months after transfusion. In the control groups, the incidence of chimerism gradually decreased and was undetectable in the majority of patients 3 months after transplantation while the marrow-transfused recipients were more likely to exhibit chimerism consistently beyond 3 months. Most important from the standpoint of the significance of chimerism was the finding that rejection episodes were significantly affected by the presence of chimerism in the recipients. Of the BM-treated recipients, 91.3% who demonstrated allogeneic chimerism were rejection free as compared with 8.7% who experienced at least one rejection. Interestingly, chimerism in the control (no BM) group correlated with rejection-free survival but the data did not reach significance. Their observation that allogeneic chimerism can occur after solid organ grafting alone (no BM infusion) was consistent with the important observation of Starzl and colleagues (1992) of donor-specific chimerism in recipients of long-term surviving liver allografts.

REFERENCES

Ascher NL, Chen S, Hoffman R, Simmons RL (1983): maturation of cytotoxic T cells within sponge matrix allografts. J Immunol 131:617.

Barber WH, Mankin JA, Laskow DA, Deierhoi MH, Julian BA, Curtis JJ, Diethelm AG (1991): Long-term results of a controlled prospective study with transfusion of donor-specific bone marrow in 57 cadaveric renal allografts recipients. Transplantation 51:70.

Billingham RE, Brent L, Medawar PB (1953): Actively acquired tolerance of foreign cells. Nature (London) 172:603.

Bishop DK, Ferguson RM, Orosz CG (1990): Differential distribution of antigen-specific helper T cells after antigenic stimulation in vivo. J Immunol 144:1153.

Bobbio SA, Wood ML, Monaco AP (1993): Significant augmentation of specific unresponsiveness by rapamycin in ALS-treated, bone marrow injected mice. Transplant 3:51.

Burnett FM (1959): "The Clonal Theory of Acquired Immunity." Cambridge: Cambridge University Press.

Caridis T, Liegeois A, Barrett I, Monaco AP (1973): ALS-treated dogs given bone marrow. Enhanced survival of canine renal allografts. Transplant Proc 5:671–674.

De Fazio SR, Hartner WC, Monaco AP, Gozzo JJ (1987a): Effect of post-transplantation administration of peripheral blood lymphocytes in skin-grafted mice treated with antilymphocyte serum plus bone marrow. Transplantation 44:70.

De Fazio SR, Hartner WC, Monaco AP, Gozzo JJ (1987b): Effect of post-transplantation administration of peripheral blood lymphocytes in skin-grafted mice treated with antilymphocyte serum plus bone marrow. Transplantation 44:70.

Gozzo JJ, Wood ML, Monaco AP (1970): Use of allogeneic, homozygous bone marrow cells for the induction of specific immunologic tolerance in mice treated with antilymphocyte serum. Surg Forum 21:281–284.

Gozzo JJ, Crowley M, Maki T, Monaco AP (1982): Functional characteristics of a Ficoll separated mouse bone marrow cell population involved in skin allograft prolongation. J Immunol 129:1584.

Hartner WC, De Fazio SR, Maki T, Markess TG, Monaco AP, Gozzo JJ (1986): Prolongation of renal allograft survival in antilymphocyte serum-treated dogs by post-operative injection of density gradient fractionated donor bone marrow. Transplantation 42:593.

Hartner WC, Markees TG, De Fazio SR, Khouri W, Maki T, Monaco AP, Gozzo JJ (1991): The effect of antilymphocyte serum, fractionated donor bone marrow, and cyclosporine on renal allograft survival in mongrel dogs. Transplantation 52:784–789.

Liegeois A, Charreire J, Brennan JL (1974): Allograft enhancement induced by bone marrow cells. Surg Forum 25:297–298.

Maki T, Gottschalk R, Wood ML, Monaco AP (1981): Specific unresponsiveness to skin allografts in ALS treated, marrow injected mice: Participation of donor marrow-derived suppressor T cells. J Immunol 127:1433–1438.

McDaniel DO, Naftilan J, Hulvey K, Shaneyfelt S, Lemons JA, Lagoo-Deenadayalan S, Hudson S, Diethelm AG, Barber WH (1994): Peripheral blood chimerism in renal allograft recipients transfused with donor bone marrow. Transplantation 57:852–856.

Monaco AP, Wood ML (1970): Studies on heterologous antilymphocyte serum in mice. VII. Optimal cellular antigen for induction of immunologic tolerance with antilymphocyte serum. Transplant Proc 2:489–496.

Monaco AP, Wood ML, Maki T, Gozzo JJ (1989): Future strategies in immunosuppression: Problems and potential for the induction of specific unresponsiveness to organ allografts in clinical transplantation. Transplant Proc 21:3939.

Monaco AP, Wood ML, Gottschalk R, Seiler FR (1991): Effect of granulocyte-macrophage colony stimulating factor on the induction of unresponsiveness by lymphoid cells. Transplantation 51:213–218.

Muraoka S, Miller RG (1980): Cells in bone marrow and in T cell colonies grown from bone marrow can suppress generation of cytotoxic T lymphocytes directed against self-antigens. J Exp Med 152:54.

Starzl TE, Trucco M, Zeevi A et al. (1992): Systemic chimerism in human female recipients of male liver. Lancet 340:876.

Streilein JW (1991): Neonatal tolerance of H-2 alloantigens: Procuring graft acceptance the old-fashioned way. Transplantation 52:1.

Streilein JW, Strome P, Wood PJ (1989): Failure of in vitro assays to predict accurately the existence of neonatally induced H-2 tolerance. Transplantation 48:630.

Takahashi T, Maki T (1990): Cloning self-major histocompatibility complex antigen specific suppressor cells from adult bone marrow. J Exp Med 172:901.

Thomas JM, Carver FM, Cunningham PRG, Olson LC, Thomas FT (1991): Kidney allograft tolerance in primates without chronic immunosuppression: The role of veto cells. Transplantation 51:198.

Thomas JM, Carver FM, Kasten-Jolly J, Haisch CE, Rebellato LM, Gross U, Vore SJ, Thomas FT (1994): Further studies of veto activity in Rhesus monkey bone marrow in relation to allograft tolerance and chimerism. Transplantation 57:101.

Tomita Y, Mayumi H, Eto M, Nomoto K (1990): Importance of suppressor T cells in cyclophosphamide induced tolerance to non-H-2 encoded alloantigen: Is mixed chimerism really required in maintaining skin allograft tolerance. J Immunol 144:463–468.

Wood ML, Monaco AP (1980): Suppressor cells in specific unresponsiveness to skin allografts in ALS treated, marrow injected mice. Transplantation 29:196.

Wood ML, Monaco AP, Gozzo JJ, Liegeois A (1971): Use of homozygous allogeneic bone marrow for induction of tolerance with antilymphocyte serum: Dose and timing. Transplant Proc 3:676–679.

Wood ML, Gottschalk R, Monaco AP (1988): The effect of cyclosporine on the induction of unresponsiveness in ALS-treated, marrow-injected mice. Transplantation 46:449.

Wood ML, Orosz CG, Gottschalk R, Monaco AP (1992): The effect of injection of donor bone marrow on the frequency of donor-reactive CTL in antilymphocyte serum-treated, grafted mice. Transplantation 54:665–671.

Chapter 16
The Veto Phenomenon and Transplantation Tolerance

Richard G. Miller

The veto hypothesis states that there are specialized antigen-presenting cells (APC) that, when recognized by a T cell, deliver signals leading to the inactivation, rather than activation, of that T cell (Fig. 1). The existence of such cells ("veto cells") can be demonstrated directly *in vitro* and there is strong indirect evidence for their activity *in vivo*. The ability to veto is a physiological property of a cell and there appear to be several different cell types possessing this ability. The normal biological function of veto cells remains speculative, but they may be involved in the maintenance of peripheral T cell tolerance and/or T cell immunoregulation. Whatever their normal function, there are promising indications they can be used to establish transplantation tolerance in a manner that makes the host specifically unresponsive to the graft with no effect on the rest of the immune system.

The first section of this chapter reviews *in vitro* experimental evidence for the existence of veto cells and describes their properties. The second section describes *in vivo* data of direct relevance to transplantation that can be explained by the veto phenomenon, but for which the exact mechanism has not been definitively established. Only a few key reference are given. For more extensive reviews of older work, see Miller (1986), Fink et al. (1988), Miller et al. (1988), and Rammensee (1989).

DEMONSTRATION OF THE VETO PHENOMENON IN AN MLR

The Basic Phenomenon

Veto cells are defined operationally. Let A and B be two MHC-different inbred mouse strains. In an A anti-B mixed lymphocyte reaction (MLR), lymphoid cells from one strain (here strain A) are cocultured with irradiated lymphoid cells from another strain (here strain B). Cytotoxic T lymphocytes (CTL) will develop from the strain A responder cells. These CTL can recognize and kill cells from strain B and from any other strain carrying the same class I MHC determinants. To search for a veto cell, one looks for a cell subpopulation from strain B that, when added to the MLR, suppresses the development of A anti-B CTL but does not suppress CTL development in a B anti-A or anti-C MLR. If these conditions are met, the added cells are specifically suppressing the development of a response against their own cell surface determinants. Next, one tests whether suppression is still observed when required growth factors [such as interleukin 2 (IL-2)] are added to the cultures. If so, it is unlikely that suppression is due to something missing from the cultures. These results by themselves do not establish that the added cells are acting as deletional APC but merely that they produce response reduction against their own de-

Transplantation Immunology, pages 267–276
© 1995 Wiley-Liss, Inc.

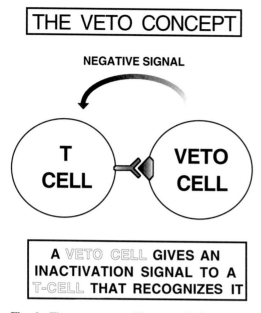

Fig. 1. The veto concept. The veto cell gives an inactivation signal to a T cell that recognizes it.

terminants by inactivating something other than required growth factors. That the added cells are acting as deletional APC is the simplest, but not the only explanation. More direct evidence that the added cells act as deletional APC will be given later.

Using the MLR assay procedure outlined above, veto activity has been demonstrated in bone marrow, thymus, and fetal liver of normal mice, and in spleen and bone marrow of athymic nude mice. Veto activity is not found on direct testing *in vitro* of such tissues as normal spleen or lymph node. Normally these tissues contain predominantly mature, resting small lymphocytes. However, mature T cells in spleen can acquire veto activity after a brief incubation *in vitro*. During this time, many of the T cells become activated and it appears that at least some, confined to the CD8$^+$ subset, simultaneously acquire veto activity. In fact it has been shown that mature CD8$^+$ CTL have veto activity against CTL precursors capable of recognizing them. Thus, cells from an established CTL line originating from strain A will, when added to an MLR, suppress the development of CTL against A or any strain sharing class I MHC with A,

independent of the specificity of the added CTL and independent of the strain of origin of the responder cells. The mechanism does not appear to involve the TCR of the CTL nor to use the cytotoxic machinery of the CTL. However, as described later, it does appear to depend upon the presence of CD8 on the added CTL.

The mechanism of the veto phenomenon is most easily explained by assuming the veto cell is triggered to suppress when its cell surface determinants are recognized. The most direct evidence for this has been obtained in an MLR in which CTL against trinitrophenol (TNP)-modified self-determinants were generated. In this assay, responder lymphoid cells from, e.g., strain A are TNP modified and put in culture. CTL develop which lyse TNP-modified target cells sharing class I MHC with A but do not lyse unmodified target cells. The CTL are TNP specific and class I MHC restricted. When veto cells from strain A [nude spleen cells in the original experiments (Miller, 1980)] are added, they suppress CTL development only if they too are TNP modified, implying they must be recognized to produce response reduction (see Table I).

Figure 2 illustrates the development of a clone of CTL from a CTL precursor (CTLp). On encountering a stimulatory or "professional" APC, it receives an activation signal. Physically, over the next 24 hr, it undergoes "blast transformation" in which it nearly doubles its volume (CTLp* in Fig. 2). Internally, many genes have been activated, one of the most critical being the IL-2 receptor α chain (p55) gene that, in combination with the constitutively expressed IL-2R receptor β and γ chains, allows the assembly of a high affinity IL-2 receptor. If IL-2 is present, the CTLp will have entered S phase of the cell cycle by 48 hr and, over the next 3 days, at least 5 cell divisions will occur to form a clone of CTL. Where in this pathway does a veto cell act? It might inactivate CTLp or reduce CTL clone size or block the action of mature CTL. As a first step in answering this question, CTLp frequencies were measured (by limiting dilution) in the presence and absence of added veto cells. The result was that CTLp frequency was reduced in the presence of veto cells. As a second step in delineating exactly where in the pathway veto cells

Table I. The Veto Cell Must Carry the Antigen Being Recognized

Responder cells	Stimulator cells	Veto cells	Response
			(A-TNP target)
A	A-TNP	0	+++
A	A-TNP	A	+++
A	A-TNP	A-TNP	+
			(A target)
B	A	0	+++
B	A	A	+
B	A	A-TNP	+

acted, they were added at varying times after MLR culture initiation and removed at varying times after addition. The result was that MLR cultures were insensitive to veto signals before 24 hr, then became maximally sensitive, but rapidly became insensitive after 48 hr. Thus the window of maximum sensitivity occurred after the CTLp had blasted but before they had actively entered cell cycle. The veto cells were equally effective during this time window, whether or not exogenous IL-2 was added. These experiments provide direct evidence that veto cells inactivate activated CTLp that recognize them.

The Role of CD8

CTL lines are very effective veto cells whereas T helper lines are not. One possibility is that the CD8 molecule, usually present on CTL lines and absent on T helper lines, can play a role in

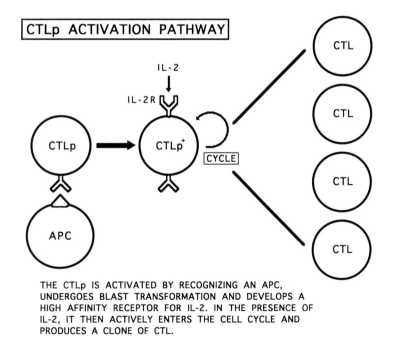

THE CTLp IS ACTIVATED BY RECOGNIZING AN APC, UNDERGOES BLAST TRANSFORMATION AND DEVELOPS A HIGH AFFINITY RECEPTOR FOR IL-2. IN THE PRESENCE OF IL-2, IT THEN ACTIVELY ENTERS THE CELL CYCLE AND PRODUCES A CLONE OF CTL.

Fig. 2. The CTLp activation pathway. The CTLp is activated by recognizing an APC, undergoes blast transformation, and develops a high affinity receptor for IL-2. In the presence of IL-2, it then actively enters the cell cycle and produces a clone of CTL.

the veto signal. To test this directly, CTL lines with or without CD8 and with the same specificity and apparent affinity were isolated from MLR cultures and tested for veto activity (Kaplan et al., 1989; Sambhara and Miller, 1991). Only the CD8+ CTL lines were active as veto cells. When anti-CD8 antibody specific for the CD8 on the veto cells (but not for the CD8 on the responder cells) was added to the cultures, the veto activity was largely eliminated. This implies a direct role for CD8 in delivering the veto signal. As a further test of this idea, CD8$^-$ myelolymphoid cell lines have been transfected with CD8 and tested for veto activity (Hambor et al., 1990; Sambhara and Miller, 1991). Such lines, initially inactive, acquire veto activity on transfection with CD8.

The CD8 molecule is expressed on the cell surface as a dimer composed either of 2 α chains or an α chain and a β chain. In the transfection experiments in which cell lines acquired veto activity on being transfected with CD8, only the α chain was transfected. Thus the α–α dimer can deliver a veto signal. The α chain has a cytoplasmic tail that can interact with the tyrosine kinase p56^{lck} and an extracellular domain that can interact with the α$_3$ domain of the class I MHC molecule. The α$_1$ and α$_2$ domains of class I MHC are highly polymorphic and form the peptide-binding groove of the class I MHC molecule. The α$_3$ domain is relatively invariant and

its principal role appears to be to form a binding site for CD8. It now seems that the CD8-class I MHC interaction has three quite different roles:

1. CD8 can act as a coreceptor in T cell recognition. When the T cell receptor (TCR) on a CD8$^+$ cell interacts with the α$_1$/α$_2$ domains of class I MHC on another cell, CD8 interacts with α$_3$ of the same MHC molecule, thus strengthening the bond and perhaps also (via p56^{lck}) generating a signal inside the recognizing T cell.

2. CD8 can generate a veto signal. When the cell being recognized carries CD8, it can interact with class I MHC on the recognizing T cell, leading to the generation of a veto signal. Figure 3 shows CD8 simultaneously playing both roles. The CD8 on the CTLp is acting as a coreceptor; the CD8 on the veto cell is acting as a veto signaller.

3. CD8 may play a role in positive selection during T cell ontogeny in the thymus. The hypothesis is that if the TCR of a CD4$^+$CD8$^+$ thymocyte can recognize a class I MHC molecule on thymic epithelium, then when CD8 (acting as a coreceptor) also recognizes class I MHC, the result is commitment of the cell to mature into a CD4$^-$CD8$^+$ T-lymphocyte.

The mechanism by which CD8 generates a veto signal is not totally clear. Either CD8 inter-

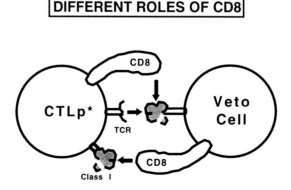

Fig. 3. Different roles of CD8. The CD8 on the CTLp is acting as a coreceptor; the CD8 on the veto cell is delivering the veto signal.

acting with class I MHC on the CTLp induces a signal directly via class I MHC that leads to inactivation of the CTLp or the CD8–α_3 interaction triggers the veto cell to produce a factor that inactivates the CTLp. There is evidence for both possibilities.

In the experiments in which cell lines acquired veto activity on being transfected with CD8α, additional experiments have been done (Hambor et al., 1990) in which a truncated CD8α lacking the cytoplasmic tail was transfected in a manner that it was anchored to the membrane via a lipid

tail. This cell line could directly deliver a veto signal. Further, monoclonal antibody supernatants specific for α_3 were found to be able to replace the need for CD8 in delivering the veto signal (Sambhara and Miller, 1991). In these latter experiments, T cells were polyclonally activated with one antibody (anti-CD3) and polyclonally vetoed with a second (anti-α_3). Since all cells were affected, it was possible to directly observe their fate. They all underwent apoptosis.

Both the truncated CD8 and anti-α_3 observations favor direct signaling of the CTLp via class

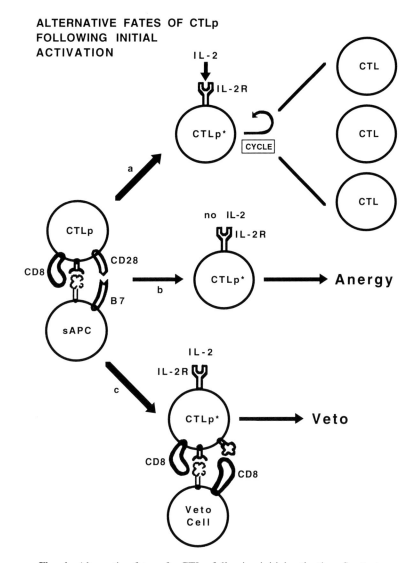

Fig. 4. Alternative fates of a CTLp following initial activation. See text.

I MHC as the veto mechanism. However, when the anti-α_3 antibodies were purified, they lost their ability to generate a veto signal, implying that some nonspecific factor in the supernatant (as yet unidentified) is also required. The cell lines used in the CD8 transfection experiments have all been of myelolymphoid origin and may be producing such a factor constitutively. Note that there is evidence that extracellular interactions with cell surface molecules anchored by a lipid tail can generate phosphorylation events within the cell (Stefanova et al., 1991).

There may be mechanisms other than CD8–α_3 class I interaction for generating a veto signal. It has been long known that cells in bone marrow possess veto activity (Muraoka and Miller, 1980). Recently, cells with veto activity that induce activated CTLp to undergo cell death have been grow from bone marrow in the presence of IL-2 (Hiruma et al., 1992). These cells are Thy-1$^+$, NK-1.1$^+$ and probably lack CD8.

Fates of a T Cell following Activation

Figure 4 summarizes much of what is known about the different pathways leading to T cell activation or inactivation. On the left, one sees a CTLp interacting with a stimulatory or professional APC (sAPC). The TCR of the CTLp is interacting with class I MHC on the sAPC and CD8 is acting as a coreceptor. This is insufficient to produce activation. A costimulatory signal is also required, here provided by an interaction between CD28 on the CTLp and B7 on the sAPC. What happens when the costimulatory signal is not present appears to depend on other variables not yet fully understood. Most frequently, it seems that nothing at all happens and the CTLp continues on its way. In other instances, it appears that the CTLp is rendered unresponsive by down-regulating its TCR, or CD8, or through other internal changes.

Given that a costimulatory signal is present, the CTLp undergoes blast transformation and develops a high affinity receptor for IL-2 (IL-2R). At least three different outcomes are now possible. In path **a** (Fig. 4, top), the activated CTLp (CTLp*) receives IL-2, enters cell cycle, and produces a clone of CTL. This is the normal activation pathway. In path **b** (Fig. 4, middle), the CTLp does not receive IL-2 and as a result is rendered "anergic," i.e., is put into a state in which it is unresponsive to appropriate activation signals. It does not die (at least not immediately) but cannot respond either. In path **c** (Fig. 4, bottom), the CTLp encounters a deletional APC (dAPC) or veto cell. The TCR of the CTLp recognizes class I MHC on the dAPC with CD8 acting as a coreceptor. In turn, the CD8 on the dAPC recognizes class I MHC on the CTLp leading to the generation of a veto signal that inactivates the CTLp in a process that appears to lead to cell death by apoptosis. Note that the CD8–class I MHC interaction is analogous to the B7–CD28 interaction, but here leads to inactivation rather than activation.

IN VIVO STUDIES

The Donor-Specific Transfusion Effect

Can veto cells be used to enhance graft survival? In principle, veto cells from the graft donor could be used to inactivate host T cells that recognize them and thus enhance graft survival. Evidence consistent with the veto hypothesis has been available for some time through independent studies using mice and in clinical studies of kidney transplantation in man. In the mouse studies, mice were injected intravenously with viable foreign lymphoid cells. When these mice were subsequently tested for their ability to generate CTL in tissue culture, it was found that the antidonor CTL response was specifically reduced (Miller and Phillips, 1976) and that this reduction was due to inactivation of host antidonor CTLp (Rammensee et al., 1984). Further, donor skin grafts could persist indefinitely in these mice (Kast et al., 1988; Heeg and Wagner, 1990; Sheng-Tanner and Miller, 1992). In parallel, it was found in clinical studies of kidney transplant recipients that prior donor-specific blood transfusion leads to enhanced kidney graft survival (Opelz et al., 1981; Lagaaij et al., 1989). The above results can be explained by assuming the infused lymphocytes act as veto cells that inactivate T cells that recognize them.

Recent mouse studies have focused on obtaining more detailed evidence on the mechanism(s) involved. Let A and B be two MHC-different inbred mouse strains. Injection of (A × B)F$_1$ viable lymphoid cells into A inactivates both CTLp (Martin and Miller, 1989) and T helper precursors (Kiziroglu and Miller, 1991) in A that can recognize B. The injected cells can be given a long-lived fluorescent label [with (fluorescein isothiocynate (FITC)]. This does not alter their biological properties and enables one to determine what happens to them *in vivo*. It was found that the injected cells rapidly enter into and equilibrate within 1 to 2 days with the recirculating lymphocyte pool of the host. Donor-reactive host T cells are inactivated in the animal within 3 days of injection of F$_1$ cells. This was shown in tissue culture using, as responder cells, a host lymphoid cell suspension from which donor F$_1$ cells had been removed by cell sorting. Recovered F$_1$ cells, but not host cells, could transfer

response reduction to a naive A recipient (see Fig. 5).

Many investigators have attributed the response reduction seen in this system to donor-specific suppressor cells developed by the host. The fact that F$_1$ cells recovered from an injected host and not host cells could transfer response reduction to a second host rules out this possibility and is consistent with the injected cells acting as veto cells that inactivate T cells that recognize them. One caveat should be added to this conclusion. The fluorescent label used in the above studies slowly disappeared and only allowed reliable separation of host and donor cells for up to about 10 days following injection, so that the possibility that donor-specific suppressor cells develop at later times cannot be excluded. Minor H-incompatible skin graft survival can be prolonged indefinitely in mice given anti-CD4 and anti-CD8 monoclonal antibodies. The host appears to establish some kind of sup-

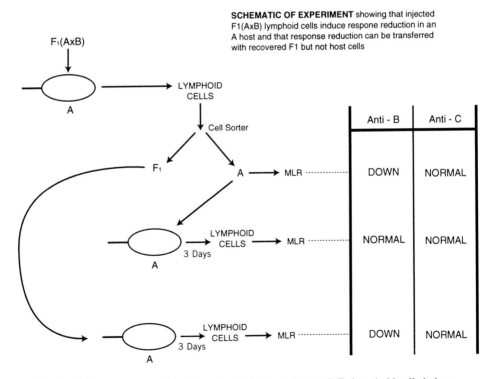

Fig. 5. Schematic of experiment showing that injected (A × B)F$_1$ lymphoid cells induce response reduction in an A host and that response reduction can be transferred with recovered F$_1$ but not host cells.

pressive state that can be transferred to a naive host at later times, but that this takes about 3 weeks to establish (Qin et al., 1993).

When an A recipient is injected with (A × B) F_1 lymphoid cells, the host antidonor response measured *in vitro* is reduced about 80% within 3 days and stays down for more than 6 weeks (Martin and Miller, 1989). Despite this residual response, an F_1 skin graft can survive indefinitely. The nature of the residual responsive cells is unclear. One possibility is that the injected F_1 cells rapidly lose their ability to inactivate donor cells. This possibility was ruled out by injecting an A host with unlabeled F_1 cells and at varying times, later injecting labeled A cells, recovering them 3 days later, and testing them *in vitro*. Their ability to respond was reduced 80% (Martin et al., 1992).

What is the fate of the donor reactive T cells? Have they been killed (deleted) or rendered unresponsive (anergic)? In normal animals, it is not possible to make this distinction as the specificity of a particular T cell can be determined only by activating it and measuring its function. This problem has been overcome with the advent of transgenic mice in which it is possible to engineer a mouse in which a large fraction of the T cells carry a particular T cell receptor of known specificity. Further, one can make a monoclonal antibody that specifically recognizes that TCR. In studies using mice carrying a transgenic TCR (tg-TCR) reactive against male antigen (H-Y) for which there is also a monoclonal antibody that recognizes the tg-TCR, it was found that injection of male lymphoid cells into female mice carrying the tg-TCR led to the disappearance of 80% of the tg-TCR$^+$ CD8$^+$ male-reactive cells (Zhang et al., 1992). To what extent these cells have been physically deleted or have down-regulated either their tg-TCR or CD8 is not fully established. The remaining 20% were fully reactive when tested *in vitro*. Male reactive cells continued to be produced in the thymus but were inactivated in the periphery. In this system, it has also been shown that CD8 on the injected cells appears to play a role in the inactivation: When cells from male mice, either normal or lacking CD4 or CD8 or both were injected, only suspensions containing CD8$^+$ cells produced in-

activation (Zhang et al., 1994). This requirement for CD8 provides further evidence that the injected cells are acting as veto cells that inactivate T cells that recognize them.

The Role of NK Cells

Most (but not all) investigators find that an injection of (A × B)F_1 lymphoid cells into A induces response reduction against B and enhances survival of a B graft. However, injection of B into A usually does not, although the arguments above predict it should. Certainly veto cells from strain B or from strain (A × B)F_1 are equally effective in vetoing an A anti-B MLR response *in vitro*. The difference appears to be that to induce response reduction and enhance graft survival *in vivo*, the injected cells must enter into and remain in the host lymphocyte recirculating pool. F_1 cells injected into A do this but B injected into A do not. Instead, they are rapidly removed by host natural killer (NK) cells (Sheng-Tanner and Miller, 1992). Unlike T cells or B cells that have receptors that recognize specific foreign determinants, NK cells appear to respond to absence of a self-marker associated with (or identical to) class I MHC. Thus (A × B)F_1 cells injected into A are poorly recognized by host NK cells because they carry A MHC. However, cells from strain B lack A MHC and are readily recognized. When NK cells of a recipient A strain mouse are in a very active state, as can be produced by infection or any other process that activates NK cells, even injected F_1 cells will be removed. Thus injection of (A × B)F_1 cells into A mediates donor-specific response reduction and enhances graft survival when NK cells are quiescent, but not when they are active. Experiments using mutant mice differing from the original strain only at a single class I or class II MHC locus show that both can enhance graft survival if they can recirculate (Sheng-Tanner and Miller, 1994). The class II-only different cells always work as they cannot be removed by NK cells. The class I-only different cells work reliably only when injected into an F_1 strain also carrying the MHC of the host.

The need for persistent recirculation of injected lymphoid cells to establish tolerance and the role of NK cells in reducing this persistence suggest some guidelines for the use of this approach in clinical transplantation.

1. The host should have a relatively low level of NK activity. In particular, the host should not be suffering from an acute virus infection as this elevates NK activity.

2. The persistence of injected cells should be monitored.

3. The injected cells should share class I MHC with the host. Transfusion of parental lymphoid cells into a child would be ideal as this mimics the $(A \times B)F_1$ into A mouse model.

4. Class II differences should be avoided as much as possible. Although class II MHC is not itself a target of NK cells, it can stimulate the host to produce interferon-γ (IFN-γ) that is a potent inducer of NK cells.

Note that the above guidelines predict empirical conclusions reached from detailed analysis of the success of the blood transfusion effect in human studies (Lagaaij et al., 1989).

Comments on Some other *in Vivo* Studies

There is an enormous literature on the induction of specific transplantation tolerance. Much of it is contradictory. No attempt will be made here to resolve the discrepancies and paradoxes. Within the narrower field of using intravenous infusion of allogenic lymphoid cells, many controversies might be resolved by taking into account the role of NK cells outlined above. If the injected cells are actively removed, they might well prime an immune response so that a cytotoxic drug given a few days after injection could well induce partial tolerance by killing all the graft-reactive cells that have been driven into cell cycle.

The NIMA phenomenon provides an interesting example of a possible role for veto cells *in vivo*. Some human patients, for varying reasons, become highly sensitized to foreign class I MHC and have circulating antibodies against most MHC specificities. Claas et al. (1988) found that this often corresponded to those class I MHC molecules present in the mother but not inherited

by the child (noninherited maternal antigens or NIMA). There is not a similar deficit in antibodies reactive against noninherited paternal antigens (NIPA). One possibility is that during pregnancy or nursing, maternal lymphocytes enter into and persist in the child where they act as veto cells, thus inactivating NIMA-reactive T cells and preventing production of antibodies against NIMA. Consistent with this, Zhang et al. (1991) found that the frequency of CTLp reactive against NIMA, but not against NIPA, was significantly reduced in about half of normal human individuals. In a mouse study, H-$2^{b/b}$ mice born of an H-$2^{b/d}$ mother often showed prolonged survival of an H-2^d skin graft. Prolonged survival correlated with the presence of circulating maternal T cells (Zhang and Miller, 1993). A preclinical transplantation model using kidneys provides a particularly promising model for establishing a role for veto cells in solid organ transplantation. In these studies (Thomas et al., 1991), rhesus monkeys had their kidneys removed, were given rabbit antithymocyte antiserum (ATG), and both bone marrow (BM) and a kidney from a full allogeneic donor. Long-term survival of the kidney graft is routinely observed, but only if both ATG and allogeneic BM are given. *In vitro* studies are fully consistent with a subpopulation of cells in the injected BM acting as veto cells.

REFERENCES

Claas FHJ, Gijbels Y, vander Velden-de Munck J, van Rood JJ (1988): Induction of B cell unresponsiveness to non-inherited maternal antigens during fetal life. Science 241:1815–1817.

Fink PJ, Shimenkovitz RP, Bevan MJ (1988): Veto cells. Annu Rev Immunol 6:115–147.

Hambor JE, Kaplan DR, Tykocinski ML (1990): CD8 functions as an inhibitory ligand in mediating the immunoregulatory activity of CD8$^+$ cells. J Immunol 145:1646–1652.

Heeg K, Wagner H (1990): Induction of peripheral tolerance to class I Major Histocompatibility Complex (MHC) alloantigens in adult mice: Transfused class I MHC-incompatible splenocytes veto clonal responses of antigen-reactive Lyt-2$^+$ T cells. J Exp Med 172:719–728.

Hiruma K, Nakamura H, Henkart PA, Gress RE (1992): Clonal deletion of portthymic T cells: Veto cells kill precursor cytotoxic T lymphocytes. J Exp Med 175:863–868.

Kaplan DR, Hambor JE, Tykocinski ML (1989): An immunoregulatory function for the CD8 molecule. Proc Natl Acad Sci USA 86:8512–8515.

Kast WM, Van Twuyver E, Mooijaart RJD, Verveld M, Kamphuis AGA, Melief CJM, De Waal LP (1988): Mechanism of shin allograft enhancement across and H-2 class I mutant difference. Evidence for involvement of veto cells. Eur J Immunol 18:2105–2108.

Kiziroglu F, Miller RG (1991): *In vivo* functional clonal deletion of recipient CD4$^+$ T helper precursor cells that can recognize class II MHC on injected donor lymphoid cells. J Immunol 146:1104–1112.

Lagaaij EL, Hennemann IPH, Ruigrok M, de Haan MW, Persijn GG, Termijtelan A, Hendriks GFJ, Weimar W, Claas FHJ, van Rood JJ (1989): Effect of one-HL-DR-antigen-matched and completely HLA-DR-mismatched blood transfusions on survival of heart and kidney allografts. N Engl J Med 321:701–705.

Martin DR, Miller RG (1989): *In vivo* administration of histoimcompatible lymphocytes leads to rapid functional deletion of cytotoxic T lymphocyte precursors. J Exp Med 170:679–690.

Martin DR, Sheng-Tanner X, Miller RG (1992): Intravenous injection of histoimcompatible lymphocytes results in both rapid and long-term changes to host cytotoxic T lymphocytes precursors reactive to donor antigens. Transplantation 54:125–129.

Miller RG, Phillips RA (1976): Reduction in the *in vitro* cytotoxic lymphocyte response produced by in vivo exposure to semiallogeneic cells: Recruitment or active suppression? J Immunol 117:1913–1921.

Miller RG (1980): An immunological suppressor cell inactivating cytotoxic T-lymphocyte precursor cells recognizing it. Nature (London) 287:544–546.

Miller RG (1986): The veto phenomenon and T cell regulation. Immunol Today 7:112–114.

Miller RG, Muraoka S, Claesson MH, Reimann J, Benveniste P (1988): The veto phenomenon in T cell regulation. Ann NY Acad Sci 532:170–176.

Muraoka S, Miller RG (1980): Cells in bone marrow and in T cell colonies grown from bone marrow can suppress generation of cytotoxic T lympho-cytes directed against their self antigens. J Exp Med 152:54–71.

Opelz G, Mickey MR, Teraski PI (1981): Blood transfusions and kidney transplants: Remaining controversies. Transplant Proc 13:136.

Qin S, Cobbold SP, Pope H, Elliott J, Kionssis D, Davies J, Waldmann H (1993): "Infectious" transplantation tolerance. Science 259:974–977.

Rammensee H-G, Fink PJ, Bevan MJ (1984): Functional clonal deletion of class I-specific cytotoxic T lymphocytes by veto cells that express antigen. J Immunol 133:2390–2396.

Rammensee H-G (1989): Veto function *in vitro* and *in vivo*. Int Rev Immunol 4:175–190.

Sambhara SR, Miller RG (1991): Programmed cell death of T cells signalled through the T cell receptor and the α_3 domain of class I MHC. Science 252:1424–1427.

Sheng-Tanner X, Miller RG (1992): Correlation between lymphocyte-induced donor-specific tolerance and donor cell recirculation. J Exp Med 176:407–413.

Sheng-Tanner X, Miller RG (1994): Correlation between lymphocyte-induced donor-specific tolerance and donor cell recirculation. Transplantation 57:1081–1087.

Stefanova I, Horejsi V, Ansotegui IJ, Knapp W, Stockinger H (1991): GPI-anchored cell-surface molecules complexed to protein tyrosine kinases. Science 25:1016–1019.

Thomas JM, Carver FM, Cunningham PRG, Olson LC, Thomas FT (1991): Kidney allograft tolerance in primates without chronic immunosuppression: The role of veto cells. Transplantation 51:198.

Zhang L, van Rood JJ, Claas FHJ (1991): The T cell repertoire is not dictated by self antigens alone. Res Immunol 142:441–445.

Zhang L, Martin DR, Fung-Leung W-P, Teh H-S, Miller RG (1992): Peripheral deletion of mature CD8$^+$ antigen-specific T cells after *in vivo* exposure to male antigen. J Immunol 148:3740–3745.

Zhang L, Miller RG (1993): The correlation of prolonged survival of maternal skin grafts with the presence aof naturally transferred maternal T cell. Transplantation 56:918–921.

Zhang L, Shannon J, Sheldon J, Teh H-S, Mak TW, Miller RG (1994): Role of infused CD8$^+$ cells in the induction of peripheral tolerance. J Immunol 152:2222–2228.

Chapter 17
The Transfusion Story and Tolerance

Kathryn J. Wood and Peter J. Morris

INTRODUCTION

The Recognition of the Transfusion Effect and Early Experimental Work

In any immune response, T cells always have to make a choice whenever they encounter antigen. Responses to alloantigens are no different. When alloantigens are encountered by a potential transplant recipient, the immune system can respond in at least three different ways. The encounter may simply be ignored and have no effect on subsequent responses to the same alloantigens. On the other hand, exposure can result in the priming of the immune system, such that the individual either becomes sensitized to a subsequent challenge by the same antigen, or the recipient may become unresponsive when exposed to the same antigen on other occasions. The outcome of any antigen encounter will vary depending on a large number of factors. These include for any antigen, the route of antigen presentation, the form of the antigen presented, and the immune status of the recipient.

As renal transplantation became more accepted as an alternative to dialysis for the treatment of patients with end-stage renal failure in the 1960s, the transplant community first became aware of the role of donor-specific cytotoxic antibodies in the phenomenon of hyperacute rejection (Morris et al., 1968; Patel and Terasaki, 1969) and as a result became concerned that dialysis patients who were repeatedly transfused because of anemia resulting from long-term dialysis would become sensitized to alloantigen and thus virtually impossible to transplant. This concern led several groups to examine graft survival in their patients in order to determine whether graft rejection was increased in patients who had received large numbers of transfusions before transplantation. To their initial surprise this did not turn out to be the case.

In a study of 29 patients, Dossetor and his colleagues (Dossetor et al., 1967) found not a negative correlation, but a clear positive association between blood transfusion and graft survival. Indeed, they found that graft survival was higher in those patients who had received the greatest number of transfusions. The patients fell clearly into two groups, the first, comprising patients who had received an average of 40 transfusions before transplantation had a mean graft survival of 33%, and a second in which patients who had received an average of 86 transfusions had a graft survival rate of 80% at 1 year (Table I).

Morris and his colleagues (Morris et al., 1968) were also able to show that previous blood transfusions did not increase the risk of graft rejection. Although their data did not show that patients who had larger numbers of transfusions had any advantage in terms of improved graft outcome than those patients receiving a smaller number of transfusions, they were among the first to suggest that deliberately exposing patients to alloantigen before transplantation may have a beneficial effect on graft outcome. Importantly, they also suggested that the apparent protective effect of pregraft blood transfusion might be a clinical manifestation of the same effect that had been reported in experimental systems, where significant graft prolongation could be achieved by pretreating the recipient with donor strain cells (e.g., Billingham et al., 1953).

Transplantation Immunology, pages 277–294
© 1995 Wiley-Liss, Inc.

Table I. Preoperative Blood Transfusion Had a Beneficial Effect on Graft Survival[a]

Group	Average number of transfusions	Mean graft survival at 1 year (%)
1	40	33
2	86	80

[a]Data taken from Dossetor et al. (1967).

There can be little doubt that the classical experiments of Billingham, Brent, and Medawar in the 1950s laid the foundation for the majority of subsequent work in the general area of antigen-induced tolerance. Their initial attempts to deliberately induce tolerance to alloantigen stemmed from observations made by Owen (1945), who noted that dizygotic cattle twins each contained red blood cells from the other twin. This prompted Billingham and his colleagues to show that the majority of these twins were tolerant of skin grafts from each other (Billingham et al., 1951) and consequently attempt to induce tolerance *in vivo* deliberately (Billingham et al., 1953). In the initial experiments, 15- to 16-day-old fetuses were injected *in utero* with cells from a genetically disparate strain of mouse (strain A). Eight weeks later, the resultant offspring were challenged with a skin graft from the same strain, A. Although two of the five animals rejected their grafts at control rates, the other three showed substantial prolongation, and two of the grafts survived indefinitely. Most importantly, they also showed that the mice with surviving grafts would accept a second skin graft from strain A donors, but not other strains, e.g., C, D, etc. without any further treatment, but if the otherwise tolerant mice were transplanted lymph nodes removed from a syngeneic mouse deliberately sensitized against strain A, the previously accepted strain A skin grafts and second grafts from the same strain were rejected. In subsequent experiments, the same authors demonstrated that alloantigen did not have to be delivered *in utero,* but could be administered intravenously (iv) to the newborn mice within 24 hr of birth (Billingham and Brent, 1959).

The work of Billingham, Brent, and Medawar clearly showed that the immune response to al-

loantigen could be modified by exposing the developing immune system to alloantigen *in vivo*. The administration of alloantigen to neonates was not regarded as having potential clinical application at the time, but now that certain congenital and other abnormalities that can be treated effectively by transplantation can be diagnosed *in utero,* this approach may be greeted with renewed enthusiasm by the transplant community. Nevertheless, the far more exacting challenge in most situations requiring transplantation was, and for that matter still is, the development of strategies for the induction of tolerance to alloantigen in the adult.

Work began in adults in the 1960s and still continues. For example, Shapiro and colleagues showed in 1961 that it was possible to induce unresponsiveness to skin grafts across an allogeneic barrier in adult mice by multiple injections of donor spleen cells before transplantation. Using a similar protocol, Gowland and Brent were able to induce tolerance by repeated injection of donor strain spleen cells into "young adult" mice, but found that the same strategy was completely ineffective when the mice grew older. It is worthy of note, as we shall return to this point later, that these early reports suggested that the persistence of donor antigen in the recipient was essential for both the induction and maintenance of the unresponsive state. In addition, Gowland also noted that during the induction of tolerance, the "young adult" mice appeared to become sensitized to the allogeneic spleen cells before the critical number of treatments required to induce tolerance had been administered. These two concepts have been redeveloped many times, and have become central to our present understanding of the requirements for the induction of peripheral tolerance to alloantigen in the adult.

These early observations in experimental models of tolerance induction combined with the later observations of Dossetor and Morris renewed interest in the possibility of inducing specific immunological unresponsiveness and ultimately tolerance to alloantigen within the transplant community. Furthermore, the development of an experimental model of a vascularized renal transplant in the rat released the transplant immunologist from "the tyranny of rodent skin graft models" for the study of tolerance induction (Fabre et al., 1971). This led to numerous studies designed to address both the specific requirements for the induction of specific unresponsiveness following exposure to alloantigen as well as the mechanisms responsible for inducing and maintaining the unresponsive state.

Donor Specific vs. Random Transfusion in Clinical Practice

The beneficial influence of blood transfusion on graft outcome was first described in a paper by Opelz and his colleagues who compared the 1 year graft survival rates in 148 recipients who had received kidney grafts from cadaver donors. Graft survival in recipients who had received more than 10 transfusions before transplantation was 66%, compared to 43% in patients who had received between 1 and 10 transfusions and only 29% in the nontransfused group (Opelz et al., 1973). This was different from the earlier studies reported, in that a substantial number of patients who had received no transfusions were included in the analysis. As a result of these reports transplant centers began to introduce deliberate transfusion policies during the 1970s, although concerns over sensitization of recipients, particularly multiparous women, following transfusions were still discussed. However, as more data emerged many clinicians felt that the potential advantages of transfusion before transplantation were more important than the potential risks involved. Data to support this intuitive approach were supported in 1980 when Opelz and Terasaki published data from a multicenter analysis of 2580 patients transplanted in North America. This analysis showed very clearly that the graft survival rates in patients who had received between 6 and 10 transfusions before transplantation was equivalent to that in recipients who had received more than 20. These data, unlike those previously, suggested that a large number of transfusions were not necessarily required to achieve the beneficial effect of pretransplant transfusions on graft survival, thereby reducing some of the risk of sensitization. Interestingly, on the basis of this study, the authors concluded that "the overall outcome of renal transplantation

is influenced to a greater degree by the effect of pre-transplant transfusions than any other variable known to us," a very dramatic statement that had a major influence on the introduction of deliberate transfusion policies at transplant centers that had not previously adopted this policy.

Clearly for recipients of cadaver grafts, there was no established genetic relationship between the blood donors and the eventual organ donor. At the same time as collation of the data for recipients of cadaver grafts, Salvatierra and his colleagues were examining the effect of donor-specific transfusions on the outcome of kidney transplants from living related donors. They also demonstrated a clear positive influence of transfusion on graft outcome (Salvatierra et al., 1983). However, clearly in these cases the blood donor and subsequent organ donor were identical. Immunologically it is easier to develop hypotheses to explain the mechanism by which blood transfusions, or more precisely exposure to donor alloantigens before transplantation, might have a beneficial effect on graft outcome if the recipient is exposed to donor alloantigen before transplantation. It could be argued that as the improvement in the survival of kidney grafts from cadaver donors was related to the number of transfusions there would be sharing of some alloantigens, particularly those that are highly represented in the population, by the cohort of blood donors and the eventual organ donor was extremely high. Indeed this hypothesis was proposed by Morris and colleagues in 1968 (Morris et al., 1968). Therefore random blood transfusion, although not deliberately exposing recipients to donor alloantigens before transplantation, may fortuitously achieve the same result for some if not all of the alloantigens of the organ donor.

Data recently published by transplant centers in The Netherlands have suggested the effect of random transfusions might be improved if information about the HLA type of the blood donors was available. They have shown that if the blood donor and recipient share at least one HLA-DR antigen the effects of transfusion before transplantation are improved compared to the effect in patients receiving transfusions from DR mismatched blood donors (Lagaaij et al., 1989, 1991; van Twuyver et al., 1991).

Although the beneficial effects of alloantigen pretreatment continue to be observed in experimental systems, the position of prior blood transfusions in clinical renal transplantation is much less clear in the cyclosporine era. The "early" clinical studies, both single and multicenter, were predominantly carried out before the introduction of cyclosporine and before the beneficial effect of matching donor and recipient for HLA-DR antigens had been described (Ting and Morris, 1978; Ting, 1988). Although results from both single (Ting and Morris, 1984) and multicenter studies published in mid-1980s showed that the transfusion effect persisted in both HLA-DR-matched and cyclosporine-treated patients, enthusiasm for transfusion before transplantation waned. Through the latter half of the 1980s the obvious influence of transfusion on graft outcome became less marked in the large multicenter studies (Opelz, 1987, 1988, 1991; Ahmed and Terasaki, 1991), and indeed some studies would suggest that at present, there is little or no beneficial influence of pretransplant transfusion on graft outcome at 1 year. These data have led many transplant units to suspend deliberate transfusion policies, for 1-year graft survival rates are now so good that the risks of sensitizing potential recipients against the alloantigens of the blood donor and of the transmission of infection outweigh the potential benefits, if any, of transfusion.

The reasons for the decline in the transfusion effect are not completely clear. Many people involved in the field have speculated as to the cause, including Opelz, one of the pioneers of the introduction of transfusion policies. He suggests that improved patient management combined with factors such as earlier diagnosis and more aggressive management of rejection episodes following transplantation have all contributed to the major improvements in graft survival achieved in nontransfused patients (Opelz, 1987). It must also be remembered that the majority of the analyses assessing the effects of preoperative blood transfusion only use short-term graft survival figures, derived 1 or 2 years posttransplant. Clearly, if 1-year graft survival rates

in cyclosporine-treated patients who receive well-matched grafts are of the order of 80–90%, irrespective of the transfusion status of the recipient, any beneficial effect of transfusion would be difficult to detect. However, if a more long-term view were taken, the benefits of transfusion might reemerge. A parallel can be drawn between this situation and the benefits of HLA matching. Although at 1 year the survival of grafts completely mismatched for HLA − A + B + DR is similar to that of matched grafts (79 and 88%, respectively), by 3 years the survival curves have diverged significantly, the matched grafts showing a survival rate of 83% compared to 62% for the mismatched grafts (Takemoto et al., 1992). Overall, the data from this multicenter study showed that the half-life of a graft with no HLA − A + B + DR mismatches was 17.3 years compared with only 7.8 years for mismatched grafts. Thus the major benefit of HLA matching is seen in the long, but not the short term. That a similar phenomenon may also exist for transfused patients has been suggested by Yang and colleagues (Yang et al., 1991). In the early posttransplant period assessment of graft function may be more informative than an evaluation of graft survival. Several studies have now shown that in nontransfused patients there is a significantly higher incidence of rejection episodes requiring treatment than in their transfused counterparts.

Thus it may not be prudent to completely write off the potential benefits of antigen pretreatment before transplantation. Clearly, more information is required. While it may be less attractive to use whole blood as the source of antigen for transfusion, other approaches that are currently being explored in experimental studies may provide an alternative strategy.

THE TRANSFUSION EFFECT IN EXPERIMENTAL MODELS

Antigen Requirements

Blood components. Cells derived from a variety of lymphoid tissues, including bone marrow, spleen (Cranston et al., 1986) and thymus, as well as whole blood transfusion (Jenkins and

Woodruff, 1971; Fabre and Morris, 1972) have been used to induce specific unresponsiveness to alloantigen in adult recipients (Fig. 1). To understand the requirements for the induction of the transfusion effect more precisely experimental and clinical studies have been carried out using the different cellular components of blood. In rodents, peripheral blood lymphocytes, erythrocytes, and platelets have all been shown to be capable of inducing unresponsiveness *in vivo* (e.g., Hibberd and Scott, 1983; Wood and Morris, 1985; Wood et al., 1985) (Table II). Furthermore, erythrocytes and platelets, which express class I, but not class II MHC antigens did not sensitize recipients to the donor alloantigens before transplantation. Other experimental studies using platelet transfusions have confirmed their efficacy, although clinical trials of platelet transfusions have produced mixed results (Chapman et al., 1986; Pouteil-Noble et al., 1991).

Studies comparing the effect of using different lymphocyte subpopulations have often produced conflicting results. For example, Lauchart and colleagues showed that only B cells were capable of inducing prolonged survival of heart allografts in rats (Lauchart et al., 1980). Whereas, in a later study using a renal allograft model, Cranston et al. (1986) found that B cells and CD4$^+$ T cells were both effective. Discrepancies of this type can almost certainly be explained by differences in the experimental systems and strain combinations used by different groups. However, comparison of all of the protocols used for this type of study reveals that the critical elements for the induction of unresponsiveness rather than sensitization following treatment with alloantigen are the route and timing of antigen administration relative to transplantation. Invariably, the intravenous delivery of antigen results in the induction of unresponsiveness and

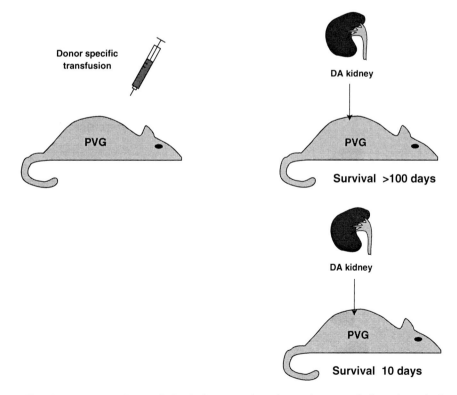

Fig. 1. Donor-specific transfusion before transplantation prolongs renal allograft survival in the rat indefinitely.

Table II. Comparison of the Capacity of Blood Components to Induced Prolonged Renal Allograft Survival in Rats[a]

Blood component	MHC and minor antigens shared	Prolonged graft survival	Sensitization
Whole blood	I + II + miH	Yes	Yes
Leukocytes	I + II + miH	Yes	Yes
Erythrocytes	I + miH	Yes	No
Platelets	I + miH	Yes	No
Plasma	None	No	No

[a]Data taken from Wood et al. (1985).

if antigen alone is used, a finite period of time after antigen administration is required for tolerance to emerge.

Sharing of major and minor histocompatibility antigens. In experimental and clinical transplantation where the organ donor is a living relative, donor-specific transfusions are used to induce specific immunological unresponsiveness. In these cases, the blood donor and organ share both major and minor histocompatibility antigens. A number of investigators have attempted to determine which antigen system contributes most to the induction of the effect. In rodents it is possible to select blood donors and organ donors from the large number of inbred strains available to ensure sharing of either major or minor antigens. The majority of studies show that the sharing of major histocompatibility antigens by the blood donor and subsequent organ donor is critical for the induction of unresponsiveness to an organ allograft (e.g., Peugh et al., 1986), but sharing of minor histocompatibility

may also contribute to the induction of the unresponsive state (Hutchinson and Morris, 1986) (Table III).

This type of analysis, which can be extended to investigate the requirements in terms of sharing of both class I and class II MHC antigens, is essential. As mentioned above, certain cell types, such as platelets, and in rodents erythrocytes, express only class I antigens, and have been shown to induce specific unresponsiveness to alloantigen. Other cells expressing class I antigens only have also been found to be effective, including hepatocytes (Foster et al., 1988). However, in the majority of cases the cells used for transfusion were derived from the organ donor and therefore in addition to the class I antigens, may also have been expressing donor minor histocompatibility antigens. MHC recombinant inbred strains of mice and rat can be used as cell donors to try and overcome this problem, so that the cell donor and organ donor share only class I or class II alloantigens, while the cell donor and recipient are matched for minor histo-

Table III. Sharing of MHC Antigens by the Blood Donor and the Organ Donor Is Sufficient to Induce Prolonged Cardiac Allograft Survival in the Mouse[a]

Blood donor	Organ donor	Antigens shared	Graft survival (days)
—	C57Bl/10 (H-2^b)	—	10
C57BL/10	C57BL/10	MHC + miH	>100
BALB.B	C57BL/10	MHC only	>100
B10.D2	C57BL/10	miH only	31

[a]C3H.He (H-2^k) recipients. Data taken from Peugh et al. (1986).

compatibility antigens. This type of system could be set up in the following way: PVG.RT1^I platelet donor, LEW.RT1^I organ donor, and PVG.FT1^c recipient. Experiments of this type are difficult to interpret as different strain combinations have to be used for each comparison. An alternative approach is to take one cell type, express different MHC antigens on the cell surface, and then use these cells to compare the efficacy of pretreatment with class I and class II antigens before transplantation. Madsen and colleagues have established just such a system using a mouse model (Fig. 2).

Cells of recipient origin, in this case a fibroblast cell line derived from C3H.He H-2^k mice, were transfected with single or multiple MHC genes from different donor strains, e.g., H-2^b. Cells expressing the allogeneic MHC molecules in a stable fashion were established *in vitro* and the integrity of the allo-MHC molecule expressed at the cell surface confirmed using serological and cellular assays. The transfected cells were then used to pretreat recipient C3H recipients intravenously before transplantation of a fully vascularized cardiac allograft from an organ donor expressing the same alloantigen as that expressed by the transfected cells, but also all of the other alloantigens associated with that donor haplotype, in other words a fully allogeneic graft, e.g., C57BL/10 H-2^b. Fibroblasts expressing either single donor class I (H-2K^b) or class II (H-2 IA^b) were both able to induce pro-

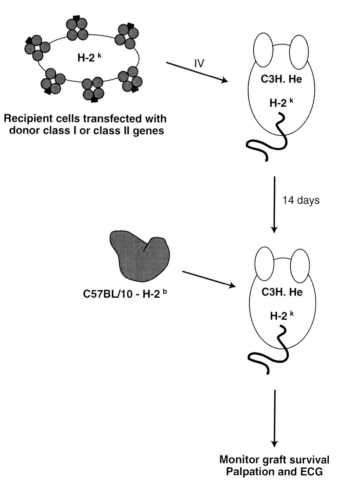

Fig. 2. Protocol for the induction of unresponsiveness using transfected cells.

longed survival of a C57 heart allograft (Madsen et al., 1988) (Fig. 3). Thus both class I and class II MHC antigens may contribute to the induction of specific unresponsiveness after donor-specific or random transfusion if these antigens are subsequently shared by the organ donor. These data provide an experimental basis for the apparent paradox noted above between the antigen specificity achieved with donor-specific transfusion and the apparent lack of donor specificity if randomly selected blood donors are used.

The data obtained in these experiments also reveal other interesting features relating to the ability of individual MHC antigens to induce specific unresponsiveness *in vivo* and suggest that the full potential of antigen pretreatment protocols for use in clinical transplantation may not have been fully explored. When the different locus products of the H-2^b haplotype were compared, the K locus class I antigens were found to be significantly more effective than the D and IA locus products. The differential capacity of the different MHC molecules to induce unresponsiveness to an H-2^b heart graft was found to be related to their individual immunogenicity in

C3H recipients (Madsen et al., 1988). Thus when C3H mice were sensitized, rather than tolerized with each of the transfectants, the cells expressing the Kb molecule were most effective at inducing accelerated graft rejection. A second factor influencing the induction of the unresponsive state was the antigen load delivered during pretreatment (Madsen et al., 1988). At sub- or supraoptimal doses of the transfected cells graft prolongation was not as marked. Assessment of the number of allomolecules on the surface of each transfectant revealed that the number of each of the transfected cells required to induce maximal graft prolongation could be predicted on the basis of the number of class I or class II molecules of donor origin expressed.

The use of recipient cells in primary culture, rather than long-term cell lines, as the vehicle for antigen delivery would allow this approach, which could be described as "gene therapy" for the induction of tolerance to alloantigens, to be adapted for use in clinical transplantation in the future. Work in this area has already begun. Preliminary data from Sykes and her colleagues have shown that a single donor MHC class I

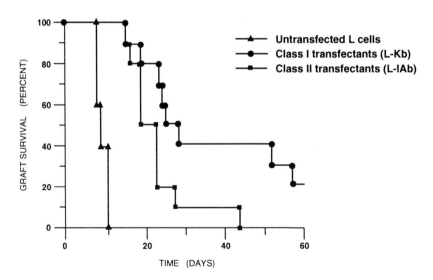

Data taken from Madsen et al (1988)

Fig. 3. Cells of recipient origin expressing donor class I or class II genes can induce specific unresponsiveness to donor alloantigens. Data taken from Madsen et al. (1988).

antigen transduced into recipient bone marrow cells can be used to induce unresponsiveness to class I disparate skin grafts (Sykes et al., 1993).

Interesting reports from two clinical centers in the Netherlands have revealed that by using HLA-typed blood donors the beneficial effects of preoperative transfusion protocols can be optimized. In both centers the data show that by matching the blood donor and the recipient for at least one HLA-DR antigen, graft survival can be improved over that obtained in recipients who receive transfusion from a DR-mismatched donor (Lagaaij et al., 1989, 1991; van Twuyver et al., 1991). The patients who received DR-matched transfusions were found to have a reduced frequency of cytotoxic cells against the class I antigens mismatched between the blood donor and the recipient (van Twuyver et al., 1991). The degree of sharing of class I and class II HLA antigens between the transfusion donor and subsequent organ donor has not yet been reported. This finding needs to be confirmed by other groups, but nevertheless provides new insights into the requirements for beneficial effect of blood transfusion in clinical transplantation.

Physical form of the antigen. The form of the antigen administered is an additional important factor in determining whether specific unresponsiveness to alloantigen is induced. It has been shown in a variety of experimental systems that soluble class I antigen is unable to induce the unresponsive state (Spencer and Fabre, 1987; Arnold et al., 1990; Foster et al., 1992). In contrast, as shown above, membrane-bound antigen is effective. Furthermore it does not appear to be necessary for the antigen to be presented by viable cells for prolonged graft survival to be induced (Foster et al., 1988; Madsen et al., 1988; Foster, 1989). Data obtained *in vitro* show that both a critical number of T cell receptors (TCRs) must be engaged by MHC and a continuous surface contact area is required for optimal interaction with responding T cells (Mescher, 1992). Soluble antigen preparations may be ineffective because they fail to meet these criteria as a result of the short half-life of the soluble material *in vivo*. To overcome this potential problem, one study described a system for the continuous infu-

sion of soluble class I antigen and showed that if the concentration of soluble antigen could be maintained at a high level graft prolongation was possible (Kamada et al., 1981) (Table IV).

As mentioned in passing above, the intravenous route is undoubtedly the most effective way to introduce antigen *in vivo* for the induction of unresponsiveness in the adult if no other form of immunosuppressive therapy is added into the system. Subcutaneous administration of antigen inocula invariably leads to sensitization. There have been reports suggesting that delivery of alloantigen into the intraportal vein is more effective than other intravenous routes (Kennick et al., 1987), but any added benefits have to be set against the added difficulty of accessing the portal vein. Recently there has been renewed interest in intrathymic injection of antigen before transplantation for the induction of tolerance. Very encouraging data have been obtained following intrathymic inoculation of islets of Langerhans, isolated glomeruli, or splenocytes, but all of these strategies have to be used in combination with antilymphocyte serum (ALS) immunotherapy to induce indefinite survival of islet, kidney, and skin grafts in rodent models (Posselt et al., 1990; Remuzzi et al., 1991). The application of this approach to larger animals is currently under investigation.

Transfusion combined with other immunosuppressive agents. Although the administration of donor antigen before transplantation in

Table IV. The Physical Form of the Antigen Administered Is Critical in Determining Whether Unresponsiveness Is Induced[a]

Form of MHC class I antigen administered (iv)	Graft prolongation
Viable cells	Yes
Nonviable cells	Yes
Membrane fragments	Yes
Purified class I antigen incorporated into micelles	Yes
Soluble class I antigen	No

[a]Data taken from Foster et al. (1988) and Foster (1989).

experimental allograft models is undoubtedly an effective strategy for inducing unresponsiveness, and, in some cases, peripheral tolerance to alloantigen given at the time of organ transplantation. However, this strategy may not result in the induction of tolerance to alloantigen in every situation. It may therefore be more effective to combine the benefits of immunological specificity achieved by using donor antigen with low levels of a less specific immunosuppressive agent, such as antilymphocyte globulin (ALG), as mentioned above for antigen administered intrathymically. This strategy has been explored in a number of different ways. Early data were produced by Monaco and his colleagues using donor bone marrow and ALG to prolong the survival of skin allografts in mice (Monaco et al., 1966). This strategy relies on the properties of the ALG to create a suitable environment for the administration of donor bone marrow cells after transplantation, allowing them to engraft and promote the induction of specific unresponsiveness to the graft in the long term. This system has been used successfully to induce tolerance to renal allografts in primates (Thomas et al., 1987) and is currently being explored in the clinical setting (see below).

ALG, as its name suggests, potentially affects the activity of all the recipient's lymphocytes, as does total lymphoid irradiation (TLI), which has also been used in combination with antigen (Myburgh, 1985). The use of monoclonal antibodies (MAbs) that specifically target subsets of cells in combination with donor antigen may allow a more subtle approach to be developed. Two research groups have shown independently that it is possible to induce long-term unresponsiveness to soluble antigen by combining antigen administration with treatment using an anti-CD4 MAb (Wofsy et al., 1985; Benjamin and Waldmann, 1986). These data suggested that anti-CD4 might be able to create an environment that facilitated tolerance induction in the adult. Restriction of the nonspecific effects of the antibody therapy to just the $CD4^+$ subset of T cells may have advantages over the use of ALG in a similar system. Our own group decided to explore this possibility in the context of the induction of tolerance to alloantigens. We have established a model

whereby it is possible to induce tolerance to an organ graft at the time of transplantation by administration of donor antigen in combination with anti-CD4 MAb. We were able to show that although anti-CD4 MAb therapy induces nonspecific immunosuppression in the first instance, recipients treated with the MAb do recover immunocompetence in a relatively short period of time (Pearson et al., 1993) (Fig. 4a). If donor antigen was administered under the cover of the anti-CD4 MAb therapy, immunocompetence to other alloantigens recovers over some weeks, as demonstrated by the ability of the recipient to reject a third-party cardiac graft, but specific unresponsiveness to the donor antigen had been induced resulting in indefinite survival of donor cardiac allografts (Pearson et al., 1992) (Fig. 4b). Thus, this strategy allows the induction of specific unresponsiveness to donor alloantigen at the time of transplantation and results in the indefinite survival of both primary and secondary grafts from the same organ donor.

MECHANISMS OF TOLERANCE INDUCTION

When T cells encounter any antigen in the periphery, a choice is made as to how they respond. Antigen reactive cells can simply ignore the presence of the antigen and no response will take place, they can become activated, a process that could lead to accelerated rejection of an organ graft sharing the same alloantigens, or the cells can be switched off following the encounter, such that when they "see" the same antigen for a second time expressed by cells of the graft they can no longer respond and tolerance will be the result. Each of these scenarios could occur after prior blood transfusion and which one occurs will depend on some of the factors discussed above.

The mechanisms responsible for the induction and maintenance of peripheral tolerance to alloantigen in adult recipients are still being investigated, particularly at the molecular level, and continue to be hotly debated. Four, nonmutually exclusive hypotheses and variations thereof have been proposed to explain the events taking place. These are, in broad terms, deletion, anergy, ig-

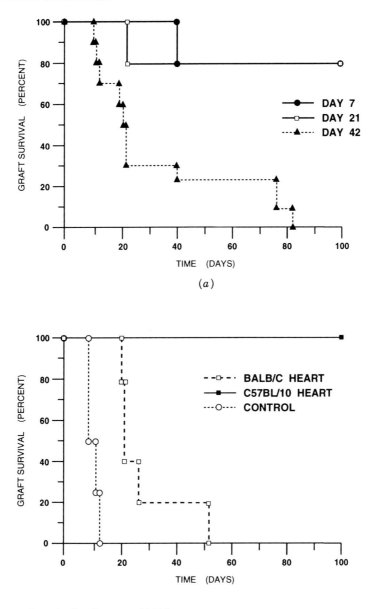

Data taken from Pearson et al (1992).

(*b*)

Fig. 4. (**a**) Nonspecific immunosuppression result-ing from treatment with anti-CD4 MAb is short-lived. Immunocompetence is recovered within 42 days. (**b**) Specific unresponsiveness to alloantigen (C57Bl/10) can be induced at the time of transplantation by com-bined treatment with donor antigen (C57BI/10 blood) and anti-CD4 MAb 42 days before transplantation. Data taken from Pearson et al. (1992).

norance, and suppression. What is clear from all studies is that tolerance induction is a dynamic process and any or all of these mechanisms may be operating at different stages of the induction and maintenance phases. What is also clear is the confusion created when different definitions for the terms are used to describe what may be the same phenomena!

Deletion

Deletion of antigen-reactive T cells has been shown to be an important mechanism for the induction of tolerance to self-antigens during development of the immune system (Kappler et al., 1987; Marrack and Kappler, 1988; von Boehmer et al., 1989). As a mechanism for the induction of peripheral tolerance to alloantigens it may be less important, but nevertheless it has been identified as the mechanism responsible for the induction of tolerance to the superantigen MIs1[a] following intravenous infusion of leukocytes into thymectomized adult mice (Webb et al., 1990). A similar series of experiments examining the mechanism of tolerance induction to MIs1[a] did not identify deletion as a mechanism (Rammensee et al., 1989), but, in this case, the adult mice were not thymectomized before the leukocyte infusion. These two studies highlight the importance of the status of the recipient in determining which mechanism is operating and suggest that there is a considerable degree of flexibility in how the immune system responds to alloantigens *in vivo*.

Ignorance

If T cells remain ignorant of an antigen that is present *in vivo* they are by definition unresponsive. The phenomenon was first described in an experimental system in mice made transgenic for a glycoprotein from the lymphocytic choriomeningitis virus (LCMV) (Ohashi et al., 1991). The transgene, which was expressed by pancreatic β cells, was ignored by the immune system. The LCMV antigen was recognized only when mice that were also transgenic for the LCMV-specific TCR were immunized with LCMV glycoprotein. Following immunization the LCMV-specific T cells destroyed the pancreatic β cells and the mice became diabetic.

Ignorance may be a feature of low affinity T cells. Work from Miller and his colleagues has shown that in transgenic mice where H-2K[b] is expressed predominantly by pancreatic β cells, high affinity T cells are deleted in the thymus as a result of low level expression of K[b] in the thymus (Heath et al., 1992). T cells that escape deletion are able to cause the rejection of skin grafts expressing K[b], but are seemingly unaware of K[b] expressed by β cells in the same mouse. Only when high levels of IL-2 are present are the β cells destroyed. These data suggest that the site of antigen expression may also play a role in determining how T cells respond to an antigen.

Anergy

The induction of anergy or the functional inactivation of alloreactive T cells is the mechanism that currently receives most support in the transplantation literature. However, the molecular mechanisms responsible for the induction of this state of T cell inactivity remain unclear.

Anergic T cells are usually identified because although they are present in a tolerant animal they are unable to respond when stimulated through their antigen receptor with either antigen or a MAb specific for the TCR they express (Lo et al., 1988; Burkley et al., 1989; Qin et al., 1989; Rammensee et al., 1989; Alters et al., 1991; Dallman et al., 1991). In some models anergy has also been shown to be associated with a down-regulation of cell surface expression of TCR and accessory molecules such as CD8 (Kisielow et al., 1988; Arnold et al., 1993).

Anergy can be induced in a variety of ways. One method might require disruption of the interaction between the APC and the T cells in some way. For example, nonprofessional APC that are able to express the appropriate MHC–peptide complex, but lack other accessory molecules, such as B7, have been shown to be very efficient inducers of T cell inactivation. In this situation, responding T cells receive signal 1, i.e., TCR engagement, but not signal 2, the interaction of the accessory molecules, B7 on the

APC and CD28 on the T cell, and are therefore inactivated (Bretscher and Cohn, 1970; Jenkins, 1992). There is evidence that this situation can arise as a result of preoperative transfusion (see below). In addition, anergy may also be a feature of T cells that interact in a suboptimal fashion with donor MHC molecules. This situation has been observed for self-reactive T cells capable of responding to a particular peptide–MHC complex, when the cells are first presented with an analogue of the antigenic peptide that binds to the same MHC molecule expressed by a live APC (Sloan-Lancaster et al., 1993). It was found that the peptide analogue–MHC complex was unable to stimulate proliferation or the production of cytokines and that the T cells became profoundly unresponsive following the encounter. Efficient contact between the APC and T cell can also be prevented by monoclonal antibodies specific for any one of the accessory molecules participating in the interaction (e.g., CD4, LFA-1, ICAM-1, CD28) and these strategies have also been shown to induce anergy in the responding T cells. The molecular mechanisms responsible for the induction and maintenance of anergic T cells are still under investigation, but some progress has already been made.

In a transplantation model, where tolerance was induced by pretreatment with donor alloantigen in the form of a blood transfusion, our own group has shown that although donor-reactive cytotoxic cells are present within the grafts of tolerant recipients (Dallman et al., 1987), the graft infiltrating cells are unable to respond to or produce functional IL-2 in vitro (Fig. 5) (Dallman et al., 1991). These data suggest that the donor-reactive cells present within these grafts are anergic. Interestingly, mRNA for IL-2 is still detectable in the graft-infiltrating population, implying that the defect in the IL-2 pathway is not at the level of gene transcription. This finding is in contrast to those reported recently using

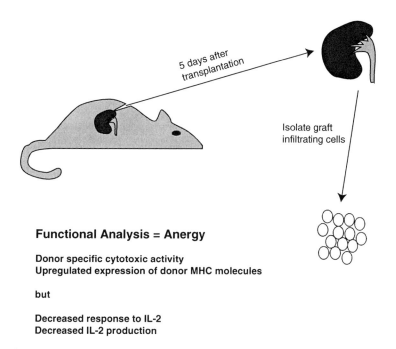

5 days after transplantation

Isolate graft infiltrating cells

Functional Analysis = Anergy

Donor specific cytotoxic activity
Upregulated expression of donor MHC molecules

but

Decreased response to IL-2
Decreased IL-2 production

Fig. 5. The induction of tolerance to alloantigen results in a defect in the IL-2 pathway leading to the induction of anergy. Functional analysis = anergy: donor-specific cytotoxic activity and up-regulated expression of donor MHC molecules but decreased response to IL-2 and decreased IL-2 production.

in vitro systems, where transcription of the IL-2 gene in anergic cells was down-regulated because of the absence of transcription factors such as AP-1 (Kang et al., 1992).

The cytokine environment may also play a role in influencing the outcome when T cells encounter antigen. It has been suggested that the cytokines, IL-4 and IL-10 that are produced by T_H2 cells, may be associated with the development of unresponsiveness (Papp et al., 1992; Takeuchi et al., 1992) or, alternatively, that a low or defective production of the T_H1 cytokines, IL-2 and interferon-γ (IFN-γ), might be responsible (Mohler and Streilein, 1989; Dallman et al., 1991; Bugeon et al., 1992). Clearly the two situations may be related. Certainly, many studies have shown that there is a difference between the pattern and kinetics of cytokine expression in rejecting and tolerant recipients (e.g., Dallman, et al., 1991; Bugeon et al., 1992). However, convincing evidence that the development of a T_H2-like environment is the critical factor for the induction of tolerance to alloantigen is still awaited and so far only associations have been demonstrated. Clear evidence supporting these ideas will likely be obtained only from studies that attempt to manipulate the cytokine environment *in vivo*. So far little has been done in this area, but studies using, for example, antibodies to IFN-γ an important T_H1 cytokine, have proved ineffective to date at both inhibiting graft rejection and inducing tolerance (Paineau et al., 1991).

Suppression

In many transplant models, including those where peroperative transfusion is used to induce tolerance to alloantigen, it is possible to adoptively transfer cells from animals bearing long-term surviving allografts to a fresh syngeneic recipient and show that these are able to modify the rejection response to a fresh graft (Hutchinson, 1986). It is important to note that suppressor cells are most frequently described in the maintenance phase of graft survival, usually 50 or more days after transplantation in rodent models. Thus it may be that the mechanisms responsible for

tolerance induction converge and become unified in the longer term after transplantation. Although there is no question that the phenomenon of active suppression can be demonstrated, the idea that suppressor cells control unresponsiveness has largely fallen into disrepute because even with advances in technology, it has proved impossible to isolate and characterize a population of cells with suppressor activity. In the recent literature suppressor or regulatory cells seem to be enjoying a revival of interest and it may not be too long before scepticism regarding their existence is finally put to rest. Perhaps the suppressor T cell is a cell that is suppressive only in a particular environment. A recent suggestion has been that cells previously defined as suppressor cells in adoptive transfer studies were responsible for creating a T_H2-like cytokine environment in the new host and, therefore, the activity of the remaining aggressive T_H1 cells that would be responsible for mediating rejection was turned off. It is interesting to note that in the majority, but not all, experimental systems for adoptive transfer studies the secondary recipient had to be modified in some way, usually by low dose irradiation, before the transfer of cells was carried out. This may have resulted in the elimination or inactivation of the majority of the T_H1 cells present in the recipient and, therefore, allowed the transferred cells to tip the balance in favor of suppression.

Another phenomenon that can be considered as fitting into the same category as active suppression is that of infectious tolerance. This again has been demonstrated in recipients bearing long-term surviving allografts, where the transfer of naive syngeneic lymphocytes to the recipient will not induce graft rejection (e.g., Billingham et al., 1956; Shizuru et al., 1987). Recent elegant experiments from Waldmann and his colleagues have shown that in mice rendered tolerant to skin grafts by treatment with anti-CD4 and anti-CD8 MAbs, a CD4$^+$ population of cells in the tolerant host is responsible for switching off the naive cells (Qin et al., 1993). Interestingly, the naive cells must be resident in the tolerant host for 14 days before they lose the capacity to reject a fresh graft. Experiments of this type may help elucidate the molecular properties of the cells responsible for maintaining tolerance to alloantigen in the long term.

Persistence of Antigen

Finally, the persistence of donor antigen has been suggested to be critical for the induction of tolerance to alloantigen *in vivo*. While graft function is maintained, donor alloantigens are continually shed into the periphery where they may be able to inactivate newly emerging T cells. In experiments where the graft has been removed and recipients are then rechallenged with alloantigen at various times later, tolerance is eventually lost. However, in most experimental systems, it takes a long time for responsiveness to return (e.g., Shizuru et al., 1990). For example, in a mouse model where tolerance was induced to a cardiac allograft using anti-CD4 MAbs, it took more than 130 days after the graft was removed for the animals to recover responsiveness to the alloantigens of the original organ donor (Hamano and Wood, unpublished observations).

In some studies it has been suggested that the development of chimerism is an important factor for the induction and maintenance of tolerance to alloantigen (e.g., Monaco et al., 1966; Thomas et al., 1987; Sykes and Sachs, 1988; Sharabi and Sachs, 1989). The development of microchimerism has recently been suggested to be important for the long-term survival of organ allografts, as in recipients who have liver or kidney grafts that have functioned for more than 20 years donor cells have been identified in recipient tissues (Starzl et al., 1992). These observations are clearly interesting, but as yet no definitive experiments addressing whether this is cause or effect have been carried out.

CONCLUSION

Treatment with alloantigen before transplantation can modify the response to a subsequent organ graft sharing some, if not all, of the same alloantigens, and result in prolonged graft survival. Blood transfusion has been the most straight-forward method for delivery of alloantigen to prospective transplant recipients and in the past has been shown to have a beneficial effect on renal allograft survival. Short-term evaluation of the effects of transfusion on graft survival may not reveal the beneficial effects, as many other improvements in the management of transplant patients have been made since the original observations were reported. New approaches for the delivery of alloantigen to transplant recipients are being investigated to overcome the problem currently associated with the use of blood products. We remain convinced that antigen pretreatment can be used effectively to down-regulate immune responsiveness before transplantation and believe that the full potential of these approaches will be realized in clinical transplantation in the future.

REFERENCES

Ahmed Z, Terasaki PI (1991): Effect of transfusions. In "Clinical Transplants 1991." Los Angeles: UCLA Tissue Typing Laboratory, pp 305–312.

Alters SE, Shizuru JA, Ackerman J, Grossman D, Seydel KB, Fathman CG (1991): Anti-CD4 mediates clonal anergy during transplantation tolerance induction. J Exp Med 173:491–494.

Arnold B, Messerle M, Jatsch L, Kublbeck G, Koszinowski U (1990): Transgenic mice expressing a soluble foreign H-2 class I antigen are tolerant to allogeneic fragments presented by self class I but not to the whole membrane-bound alloantigen. Proc Natl Acad Sci USA 87:1762–1766.

Arnold B, Schonrich G, Hammerling GJ (1993): Multiple levels of peripheral tolerance. Immunol Today 14:12–14.

Benjamin RJ, Waldmann H (1986): Induction of tolerance by monoclonal antibody therapy. Nature (London) 320:449–451.

Billingham RE, Brent L (1959): Quantitative studies on tissue transplantation immunity. IV. Induction of tolerance in newborn mice and studies on the phenomenon of runt disease. Phil Trans R Soc (London) Ser B 242:439–477.

Billingham RE, Brent L, Medawar PB (1956): Quantitative studies on tissue transplantation immunity. III. Actively acquired tolerance. Phil Trans R Soc (London) Ser B 239:357–412.

Billingham RE, Lampkin GH, Medawar PB, Williams HL (1951): Tolerance to homografts, twin diagnosis, and the freemartin condition in cattle. Heredity 6:201–212.

Billingham RE, Brent L, Medawar PB (1953): Actively acquired tolerance of foreign cells. Nature (London) 12:603–606.

Bretscher P, Cohn M (1970): A theory of self-nonself discrimination. Science 169:1042–1049.

Bugeon L, Cuturi M-C, Hallet J, Paineau J, Chabannes D, Soulillou J-P (1992): Peripheral tolerance of an allograft in adult rats—characterisation by low interleukin-2 and interferon-γ mRNA levels and by strong accumulation of major histocompatibility complex transcripts within the graft. Transplantation 54:219–225.

Burkley LC, Lo D, Kanegawa O, Brister RL, Flavell RA (1989): T-cell tolerance by clonal anergy in transgenic mice with nonlymphoid expression of MHC class II I-E. Nature (London) 342:564–566.

Chapman JR, Ting A, Fisher M, Carter NP, Morris PJ (1986). Failure of platelet transfusion to improve human renal allograft survival. Transplantation 41:468–473.

Cranston D, Wood KJ, Carter NP, Morris PJ (1986): Pretreatment with lymphocyte subpopulations and renal allograft survival in the rat. Transplantation 43:809–813.

Dallman MJ, Wood KJ, Morris PJ (1987): Specific cytotoxic T cells are not found in the non-rejected kidneys of blood transfused rats. J Exp Med 165:566–571.

Dallman MJ, Shilo O, Page TH, Wood KJ, Morris PJ (1991): Peripheral tolerance to alloantigen results from altered regulation of the interleukin-2 pathway. J Exp Med 173:79–87.

Dossetor JB, MacKinnon KJ, Gault MH, MacLean LD (1967): Cadaver kidney transplants. Transplantation 5:844–853.

Fabre JW, Morris PJ (1972): The effect of donor strain blood pretreatment on renal allograft rejection in rats. Transplantation 14:608–617.

Fabre J, Lim S, Morris P (1971): Renal transplantation in the rat: Details of a technique. Aust NZ J Surg 41:69.

Foster, S (1989): "Induction of Specific Unresponsiveness by Class I MHC Antigen: A Study in a Rat Renal Allograft Model." Oxford: University of Oxford.

Foster S, Cranston D, Wood KJ, Morris PJ (1988): Pretreatment with viable and non-viable hepatocytes or liver membrane extracts produces indefi-

nite renal allograft survival in the rat. Transplantation 45:228–231.

Foster S, Cranston D, Wood KJ, Morris PJ (1992): The effectiveness of pretreatment with soluble or membrane bound donor class I MHC antigens in the induction of unresponsiveness to a subsequent rat renal allograft. Transplantation 53:1322–1328.

Heath WR, Allison J, Hoffman MW, Schonrich G, Hammerling G, Arnold B, Miller JFAP (1992): Autoimmune diabetes as a consequence of locally produced interleukin-2. Nature (London) 359:547–549.

Hibberd AD, Scott LJ (1983): Allogeneic platelets increase survival of rat renal allografts. Transplantation 35:622–624.

Hutchinson IV (1986): Suppressor T cells in allogeneic models. Transplantation 41:547–555.

Hutchinson IV, Morris PJ (1986): The role of major and minor histocompatibility antigens in active enhancement of rat kidney allograft survival by blood transfusion. Transplantation 41:166–170.

Jenkins MK (1992): The role of cell division in the induction of clonal anergy. Immunol Today 13:69–73.

Jenkins A, McL, Woodruff MFA (1971): The effect of prior administration of donor strain blood or blood constituents on the survival of cardiac allografts in rats. Transplantation 12:57–60.

Kamada N, Davies HS, Roser BJ (1981): Reversal of transplantation immunity by liver grafting. Nature (London) 292:840–842.

Kang S-M, Beverly B, Tran A-C, Brorson K, Schwartz RH, Lenardo MJ (1992): Transactivation by AP-1 is a molecular target of T cell clonal anergy. Science 257:1134–1138.

Kappler JW, Roehm N, PM (1987): T cell tolerance by clonal elimination within the thymus. Cell 49:273–280.

Kennick S, Lowry RP, Forbes RDC, Lisbona R (1987): Prolonged cardiac allograft survival following portal venous inoculation of allogeneic cells. What is hepatic tolerance? Transplant Proc 19:478–480.

Kisielow P, Bluthmann H, Staerz UD, Steinmetz M, von Boehmer H (1988): Tolerance in T-cell-receptor transgenic mice involves deletion of nonmature CD4⁺8⁺ thymocytes. Nature (London) 333:742–746.

Lagaaij EL, Hennemann IPH, Ruigrok M, de Haan MW, Persijn GG, Termijtelen A, Hendriks GFJ, Weimar N, Class FHJ, van Rood JJ (1989): Effect of one-HLA-DR antigen matched and completely HLA-DR-mismatched blood transfusions on survival of heart and kidney allografts. N Engl J Med 321:701–705.

Lagaaij EL, Ruigrok MB, van Rood JJ, Hendriks GFJ, van der Woude F, Weimar W, Van Houwelingen HC, Goulmy E (1991): Blood transfusion induced changes in cell-mediated lympholysis: To immunise or not to immunise. J Immunol 147:3348–3352.

Lauchart W, Alkins BJ, Davies DAL (1980): Only B lymphocytes induce active enhancement of rat cardiac allografts. Transplantation 29:259–261.

Lo D, Burkly LC, Widera G, Cowing C, Flavell RA, Palmiter RD, Brinster RL (1988): Diabetes and tolerance in transgenic mice expressing class II MHC molecules in pancreatic β cells. Cell 53:159–168.

Madsen JC, Superina RA, Wood KJ, Morris PJ (1988): Immunological unresponsiveness induced by recipient cells transfected with donor MHC genes. Nature (London) 332:161–164.

Marrack P, Kappler J (1988): The T cell repertoire for antigen. Immunol Today 9:308–315.

Mescher MF (1992): Surface contact requirements for activation of cytotoxic T lymphocytes. J Immunol 149:2402–2405.

Mohler KM, Streilein JW (1989): Lymphokine production by MLR-reactive reaction lymphocytes obtained from normal mice and mice rendered tolerant of class II MHC antigens. Transplantation 47:625–633.

Monaco AP, Wood ML, Russel PS (1966):Studies on heterologous anti-lymphocyte serum in mice: III. Immunologic tolerance and chimerism produced across the H-2 locus with adult thymectomy and anti-lymphocyte serum. Ann NY Acad Sci 129:190–206.

Morris PJ, Ting A, Stocker JW (1968): Leucocyte antigens in renal transplantation. The paradox of blood transfusion in renal transplantation. Med J Aust 2:1088–1090.

Myburgh JA (1985): Total lymphoid irradiation and transplantation tolerance. Progress in Transplantation 16–43.

Ohashi PS, Oehen S, Buerki K, Pircher H, Ohashi CT, Odermatt B, Malissen B, Zinkernagel RM, Hengartner H (1991): Ablation of "tolerance" and induction of diabetes by virus infection in viral antigen transgenic mice. Cell 65:305–317.

Opelz G (1987): Improved kidney graft survival in nontransfused recipients. Transplant Proc 19:149–152.

Opelz G (1988): Blood transfusions and renal transplantation. In "Kidney Transplantation. Principles and Practice," 3rd ed. Philadelphia: W.B. Sanders, pp 417–438.

Opelz G (1991): The role of HLA matching and blood transfusions in the cyclosporine era. Transplant Proc 21:609–612.

Opelz G, Senger DPS, Mickey MR, Terasaki PI (1973): Effect of blood transfusions on subsequent kidney transplants. Transplant Proc 5:253–259.

Owen RD (1945): Immunogenetic consequences of vascular anastomoses between bovine twins. Science 102:400–401.

Paineau J, Priestley C, Bergh J, Tengblad A, Hallgren R (1991): Effect of recombinant interferon-γ and interleukin-2 and of a monoclonal antibody against interferon gamma on the rat immune response against heart allografts. J Heart Lung Transplant 10:424–30.

Papp I, Wieder KJ, Sablinski T, O'Connell PJ, Milford EL, Strom TB, Jw K-W (1992): Evidence for functional heterogeneity of rat CD4+ T cells in vivo. Differential expression of IL-2 and IL-4 mRNA in recipients of cardiac allografts. J Immunol 148:1308–14.

Patel R, Terasaki PI (1969): Significance of the positive crossmatch test in kidney transplantation. N Engl J Med 288:735–739.

Pearson TC, Madsen JC, Larsen C, Morris PJ, Wood KJ (1992): Induction of transplantation tolerance in the adult using donor antigen and anti-CD4 monoclonal antibody. Transplantation 54:475–483.

Pearson TC, Darby C, Bushell AR, West L, Morris PJ, Wood KJ (1993): The assessment of transplantation tolerance induced by anti-CD4 monoclonal antibody in the murine model. Transplantation 55:361–367.

Peugh WN, Superina RA, Wood KJ, Morris PJ (1986): The role of H-2 and non-H2 antigens and genes in the rejection of murine cardiac allografts. Immunogenetics 23:30–37.

Posselt AM, Barker CF, Tomaszewski JE, Markmann JF, Choti MA, Naji A (1990): Induction of donor-specific unresponsiveness by intrathymic islet transplantation. Science 249:1293–1295.

Pouteil-Noble C, Betuel H, Raffaele P, Robert F, Dubernard JM, Touraine JL (1991): The value of platelet transfusions as preparation for kidney transplantation. Transplantation 51:777–781.

Qin S, Cobbold S, Benjamin R, Waldmann H (1989): Induction of classical transplantation tolerance in the adult. J Exp Med 169:779–794.

Qin S, Cobbold SP, Pope H, Elliott J, Kioussis D, Davies J, Waldmann H (1993): Infectious transplantation tolerance. Science 259:974–977.

Rammensee H-G, Kroschewski R, Frangoulis B (1989): Clonal anergy induced in mature Vβ6$^+$ T lymphocytes on immunising MIs-1^b mice with MIs-1^a expressing cells. Nature (London) 339: 541–544.

Remuzzi G, Rossini M, Imberti O, Perico N (1991): Kidney allograft survival in rats without immunosuppressants after intrathymic glomerular transplantation. Lancet 337:750–752.

Salvatierra O, Vincenti F, Amend W (1983): Four year experience with donor-specific blood transfusions. Transplant Proc 15:924–931.

Sharabi Y, Sachs DH (1989): Mixed chimerism and permanent specific transplantation tolerance induced by a nonlethal preparative regimen. J Exp Med 169:493–502.

Shizuru JA, Gregory AK, Chao CT-B, Fathman CG (1987): Islet allograft survival after a single course of treatment of recipient with antibody to L3T4. Science 237:278–280.

Shizuru JA, Seybel KB, Flavin TF, Wu AP, Kong CC, Hoyt EG, Fujimoto N, Billingham ME, Starnes VA, Fathman CG (1990): Induction of donor-specific unresponsiveness to cardiac allografts in rats by pretransplant anti-CD4 monoclonal antibody therapy. Transplantation 50:366–373.

Sloan-Lancaster J, Evavold BD, Allen PM (1993): Induction of T cell anergy by altered T cell receptor ligand on live antigen presenting cells. Nature (London) 363:156–159.

Spencer SC, Fabre JW (1987): Bulk purification of a naturally occurring soluble form of RT1A class I major histocompatibility antigens from DA rat liver and studies of specific immunosuppression. Transplantation 44:141.

Starzl TE, Demetris AJ, Murase N, Ildstad S, Ricordi C, Trucco M (1992): Cell migration, chimerism and graft acceptance. Lancet 339:1579–1582.

Sykes M, Sachs DH (1988): Mixed allogeneic chimerism as an approach to transplantation tolerance. Immunol Today 9:23–27.

Sykes M, Sachs DH, Nienhuis AW, Pearson DA, Moulton AD, Bodine DM (1993): Specific prolongation of skin graft survival following retroviral transduction of bone marrow with an allogeneic major histocompatibility complex gene. Transplantation 55:197–202.

Takemoto S, Terasaki PI, Cecka JM, Cho YW, Gjertson DW, Registry FtUSRT (1992): Survival of nationally shared, HLA-matched kidney transplants from cadaveric donors. N Engl J Med 327:834–839.

Takeuchi T, Lowry RP, Konieczny B (1992): Heart allografts in murine systems—The differential activation of TH2-like effector cells in peripheral tolerance. Transplantation 53:1281–1294.

Thomas JM, Carver M, Cunningham P (1987): Promotion of incompatible allograft acceptance in rhesus monkeys given posttransplant anti-thymocyte globulin and donor bone marrow. I. In vivo parameters and immunohistologic evidence suggesting microchimerism. Transplantation 43:332–338.

Ting A (1988): HLA matching and crossmatching in renal transplantation. In "Kidney Transplantation Principles and Practice," 3rd ed. Philadelphia: W.B. Saunders, pp 183–214.

Ting A, Morris PJ (1978): Matching for B-cell antigens of the HLA-DR series in cadaver renal transplantation. Lancet I:575.

Ting A, Morris PJ (1984): The influence of HLA-A,B and -DR matching and pregraft blood transfusions on graft and patient survival after renal transplantation in a single centre. Tissue Antigens 24:256–264.

van Twuyver E, Mooijaart RJD, ten Berge IJM, van der Horst AR, Wilmink JM, Kast WM, Melief CJM, de Waal LP (1991): Pretransplantation blood transfusion revisited. N Engl J Med 325:1210–1213.

von Boehmer H, Teh HS, Kisielow P (1989): The thymus selects the useful, neglects the useless and destroys the harmful. Immunol Today 10:57–61.

Webb S, Morris C, Sprent J (1990): Extrathymic tolerance of mature T cells; clonal elimination as a consequence of immunity. Cell 63:1249–1256.

Wofsy D, Mayes DC, Woodcock J, Seaman WE (1985): Inhibition of humoral immunity in vivo by monoclonal antibody to L3T4: Studies with soluble antigens in intact mice. J Immunol 135:1698–1701.

Wood KJ, Morris PJ (1985): The blood transfusion effect: Suppression of renal allograft rejection in the rat using purified blood components. Transplant Proc 17:2419–2420.

Wood KJ, Evins J, Morris PJ (1985): Suppression of renal allograft rejection in the rat by class I antigen on purified erythrocytes. Transplantation 39:56–62.

Yang HC, Weaver AS, Gilford RRM (1991): Transfusion effect still present with quadruple immunosuppression of recipients of renal transplants. Transplant Proc 23:1247–1248.

Chapter 18
Antigen-Presenting Cell Regulation of T Cell Activation and Anergy Induction

Marc K. Jenkins

INTRODUCTION

The effectiveness of the adaptive vertebrate immune response can be attributed to the generation of a vast number of T- and B-lymphocyte clones each expressing a different antigen receptor and thus each capable of binding a different foreign antigen. Although the diversity of antigen receptors generated by a relatively random gene rearrangement process (Davis, 1990) allows the host respond to almost any foreign protein, this diversity also creates a problem for the host in that antigen receptors specific for the host's own (self) proteins are also generated. Therefore, the immune system must have mechanisms to rid itself of T and B cells that produce self-reactive antigen receptors [TCR and surface immunoglobulin (Ig), respectively]. Because T and B cells recognize antigen differently, the types of self-molecules that each must tolerate are different. Ig molecules recognize the three-dimensional structure of intact protein antigens, and thus, B cells specific for intact self-antigens must be silenced; whereas TCRs recognize antigenic peptides bound to major histocompatibility complex (MHC)-encoded molecules on the surface of another cell, the antigen-presenting cell (APC), and thus, T cells specific for self-peptide/MHC complexes must be silenced. As described below, tolerance can be attributed to several cellular mechanisms, one of which, clonal anergy, will be discussed in detail here. Although this mechanism is operative in both the T and B cell (Nossal, 1992) compart-ments, this chapter will focus primarily on T cell anergy.

SELF-TOLERANCE: DEFINITIONS

Historically, immunologists have considered three potential mechanisms for the maintenance of T cell self-tolerance: clonal deletion, clonal anergy, and suppression (Schwartz, 1989). Clonal deletion is defined as the physical elimination of self-reactive lymphocytes, generally at the sites of lymphocyte development, the thymus for T cells and the bone marrow for B cells. Immature pre-T cells that generate and express TCRs with a high affinity for self-peptide/MHC complexes on thymic APCs, and thus have the potential to mediate autoimmunity, are physically eliminated in the thymus. It is thought that immature self-reactive $CD3^{lo}CD4^+8^+$ T cells increase their cytoplasmic free calcium concentration in response to self-peptide/MHC complexes and that this activates an endonuclease which cleaves DNA between nucleosomes resulting in the death of the cells. Susceptibility to intrathymic clonal deletion is, therefore, a function of the maturational state of the responding thymocyte, with immature T cells being more susceptible than mature T cells. Self-antigen presentation by thymic bone marrow-derived APC appears to be most the effective means of inducing deletion of immature T cells, although non-bone marrow-derived thymic epithelial cells are also competent. Intrathymic clonal deletion

Transplantation Immunology, pages 295–304
© 1995 Wiley-Liss, Inc.

has been shown to be an important tolerance mechanism in normal mice for products of endogenous retroviruses and in TCR transgenic mice that express the antigen the transgenic TCR is specific for in the thymus.

Suppression is defined as a state in which self-reactive lymphocytes are physically present but are inhibited from functioning by suppressor T cells. Although this idea was very popular in the 1970s and early 1980s, experiments where molecular techniques have been applied to the study of tolerance have failed to provide evidence for suppression. For example, T cells from various transgenic mouse strains that express a single TCR specific for a self-antigen are either deleted or rendered anergic *in vivo* without evidence of suppression (see below). Because little molecular evidence exists for a role for suppression in self-tolerance, this mechanism will not be discussed further.

Clonal anergy is defined as a state in which self-reactive lymphocytes are physically present but are functionally unresponsive to antigen. By definition anergy is induced in the responding T cell as a direct consequence of TCR signaling and not by a suppressive population of regulatory T cells. Although it can be induced in the thymus, anergy has been shown to be primarily a peripheral tolerance mechanism, i.e., it is induced in mature peripheral T cells.

IN VIVO CLONAL ANERGY MODELS

Clonal deletion of immature thymocytes would be expected to be an effective tolerance mechanism for antigens expressed in the thymus on bone marrow-derived APC. It is less clear how tolerance would be induced to antigens expressed outside of the thymus, for example, membrane molecules that are expressed in a highly tissue-specific fashion or secreted proteins that are present at too low a concentration to be effectively presented in the thymus. In addition, intrathymic clonal deletion would not be expected to be effective for developmentally regulated proteins that appear in the periphery only after the peripheral T cell repertoire has been established. Several lines of evidence suggest that clonal anergy may be responsible for tolerance to some of these antigens (Lo et al., 1991). T cells from mice expressing a class II MHC transgene only in the β cells of the pancreas become tolerant to the transgene product by an anergy mechanism, i.e., T cells expressing TCRs specific for the transgenic MHC molecule are present but do not proliferate in response to that molecule expressed on splenocytes or in response to anti-TCR antibodies. When analyzed *in vitro,* purified transgene-expressing β cells do not stimulate antigen-specific T cell clones to proliferate, but instead make the T cells anergic. Tolerance to transgenic class I MHC molecules expressed only on pancreatic β cells may also be maintained by anergy induction in the interleukin 2 (IL-2)-producing subset of transgene-specific $CD8^+$ T cells although recent studies suggest that this tolerance may instead be explained by deletion of high affinity T cells leaving a low affinity population that ignores the transgenic class I molecules (Heath et al., 1992).

Anergy appears to be particularly important for $CD8^+$ T cells because most tissues express class I MHC and are constantly presenting endogenous self-proteins, some of which are specific only to that tissue and thus are not presented in the thymus. Hammerling and co-workers (Arnold et al., 1993) have studied peripheral tolerance for $CD8^+$ T cells in transgenic mice that express a class I MHC molecule (K^b) under the control of the albumin, keratin IV, or glial fibrillary acidic protein promoters that direct K^b expression only to hepatocytes, keratinocytes, and neuroectodermal cells, respectively. In each case K^b-specific tolerance is induced as evidenced by the fact that the transgenic mice do not respond to the tissue where the K^b molecules are expressed, and the fact that they accept skin grafts expressing K^b molecules. The cellular mechanism of tolerance can be studied in the offspring of crosses between the aforementioned transgenic mice and transgenic mice that express on most of their T cells a K^b-specific TCR. In these mice the K^b-specific T cells can be physically monitored with a monoclonal antibody specific for the transgenic TCR. In each of the three cases of tissue-specific K^b expression described above, the K^b-specific T cells are not deleted suggesting that they are anergic *in vivo*.

When mature T cells are chronically exposed to retroviral products in normal mice (Webb et al., 1990) or when TCR transgenic T cells are injected into a host that expresses their antigen (Rocha and von Boehmer, 1991), the T cells first become activated and proliferate, but then many cells die and the remaining cells become unresponsive. This could be what happens when a developmentally regulated self-protein begins to be secreted after birth (e.g., during puberty). In this case the T cell repertoire present at that time would have been established in the absence of the protein, and thus would be expected to contain clones specific for peptides generated from the protein.

The molecular basis for the unresponsiveness observed in these various systems appears to differ for reasons that are not understood. In some systems the T cell unresponsiveness can be demonstrated *in vitro*. In a subset of these cases, the anergic T cells fail to proliferate or produce IL-2 in response to antigen (Lo et al., 1990; Arnold et al., 1993) *in vitro* despite normal TCR and accessory molecule expression and IL-2 receptor function; whereas in others unresponsiveness is accompanied by reduced TCR or accessory molecule expression, unresponsiveness to exogenous IL-2, or reduced TCR-mediated increases in intracellular calcium. In certain transgenic systems where MHC molecules are expressed only on a peripheral tissue, *in vitro* reactivity to splenic APC expressing that MHC molecule is demonstrable, despite the fact that the animals fail to respond to the tissue even after priming with the antigen on bone marrow-derived APC. This discrepancy could be explained by the fact that the T cells specific for peptide/MHC complexes expressed only on the tolerated tissue may actually be unresponsive but the T cells specific for spleen-specific peptide/MHC complexes are not. This possibility suggests that MLR reactivity should be interpreted with caution as a sign of lack of *in vivo* tolerance. It should be noted that although these elegant transgenic experiments demonstrate that that anergy can be a tolerance mechanism, to date it has not been possible to unequivocally determine whether clonal anergy is a tolerance mechanism for self-peptide antigens in unmanipulated animals because it is not possible with current methods to physically track T cells of known self peptide/MHC specificity *in vivo*.

The situations in which T cell anergy is demonstrable *in vivo* and/or *in vitro* are in contrast to several reports in which T cells in transgenic mice that express viral antigens only on pancreatic β cells do not respond to the β cells but are also not rendered tolerant, i.e., the antigen appears to be ignored (Arnold et al. 1993). Although the pancreas is not normally rejected in these animals, priming with bone-marrow-derived APC bearing the antigen results in a destructive β cell-specific immune response. Whether a tissue-specific antigen induces anergy or is ignored may depend on the amount of antigen expressed and the affinities of the responding TCRs for the relevant peptide/MHC complexes. For example, if the number of peptide/MHC complexes expressed on a peripheral tissue is very low, or if only low affinity T cells are present, then these complexes might be ignored unless the T cells are primed by professional APC.

IN VITRO CLONAL ANERGY MODELS

The theoretical paradox that must be explained by the *in vivo* peripheral tolerance models is: "how can self-antigen recognition by mature T cells in the periphery inactivate these T cells when their normal response is to be activated by foreign cells and molecules?" Clues as to how this could occur can be found in experiments on the immunogenicity of foreign antigens. It has long been known that the immunogenicity of soluble proteins for T cells is dependent on the form and route of antigen administration. Antigen aggregation and subcutaneous administration in complete Freund's adjuvant (CFA) promote immunogenicity whereas deaggregation and intravenous, oral, or intraperitoneal administration without adjuvant do not (Mueller et al., 1989). In fact, the latter conditions often induce unresponsiveness to subsequent subcutaneous antigen administration in CFA. Antigens covalently coupled to lymphoid cells with chemical cross-linkers or antigens targeted to resting B cells are also tolerogenic *in vivo* following intravenous injection. Because the "foreign-ness" of the antigen is not affected by these treatments, it is likely that they instead affect the environment in which the responding T cells recognize peptide/MHC complexes. Lafferty and co-workers (Lafferty et al., 1983) proposed that to support maximal T cell activation, APC must not only present peptide/MHC complexes but also provide essential nonspecific costimulatory signals. Bretscher and Cohn (1970) further hypothesized that lymphocytes that recognize antigen in the absence of the costimulatory signal become refractory to further stimulation. Putting these ideas together one can construct a model in which T cells must both recognize peptide/MHC complexes and receive costimulatory signals from APC to become activated (Mueller et al., 1989). If only peptide/MHC recognition occurs then the T cells become unresponsive (Mueller et al., 1989).

Results from *in vitro* experiments have provided additional support for this model (Schwartz, 1990). To produce IL-2 maximally *in vitro*, T cells must receive two different sets of signals from APC, one set transduced through the TCR/CD3 complex and the other through receptors for costimulatory molecules. TCR perturbation by peptide/MHC complexes or anti-TCR or -CD3 antibodies rapidly leads to the activation of tyrosine kinases and phosphorylation of phospholipase-Cγ1. This enzyme then cleaves phosphatidylinositol-4,5-bisphosphate in the T cell membrane to produce inositol trisphosphate and diacylglycerol, which in turn stimulate increases in intracellular calcium and protein kinase C activation, respectively. Although necessary, TCR occupancy and its biochemical consequences alone do not induce proliferation by most normal T cells unless a costimulus is provided. IL-1 serves this function for some IL-4-producing CD4$^+$ T cell clones (known as Th2 in the mouse) by allowing these cells to respond to the IL-4 they produce. In contrast, cytokines do not provide costimulation to IL-2-producing T cell clones (known as Th1 in the mouse) or freshly purified T cells; instead an APC-derived surface molecule(s) is involved. The requirement for this costimulatory signal is illustrated by the observations that murine or human IL-2-producing T cell clones do not proliferate or produce IL-2 in response to peptide-pulsed, metabolically inactive fixed APC or purified MHC molecules in artificial membranes. The missing costimulatory function can be provide by viable splenocytes that cannot be recognized by the TCR on the T cells if the splenocytes are allowed to contact the T cells. Costimulatory activity operates via a biochemical pathway distinct from inositol phospholipid hydrolysis. The molecules involved are inducible and differentially expressed by various APC, e.g., dendritic cells, macrophages, and activated B cells are potent costimulators whereas resting B cells are poor costimulators. The inducibility of costimulatory molecules probably explains the effect of fixation, i.e., fixed APC are unable to induce the costimulatory molecules upon cognate interaction with T cells.

Recent results have provided convincing evidence that the T cell-specific surface molecule CD28 is a T cell receptor that transduces a costimulatory signal (June et al., 1990). CD28 is a 44-kDa homodimeric integral membrane protein encoded by an immunoglobulin-like gene. CD28 is expressed exclusively on T cells, all CD4$^+$ cells, and most CD8$^+$ cells. Another molecule called CTLA4 is highly homologous to CD28 and appears to be induced in T cells upon activation. Both CD28 and CTLA4 bind to another immunoglobulin gene superfamily member called B7. The level of B7 expression correlates quantitatively with the costimulatory potency of different APC, i.e., dendritic cells $>$ activated B cells $\gg$ resting B cells. B7-transfected cells or cross-linked anti-CD28 monoclonal antibodies greatly enhance the amount of IL-2 and other lymphokines produced by purified T cells in response to TCR stimulation whereas anti-B7 antibodies or uncross-linked anti-CD28 mAb block T cell activation in response antigen presentation by APC. Finally, like the APC-derived costimulatory signal, CD28 signal transduction does not augment inositol phosphate production or calcium increase. Although the biology of CD28/B7 interaction most closely resembles that of APC-derived costimulation, it should be noted that other adhesion receptor/ligand pairs probably deliver additional costimulatory signals (van Seventer et al., 1991).

For most murine and human IL-2 producing $CD4^+$ T cells, TCR occupancy in the absence of costimulatory signals *in vitro* results in the induction of a long-lasting state of anergy (Mueller et al., 1989; Schwartz, 1992; Jenkins, 1992). This generally involves situations where the TCR is stimulated in the absence of viable bone marrow-derived APC. Under these conditions, TCR occupancy occurs but IL-2 is not produced, the T cells do not proliferate, and instead are subsequently unable to produce IL-2 when re-challenged with splenic APC plus antigen. Increases in intracellular calcium and new protein synthesis are critical for anergy induction. Anergy is maintained by a defect in TCR-mediated IL-2 mRNA accumulation, not by TCR, CD4, or IL-2 receptor modulation. Responsiveness to exogenous IL-2 is maintained. Anergic T cells fail to initiate transcription from a heterologous promoter controlled by the 5' IL-2 gene enhancer or by a multimer of the AP-1 sequence present within the enhancer (Kang et al., 1992). In addition, the protein complex that binds the AP-1 sequence, presumably a c-*fos*/c-*jun* heterodimer, is induced slowly in anergic T cells upon restimulation. Therefore, the simplest explanation that takes into account all of these results, including the requirement for new protein synthesis, is that an AP-1-binding repressor is made under conditions that result in anergy. Anergic Th1 cells also appear to contain reduced levels of the $p56^{lck}$ and $p59^{fyn}$ tyrosine kinases, suggesting that these cells may also have proximal signaling defects (Quill et al., 1993).

Provision of costimulatory signals in the form of B7-expressing viable accessory cells or cross-linked anti-CD28 monoclonal antibody (MAb) interferes with anergy induction (Schwartz, 1992). however, the antagonistic relationship between costimulation and anergy induction appears to be indirect (Jenkins, 1992). T cell clones preincubated with viable APC, antigen, and anti-IL-2/IL-2 receptor antibodies, conditions where costimulation is provided and IL-2 is produced but where proliferation is blocked, are unresponsive to subsequent restimulation with antigen. Furthermore, T cell clones become anergic following chronic stimulation with anti-CD3 antibody plus viable APC, another situation where costimulation is provided but subsequent cell division is inhibited by chronic TCR signaling. These results together with the earlier results on anergy induction suggest that unresponsiveness is induced as result of TCR signaling in the absence of cell division. This can occur when costimulation is not provided and IL-2 is not produced or when costimulation is provided and IL-2 is produced but subsequent cell division is prevented. Therefore the ability of viable accessory cells to prevent anergy is likely explained by the fact that the costimulation they provide enhances the amount of IL-2 the T cells produce, promoting multiple rounds of cell division, allowing the T cells to inactivate or dilute out the repressor protein. The observation that cycling anergic T cells in exogenous IL-2 results in recovery of their antigen responsiveness is consistent with this idea (Jenkins, 1992).

In many of the *in vivo* models the experimental "self"-antigen is presented on cells known to be poor providers of costimulatory signals (pancreatic β cells or epithelial cells), a situation that results in anergy *in vitro*. Antigen-bearing splenocytes treated with chemical fixation or ultraviolet irradiation, or normal resting B cells are all inefficient providers of costimulatory signals *in vitro* and induce T cell unresponsiveness *in vitro* and *in vivo*. Furthermore, the inflammation induced by CFA is likely to up-regulate expression of costimulatory molecules like B7 on APC favoring T cell priming whereas antigen administration in the absence of inflammation and B7 induction could explain why T cells are tolerized under these conditions. In addition, in several, but not all, of the *in vivo* anergy models the unresponsiveness is due mainly to an IL-2 production defect, not an IL-2 responsiveness defect (Jenkins, 1992). Therefore, the *in vitro* model appears to describe well the conditions that induce anergy *in vivo* and, at least for a subset of cases, describes the maintenance of the *in vivo* anergic state.

COSTIMULATION AND ANERGY IN TRANSPLANTATION BIOLOGY

Lafferty and colleagues championed the idea that the capacity of allogeneic tissue to be rejected is related to the number of professional bone marrow-derived APC present in that tissue (Lafferty et al., 1983). This hypothesis was based on the observation that depletion of "passenger leukocytes" from pancreatic islet grafts reduced their immunogencity *in vivo*. It is therefore possible that allograft rejection is initiated by direct recognition of alloantigen on the surface of graft-borne APC either in the graft itself or in the draining lymph node (Fig. 1). In support of the latter possibility, it appears that resident dendritic cells leave grafted tissues and migrate to the draining lymph node where they acquire potent T cell-activating properties (Larsen et al., 1990). Allogeneic dendritic cells could activate alloantigen-specific lymph node T cells, which could then recirculate back to the graft where they could be activated further by remaining dendritic cells. Although unlikely for naive T cells, it is also possible that T cells recently activated by alloantigen presentation by dendritic cells may also be able to respond to the parenchymal graft tissue itself. The latter recognition event would be facilitated for $CD4^+$ T cells by induction of class II MHC molecules on parenchymal cells by interferon-γ produced in response to alloantigen presentation by dendritic cells. Based on this type of model, grafts initially devoid of resident dendritic cells would be incapable of initiating the graft rejection process. This model is supported by the finding that mice that express transgenic allogeneic MHC molecules only on their pancreatic β cells do not develop insulitis and instead become immunologically tolerant to the transgenic product (Lo et al., 1991).

Expression of costimulatory ligands could determine tissue immunogenicity. Most parenchymal cell types even when induced to express class II MHC molecules are poor stimulators of freshly isolated T cells or resting T cell clones (Schwartz, 1992), and thus would be expected to be poor initiators of graft rejection, although they might be able to further stimulate already activated T cells. In contrast, dendritic cells are the most stimulatory APC. *In vitro* culture of Langerhans cells, immature dendritic cells of the skin, is thought to mimic the acquisition of potent accessory function by dendritic cells following migration to the lymph node. Interestingly, freshly isolated Langerhans cells do not express B7 and are poor accessory cells, whereas cultured Langerhans cells express high levels of B7 and are potent accessory cells (Larsen et al., 1992).

Further support for the role of costimulation by passenger leukocytes during graft rejection is provided by the finding that CTLA4–Ig, a fusion protein composed of the extracellular portion of CTLA4 fused to human IgG_1 Fc, inhibits rejection of allogeneic heart grafts (Turka et al., 1992) and xenogeneic pancreatic islet grafts (Lenschow et al., 1992). In the latter case, mice grafted with human islets did not reject their grafts following treatment with either human CTLA4–Ig or anti-human B7 antibody. Although the CTLA4–Ig is capable of binding both murine and human B7, the anti-B7 antibody is specific only for the human molecule. Therefore, the antibody must have interfered with stimulation of murine T cells by alloantigen expressed on human bone marrow-derived cells (as these are the cells that express B7) present in the graft. It should be noted, however, that the anti-B7 antibody was less effective than the CTLA4–Ig at blocking rejection. This could be explained by the fact that murine $B7^+$ APC are involved in xenograft rejection by picking up, processing, and presenting xenoantigens to T cells. The ability of CTLA4–Ig to block graft rejection could be explained by a blockage of lymphokine production by $CD4^+$ T cells or by blockage of precursor cytotoxic T cell (CTL) differentiation, which has been shown *in vitro* to be augmented by B7.

CTLA4–Ig-treated xenograft recipients are unable to reject a second xenograft from the original donor even after the CTLA4–Ig is no longer present (Lenschow et al., 1992). This is a specific effect in that these animals reject third-party grafts. This result suggests that as in the *in vitro* system, foreign antigen recognition in the absence of the CD28 signal results in T cell unresponsiveness. It should be noted, however, that

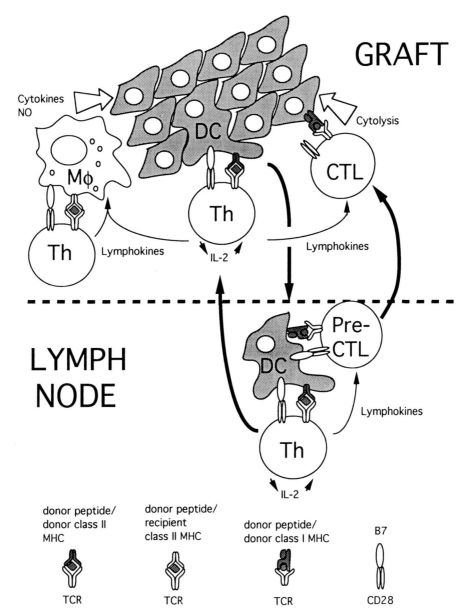

Fig. 1. Antigen presentation during graft rejection. In this model, graft rejection is initiated by dendritic cells (DC). Graft parenchymal cells are not capable of the stimulating T helper cells (Th) because they do not express class II MHC or B7 molecules. Graft DCs activate recipient Th cells by presenting to them alloantigenic peptide/class II MHC complexes and B7 molecules in the graft itself, or in the draining lymph node. Once activated, the Th cells migrate to the graft site where they secrete lymphokines that facilitate the differentiation of macrophages (Mϕ) and cytolytic T cells (CTL) specific for alloantigenic peptide/class I MHC complexes expressed by the parenchymal cells. The activated Mϕs and CTL destroy the graft. If the recipient is preinjected with resting B cells that express alloantigenic peptide/class II MHC complexes but not B7 molecules, then anergy is induced in the Th cells preventing the entire process. A similar result would be predicted in recipients injected with agents that interrupt the CD28/B7 interaction.

long-term tolerance is not achieved in the rat heart allograft model even though allograft rejection is greatly delayed by the CTLA4–Ig treatment. This could be related to fact that human CTLA4–Ig probably does not bind as well to rat B7 as it does to human B7. Interference with the LFA-1/ICAM-1 interaction also prevents heart allograft rejection and results in the long-term tolerance (Isobe et al., 1992), suggesting that these molecules play a role in costimulation *in vivo*. In neither of the cases where long-term tolerance is achieved is it possible to determine whether the mechanism underlying the unresponsiveness is clonal anergy. However, in a case where class II MHC-specific T cells can be physically monitored, mice treated with anti-CD4 antibody at the time they receive allogeneic pancreatic islets become tolerant to the graft because of anergy induction in the responding T cells (Alters et al., 1991).

Another strategy to inhibit allograft rejection is to inject the eventual graft recipient with APC that express the MHC molecules of the graft but that do not express costimulatory molecules with the hope of inducing unresponsiveness in the responding T cells. Resting B cells are ideally suited for this purpose. They express high levels of class I and II MHC molecules but not B7 molecules, and have been shown to be inefficient providers of costimulation *in vitro* (Mueller, 1989). Mice infused with allogeneic resting B cells fail to reject skin grafts from the strain that donated the B cells (Hori et al., 1989), and female mice injected with resting B cells from male mice fail to reject male skin grafts or generate antimale antigen-specific CTLs (Fuchs and Matzinger, 1992). In contrast, injection of female mice with male dendritic cells leads to enhanced rejection of male skin grafts. Finally, antigen presentation to precursor CTLs in the absence of signals from CD4+ helper T cells results in the functional inactivation of the former population (Guerder and Matzinger, 1989; Rees et al., 1990). Therefore, it is conceivable that alloantigen-specific CD4+ T cells are rendered unresponsive in the mice injected with allogeneic resting B cells and are unable to provide helper signals to precursor CTL resulting in their functional inactivation.

The ability of resting B cells to induce transplantation tolerance is supported by studies of soluble protein antigen-specific T cell responses. Targeting antigens to resting B cells *in vivo* not only fails to induce a T cell response, but instead induces unresponsiveness to the same antigen injected in adjuvant (Eynon and Parker, 1992). Although it is tempting to conclude that anergy is the mechanism underlying all of these unresponsive states because resting B cells are costimulation-deficient APC, it should be noted that none of the studies performed to date distinguishes between functional inactivation and physical deletion of the responding T cells.

CONCLUSION

In summary, intrathymic clonal deletion of immature T cells is likely to be the major tolerance mechanism for proteins produced in the thymus or present in the serum at high enough concentration to be taken up and presented by thymic APC. In contrast, tolerance to proteins expressed only by specific extrathymic tissues could be maintained by T cell ignorance or anergy. Antigens could be ignored by all T cells if they are poorly expressed or by CD4+ T cells if they are expressed on a tissue that does not express class II MHC molecules, as is the case for most noninflamed parenchymal tissues. Anergy could be particularly important for CD8+ T cells because most tissues express class I MHC, but not B7, and are constantly presenting endogenous self-proteins, some of which are specific only to that tissue. Anergy could also be important for soluble proteins that are present at too low a concentration to be taken up and presented by nonspecific thymic APC but could be taken up and presented effectively by resting, costimulation-deficient B cells whose surface Ig molecules are specific for that self-protein. Anergy could also be important for developmentally regulated proteins that are expressed in the periphery after the mature T cell repertoire has been established.

This model also makes predictions about graft rejection. Costimulatory APC expressing molecules like B7 should be critical for the initiation of graft rejection. In addition, if graft-borne alloantigens are presented in the absence of costimulatory signals then long-term tolerance should ensue. Although the preliminary experiments described above suggest that these predictions are correct, additional work will be required to determine if these are general concepts and to identify the mechanism involved.

REFERENCES

Alters SE, Shizuru JA, Ackerman J, Grossman D, Seydel KB, Fathman CG (1991): Anti-CD4 mediates clonal anergy during transplantation tolerance induction. J Exp Med 173:491–494.

Arnold B, Schonrich G, Hammerling GJ (1993): Multiple levels of peripheral tolerance. Immunol Today 14:12–14.

Bretscher P, Cohn M (1970): A theory of self-nonself discrimination: Paralysis and induction involve recognition of one and two determinants on an antigen, respectively. Science 169:1042–1049.

Davis, MM (1990): T cell receptor gene diversity and selection. Annu Rev Biochem 59:475-496.

Eynon EE, Parker DC (1992): Small B cells as antigen-presenting cells in the induction of tolerance to soluble protein antigens. J Exp Med 175:131–138.

Fuchs EJ, Matzinger P (1992): B cells turn off virgin but not memory T cells. Science 258:1156–1159.

Guerder S, Matzinger P. (1989): Activation versus tolerance: A decision made by T helper cells. Cold Spring Harbor Symp Quant Biol 54:799–805.

Heath WR, Allison J, Hoffmann MW, Schonrich G, Hammerling G, Arnold B, Miller JFAP (1992): Autoimmune diabetes as a consequence of locally produced IL-2. Nature (London) 359:547–549.

Hori S, Sato S, Kitagawa S, Azuma T, Kokudo S, Hamaoka T, Fujiwara H (1989): Tolerance induction of allo-class II H-2 antigen-reactive L3T4+ helper T cells and prolonged survival of the corresponding class II H-2-disparate skin graft. J Immunol 143:1447–1452.

Isobe M, Yagita H, Okumura K, Ihara A (1992): Specific acceptance of cardiac allografts after treatment with antibodies to ICAM-1 and LFA-1. Science 255:1125–1129.

Jenkins MK (1992): The role of cell division in the induction of clonal anergy. Immunol Today 13:69–73.

June CH, Ledbetter JA, Linsley PS, Thompson CB (1990): Role of the CD28 receptor in T cell activation. Immunol Today 11:211–216.

Kang SM, Beverly B, Tran AC, Brorson K, Schwartz RH, Lenardo MJ (1992): Transactivation by AP-1 is a molecular target of T cell clonal anergy. Science 257:1134–1138.

Lafferty KJ, Prowse SJ, Simeonovic CJ (1983): Immunobiology of tissue transplantation: a return to the passenger leukocyte concept. Annu Rev Immunol 1:143–173.

Larsen CP, Steinman RM, Witmer-Pack M, Hankins DF, Morris PJ, Austyn JM (1990): Migration and maturation of Langerhans cells in skin transplants and explants. J Exp Med 172:1483–1493.

Larsen CP, Ritchie SC, Pearson TC, Linsley PS, Lowry RP (1992): Functional expression of the costimulatory molecule, B7/BB1, on murine dendritic cell populations. J Exp Med 176:1215–1220.

Lenschow DJ, Zeng Y, Thistlewaite JR, Montag A, Brady W, Gibson MG, Linsley PS, Bluestone JA (1992): Long term survival of xenogeneic pancreatic islets induced by CTLA4Ig. Science 257:789–792.

Lo D, Freedman J, Hesse S, Brinster RL, Sherman L (1991): Peripheral tolerance in transgenic mice: tolerance to class II MHC and non-MHC transgene antigens. Immunol Rev 122:87–102.

Mueller DL, Jenkins MK, Schwartz RH (1989): Clonal expansion versus functional clonal inactivation: A costimulatory signalling pathway determines the outcome of T cell antigen receptor occupancy. Annu Rev Immunol 7:445–480.

Nossal GJV (1992): Cellular and molecular mechanisms of B lymphocyte tolerance. Adv Immunol. 52:283–327.

Quill H, Riley MP, Cho EA, Casnellie JE, Reed JC, and Torigoe T (1992): Anergic Th1 cells express altered levels of the protein tyrosine kinases p56lck and p59fyn. J Immunol 149:2887–2893.

Rees MA, Rosenburg AS, Munitz T, Singer A (1990): In vivo induction of antigen-specific transplantation tolerance to Qa1a by exposure to alloantigen in the absence of T-cell help. Proc Natl Acad Sci USA 87:2765–2769.

Rocha B, von Boehmer H (1991): Peripheral selection of the T cell repertoire. Science 251:1225–1228.

Schwartz RH (1989): Acquisition of immunologic self-tolerance. Cell 57:1073–1081.

Schwartz RH (1990): A cell culture model for T lymphocyte clonal anergy. Science 248:1349–1356.

Schwartz RH (1992): Costimulation of T lymphocytes: the role of CD28, CTLA-4 and B7/BB1 in IL-2 production and immunotherapy. Cell 71: 1065–1068.

Turka LA, Linsley PS, Lin H, Brady W, Leiden JM, Wei RQ, Gibson ML, Zheng XG, Myrdal S, Gordon D, Bailey T, Bolling SF, Thompson CB (1992): T-cell activation by the CD28 ligand B7 is required for cardiac allograft rejection in vivo. Proc Natl Acad Sci USA 89:11102–11105.

van Seventer GA, Shimizu Y, Shaw S (1991): Roles of multiple accessory molecules in T-cell activation: Bilateral interplay of adhesion and costimulation. Curr Opin Immunol 3:294–303.

Webb S, Morris C, Sprent J (1990): Extrathymic tolerance of mature T cells: Clonal elimination as a consequence of immunity. Cell 63:1249–1256.

Chapter 19
Xenotransplantation

Fritz H. Bach, Hugh Auchincloss, and Simon C. Robson

INTRODUCTION

Xenotransplantation refers to the surgical grafting of organs from a member of one species to a member of another species and is frequently classified into two main categories: concordant and discordant according to the presumptive immunological barriers to graft acceptance (Calne, 1970). Concordant transplants are performed between species that are relatively closely related phylogenetically such as baboon to human; in such species combinations, hyperacute rejection (HAR) is not observed. (Starzl et al., 1993).

Transplantation between members of discordant or distantly related species, on the other hand, such as pig to human, results in hyperacute rejection in unmodified recipients. Hyperacute rejection can take place in just 10–15 mins in a discordant xenograft from guinea pig to rat, for instance, or in approximately 1–2 hr if a pig heart is transplanted to a baboon or a rhesus monkey. This extremely rapid rejection process is associated with codeposition of recipient xenoreactive natural antibodies (XNA) and complement (C) on the endothelium of the donor organ (Bach et al., 1992, 1993).

There are fundamental pathophysiological differences between the transplantation of an immediately vascularized organ, such as heart, kidney, liver, or pancreas, where the grafted endothelium is immediately exposed to the recipient's circulating blood and thus to the XNA and C, and transplantation of neovascularized tissues, such as in the case of pancreatic islets, in which blood vessels from the host grow over days into the transplanted tissues. The endothelium is a single cell layer that lines the inside of the blood vessels and forms the barrier between the circulating blood and the tissue fluid of the organ. In the immediately vascularized organ, the endothelium of the transplanted vasculature persists in very large measure as donor type, and thus remains foreign to the recipient. In the case of transplanted islets of the pancreas, it is host endothelium that grows into the transplanted tissues (Bach, 1993). If endothelial cells (EC) are damaged, it is not clear whether they would be replaced by other donor EC or by host EC.

HAR occurs in untreated recipients and involves EC activation. This model posits that following transplantation and establishment of blood flow from the recipient to the transplanted organ, recipient xenoreactive natural antibodies attach to donor endothelial cells. Natural antibodies are in significant measure IgM, and thus fix complement. The combination of the recipient's natural antibodies plus the activated complement leads to activation of the endothelial cells lining the vessels of the donor organ. Progressive EC activation is a central event that leads to complications associated with xenograft rejection.

In the very few minutes that it takes for an organ to be destroyed in HAR in some discordant species combinations, there is no time for gene up-regulation and synthesis of new proteins. In contrast, in delayed xenograft rejection (DXR), which takes place if the recipient is pretreated in one or another way to ameliorate the initial events, the rejection process may take place over a matter of hours, or even days, permitting gene up-regulation and its consequences. Given pre-

Transplantation Immunology, pages 305–338
© 1995 Wiley-Liss, Inc.

sent treatments, DXR in a guinea pig to rat transplant can occur in many hours or a few days, as compared with HAR, which takes 10–15 min; in the pig to primate transplant, DXR takes place after several days or even a very few weeks. These potential differences in mechanisms involved in HAR and DXR may relate to the following. The events that occur when EC are stimulated can be divided into those that occur very rapidly and do not require protein synthesis, and those that do require protein synthesis and take longer to manifest. These have been referred to as EC stimulation and EC activation, respectively (Cotran and Pober, 1989). To avoid the problem of using the term "stimulation" both for the action of stimuli that lead to activation of the EC, and for a part of that activation response, we have used the terms "Type I" and "Type II" activation, and grouped both types of responses as "EC activation." It is likely that HAR involves the consequences of events that constitute type I EC activation, whereas DXR likely involves the consequences of type II EC activation as well. From a clinical perspective, it is the problem of DXR with which we have to deal given that we can already reliably postpone rejection of a pig heart or kidney in a primate for at least some days given the current interventions that remove XNA and C.

Discussed below are each of the major components that are thought to be involved in rejection, hyperacute or delayed, or an immediately vascularized organ. These include (1) recipient xenoreactive natural antibodies (XNA), (2) recipient complement (C), (3) donor endothelial cells that interact with the recipient's blood cells, which themselves likely play a significant role in the rejection response, and (4) the recipient's coagulation system. It seems probable that other factors play a role as well.

This chapter will therefore restrict itself to the discussion of immediately vascularized xenografts and will include both a discussion of the mechanisms involved in rejection of a xenograft as it occurs consequent to XNA and C, as well as of the cellular mechanisms that are involved, including T cell-mediated rejection. In the first part of the chapter, the focus is on those events that precede the T cell-mediated rejection. As

such, both HAR and DXR refer to these non-T cell-mediated forms of rejection.

XENOREACTIVE NATURAL ANTIBODIES (XNA)

The term "natural antibodies" has been used, at least in part, to refer to antibodies that are present without overt stimulation, such as the ABO isohemagglutinins and XNA. In fact, for both of these types of antibodies, there is evidence that they are not just "naturally" present, as though there are genetically programmed B cells that produce the antibodies irrespective of the immunological exposure of the animal. Rather, it seems likely that the XNA are elicited in response to carbohydrates, in the case of XNA involving terminal galactose moieties (Cooper et al., 1994) present on surface molecules of organisms in the gastrointestinal tract and other sites.

There seems to be general agreement that IgM can function as XNA, resulting in the fixation and activation of complement at the surface of EC. There is less information about the role of IgG in rejection. Some studies of the immunopathology of rejecting pig hearts in rhesus monkeys showed primarily, if not solely, IgM deposition on the endothelium of the donor organ. IgG, when found, appeared to have the same distribution as albumin, and was thus interpreted to be present secondary to loss of vascular integrity and diffusion from the intravascular space into the subendothelial tissues as endothelium responds to the insult of the transplant situation (see below) (Platt et al., 1991; Bach et al., 1992). Other studies show that IgG "binds" to xenogeneic target cells; however, there is controversy whether such binding is via the paratope (i.e., whether it is the antigen-combining site of the IgG molecule that binds) and thus whether the IgG molecule could either contribute a signal to the EC, or bind complement (Bach et al., 1991a,b).

However, there is also direct evidence for a role for IgG in some discordant models. Human IgG binds to pig EC *in vitro*. Importantly, Inveradi and his co-workers have shown that human IgG binds to rat EC *in vitro,* and serves to promote natural killer (NK) cell-mediated antibody-dependent cytotoxicity (ADCC) directed at the EC (Inverardi et al., 1993). The IgG molecule presumably binds targets on the EC via its antigen-combining site (the paratope); this interaction allows the Fc portion of the IgG to interact with the Fc receptor III on the NK cells, which is referred to as CD16. This overall finding may take on additional importance in view of some of our recent observations that activated NK cells and activated monocytes are prominent in guinea pig hearts rejected after approximately 3 days in rats treated with cobra venom factor to activate and thus deplete the complement system (Blakely et al., 1993).

It is important to note that in addition to preexisting natural antibodies, there can be an immune response of the recipient to the donor tissues, which results in the presence of elicited antibodies directed at targets on endothelial cells. Elicited antibodies are of central importance in the rejection of at least some concordant transplants, and will likely be an issue in discordant ones with prolonged survival as well.

The titers of XNA that are of the IgM isotype (IgM-XNA) in different humans vary widely. Vanhove and Bach (1993), studying 50 apparently healthy volunteers, found that the titers of serum XNA measured in an anti-porcine EC ELISA varied more than 400-fold between individuals with the highest and lowest tiers. In our previous studies of a smaller panel of control human sera, we found that this variation in titer did not correlate with either the total amount of IgM in the serum or the titers of the ABO isohemagglutinins. To help plan therapeutic strategies aimed at removing, or blocking, XNA, several other issues were investigated by Vanhove and Bach. From the data, it appeared that XNA derived from individuals with the relatively higher titers of these antibodies represented approximately only 0.1% of the total IgM, but that about 100,000 IgM molecules can deposit on each EC *in vitro* and that the dissociation constant of the XNA is of the order of $1 \times 10^{-9} M$. While these results may be dependent on the methods used to obtain the XNA and the porcine endothelial cells, they provide a general guideline for potential therapeutic manipulations.

Methods to Remove or Block XNA

The two most common methods that have been used to deplete XNA from a prospective recipient are plasmapheresis and organ absorption (reviewed in Bach et al., 1991). Plasmaphereses consist of having the individual's blood flow through a plasmapheresis machine in which plasma is separated from the whole blood and exchanged for plasma substitutes such as albumin. Thus, in addition to XNA, other factors of importance in vascular rejection, such as complement and coagulation factors, are also depleted by this approach.

Plasmaphereses. This is an excellent intervention for removing high concentrations of preformed antibodies (prophylactically) or immune complexes (therapeutically) with repeated plasma exchanges. On the other hand, plasmapheresis is not particularly good at lowering the level of a given substance such as XNA already present in low concentrations to exceedingly low levels, or removing the last measurable traces of such a substance.

Organ absorption. Absorption of XNA on endothelial cells lining the vessels of an organ of the donor species, such as by passaging the potential recipient's blood through a pig kidney or liver, is very effective at removing small residual amounts. However, the total amount of XNA removed is limited by the number of EC available in that organ for absorption. In our experience, perfusion of two pig kidneys by primate blood sequentially, each for approximately 30 mins, reduces XNA levels significantly, and in some cases to below the detectable level in the ELISA assay described above. The first kidney starts to be rejected during the perfusion period; the second less so. Activation of complement on the endothelial lining of the perfused organs may, however, lead to inflammatory processes in the recipient and the possibility of sensitization is a concern. Sensitization of recipients by prior exposure to xenogeneic endothelium is obviously undesirable in terms of future transplantation. Although it is not yet known to what extent such sensitization occurs by organ absorption, there is the hope that the use of anti-B cell immunosuppressants (see below) will help avoid sensitization.

Column absorption. Another approach with the same goals would consist of the following intervention. If the target antigenic epitopes, presumably sugars, that are recognized by the XNA are better defined, those moieties could be linked to a solid phase, e.g., beads on a column. Subsequently, the recipient's plasma could be filtered through the column, thus removing the XNA from the circulation. Such columns exist to remove anti-AB antibodies from patients prior to their receiving an AB incompatible transplant. Usually there are two columns. First, the targetted/offending antibodies are removed on one column; when that column is saturated with bound antibodies, the apparatus switches so that the second column is used for further depletion, while the first column is regenerated for reuse.

Blocking XNA binding *in vivo*. While not a method to remove antibodies, if the target epitopes for the XNA were known, those substances could also be administered in a soluble form *in vivo* in an attempt to block the binding of the XNA to their targets on the EC. (See above and Chapter 5 for a discussion of how this has been done for AB-incompatible transplants.) Substituted sugar moieties containing terminal galactose or other residues may have a role in this context.

Although both plasmaphereses and organ absorption are effective and the other techniques mentioned above may have technological advantages, XNA rapidly return to the circulation. Thus, in the last few years, additional approaches with adjunctive therapies have been evaluated.

Anti-B cell immunosuppressants. Most immunosuppressive drugs developed for transplantation have been chosen based on their anti-T cell activity. This has been motivated by the presumption that allografts are rejected by T cells. Recently several agents have been developed that are effective at preventing the synthesis of elicited antibodies as well as suppressing T cells. These agents include mycophenolate mofetil (RS61443), rapamycin, brequinar, and 15-deoxy-

spergualin. We have shown that all of these are effective at suppressing XNA as well as the elicited antibodies. Several of these agents are also effective at suppressing T cell responses, a problem that will become more evident in discordant xenografts where rejection can be postponed for a period long enough to allow T cell rejection responses to be generated. These agents may thus be useful in maintaining lowered levels of XNA and in the prevention of the generation of elicited antibody responses, as well as providing anti-T cell activity (Leventhal et al., 1992; Figueroa et al., 1993).

Anti-μ chain MAb. It has been known for many years that administration of an anti-μ chain antibody in the neonatal period results in prolonged suppression of IgM synthesis. Bazin and we thought that this might also be applicable in adult life, and have used a mouse anti-rat μ chain monoclonal antibody (MAb) to suppress IgM and IgM-XNA levels in adult rats (Latinne et al., 1994). There are several concerns about using such an approach clinically. First, the general use of MAb of xenogeneic origin will likely lead to antibody production against the administered antibody; this is a general problem to which certain "solutions" have been offered, such as the molecular "humanization" of the antibody. In this case, since anti-B cell immunosuppressive agents would likely be administered concurrently with the MAb, there may be added protection. Second, there is the concern that the administered MAb will complex with remaining IgM in the circulation, which could lead to immune complex disease. Whether XNA levels can be maintained at essentially low enough levels for the duration of the administration of the anti-μ reagent so that this does not become a problem is also a matter for future experimentation. However, to date, anti-μ treatment in rats has resulted in the most profound depletion of XNA in the peripheral blood of any procedure available: up to $2^{1}/_{2}$ to 4 weeks of undetectable levels of XNA. Further, none of the other approaches has, except for a 1- to 2-day period in the case of organ absorption, lowered the XNA levels to such a great extent.

In an attempt to avoid the needed use of multiple doses of anti-μ antibody, we have combined the use of a few doses of anti-μ with pharmacological anti-B cell immunosuppressants in rats. As shown in Figure 1, in the relatively short-term experiments done to date, the pharmacological anti-B cell immunosuppressants can be used to maintain the undetectable levels of IgM-XNA achieved by the abbreviated anti-μ treatment.

Splenectomy. Most experimental animals used as recipients of a xenotransplant are splenectomized prior to transplantation. We have shown that splenectomy in rats leads to lowered levels (by about 50%) of XNA (Bach et al., 1993). In addition, it may be that splenectomy is associated with a reduction of B and NK cells, since the spleen is a major source of these cells.

Assays for XNA

Classically, the presence of XNA in serum has been quantitated by hemagglutination or lymphocytotoxicity assays. We reasoned that since the biologically important target for XNA *in vivo* is probably EC, we could measure XNA in an ELISA using EC of the potential donor species as the target cells. A variation of this assay is to use isolated membrane target antigens from the EC, or from platelets, which seem to share major targets with the EC, as the target antigens in the ELISA (see Fig. 1). This assay is at least as sensitive as previously used assays, and may

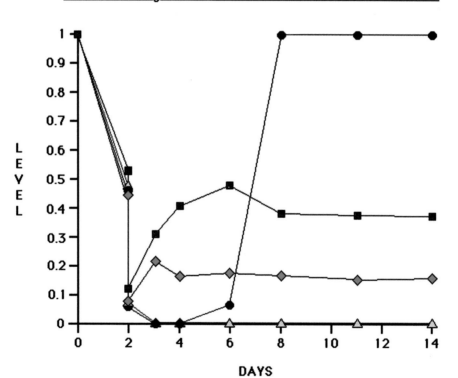

RELATIVE IgM-XNA LEVEL VS. TREATMENT DAY

Fig. 1. IgM-XNA levels as determined by ELISA. IgM-XNA levels were determined by ELISA using guinea pig platelet extract as the target. Lewis rats underwent splenectomy on day 0, plasmapheresis on day 2, and received one of four different treatment regimens from day 0 to 14: control (no further treatment) (square), rapamycin and cyclosporine A (diamond), anti-μ monoclonal antibody (circle), and rapamycin plus cyclosporine A and anti-μ.

provide quantitation that is more meaningful in terms of xenotransplantation, although this is, at least for the present, a theoretical point (Platt et al., 1990).

Targets of XNA

These must be considered at two levels: first, the (glyco)proteins and other molecules in the membranes of EC to which the XNA bind, and second, the carbohydrates epitopes on those molecules that are actually recognized by the XNA.

There are a number of molecules on pig EC and platelets to which XNA bind. These include a triad of glycoproteins with molecular weights 115,000, 125,000, and 135,000 (referred to as gp115–135) (Platt et al., 1990), and a number of other prominent targets with molecular weights in the range of 45,000 to 200,000 (Hofer-Warbinek et al., 1993). For the most part, the target molecules recognized by human XNA on porcine cells have been defined based on their relative molecular mass as analyzed on SDS–polyacrylamide gels (SDS–PAGE), with the antigens detected by Western blotting techniques. Of those studied, it appears that the XNA recognize carbohydrate moieties of the glycoproteins as the epitopes, some of which have recently been identified as discussed above.

As is likely clear from the above discussion, there are at least two reasons why it is important to define the carbohydrates recognized by XNA for potential therapeutic purposes. Administration of those sugars *in vivo* may block reactivity of XNA with target EC on the transplanted organ, as already discussed above for ABO-incompatible allotransplants. There is evidence that administration *in vivo* of the carbohydrate target moieties recognized by the anti-AB antibodies may block access of those antibodies to the endothelium and may thus prolong survival of ABO-incompatible allografts. Alternatively, the sugars could be bound to a matrix on appropriate columns; passage of the plasma of the potential recipient through such columns might, as has been done for the anti-AB antibodies, remove the XNA from the recipient, at least temporarily.

Molecules of different sizes are recognized as the predominant targets on different cells. In our own studies, the gp115–135 complexes were not detected on lymphocytes of red blood cells or lymphocytes, even though all the XNA reactive with EC could be absorbed from human serum by RBC or lymphocytes. This finding is consistent with the fact that XNA react with carbohydrate moieties, and that the same, or cross-reactive, sugars are present on different molecules on the different cells.

COMPLEMENT

There are two pathways by which complement can be activated, which are depicted in Figure 2. The classical pathway is initiated by antibodies that can bind to the first component, C1q, of the classical pathway of complement, from which event a cascade of reactions takes place that eventually leads to formation of the membrane attack complex (MAC), the terminal components of which (poly-C9) insert into the membrane of cells. The second pathway of complement activation is referred to as the alternative pathway. Antibody is not involved in this pathway. As shown in the figure, the two pathways meet at the level of C3, after which the events are identical regardless of the pathway with which the complement cascade was initiated. At various stages of the pathway, mediators are generated that can play important roles in inflammation. Among these are C3a and C5a.

An issue of some import in terms of helping define how to intervene in the complement reaction is the determination of which components of complement are involved in selected aspects of endothelial cell activation; some aspects of EC activation have been shown not to require the entire C cascade.

Whether the alternative pathway of complement is activated in xenotransplantation appears to depend to some extent on the species combination being studied. Following transplantation of guinea pig organs to rats, or the transplantation of rabbit organs to pigs lacking XNA, the alternative pathway is activated (Johnston et al., 1992). However, in the transplantation of pig organs to primates, there is no clear *in vivo* evi-

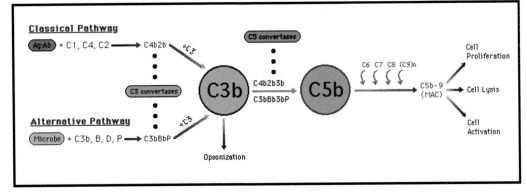

Fig. 2. Complement pathways. There are two mechanisms of complement activation as detailed in the figure that have in common a final common pathway leading to generation of the membrane attack complex (see text for further details).

dence of alternative pathway activation; there is codeposition of components of the classical pathway (C2 and C4) with antibody, but no evidence for activation of components of the alternative pathway such as factor B, although this area also needs more study. It is still controversial whether there is alternative pathway activation *in vitro*. This can be a critical issue in terms of planning therapy. A major approach to control HAR is to remove XNA from the potential recipient. If the alternative pathway of complement is activated, then removal of XNA will not prevent the activation of complement, although the magnitude of activation may be less. XNA may, as discussed above, have a role in xenograft rejection in addition to the activation of complement.

Methods to Inhibit Complement Action

The inhibition of complement activation has posed a major problem for clinical medicine. Few methods exist that are considered clinically applicable. The stimulus provided by xenograft rejection, with the special opportunity afforded by having a donor animal that might be genetically manipulated, has revitalized interest in potential methods to inhibit complement.

Cobra venom factor (CVF). This viperid equivalent and functional analogue of C3, which forms a physicochemically stable CVF-Bb complex, has been used in experimental animals for many decades. Indeed, the work done in xenotransplantation more than three decades ago demonstrated that administration of CVF, and the consequent inhibition of complement, did prolong survival of xenografts. More recently, CVF has again been used, in part in a more purified form, eliminating the associated venom proteases and toxins, and shown its efficacy. The most undesirable aspect of the use of CVF, aside from its potential toxicity, is that it works by initially activating rather than inhibiting complement. As such, it is necessary to administer it with great care in terms of dose and rapidity of administration, as activated products of complement may precipitate severe and undesirable side effects such as shock and pulmonary hemorrhage. Whether recipients will make antibodies to the CVF and thus neutralize the administered material after a few days remains a moot point. Nonetheless, certain investigators are considering the use of a highly purified form of CVF, presumably with anti-B cell immunosuppressive agents to prevent antibody production against the CVF, for potential application to humans, primarily because of the relative paucity of other approaches (Bach, 1993).

Soluble Complement Receptor 1 (sCR1). A much more satisfying approach, from a conceptual point of view, is the use of soluble CR1. Initiated by the work of Douglas Fearon and his colleagues (Hebell et al., 1991), it has been shown that the administration of sCR1 effectively inhibits complement and permits prolongation of xenograft survival. The attractive part of this approach is that it inhibits complement activation rather than depleting complement by activating it, as does CVF. A major limiting factor in the initial application of sCR1 may relate to the potential cost of this novel recombinant protein, as was initially the case of OKT3, an immunosuppressive agent.

Membrane-associated inhibitors of complement. Among the most exciting approaches to inhibit complement involves the use of membrane-associated inhibitors of complement as therapeutic modalities. There are a number of different membrane-associated molecules that inhibit different parts of the complement cascade. These include decay accelerating factor (DAF, CD55) and membrane cofactor protein (MCP, CD46), both of which inhibit at the C3 stage, and thus interfere with both the alternative and classical pathways. In addition, there are homologous restriction factor and CD59, which inhibit the very late stages of complement, at the C8–C9 level (Rooney et al., 1993).

Bach et al. and Dalmasso et al. introduced human forms of membrane-associated inhibitors of complement into porcine EC to inhibit complement action *in vitro*. This approach was based on two concepts. First, it has been shown for certain of these inhibitors that there is species specificity; thus, the pig inhibitor in the EC of the donor organ may not be particularly effective at inhibiting human complement. Second, by genetically engineering the pig EC, it may be possible to express the complement-inhibitory factors at a higher density than normally found, and thus achieve greater inhibition. It has now been demonstrated *in vitro* that such an idea has validity (Dalmasso et al., 1991; Bach et al., 1991a,b; White et al., 1992). In addition, White and his colleagues have recently produced pigs transgenic for human DAF. Those pigs express the human DAF product and their lymphocytes are lysed to a lesser extent than are control lymphocytes by human serum (personal communications). It is the goal of this group and other groups to derive a transgenic pig that expresses

high levels of several human inhibitors of complement, possibly including DAF, CD46, and CD59, at the endothelial interface.

A number of other substances can be used to inhibit complement, such as a nonanticoagulant form of heparin. None of these other methods studied to date has been shown to have sufficient efficacy to warrant serious consideration of them as therapeutic agents in xenotransplantation at this time.

A critical issue that is not yet resolved is whether DXR, mediated by factors other than T cells, would be averted or adequately treated if complement action could be blocked completely. Furthermore, if transgenic pigs are produced that express human DAF and other complement inhibitory proteins on their membranes, so that complement action is completely blocked, would a pig heart transplanted to a human be able to survive in the long term given the inability to generate a complement reaction on the endothelium under circumstances in which complement would normally be activated. If problems such as these arise, it may be that the expression of DAF or other inhibitors could eventually be expressed only when needed (see Chapter 21).

ENDOTHELIAL CELL ACTIVATION

A great deal is known about EC activation, largely based on *in vitro* studies in which the EC are stimulated by interleukin 1 (IL-1), tumor necrosis factor (TNF), or lipopolysaccharide (LPS) (Mantovani et al., 1992; Pober and Cotran, 1990). The discussion below is in large measure based on the information accumulated in those systems, although we and others have now shown that many of the changes in EC as they are activated in those other systems are also present when human serum, containing XNA + C, is used for activation *in vitro* of porcine EC. In addition, there is evidence that EC are activated *in vivo* as well, both in HAR and in the course of DXR. (It seems likely that in part there will be injury to the EC leading to cell death under some circumstances.) The presence of activated complement in the models of xenotransplantation leads to responses and interactions that are special for this system: e.g., deposition on donor organ EC of iC3b, which serves as a ligand for neutrophils and monocytes via CD11b–CD18 (Vercelloti et al., 1991).

Role of EC

Figure 3, which is a diagrammatic representation of discordant xenograft rejection, depicts several of the features associated with quiescent and activated EC. Quiescent EC perform several functions. First, because they are tightly juxtaposed, each touching its neighbors, they maintain a barrier that keeps cells and proteins of blood in the intravascular space and prevents leakage into the extracellular fluids of the organ. Second, the EC have on their surface a number of molecules that help to maintain anticoagulation and perform other functions. Two of the most important of these are heparan sulfate, a proteoglycan, and thrombomodulin, both of which are lost from the surface of the EC with EC activation (see later).

Heparan sulfate consists of a protein core with glycosaminoglycan chains attached to it. Antithrombin III (ATIII) binds to appropriately substituted residues on the glycosaminoglycan chains. When ATIII attaches to the heparan sulfate, it is activated and becomes a very powerful anticoagulant, interfering with the action of thrombin, a key component of the coagulation cascade, as well as other factors. Also associated with the heparan sulfate are superoxide dismutases (SOD), which break down oxygen radicals (O_2^-) that are produced, for instance, by activated neutrophils that attach to the activated EC (Balla et al., 1992; Esmon, 1993).

Thrombomodulin, present on the surface of quiescent EC, binds thrombin. As a consequence of that interaction, protein C (PC), which is present in blood, is converted to activated protein C (APC). Together with protein S, another component of blood, APC interferes in the coagulation cascade by splitting clotting factors VA and VIIIa, and thus interfering with thrombosis, i.e., having an anticoagulant effect (Esmon, 1993).

Functions of activated EC. When endothelial cells are activated they respond in many ways. The responses can be arbitrarily divided into four categories.

First, there is a loss of vascular integrity in that the EC retract from one another, initially exposing the subendothelial matrix and then allowing cells and proteins to pass from the intravascular space into the tissues of the organ, resulting in hemorrhage and edema.

Second, a series of cell surface adhesion molecules are up-regulated; some of these, such as E-selectin, are not expressed on the quiescent EC but appear on the surface when the EC are activated, while others are present even on the resting EC but are further up-regulated with EC activation. A major function of some of these ligands is to bind cells of blood, including neutrophils, monocytes, and lymphocytes, which express their own cell surface ligands that have affinity for E-selectin, ICAM-1, etc. on the activated EC. When EC are activated with xenogeneic serum, as occurs in the combination of human serum added to pig EC, the deposition of iC3b on the EC appears to be the most important ligand to promote neutrophil adhesion early after activation (Vercellotti et al., 1993). In addition to the ligands shown, EC up-regulate class I and class II molecules of the MHC under certain conditions. The cells that bind to the activated EC also participate in the inflammatory process. Neutrophils activated by C5a and platelet-activating factor (PAF) secrete reactive oxygen species; monocytes activated by IL-1 and other factors secrete IL-1 and TNF, both of which can act on the EC, as well as expressing tissue factor that contributes to the procoagulant environment (Murphy et al., 1992).

Third, the activated EC secrete a number of cytokines and other molecules, including IL-1, IL-6, and IL-8 as well as PAF. IL-1 is likely stimulatory to the EC in an autocrine loop, as well as functioning to activate cells of blood, such as monocytes. IL-8 is a chemoattractant for leukocytes and has some of the functions discussed for C5a above. PAF serves to activate neutrophils as well as taking part in the fourth area associated with EC activation, i.e., promotion of clotting (see below).

In the fourth category, there are at least six mechanisms that affect the balance of anticoagulation (associated with, and actively promoted by, quiescent EC) and procoagulation (associated with activated EC). (1) The action of

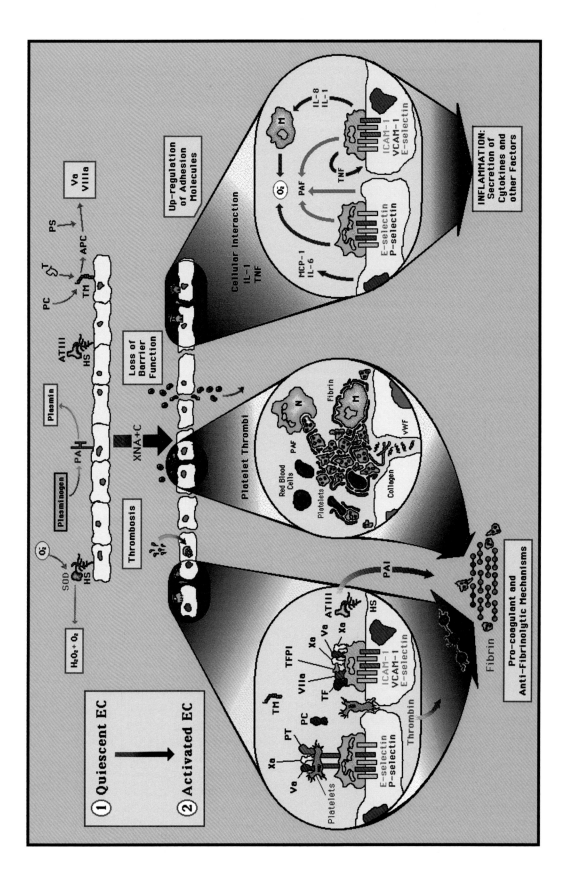

PAF in this context is to promote the activation of platelets and thus the formation of platelet thrombi. (2) Loss of HS, induced with EC activation, results in a loss of the anticoagulant contribution of ATIII. (3) Loss of thrombomodulin results in the loss of the ability to bind thrombin, and consequently of the generation of APC. (4) Secretion of plasminogen activator inhibitor (PAI-1) inhibits the naturally occurring action of plasminogen activator, which helps to break down fibrin clots: thus, there is again a net procoagulant effect associated with PAI-1 production. (5) Membrane vesicles break off from the activated EC containing components of the membrane attack complex (MAC, C5b-

C9), which activate the prothrombinase complex, leading to clotting. (6) Perhaps most important, and apparently the major pathway of induced clotting when EC are stimulated with XNA + C, is based on the production of tissue factor by the EC leading to conversion of factor VII to factor VIIa, and then the consequent clotting cascade. The area of coagulation is considered so important in the rejection of a xenograft, that it is dealt with in greater detail below, including discussion of platelet activation and aggregation.

In addition to these events, there are many others, most of which are not included in this brief discussion. One that is particularly impor-

---

Fig. 3. Hyperacute rejection in a discordant xenograft model. The figure presents a model of proposed major pathogenetic events leading to hyperacute rejection in a discordant xenograft. It is proposed that XNA and complement of the recipient activate donor organ EC as the basic event leading to rejection. Quiescent EC, which are tightly juxtaposed, maintain a barrier that keeps cells and proteins of blood in the intravascular space. Quiescent EC express heparan sulfate (HS) and thrombomodulin (TM) on their surface; HS binds both antithrombin III (ATIII), which functions as an anticoagulant, as well as superoxide dismutase (SOD), which breaks down superoxide (O_2^-). TM binds thrombin, leading to the generation of activated protein C (APC), which also has an anticoagulant effect. As a result of EC activation, there is a loss of vascular integrity as the EC retract from one another, resulting in hemorrhage and edema. Second, there is up-regulation and appearance on the EC surface of P-selectin, E-selectin, ICAM-1, and VCAM-1, which can function as ligands to bind neutrophils, monocytes, and lymphocytes of blood. When pig EC are activated with human XNA + C, the deposition of iC3b is an important ligand for neutrophils. In addition to the ligands shown, the activated EC up-regulate class I and II antigens of the MHC. Third, the activated EC secrete IL-1, IL-6, and IL-8 as well as platelet-activating factor (PAF). IL-1 is likely stimulatory to the EC in an autocrine loop, as well as functioning to activate cells of blood, such as monocytes. IL-8 is a chemoattractant for leukocytes and has some of the functions discussed for C5a below. PAF serves to activate neutrophils and platelets. Fourth, activated EC tip the balance from anticoagulation (promoted by quiescent EC) to procoagulation. Secreted PAF promotes the formation of platelet

thrombi; loss of HS and TM results in loss of the anticoagulant mechanisms discussed for quiescent EC; secretion of plaminogen activator inhibitor (PAI-1) inhibits the naturally occurring action of plasminogen activator; membrane vesicles break off from the activated EC containing components of the membrane attack complex (MAC, C5b-C9), which activate the prothrombinase complex leading to clotting; and the activated EC (as well as activated monocytes) produce tissue factor, perhaps the most powerful stimulus to coagulation. In addition to these events, there are others that likely impact HAR. Components of the activated complement system probably deliver a signal(s) to the EC, aiding in the full activation of the EC. In addition, split products of complement, such as C5a, can function, as does IL-8, to induce chemotaxis, chemokinesis, degranulation, and respiratory bursts in neutrophils, as well as increasing neutrophil integrin affinity for ligands on EC, and participating in the loss of heparan sulfate from the activated EC. C5a also likely stimulates macrophages and mast cells to release TNF and/or IL-1, which can then activate EC. The cells that bind to the activated EC also participate in the inflammatory/rejection process. Neutrophils activated by C5a and PAF secrete reactive oxygen species. The production of superoxide by activated cells bound to the activated EC as well as by the EC themselves are likely major players in the overall response, perhaps primarily by activation of NFκB; the loss of SOD aggravates these complications. Other factors of note produced by quiescent EC are endothelial derived relaxing factor (EDRF) (which leads not only to relaxation of the vessels but also prevents platelet thrombi), ADPases, prostacyclines, and tissue plasminogen activator; the latter is countered by PAI-1, as shown.

tant involves the superoxide dismutase that is attached to heparan sulfate and that, as noted above, serves to convert superoxide species to hydrogen peroxide and oxygen. The loss of heparan sulfate with EC activation leads to a diminution in this mechanism of defense. Heparan sulfates also bind proinflammatory cytokines such as IL-8. Others would include the production by EC of endothelial-derived relaxing factor (EDRF), which leads not only to relaxation of the vessels but also prevents platelet thrombi, and production of tissue plasminogen activator, which is countered by PAI-1.

Methods to Interfere with the Consequences of EC Activation

Blocking of adhesion molecules. One approach that is actively being pursued to abrogate undesirable consequences of EC stimulation/ activation is to block the adhesion molecules expressed on activated EC. Monoclonal antibodies to E-selectin, ICAM-1, and others prevent attachment of neutrophils and monocytes to the EC and thus inhibit the stimulus provided by products of these cells to the EC. Monoclonal antibodies are aimed either at the molecule expressed on the activated EC or on the neutorphils or other cells to prevent attachment of the cells to the activated endothelium. Antibodies to other cell surface antigens (e.g., tissue factor when expressed), or peptides that bind those same molecules, are being tested to block those molecules (Inverardi et al., 1993).

Inhibition of EC activation. Methods that would inhibit EC activation in general, or specific aspects thereof, are still very much in developmental stages. At present the approaches fall into two categories. First, there are a number of drugs, or other inhibitory agents, that interfere with one or another aspect of EC activation. Most of these drugs are selective in that they prevent expression of some aspects of EC activation but not others. Included in this list are agents that interfere with expression of adhesion molecules, with aspects of procoagulation and others. Efforts are underway to find new agents that might be useful in this regard. Second, there are efforts to manipulate pig EC genetically to avoid,

or counteract, some of the undesirable consequences of EC activation. These include expression of new molecules in the EC as well as preventing the expression of certain molecules (such as tissue factor). The various approaches that can be used at the molecular level to block expression of various genes are discussed in Chapter 21.

COAGULATION AND HEMOSTASIS IN XENOTRANSPLANTATION

The activation of clotting appears to be closely related to host immune responsiveness *in vivo* (Esmon, 1993). Fibrin deposition and platelet aggregation in vascularized xenografts are likely a consequence of the immune and inflammatory responses observed during the complex process of rejection (Hunt and Rosenberg, 1993). Some products of the coagulation pathway, such as fibrin, participate in immunologically mediated tissue damage and degradation products of fibrin may modify the function of cells of the immune system (Mosesson, 1992; Robson et al., 1993). In a reciprocal fashion, stimulation of the immune system with complement activation is crucial to several key events in blood coagulation, which include thrombin generation and platelet aggregation (Sims and Wiedmer, 1991).

Blood coagulation requires the sequential activation of a series of proteases that must combine with membrane-associated protein cofactors that serve to accelerate the process (Furie and Furie, 1992; Esmon, 1993). Specific regulators, anticoagulants, and fibrinolytic agents are primarily localized to the endothelium. The functional expression of these factors may be modified by the inflammatory response that results in vascular injury (Butcher, 1991; Edwards and Rickles, 1992; Altieri, 1993; Languino et al., 1993). Inappropriate initiation of coagulation or disordered regulation of the process, enhanced by the inflammatory response, could result in the extensive intravascular thrombosis seen in acute xenograft rejection (Hunt and Rosenberg, 1993).

A great deal of attention has been given to the molecular incompatibilities that exist between membrane-associated inhibitors of complement, such as decay accelerating factor (see section on complement above) across species barriers as in the case of pig to primate. In the context of coagulation, we must consider that there are potentially similar molecular, and thus functional, incompatibilities in both coagulation pathways and anticoagulant mechanisms. Our review of this area below is based on current knowledge without considering these potential incompatibilities.

Coagulation Pathways and Platelet Activation

Recent advances have allowed the reinterpretation of the cascade (or waterfall) hypothesis of coagulation, which proposed a sequential assembly process, involving coagulation factors of both the intrinsic and extrinsic pathways, enhanced by cell membrane-associated phenomena and ionized calcium (Furie and Furie, 1992; Esmon, 1993). The interaction of blood with foreign surfaces had been known for some time to initiate factor XII activation *in vitro*. However, more recent evidence has suggested that the early "contact" components of the intrinsic pathway, e.g., factor XII, prekallikrein, or high-molecular-weight kininogen, are not critical for effective hemostatsis *in vivo*. Certainly, individuals with deficiencies of these factors do not have significant episodes of hemorrhage (Broze, 1992). A further crucial observation was that the factor VIIa/tissue factor (Tf) catalytic complex was capable not only of activating factor X, but also of associating with factor IX to generate the IXa–VIIIa "tenase" complex (Nemerson, 1988; Furie and Furie, 1992; Esmon, 1993). Finally, the (re)discovery of the coagulation regulator, tissue factor pathway inhibitor (TFPI), which produces factor Xa-dependent feedback inhibition of the factor VIIa/Tf complex, gave further impetus to the formulation of a theory of clotting that could integrate the convergent classical pathways (Broze, 1992).

The initiation of clot formation, in the context of blood vessel damage, involves the exposure of membrane Tf, associated with the subendothelium (or with activated endothelial cells) to factor VII or VIIa, to form a highly effective catalytic complex that is a potent activator of factors Xa and IXa. However, hemostasis is not necessarily achieved following the activation of factor X to Xa, and hence prothrombin to thrombin, which then converts fibrinogen to fibrin. In fact, the early generation of factor Xa is associated with the inhibitory effect of TFPI, which forms a quaternary complex (TFPI–VIIa–Xa–Tf) that blocks further production of factors Xa and IXa. Under these circumstances, with the additional removal of activated clotting factors by the effects of blood flow, their inactivation by protease inhibitors and the antagonistic process of fibrinolysis, the initial coagulation response must be consolidated or amplified by the progressive, localized generation of Xa and thrombin for adequate hemostasis to result. Several proteases (including factors Xa, IXa, XIIa, thrombin, and VIIa) can generate further factor VIIa in plasma, which then binds avidly to Tf. Additional factor Xa can then be produced by the alternative (or amplification) pathway, involving factors IXa and VIIIa (Fig. 4). Here the factor IXa is formed as a result of the action of the factor VIIa/Tf complex and by factor XIa, an ancillary coagulation factor (Broze, 1992).

Functional Tf is not normally present on endothelial cells but is found associated with the subendothelial matrix. Upon EC activation, there is an increase in Tf associated with the matrix as well as new expression on the surface of the activated cells; Tf-dependent coagulation would thus be initiated under these circumstances (Bach, 1988). The membrane assembly of the prothrombinase complex, including factors Xa, Va, and prothrombin (PT) (Fig. 5), is dependent upon the association with factor Va, which then accelerates the conversion of prothrombin to thrombin. Thrombin then cleaves the fibrinopeptides A and B from the intact fibrinogen protein to form fibrin monomers, which associate and are cross-linked by factor XIIIa to form polymeric fibrin (Furie and Furie, 1992).

The Tf–VIIa complex also converts factor IX to IXa, which then binds to activated factor VIIIa causing increased generation of the prothrombinase complex. Factor X can be proteolytically cleaved to Xa by both the Tf–VIIa and the IXa–VIIIa complexes. The generation of Xa, and

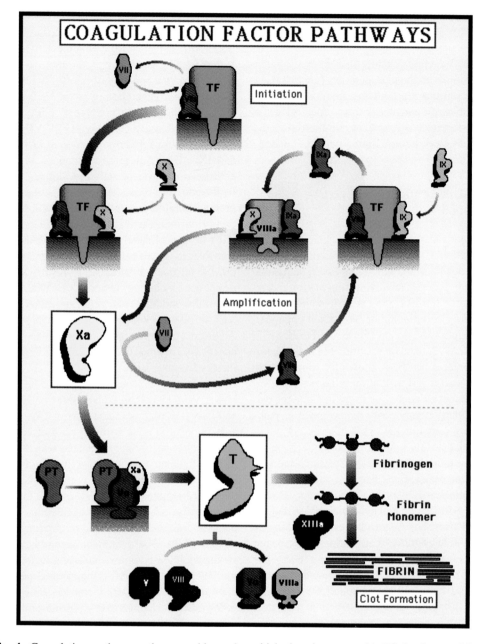

Fig. 4. Coagulation pathways, the assembly and function of coagulation complexes. Inactive coagulation factors or zymogens interact on negatively charged cell membranes (the outer leaflet must contain aminophospholipid) with activation complexes comprising serine proteases, regulatory (activated) cofactors, and calcium. In the initiation reaction, the Tf–factor VIIa complex generates factor Xa. Even though the protease factor VII may interact with Tf, human factor VII must be activated to attain function. Factors Xa and VIIa can generate more factor VIIa, which then interacts with Tf. In the amplification pathways, the Tf–VIIa complex binds IX and forms IXa, which then binds to the activated cofactor VIIIa. This complex then generates functionally competent factor Xa, which augments that formed by the initial Tf–VIIa complex. The prothrombinase complex comprises the active cofactor Va, the protease factor Xa, and the zymogen prothrombin. The generated thrombin cleaves the fibrinopeptides A and B from fibrinogen proteins to form fibrin monomers, which then interact and are cross-linked by the trans-

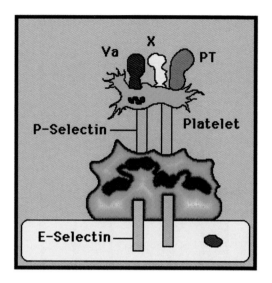

Fig. 5. Cellular components of coagulation. Neutrophils (or monocytes) bind to endothelial cells by virtue of the leukocyte adhesion receptors, the selectins, and integrins (not shown for simplification), which interact with carbohydrate moieties, the intercellular adhesion molecules (ICAM-1 and 2), and peptide sequences in matrix proteins and fibrin. Platelets interact with leukocytes and serve as additional loci for the formation of the prothrombinase complex, thrombin generation, and fibrin formation. The fibrinogen (and other coagulation factor) content of platelets serves to further localize or focus clot formation.

hence thrombin, leads to accelerated coagulation by virtue of the ability of these proteases to activate a number of earlier coagulation factors. In particular, thrombin can activate both factors V and VIII to form Va and VIIIa, as part of a positive feedback pathway (Fig. 4) (Furie and Furie, 1992; Esmon, 1993).

Activated monocytes, which also express tissue factor, may interact with the endothelium and platelets by cell surface adhesion molecules and also create loci for the initiation of coagulation (see later and Fig. 5) (Edwards and Rickles, 1992; Esmon, 1993). The endothelial cell is crucial for the coordination of these processes; in turn, the degradation products of fibrin(ogen) generated during these reactions impacts on the EC (Ge et al., 1993).

Anticoagulatory Mechanisms and Fibrinolysis

There are three major (anticoagulatory) systems in the blood that modulate the cell-mediated events that initiate and control coagulation. These include (1) the vitamin K-dependent factors, proteins C and S, (2) the tissue factor pathway inhibitor, and (3) antithrombin, the activity of which is potently enhanced by heparin (Fig. 6).

Thrombomodulin, expressed on vascular endothelial cells, is known to bind thrombin with high affinity and capacity. Once bound and stabilized, the thrombomodulin interaction alters the specificity of thrombin leading to enhanced activation of protein C (Esmon, 1993). Activated protein C binds protein S to form membrane-bound complexes on the endothelium (and platelets) that result in the inhibition of further thrombin generation by the specific inactivation of factors Va and VIIIa. Protein S circulates both in a free and active form or complexed to C4bBP, an inhibitory protein of the classical complement pathways. After complex formation, the activated protein C is inactivated either by α_1-protease inhibitor or a specific protein C inhibitor. This latter inhibitory reaction is enhanced by heparin and other glycosaminoglycans (Walker and Fay, 1992).

TFPI is a plasma protein with potent and selective inhibitory activity for factor Xa, which is associated with the Tf–VIIa complex. A pool of this inhibitor is also associated with endothelial

---

glutaminase XIIIa. Note that thrombin also activates the pro-cofactors V and VIII, which then permits their binding function as described above. The integrated "to and fro" pathways depicted in the figure suggest that the initiation process is consolidated by the amplification pathways and that low levels of thrombin activation are crucial for the activation of the cofactors V and VIII. See text for more detailed discussion. TF, tissue factor; PT, prothrombin; T, thrombin. Factor is deleted before the Roman numerals for convenience.

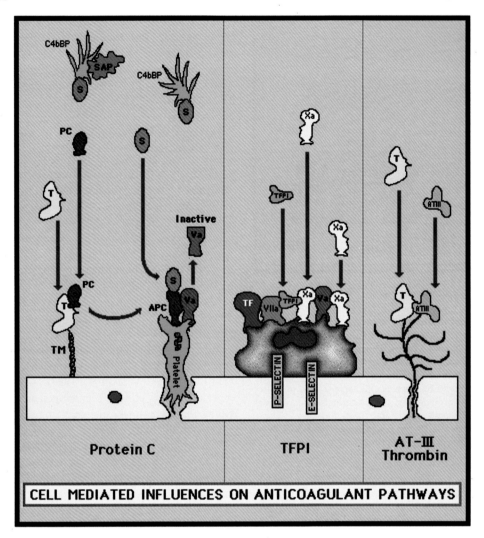

Fig. 6. Anticoagulant proteins: protein C and S, TFPI, and antithrombin III. The major anticoagulant pathways are illustrated above. Protein C is activated by thrombin bound to thrombomodulin, which is depicted as a elongated multidomain protein on the endothelial cell surface. The activated protein C interacts with uncomplexed protein S and the new complex is bound by platelets or endothelial cells where the complex is responsible for the inactivation of factor Va. Only free protein S is an active anticoagulatory protein and the circulating protein S may be complexed to C4bBP, an inhibitory protein of the classical complement pathways. TFPI has three inhibitor domains, one of which interacts with factor Xa and inhibits it. The resultant complex of Xa–TFPI interacts with the Tf–VIIa complex and results in reversible inhibition of its catalytical function. One the right-hand side of the monocyte membrane, factors Xa and Va are preparing to bind prothrombin to form the prothrombinase complex. The balance of these opposing processes on the cell surface is influence by the circulating and endothelial-associated TFPI and its activation by factor Xa. Finally, the antithrombin activity may be localized on either thrombomodulin or on the heparin-like proteoglycans, depicted as an arboreal structure on the endothelial cell. Interestingly, antithrombin III when complexed to heparin is also capable of inhibiting the Tf–VIIa complex but not free VIIa (not shown). TF, tissue factor; TFPI, tissue factor pathway inhibitor; PT, prothrombin; T, thrombin; C4bBp, C4b binding protein; SAP, serum amyloid P; PC, protein C; APC, activated protein C; S, protein S; Tm, thrombomodulin; ATIII, antithrombin. Factor is deleted before the Roman numerals for convenience.

cells and platelets and may be released by heparin infusion (Broze, 1992).

Antithrombin irreversibly inhibits the serine protease components thrombin, Xa, and IXa. Heparin-like activity, crucial for the interaction of antithrombin and thrombin, is associated with the proteoglycans of the endothelium and also the chondroitin sulfate linked to thrombomodulin (Esmon, 1993).

Other inhibitors exist. Endothelial cells produce the protease nexin, a serine protease inhibitor that binds thrombin. Heparanoids associated with the subendothelial matrix also potentiate the inhibitory activity of another thrombin inhibitor termed heparin cofactor 2 (Esmon, 1993).

In addition to specific inhibitors of coagulation, endothelial cells also influence the process of fibrinolysis by the regulated secretion of plasminogen activators and their specific inhibitors. Endothelial cells also release thrombospondin, a large adhesion molecule that modulates plasmin generation and hence fibrinolysis (Li et al., 1993; Anonick et al., 1993).

Platelet Aggregation and Activation

A rapid and efficient clotting process is dependent upon platelet activation and aggregation (see Fig. 7a, b, and c). Thrombi that develop under conditions of high shear, as in the arterial system, contain large numbers of activated platelets and may be pathologically designated as white thrombi (Roth, 1992). The participation of platelets in the coagulation process is modulated by other blood cells and the endothelium in a process termed thromboregulation (Marcus and Safier, 1993).

Platelets are essential to the integrity of the endothelial monolayer and release substances essential for this process (Kobayashi, 1992; Marcus and Safier, 1993). Platelet adhesion and activation responses are governed by their interaction with various components of the subendothelial matrix in the context of shear stresses generated by blood flow (Chow et al., 1992). As shear is dependent upon both flow and inversely related to vessel diameter, high rates of stress are generated predominantly in the arterioles and microvasculature, where the thrombotic insults

seen in early xenograft rejection are thought to be localized (Hunt and Rosenberg, 1993).

Two receptors are principally involved in platelet binding to endothelium and fibrin(ogen), the latter leading to the formation of platelet-fibrin hemostatic plugs (Fig. 7a) (Savage et al., 1992). The initial binding of platelets to the "endothelium" is dependent on the interaction of platelet receptor GPIb with von Willebrand factor (vWF), which is expressed and bound to the subendothelial matrix; this receptor interaction is highly dependent on shear stress (Roth, 1992; Ruggeri and Ware, 1993). This process is also modulated by the other adhesive protein receptors on the platelet surface that bind collagen and fibronectin in the subendothelial matrix (Roth, 1992; Hynes, 1992). Activation signals generated by these interactions act in concert with thrombin to enhance expression and affinity of GPIIbIIIa and P-selectin on the platelets (Kroll et al., 1991; Smyth et al., 1993). The important platelet integrin, GPIIbIIIa, binds to both vWF (at a different site to that of GPIb) and fibrin(ogen), promoting platelet aggregates (Ruggeri and Ware, 1993). Selectin expression by platelets and leukocytes promotes cellular adhesion to the area of injury (Furie and Furie, 1992).

The assembly of coagulation factors on the platelet surface is facilitated by several events. First, there is expression of specific receptors for coagulation favor V, which are up-regulated as a consequence of platelet activation. Second, the platelet membrane aminophospholipids are exposed as a result of microparticle formation, which enhances the binding and assembly of the prothrombinase complex (Furie and Furie, 1992; Esmon, 1993). Third, platelets contain in their α granules high concentrations of fibrinogen and other coagulation proteins that, when expressed on the cell surface or secreted into the extracellular environment, promote local fibrin deposition (Harrison and Martin Cramer, 1993).

The process of platelet aggregation comprises an initiation trigger (thrombin, exposure to collagen etc.) amplified by the release of ADP and serotonin. The generation of thrombin serves as a potent positive feedback step. Platelet aggregation is influenced by other factors. Erythrocytes promote platelet aggregation and hemostatic

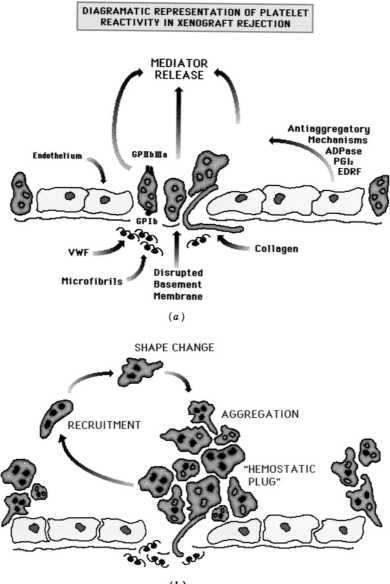

DIAGRAMATIC REPRESENTATION OF PLATELET REACTIVITY IN XENOGRAFT REJECTION

(a)

SHAPE CHANGE

RECRUITMENT

AGGREGATION

"HEMOSTATIC PLUG"

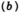

(b)

Fig. 7. Diagrammatic representation of platelet reactivity in xenograft rejection: a hypothesis. (**a**) Platelets circulate in the blood in an inactive state. Following tissue injury, platelets adhere to and spread on the subendothelial matrix by the interaction of GPIb and von Willebrand factor (vWF), which is facilitated by shear stress (see text). It is feasible that xenogeneic vWF may have increased affinity for GPIb in the apparent absence of stress or vascular injury. The activation of platelets with increased expression of P-selectin and GPIIbIIIa is accompanied by mediator release, further recruitment, and the promotion of the coagulation process. This process can be antagonized by the endothelial cell antiaggregatory mechanisms, which include the ADPase systems, the synthesis of the prostacycline PGI2 and nitric oxide or endothelial cell-derived relaxing factor (EDRF). (**b**) Recruitment is accompanied by platelet activation with the shape changes and aggregation associated with this process. Platelet aggregates colocalize with the initial adherent platelets to form the early hemostatic plugs of platelet deposition. (**c**) Thrombosis is a multicellular process. Both bound neutrophils and monocytes may participate in the inflammatory process (release of cytokines) and platelet activation (platelet-activating factor) associated with the vascular injury. Monocytes, in particular, promote the local process of thrombogenesis by the expression of Tf. Red blood cells modulate platelet activation and are also incorporated into the clot. The endothelial surface loses its barrier function and extravasation begins. vWF, von Willebrand factor; this and other explained in legend.

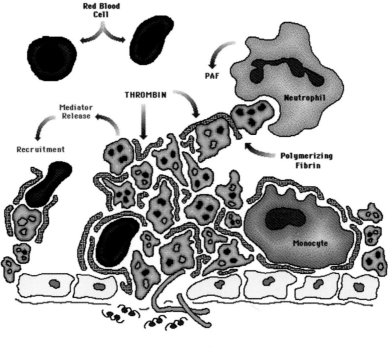

(c)

Fig. 7. (*Continued*)

plugs by coexpression of adhesion receptors, such as for thrombospondin, a large adhesion molecule, and by modulating the eicosanoid formation by platelets (Marcus ad Safier, 1993).

Endothelial cells inhibit platelet aggregation by at least three mechanisms. These include the release of prostacyclines, the generation of nitric oxide, and the action of the ecto-ADPase, which efficiently binds and degrades platelet-derived ADP, thus inhibiting amplication pathways that result in platelet plug formation (Marcus and Safier, 1993). Thrombomodulin expressed by the vascular endothelium is also capable indirectly of abrogating platelet responses to thrombin by virtue of high affinity binding by thrombomodulin of thrombin (Esmon, 1993). Finally, neutrophils are considered to have both a negative or positive overall influence on platelet hemostatic function; this negative action occurs despite the release of PAF by activated cells (Zhou et al., 1992). This action of neutrophils is enhanced when platelets and neutrophils are not adherent to each other and could be related to the

release of metalloproteases and serine proteases, which are capable of rapid fibrin degradation and fibrinogen modification *in vitro*. One possibility is that P-selectin expressed on platelets reverses the neutrophil inhibition of platelet reactivity (Faint, 1992; Marcus and Safier, 1993). Neutrophil-generated superoxides and radicals are also capable of activating platelets (Practico et al., 1993).

Coagulation and Platelet Aggregation as Related to Xenograft Rejection

The localization of leukocytes to activated endothelium by adhesion receptors, both selectins and integrins, promotes fibrin deposition at inflammatory sites (Fig. 5) (Hynes, 1992; Edwards and Rickles, 1992; Esmon, 1993). The formation and accumulation of fibrin at the site of an inflammatory response are dependent on both the initiation of a procoagulant stimulus and the inhibition of fibrinolysis (Furie and Furie, 1992).

The monocyte is capable of expressing Tf and under certain circumstances, a prothombinase complex. By directly binding factors X, V, fibrinogen, and XIII, these cells can coordinate the assembly of coagulation factors resulting in the generation of cross-linked fibrin (Edwards and Rickles, 1992; Altieri, 1993). Proinflammatory cytokines such as IL-1, released by these cells and by activated endothelial cells, can upregulate endothelial cell Tf activity, reduce the surface expression of thrombomodulin (Labarrere et al., 1992), and inhibit fibrinolysis by the reduced secretion of tissue-plasminogen activator and by the generation and release of plasminogen activator inhibitors type-1 (Esmon, 1993). Under certain circumstances the neutrophil may also play a role in the mediation of procoagulant responses, facilitated by the expression of the CD11b CD18 fibrinogen receptor (Edwards and Rickles, 1992).

Complement components augment thrombosis by interacting with platelets, leukocytes, and endothelium. Terminal components of the complement system, C5b–C9 have potent platelet aggregatory effects and promote microparticle release (Sims and Wiedmer, 1991). The increased vesiculation seen on endothelial cells following the binding of activated complement has an end-result comparable to that of platelet microparticle formation viz increased expression of aminophospholipid moieties with enhanced interactions with coagulation factors (Esmon, 1993).

Inappropriate coagulation processes in the context of xenografting. The extensive thrombosis seen during xenograft rejection may be in part triggered by the activation of the complement cascade, which can initiate coagulation and platelet aggregation in its own right. It is therefore difficult to determine the contribution of primary initiators of coagulation *in vivo*. Platelet activation may be facilitated by unusual interactions of GPIb with vWF (in the fluid phase or associated with endothelial cells) across species barriers; for instance, porcine vWF, as a contaminant of factor VIII preparations, following "therapeutic" infusion for hemophiliac patients, has the ability to bind human GPIb in the appar-

ent absence of shear stress. These forms of interactions that occur because of the species barrier could result in platelet activation and thrombocytopenia *in vivo* (Hunt and Rosenberg, 1993).

Mechanisms to Interfere with the Consequences of the Activation of Coagulation and Platelet Aggregation in Xenograft Rejection

Therapeutic approaches to interfere with the clotting process seen in xenograft rejection are confounded by the current inability to determine the initiation and amplification events that occur prior to, concurrently with, or independently of the associated inflammatory response *in vivo*. The current modalities of anticoagulant and antithrombotic therapy are summarized in Table I (modified from Fareed et al., 1993). Recent advances in the therapy of thrombosis have been brought about by molecular biological techniques and the production of recombinant modified anticoagulant proteins such as protein C (Walker and Fay, 1992; Dichek, 1993).

The use of antagonists of PAF in the situation of xenotransplantation has resulted in some improvement in survival times, suggesting a role for platelet activation by this phospholipid in the process of hyperacute xenograft rejection (Makowka et al., 1990). In a similar fashion, the use of snake venom proteases with defibrinating properties in carefully titrated doses may allow for partial depletion of certain crucial coagulation factors and fibrinogen prior to grafting and still allow adequate hemostasis at the time of surgery.

There are many potential candidate drugs to consider in the context of abrogating the thrombotic component of xenograft rejection. As the generation of thrombin would appear to be a central event in this process, modulation of this process may yield some success in prolonging xenograft survival. Thrombin is crucial to both the amplification pathways of the coagulation process and platelet aggregation (Furie and Furie, 1992; Esmon, 1993). This suggests that the selective and controlled inhibition of thrombin activity, either by binding and inactivation

Table I. Classification of Potential Antithrombotic Interventions in Xenografting Procedures

Heparin-related drugs	Low, medium, and high M_r heparins, heparans, dermatans, antithrombotic oligosaccharides, etc.
Antiplatelet agents	Prostenoid modulators, eicosanoids, and omega-3 fatty acids, phosphodiesterase inhibitors, ticlopidine, clopidogrel, etc.; specific GPIIbIIIa antagonists including peptides and antibodies
Antitissue factor agents.	Dexamethazone, antibodies.
Endothelial lining modulators	DDAVP, nucleic acid derivatives (defibotide)
Vicosity modulators	Pentoxifylline, venoms, and polymers
Biotechnology-based proteins	Tissue plasminogen activators and mutants, hirudin and derivatives, protein S and C, thrombomodulin and protease-specific inhibitors, etc.
Antithrombin agents	D-Me-Phe-Pro-Arg-derived antithrombotics, hirulogs, hirudisins, etc.
Combinations of therapies	Heparin/antiplatelet agents; hirudin/antithrombotics/thrombolytics; etc.
Novel delivery systems	Oral, intrapulmonary, organ infusions via catheter, target-specific and sustained release preparations

(thrombomodulin, hirudin, etc.), by thrombin antagonists (D-Phe-Pro-Arg-CH$_2$Cl or PPACK) or by the blockage of the specific thrombin receptor with the newly developed "tethered receptor" peptide analogues (Maraganore, 1993), may control the local thrombotic manifestations of xenograft rejection. The combination of this approach with that of GPIIbIIIa antagonists may have additional benefits in the possible reduction of the dose of antithrombin agents.

Heparin-related compounds have a new advantage in that the low-molecular-weight variants that are beginning to enter clinical practice are associated with less bleeding complications (Fareed et al., 1993). All heparinoids, in addition to their well-described interaction with antithrombin, also induce tissue factor pathway inhibitor release, a potent antagonist of the initial coagulation process (Broze, 1992). The major disadvantages of heparin therapy relate to the inability to completely prevent rethrombosis in several models. This may be secondary to the inability of heparin-antithrombin to neutralize factor Xa contained within the prothrombinase complex and the inactivation of heparin by platelet factor 4 (Zwaginga et al., 1990; Maraganore, 1993).

Antiplatelet agents currently in clinical use are disadvantaged by their side-effects, ineffectiveness under certain circumstances, and lack of selectivity (Marcus and Safier, 1993). Newer GPIIbIIIa antagonists, both peptides and anti-

bodies, may be more selective and more potent (Gould et al., 1990). Fibrinolytic agents will have minimal utility if used in their current manner, but if administered in low dose or by local infusion as part of a prophylactic intervention may potentiate the benefit of the above agents. Bleeding will obviously remain a major concern in the setting of the xenografting or any major surgical procedure. Endothelial cell modulators, such as vasopressin analogues (1-desamino-8D-arginine vasopressin or DDAVP) and defibrotide (nucleic acid derivative) or viscosity modulators (polymers and defibrinating venoms) (Fareed et al., 1993) may have an adjunctive role, but there are few current data available on their use in this context.

Combinations of the above therapeutic modalities and the evolution of more rational drug delivery systems will provide many avenues for therapeutic trials. These could include the application of intrapulmonary nebulized heparin (low M_r) or the infusion and concentration of pro-urokinase in platelets. Increased understanding of the potential use of the "biotechnology"-based products, such as the hirudin and disintegrin (GPIIbIIIa antagonist) constructs termed hirudisins (Knapp et al., 1992), may lead to the development of novel interventional strategies. The expression of these peptides, thrombomodulin, tissue plasminogen activators, or other immunomodulatory factors may well be evaluated in the not too distant future (Dichek, 1993).

AN *IN VITRO* MODEL OF EC ACTIVATION RELATING TO XENOTRANSPLANTATION

Porcine EC, either from the aorta or from the vessels of the microvasculature, at which site the manifestations of vascular rejection primarily occur, can be grown in monolayer cultures. The EC not only have a characteristic morphology, but also can be characterized, for instance by staining with low-density lipoprotein (LDL), for which the cells have receptors, to ensure that one is culturing EC and not smooth muscle or other cells. Addition of human serum to the EC, as a source of xenoreactive natural antibodies and complement, results in changes in the EC that appear to mimic what occurs *in vivo* when blood flow to a transplanted organ is established.

Responses of EC under the established *in vitro* conditions that are of interest include the following. The EC retract from one another, accompanied by changes in their actin filaments, resulting in increased permeability to molecules of various sizes, presumably mimicking the leakiness that occurs *in vivo*.

Both heparan sulfate and thrombomodulin are lost from the surface of the EC upon stimulation with human serum; thrombomodulin loss is also seen when EC are stimulated with cytokines. Loss of the heparan sulfate requires XNA plus complement. However, the entire complement cascade is not involved in this process; XNA + C5a are sufficient to mediate loss. Loss of thrombomodulin is dependent on generation of the entire complement cascade as poly-C9 formation is needed to effect release of thrombomodulin.

In addition to these findings, a number of the genes that are up-regulated *in vitro* following EC activation with classical stimuli such as IL-1 and TNF are also up-regulated by human serum that is added to the EC monolayer. There is now evidence that the protein products of several of these genes is also stimulated to appear *in vivo* when EC are activated (Vanhove et al., 1993). An important aspect of EC activation is the development of a net procoagulation effect. Addition to the EC *in vitro* of either a classical activating substance such as IL-1 or LPS, or the addition of human serum, presumably as a source of XNA and complement, mimics the *in vivo* situation by inducing more rapid clotting of the human plasma.

In vivo, EC are in close contact with cells below them (in the context of the vessel lumen). These substratum cells (smooth muscle or pericytes) interact with the EC and modify the reactions of the EC. To which degree such an *in vitro* model is misleading because the EC are studied without the presence of smooth muscle cells or pericytes is not known. In part to address this issue, an alternative model to study the reaction of EC to xenogeneic blood components is to use "perfusion models" in which, for instance, a pig organ is perfused with human blood or components thereof.

IN VIVO MODELS OF DISCORDANT XENOGRAFTING

The two models most commonly used for discordant xenografting are guinea pig to rat and pig to primate (baboon, rhesus, and cynomologus monkeys have been the species used most commonly) (Latinne et al., 1993). Other species combinations have been studied and can appropriately be considered discordant in that hyperacute rejection occurs in the unmodified recipient in minutes to only 1 or 2 hr, and natural antibodies in the recipient can easily be demonstrated to react with donor cells. In part, our knowledge has been increased by using animal strains that have genetic deficiencies, such as of the complement system (e.g., C6-deficient rats).

The Role of XNA and Complement in Discordant Xenograft Rejection

In certain species combinations, such as guinea pig to rat, the alternative pathway of complement is activated and thus there is no requirement for binding of XNA to initiate HAR. However, when present, the XNA almost certainly contribute to the rejection process by stimulating the classical pathway of complement. In the pig to primate combination, it does not appear that the alternative pathway is involved, at least to any great extent. Thus, it is the XNA that initiate the reaction. It appears that XNA function not only as passive molecules on the surface of the EC that bind complement and thus allow the complement cascade to proceed, but actually themselves provide a stimulus to the EC. Whether the total removal of XNA will result in the abrogation of vascular rejection and thus the survival of a discordant xenograft (ignoring the cell-mediated rejection mechanism, which would have to be dealt with separately) must still be tested.

Complement plays a key role in rejection, likely from several perspectives. To the extent that EC activation is important in generating reactions that contribute to HAR, components of the activated complement system probably deliver a signal(s) to the EC, aiding in the full activation of the EC. In addition, split products of complement, such as C5a, can function to induce chemotaxis, chemokinesis, degranulation, and respiratory bursts in neutrophils, as well as increasing neutrophil integrin affinity for ligands on EC. C5a also likely stimulates macrophages and mast cells to release TNF and/or IL-1, which can then activate EC. Attachment of these cells in an activated form to the EC further aggravates the rejection response.

It should be noted that factors in serum other than XNA and complement may well act on EC. Addition of exogenous, pooled α-globulins of human serum to porcine EC *in vitro* inhibits the up-regulation of E-selectin, ICAM-1, and VCAM-1, while at the same time not inhibiting certain other genes (Stuhlmeier et al., 1993).

In part, our knowledge regarding precise mechanisms is based on the effects of various drugs, or other manipulations, aimed at prolonging xenograft survival. The information gained from such studies, however, is difficult to interpret due to the pleiotropic affects that many manipulations and/or drugs have. Immunosuppressive agents, for instance, which are known to be effective in terms of suppressing T-lymphocytes and B-lymphocytes, may also block endothelial cell activation, or some components thereof. Mycophenolate mofetil (RS61443) inhibits smooth muscle proliferation (a component of certain forms of microvascular injury) while blocking antibody production and T cell responses. Physical depletion of natural antibodies, while clearly lowering the levels of those antibodies, in most protocols likely lowers complement factors and, in the case of physical removal as by plasmapheresis, lowers coagulation factors and other molecules as well.

ACCOMMODATION: A WORKING MODEL FOR XENOGRAFT SURVIVAL

Given the importance of XNA and complement in initiating vascular rejection, many investigators have focused on methods that would inhibit one or both of these factors for the hoped-for lifetime of the graft. If successful, the inhibition of recipient complement by membrane-associated inhibitors of complement placed in the ECs of the donor organ by transgenic or other methodology might achieve this for complement. There are also potential approaches that would achieve long-term depletion for XNA; two examples include (1) B cells producing the XNA might be selectively eliminated by immunotoxins attached to antibodies recognizing the idiotypes that characterize the XNA, or (2) tolerance to the xenoantigens recognized by XNA and elicited antibodies might be achieved. However, these approaches to lower XNA and elicited antibodies for years are far from reality at this time.

It may not be necessary to remove XNA and compromise the complement system for the lifetime of the graft to prevent vascular rejection (Bach et al., 1991). Based on findings in allotransplantation across the ABO barrier, it may transpire that if XNA and complement are depleted, and perhaps other factors are compromised for some time after the transplant is in place, at a later time it may be possible to let XNA, C, and other factors return to normal without evoking EC activation to the extent that rejection occurs (Bach et al., 1993). We envision that during the time that the graft is in place in the "absence" of XNA etc., the EC of that graft will have time to "heal in" and recover from the trauma of having been exposed to relative hypothermia and low oxygen tensions, with subsequent reperfusion. We have referred to the survival of a graft under such circumstances as "accommodation," and have discussed possible reasons why accommodation may be achieved.

In brief, these include possible changes in the antibodies that return after depletion, including the possibility that non-complement-fixing antibodies block the target sites on the EC, and/or that the targets themselves change, such as addition of terminal sialic acids to the target carbohydrates, thus protecting them from XNA binding. However, we regard it as most likely that accommodation is based on changes in the EC, as discussed below, including transformations such as up-regulation of inhibitors of complement as part of the accommodation process.

Based on the data described in the section on XNA above (Vanhove and Bach, 1993), one might consider the following. In the nontreated recipient, as soon as blood flow is established to the donor organ, there is a sudden and massive onslaught against the EC of that organ as potentially as many as 100,000 molecules of XNA are deposited on each EC in combination with the consequent deposition of complement. This would occur within seconds to minutes. The reaction that might be evoked under those circumstances might be quite different from the one in which XNA and complement are depleted prior to transplantation, and then only allowed to return slowly some time after the EC in the transplanted organ have had the opportunity to "heal in" without any such massive insult against them. We hypothesize that in the latter circumstances, the EC will accommodate, i.e., not respond, so as to lead to rejection of the graft.

It seems possible that in response to certain stimuli, such as the slow return of XNA after the "healing in" period, EC will actively develop mechanisms that interfere with aspects of the EC response that might contribute to HAR. Two recent findings are consistent with such a line of thinking.

First, an exceedingly early event following stimulation of EC is activation of the transcription factor, NFκB, which appears to play a prominent role with respect to up-regulation of a number of genes, including E-selectin and tissue factor, that are characteristic of EC activation. Work from our laboratories (de Martin et al., 1993) has recently shown that following EC activation, there is not only rapid activation of NFκB, but also up-regulation of a gene coding

for an IκB (inhibitor of NFκB)-like molecule. The IκB protein binds to and inhibits the function of NFκB. To the extent that this occurs, there would be decreased NFκB function; thus, several of the genes that are dependent on NFκB for up-regulation, and the products of which are likely participants in HAR, would *not* be up-regulated. One could imagine that under certain conditions (i.e., those leading to accommodation), IκB activity would be dominant over NFκB, and thus full EC activation would be prevented, leading to accommodation rather than HAR.

Second, Vercellotti and colleagues have shown that a given stimulus to EC can, dependent on the conditions, induce either sensitization of the EC to a subsequent toxic challenge, or what might be considered accommodation to that same toxic challenge. Stimulation of EC for an hour with heme leads to an increased sensitivity of the EC with regard to lysis by activated neutrophils. However, if the EC are stimulated with heme for 1 hr, and then left for approximately 16 hr, the cells up-regulate certain metabolic pathways and synthesize ferritin. This active response of the EC apparently protects the EC from oxidative damage by activated neutrophils or H_2O_2 (Balla et al., 1992). In both of these examples, the EC respond actively by up-regulating genes that could, under the right circumstances, contribute to achieving accommodation.

In addition to the active development of defense mechanisms, we suggest that normally occurring inhibitory factors, such as the α-globulins, which, as pointed out above, inhibit up-regulation of E-selectin and other cell surface ligands, may play a role in accommodation. Clearly the presence of the α-globulins *in vivo* does not prevent up-regulation of E-selectin under at least some circumstances (Stuhlmeier et al., 1993). We view the potential function of the α-globulins rather as inhibitory factors that prevent response to low-level stimulation that, from an evolutionary point of view, would be undesirable. In this context, they might behave rather like the membrane-associated inhibitors of complement, such as DAF, discussed above. If XNA return very slowly, the stimulus to the EC may be quite weak, and thus these naturally occurring inhibitors might function to protect the graft.

There are now at least some experimental models showing that accommodation can be achieved in xenotransplantation. We have studied one rhesus monkey recipient of a pig heart in which case accommodation was achieved. More recently, White and his colleagues have attained what appears to be accommodation in hamster to rat heart transplants (Hassan et al., 1992). These findings at least encourage further studies to make accommodation a potential therapeutic goal for xenotransplantation.

CONCORDANT XENOGRAFTS

By definition, any xenograft that is not hyperacutely rejected in the unmodified recipient is a concordant graft. One experimentally important question, however, is which combination of species as donor and recipient is a good one to predict what will happen in the concordant, clinically relevant baboon to human transplant, the most likely concordant graft that is being, and would be, attempted clinically (Starzl et al., 1993). Without lengthy comment, it is simply not clear at present which of the concordant experimental grafts would be a good model for baboon to human transplants, although all fit the definition of concordant xenografts.

The most commonly used model of concordant xenografts uses hamsters as donors and rats as recipients. Hamster hearts transplanted to rats are rejected after 3 to 4 days. Following transplantation of a hamster heart into a rat, the recipient rats produces anti-hamster antibodies that are first detected by day 2 and reach high titers by day 3. There is accumulating evidence that rejection is mediated by the elicited antibodies plus complement: inhibition of antibody production or inhibition of complement activation results in prolonged survival of such grafts. Transplantation between different species of nonhuman primates is also used as a model for transplantation from baboon to human.

Based on these facts, it would appear that a concordant xenograft, at least as represented by the hamster to rat model, resembles the discordant model in concept, i.e., with recipient antibodies plus complement initiating the rejection response. It is elicited antibodies that initiate the response, whereas in the discordant model, the preexisting natural antibodies can function in this capacity. There is some argument whether there are low titers of preexisting antibodies present in a rat that are reactive with hamster tissues; if such antibodies are present, they are not sufficient to elicit an HAR response.

CELL-MEDIATED XENOGRAFT REJECTION

Consideration of cell-mediated xenograft rejection is of secondary importance compared to the discussion of humoral rejection mechanisms above. The strength of the humoral response is the critical feature that distinguishes xenogeneic from allogeneic transplantation and the extraordinary power of the humoral mechanisms that cause early xenograft destruction, both by preformed natural antibodies and by induced antibodies, has made it difficult even to examine the later cellular mechanisms that might be involved. Nevertheless, control of cellular immunity will eventually be necessary to achieve long-term xenograft survival, and thus it is worth considering the features that might distinguish the cellular immune responses to tissues of another species from the allogeneic response.

When considering the cell-mediated xenograft rejection, one should beware of three simple, but perhaps inaccurate assumptions: (1) that cellular xenoreactivity is qualitatively similar to alloreactivity, (2) that this cellular response is likely to be quantitatively stronger than to alloantigens, and (3) that the quantitative difference is likely to reflect the phylogenetic distance between the donor and recipient species. These assumptions arise from the view that xenotransplantation is simply a variant of allotransplantation, with the problems getting larger as the genetic differences expand. Since the clinical outcome for organ transplantation is best when genetically matched combinations are used and somewhat less good when less well-matched cadaver donors are used, it seems reasonable to conclude that the rejection response will be even stronger when organs are selected from animal donors with still larger numbers of genetic disparities. Although this conclusion may be true in some cases, the purpose of this chapter is to describe the experimental findings suggesting that it is not always true and to indicate that such simple assumptions are likely to obscure certain aspects of xenogeneic cellular immunity that will be important in our efforts to modify and control this response.

Cellular Responses *in Vitro*

One way to consider the nature of the cell-mediated immune response to xenoantigens is to start by considering why it is that the cell-mediated response to allogeneic MHC antigens is so strong. This issue has been mentioned earlier in this book (Chapter 3) and is a dominant feature of transplantation immunology. The measured precursor frequency of T cells for allogeneic MHC antigens is roughly 100-fold higher than for ordinary environmental pathogens, even though there is no apparent physiologic reason for our ability to reject transplanted organs. Current theories to explain the strength of alloreactivity are based, first, on the observation that the T cell repertoire is selected in the thymus to enrich for cells able to recognize modified self-MHC antigens; second, on the finding that T cells able to recognize modified self-MHC molecules are also able to recognize allogeneic MHC antigens "directly" (without the usual requirement that these antigens be presented as peptides by self-MHC molecules); and, third, on the belief that allogeneic MHC antigens expressed on donor antigen-presenting cells (APCs) provide both a high frequency and/or density of novel determinants compared to self-APCs presenting peptide antigens. Two features are central to this model: first, that direct recognition of allogeneic MHC antigens (which is required for the special strength of the response) depends on the similarity of the allogeneic MHC antigens to self-MHC antigens, and second, that the strength of alloreactivity depends on the capacity of donor APCs to function as efficiently as self-APCs. Considering the strength of alloreactivity in this way, it is apparent that cell-mediated xenogeneic responses may

not be as strong as allogeneic responses if either the xenogeneic MHC antigens are too dissimilar from self-MHC molecules or the xenogeneic APCs fail to function efficiently with T cells of a different species. Numerous *in vitro* studies have been performed in many laboratories to test the ability of T cells from animals of one species to recognize MHC antigens of another species directly (see Chapter 3 for a discussion of direct versus indirect recognition) (Moses, 1991). These assays have included mixed lymphocyte reactions (MLR) and IL-2 production assays to measure T cell helper function and CTL assays to measure the function of cytotoxic T cells. The helper cell assays have included efforts to deplete APCs of the stimulator and of the recipient to determine whether direct or indirect pathways were involved.

The results of these studies have been variable, depending primarily on the species combination and the T cell function being tested. On one end of the spectrum, results from some of the most clinically relevant species combinations (such as human responses to non-human primate or pig stimulators) have shown that direct recognition of xenogeneic MHC antigens can occur. On the other end of the spectrum, results from combinations involving mouse responses to various discordant stimulators have suggested that little if any direct stimulation occurs, especially for helper responses. Even after skin graft rejection, murine T cells have been shown to respond to primate stimulation only by recognition of donor antigens presented in association with APCs of the mouse. On the other hand, the direct response by human T cells to stimulators of pig donors has not yet been quantitatively examined to determine whether there are subtle differences in strength compared to allogeneic stimulation.

Factors Responsible for Diminished Direct Recognition

As diagrammed in Figure 8, direct T cell stimulation by an APC involves several different interactions between the two cells, including the recognition of the donor MHC antigen by the T cell receptor, the interaction of several different accessory, adhesion, and costimulatory mole-

Functions of an Antigen
Presenting Cell

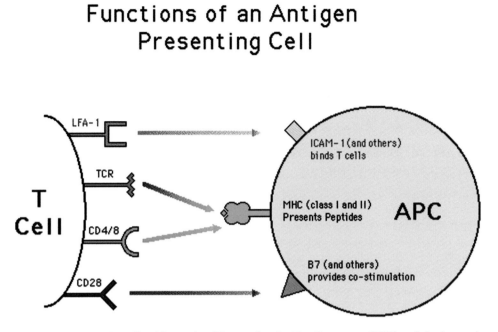

Fig. 8. Activation of cell-mediated immunity. Direct T cell stimulation by an antigen-presenting cell (APC) involves multiple separate interactions between the two cells viz the recognition of donor MHC by the T cell receptor (TCR) and the interaction of several accessory, adhesion, and costimulatory molecules including the various cytokines.

cules with their ligands, and the ability of lymphokine receptors to bind the lymphokines produced by the other cell. Based on this picture, one can see that several factors might potentially account for diminished direct cellular recognition of xenogeneic stimulators, including the possibility that xenogeneic MHC molecules might be too dissimilar to self MHC molecules or the possibility that there might be incompatibilities between the molecules involved in adhesion and costimulation when the T cells and stimulating cells come from different species.

The role of these potential factors in some of the species combinations where direct cellular recognition is absent has been examined by exogenously replacing some of the factors produced by APCs or by manufacturing APCs that are partly allogeneic and partly xenogeneic (using techniques of molecular biology) (Moses et al., 1992). For example, the weak human direct response to murine stimulators has been reconstituted by adding human IL-1 to *in vitro* cultures, suggesting that the murine IL-1 produced by the mouse stimulating cells may not be able to function with human T cells (Alter and Bach, 1990). On the other hand, the absent murine direct response to discordant xenogeneic stimulators has not been reconstituted by adding mouse IL-1, by using mouse APCs that express xenogeneic MHC antigens, or by using xenogeneic APCs that express allogeneic MHC antigens. These results suggest that multiple different factors may be responsible for diminished direct recognition of xenogeneic stimulating cells and that the particular factors of importance are different, depending on the species combination that is involved. In some cases the ability of T cells to respond to lymphokines produced by xenogeneic stimulators appears to be the principal factor, while in others, binding of CD4 and/or CD8 coreceptors to their respective ligands as well as defective interactions between surface accessory molecules appear to be important. In no case, however, has the dissimilarity of xenogeneic MHC molecules compare to self-MHC molecules been shown to be a factor in diminished direct recognition of xenogeneic stimulators. In fact, evidence suggests that there is an extraordinary similarity in the hypervariable regions of MHC molecules of different species and that the strength of T cell xenoreactivity is not likely to be altered by a defective T cell receptor repertoire for recognition of xenogeneic MHC antigens (Gustafsson, 1990).

Possible Altered Cellular Immunity Even When Direct Recognition Is Present

Relatively few studies have so far examined the nature of the cellular immune response in those species combinations where direct recognition of xenogeneic stimulators appears to be intact. It is quite possible, however, that not all of the components of T cell activation are fully functional in some of these combinations. If there are redundancies in the adhesion or costimulatory molecules involved in T cell activation, then apparently normal *in vitro* responses might be obtained even if some of the molecular interactions could not function across species barriers. These defects might be revealed by finding that particular reagents could block xenogeneic responses but not allogeneic responses (where redundant stimulatory mechanisms could overcome the blocking reagent).

Hidden defects in direct T cell stimulation may explain the finding that the outcome of T cell stimulation is sometimes different in xenogeneic compared to allogeneic combinations. While allogeneic MLRs tend to generate cytokine production typical of Th1 cells, some experiments have suggested that xenogeneic cultures sometimes generate cytokines more typical of Th2 responses (Wren, 1993). Perhaps weaker stimulation of the Th1 subpopulation is caused by defective function of some elements of direct activation. Even though the direct T cell response is still intact in these species combinations, the altered cytokine production detected in these experiments could have important effects in changing the nature of the rejection process.

Cellular Xenograft Rejection *in Vivo*

The discussion above has tended to emphasize the ways in which xenogeneic cellular responses are different from and weaker than allogeneic responses. This discussion should not be taken to suggest that cell-mediated rejection of xenografts is not a powerful process. Indeed, the overwhelming majority of studies that have attempted to assess cellular xenograft rejection *in vivo* have demonstrated faster xenograft than allograft rejection under comparable circumstances and better prolongation of allograft compared to xenograft survival by almost every known form of immunosuppression (Auchincloss, 1988). Thus, the bulk of the evidence continues to suggest that cell-mediated rejection of xenografts is another important obstacle to their successful clinical transplantation.

Part of the difficulty in assessing these studies of cellular xenograft rejection *in vivo* is that it is hard to be certain that humoral responses are not the primary cause of rejection. Even in concordant combinations, induced antibody production after transplantation has been shown to be an important cause of xenograft destruction. As a result of this concern, many studies of cellular xenoresponses *in vivo* have used mice as recipients of xenogeneic skin grafts since skin is unusually resistant to antibody-mediated rejection (Winn et al., 1973). This has the disadvantage that these species combinations show the most profound lack of direct cellular recognition, which may not be representative of the responses in more clinically relevant species combinations. On the other hand, these experiments have the advantage of highlighting the differences between xenogeneic and allogeneic graft rejection.

Even using murine recipients, most studies of the effectiveness of standard immunosuppressive agents have shown them to be less effective for prolonging xenograft compared to allograft survival. There are, however, two exceptions to this generalization. First, depletion of CD4+ T cells from mice by treatment with anti-CD4 antibody prolongs the survival of primate skin grafts while having little effect on MHC-mismatched murine allografts on the same recipients (Pierson et al., 1989). Second, anti-human B7 antibody treatment to block the function of one of the components of the "second signal" (see Chapter 3) allows indefinite survival of human islets in mice but not of allogeneic islets (Lenschow et al., 1992). These two results, showing better xenograft than allograft survival, indicate that some features of the two responses are different and that, under certain circumstances, the xenogeneic cellular response is actually weaker.

The Mechanisms of Cellular Xenograft Rejection *in Vivo*

The demonstration that xenograft survival can sometimes be prolonged better than allograft survival indicates that under some circumstances the mechanisms of xenograft rejection *in vivo* may be different from those for allograft destruction. Exactly what these differences are, however, and whether they suggest that unique mechanisms for xenograft destruction are available remain unclear.

The special importance of CD4+ cells in xenogeneic skin graft rejection may simply reflect a weaker function of CD8+ cells that are CD4 (helper cell) independent. However, adoptive transfer studies in mice have shown that CD4+ cells without CD8+ cells or B cells can cause xenograft rejection even though the *in vitro* evidence suggests that the CD4+ cells respond to the xenoantigens only when they are presented by recipient APCs. This has suggested the possibility that effector cells that do not recognize any determinants expressed in the graft may be capable of causing xenograft destruction by some indirect effector function. As discussed earlier in this book, the evidence at this point suggests that such indirect effector mechanisms cannot generally cause allograft rejection and that specific recognition of determinants expressed in the donor graft (probably by cytotoxic T cells) is essential for graft destruction (see Chapter 5).

The possibility that indirect effector mechanisms may be especially important in xenograft rejection has led many investigators to suggest that some other cell population besides cytotoxic T cells may play an important role. Often, NK cells have been suggested as likely candidates, perhaps recognizing the absence of their own species' MHC antigens. Immunohistologic studies of the cellular infiltrate in xenogeneic grafts have shown a large component of NK cells. However, no study has convincingly demonstrated that depletion of NK cells can delay cell-mediated xenograft rejection. Other investigators have suggested that cytokines might be especially important in xenograft rejection, by direct cytolytic effects, or by activating macrophages causing a DTH-type of response. These possibilities, however, remain pure speculation at this time.

The possibility that unique mechanisms for cell-mediated xenograft rejection exist, that cannot cause allograft rejection, would explain the extremely rapid rejection of xenografts by unmanipulated recipients and would explain the finding that all standard forms of exogenous immunosuppression (such as cyclosporine or antithymocyte globulin) prolong xenograft survival less well than allograft survival. Alternatively, the strength of cellular xenograft rejection may be simply a quantitative, not a qualitative outcome, reflecting the larger number of protein disparities between members of different species, providing a larger number of peptides to activate T cells. The distinction is important because those who believe that unique mechanisms can cause xenograft rejection will be inclined to search for new immunosuppressive agents to block these particular pathways, while those who see the problem as quantitative will be inclined to see the future of xenogeneic transplantation as depending on strategies to induce tolerance to all donor antigens, thereby equalizing the outcome of allogeneic compared to xenogeneic transplantation.

Not all of the *in vivo* studies have suggested that xenograft rejection occurs without direct recognition of determinants in the graft. Even in mice, where the *in vitro* evidence showing a lack of direct recognition of discordant APCs is most clear, some studies suggest that direct recognition is required for xenograft rejection. For example, the ability of anti-human B7 antibody to prolong human islet graft survival in mice has suggested that direct recognition of antigens on human cells is involved in islet rejection (Lenschow, 1992). Since this antibody works for xenogeneic islets while a similar antibody does not work for allogeneic islets, it is possible that some alternative costimulatory molecules that are available in allogeneic responses are not functional in xenogeneic combinations. Thus the xenogeneic response may be particularly dependent of the function of the B7 molecule.

Future Directions in the Study of Cell-Mediated Xenograft Rejection

The investigation of cellular responses to xenografts thus far has demonstrated that these responses are not precisely the same as allogeneic responses in some species combinations and that defects in the function of some of the elements involved in T cell activation account for some of these differences. These observations, however, provide only a starting point for the analysis of cellular mechanisms of xenograft rejection and several important issues remain to be studied.

Studies of cellular immunity in mice responding to pigs are of interest biologically and have given us insight into some important principles. They cannot, however, be used to predict the nature of defects that may exist when human T cells are stimulated by pig cells, which obviously represents the more relevant species combination. While several studies have suggested that direct human responses to pig stimulators can occur, there may still be particular defects in the interactions of some of the molecules involved in T cell activation. Such defects may make human responses to pig stimulators more susceptible to blocking residual compensatory elements of activation than allogeneic responses would be. As a hypothetical example, perhaps human CD28 interacts well with pig B7 but human CTLA-4 fails to interact with a second costimulatory molecule (see Chapter 3). Under these circumstances direct T cell activation might appear normal *in vitro* but be more susceptible to blocking of the B7 molecule than a human allogeneic response might be. A careful analysis of the human T cell response to pig stimulators would therefore be useful to identify those immunosuppressive strategies most likely to be useful for pig organ transplantation to humans.

It would also be useful to determine whether there are particular species that might have an especially large number of important defects in the stimulation of human cellular responses. The study of xenogeneic transplantation has frequently assumed that pigs would be the ideal donor for humans in the long run. However, sheep or cows or some other species may have critical defects in the interactions leading to T cell activation such that they would actually be better donors.

The issue remains open at this time whether differences between allogeneic and xenogeneic cell-mediated rejection are simply quantitative, involving greater numbers of antigenic differences and perhaps greater reliance on indirect sensitization of helper cells in xenogeneic responses, or whether there are truly unique mechanisms of cellular xenograft rejection that are not available for allografts. Despite the clinical irrelevance of mouse recipients, this question is still well addressed in rodent models where the data suggesting such unique responses have been most obvious and where the reagents and tools to manipulate immune responses are most powerful. If such unique xenogeneic mechanisms are identified, then it will be necessary to test the immunosuppressive strategies designed to cope with these responses in larger animals.

One of the relative advantages of animal compared to human organs for clinical transplantation would be the greater ability to alter animal donors genetically so that their tissues elicit weaker immune responses. Some of the efforts to insert genes to diminish humoral rejection of xenografts have been discussed above. Similar efforts to modify cellular responses have only just begun.

As is discussed in more detail in Chapter 21, there are basically two ways that genetic engineering can be used to alter donor animals. First, transgenic technology can be used to insert new genes into animals, sometimes controlling the expression of these genes by incorporating specific promotors. Second, the technique of homologous recombination can be used to replace normal genes with new ones that may be unable to be expressed or that may be expressed in an altered form. The first technique is already in use in larger animals while the second is available only for mice at this time.

Deciding exactly which genes to insert or to remove will depend on the outcome of the studies described above analyzing the particular defects in cellular xenogeneic responses and examining the mechanisms of xenograft rejection. For example, if several adhesion molecules do not function across a particular species combination, but cellular responses remain intact because of remaining compensatory interactions, then obviously alterations in the remaining interactions will be more useful than efforts to modify interactions that do not work anyway. Similarly, a better knowledge of the mechanisms of xenograft destruction may suggest particular genetic manipulations to diminish these responses.

The ultimate solution to the vigorous rejection of xenografts, both cellular and humoral, will be to induce tolerance to the donor antigens. Strategies to induce tolerance to allografts have already been discussed in this book and similar strategies may be considered for xenografts as well. However, application even in rodents of the many strategies that work so well for allografts have been much less successful for xenografts (Auchincloss, 1988). Some of this difficulty may reflect the strength of immunologic barriers to xenogeneic engraftment, but, in addition, physiologic barriers preventing the growth and differentiation of xenogeneic cells may be particularly important, especially when bone marrow chimerism is the approach used to induce xenogeneic tolerance. Therefore, a particular feature of research to induce tolerance to animal antigens is the need to determine the factors and environmental requirements for long-term survival and differentiation of xenogeneic stem cells.

REFERENCES

Alexandre GPJ, Latinne D, Gianello P, Squifflet JP (1991): Preformed cytotoxic antibodies and ABO-incompatible grafts. Clin Transplant 5:583–594.

Alter B, Bach FH (1990): Cellular basis of the proliferative response of human T cells to mouse xeno-antigens. J Exp Med 171:333–338.

Altieri DC (1993): Coagulation assembly on leukocytes in transmembrane signalling and cell adhesion. Blood 267:8571–8576.

Anonick PK, Yoo JK, Webb DJ, Gonias SL (1993): Characterisation of the antiplasmin activity of human thrombospondin-1 in solution. Biochem J 289:903–909.

Auchincloss H Jr. (1988): Xenogeneic transplantation. A review. Transplantation 46:1–20.

Bach FH (1993): Xenotransplantation: A view to the future. Transplant Proc 25:25–29.

Bach FH, Platt JL, Cooper D (1991a): Accommodation: The role of natural antibody and complement in discordant xenograft rejection. In Cooper D, Kemp E, Reemtsma K, White DJG (eds): "Xenotransplantation—The Transplantation of Organs and Tissues Between Species." Heidelberg: Springer-Verlag, pp. 81–100.

Bach FH, Turman MA, Vercellotti GM, Platt JL, Dalmasso AP (1991b): Accommodation: A working paradigm for progressing toward clinical discordant xenografting. Transplant Proc 23:205.

Bach FH, Dalmasso G, Platt JL (1992): Xenotransplantation: A current perspective. Transplant Rev 6:1–7.

Bach FH, Blakely ML, van der Werf M et al. (1993): Discordant xenografting: A working model of problems and issues. Xeno 1:8–15.

Bach RR (1988): Initiation of coagulation by tissue factor. Crit Rev Biochem Mol Biol 23:339–368.

Balla G, Jacob HS, Balla J, Rosenberg M, Nath K, Apple F, Eaton JW, Vercellotti GM (1992): Ferritin: A cytoprotective antioxidant stratagem of endothelium. J Biol Chem 267:18148–18153.

Blakely ML, Van der Werf WJ, Hancock WW, Bach FH (1993): Rejection of guinea pig cardiac xenografts post-cobra venom factor therapy is associated with endothelial cell activation and mononuclear cell infiltration. Surg Forum XLIV:399–401.

Blakely ML, Van der Werf WJ, Hancock WW, Bach FH (1994): Prolonged suppression of xenoreactive natural antibodies and elimination of hyperacute rejection in a discordant xenotransplantation model. Submitted.

Broze GJ (1992): The role of tissue factor pathway inhibitor in a revised coagulation cascade. Semin Hematol 29:159–169.

Butcher EC (1991): Leukocyte-endothelial cell recognition: Three (or more) steps to specificity and diversity. Cell 67:1033–1036.

Calne RY (1970): Organ transplantation between widely disparate species. Transplant Proc 2:550.

Chow TW, Hellums JD, Moake JL, Kroll MH (1992): Shear stress induced von Willebrand factor binding to platelet glycoprotein Ib initiates calcium influx associated with aggregation. Blood 80:113–120.

Cooper DKC, Koren E, Oriol R (1994): Natural antibodies, α-galactosyl oligosaccharides and discordant xenografting. Xeno 2:22–25.

Cotran RS, Pober JS (1989): Endothelial activation and inflammation. Prog Immunol 8:747–753.

Dalmasso AP, Vercellotti GM, Platt JL, Bach FH (1991): Inhibition of complement-mediated endothelial cell cytotoxicity by decay accelerating factor: Potential for prevention of xenograft hyperacute rejection. Transplantation 52:530–533.

de Martin R, Vanhove B, Cheng Q, Csizmadia V, Hofer E, Winkler H, Bach FH (1993): Cytokine-inducible expression of IκB involves NFκB regulatory circuit for transient gene transcription. EMBO J 12:2773–2779.

Dichek DA (1993): Gene therapy in the treatment of thrombosis. Thromb Haemostasis 70:198–201.

Edwards RL, Rickles FR (1992): The role of leukocytes in the activation of blood coagulation. Semin Hematol 29:202–212.

Esmon CT (1993): Cell mediated events that control blood coagulation and vascular injury. Annu Rev Cell Biol 9:1–26.

Faint RW (1992): Platelet-neutrophil interactions: Their significance. Blood Rev 6:83–91.

Fareed J, Hoppensteadt MS, Walenga JM (1993): Current perspectives on low molecular weight heparins. Semin Thromb Hemostasis 19:1–11.

Figueroa J, Fuad SA, Kunjummen BD, Platt JL, Bach FH (1993): Suppression of synthesis of natural antibodies by mycophenolate mofetil (RS-61443). Transplantation 55:1371–1374.

Furie B, Furie BC (1992): Molecular and cellular biology of blood coagulation. N Engl J Med 326:800–806.

Ge M, Tang G, Ryan TJ, Malik AB (1993): Fibrinogen degradation product D induces endothelial cell detachment by activation of cell-mediated fibrinolysis. J Clin Invest 90:2508–2516.

Gould RJ, Polokoff MA, Friedman PA et al. (1990): Disintegrins: A family of integrin inhibitory proteins from viper venoms. Proc Soc Exp Biol Med 195:168–171.

Gustafsson K, Germana S, Hirsch F, Pratt K, LeGuern C, Sachs DH (1990): Structure of miniature swine class II DRB genes: Conservation of hypervariable amino acid residues between distantly related mammalian species. Proc Natl Acad Sci USA 87:9798–9802.

Harrison P, Martin Cramer E (1993): Platelet alpha granules. Blood Rev 7:52–62.

Hassan R, Van den Bogaerde, Forty J, Wright L, Wallwork J, White DJG (1992): Xenograft adaptation is dependent on the presence of antispecies antibody, not prolonged residence in the recipient. Transplant Proc 24:531.

Hebell T, Ahearn JM, Fearon DT (1991): Suppression of the immune response by a soluble complement receptor of B lymphocytes. Science 254(5028): 102.

Hunt BJ, Rosenberg RD (1993): The essential role of haemostasis in hyperacute rejection. Xeno 1:16–20.

Hynes RO (1992): Integrins: Versatility, modulation and signalling in cell adhesion. Cell 69:11–25

Inverardi L, Socci C, Pardi R (1993): Leukocyte adhesion molecules in graft recognition and rejection. Xeno 1:35–39.

Johnston PS, Wang MW, Lim SM, Wright LJ, White DJ (1992): Discordant xenograft rejection in an antibody-free model. Transplantation 54:573–577.

Knapp A, Degenhardt T, Dodt J (1992): Hirudisins. Hirudin-derived thrombin inhibitors with disintegrin activity. J Biol Chem 267:24230–24234.

Kobayashi M, Shimada K, Ozawa T (1992): Human platelet-derived transforming factor beta stimulates synthesis of glycosaminoglycans in cultured porcine endothelial cells. Gerontology 38:36–42.

Kroll MH, Harris TS, Moake JL, Handin RI, Schafer AI (1991): von Willebrand factor binding to platelet GpIb initiates signals for platelet activation. J Clin Invest 88:1568–1573.

Labarrere CA, Pitts D, Halbrook H, Faulk WP (1992): Natural anticoagulant pathways in normal and transplanted human hearts. J Heart Lung Transplant 11:342–347.

Languino LR, Plescia J, Duperray A, Brian AA, Plow EF, Geltosky JE, Altieri DC (1993): Fibrinogen mediates leukocyte adhesion to vascular endothelium through an ICAM-1-dependent pathway. Cell 73:1423–1434.

Latinne D, Gianello P, Smith CV, Nickelett V, Kawai T, Beadle M, Haug C, Sykes M, Lebowitz E, Bazin H, Colvin R, Cosimi AB, Sachs DH (1993): Xenotransplantation from pig to cynomolgus monkey: Approach toward tolerance induction. Transplant Proc 25:336–338.

Latinne D, Soares M, Havaux X, Cormont F, Lesnikoski B, Bach FH, Bazin H (1994): Depletion of IgM xenoreactive natural antibodies by injection of anti-μ monoclonal antibodies. Immunological Reviews 141:95–125.

Legrand C, Thibert V, Dubernard V, Begault B, Lawler J (1992): Molecular requirements for the interaction of thrombospondin with thrombin activated human platelets: Modulation of platelet aggregation. Blood 79:1995–2003.

Lenschow DJ, Zeng Y, Thistlethwaite JR, Montag A, Brady W, Gibson MG, Linsley PS, Bluestone JA (1992): Long-term survival of xenogeneic pancreatic islet grafts induced by CTLA4Ig. Science 257:789–92.

Leventhal J, Flores H, Gruber S, Figueroa , Platt JL, Manivel J, Bach FH, Matas AJ, Bolman RM III (1992): Natural antibody production can be inhibited by 15-deoxyspergualin in a discordant xenograft model. Transplant Proc 24:714–716.

Li WX, Howard RJ, Leung LL (1993): Identification of SVTCG in thrombospondin as the conformation-dependent, high affinity binding site for its receptor, CD36. J Biol Chem 268:16179–16184.

Makowka L, Chapman FA, Cramer DV, Qian S, Sun H, Starzl TE (1990): Platelet-activating factor and hyperacute rejection. The effect of a platelet-activating factor antagonist, SRI 63-441, on rejection of xenografts and allografts in sensitised hosts. Transplantation 50:359–365.

Mantovani A, Bussolino F, Dejana E (1992): Cytokine regulation of endothelial cell function. FASEB J 6:2591–2599.

Maraganore JM (1993): Thrombin, thrombin inhibitors and the arterial thrombotic process. Thromb Haemostasis 70:208–211.

Marcus AJ, Safier LB (1993): Thromboregulation: Multicellular modulation of platelet reactivity in hemostasis and thrombosis. FASEB J 7:516–522.

Moses RD, Auchincloss H Jr (1991): Mechanisms of cellular xenograft rejection. In Cooper DKC, Kemp E, Reemstma K, White DJG (eds): "Xenotransplantaiton: The Transplantation of Organs Between Species." Berlin: Springer-Verlag, pp 101–120.

Moses RD, Winn HJ, Auchincloss H Jr (1992): Evidence that multiple defects in cell-surface molecule interactions across species differences are responsible for diminished xenogeneic T cell responses. Transplantation 53:203–209.

Mosesson MW (1992): The roles of fibrinogen and fibrin in hemostasis and thrombosis. Semin Hematol 29:177–188.

Murphy HS, Shayman JA, Till GO, Mahrougui M, Owens CB, Ryan US, Ward PA (1992): Superoxide responses of endothelial cells to C5a and TNF alpha: Divergent signal transduction pathways. Am J Physiol 263:L51–L59.

Nemerson Y (1988): Tissue factor and hemostasis. Blood 71:1–8.

Pierson RN, III, Winn HJ, Russell PS, Auchincloss H Jr. (1989): Xenogeneic skin graft rejection is especially dependent on CD4+ T cells. J Exp Med 170:991–996.

Platt JL, Lindman BJ, Chen H, Spitalnik SL, Bach FH (1990): Endothelial cell antigens recognized by xenoreactive human natural antibodies. Transplantation 50:817–822.

Platt JL, Lindman BJ, Geller RL, Noreen HJ, Swanson J, Dalmasso AP, Bach FH (1991a): The role of natural antibodies in the activation of xenogeneic endothelial cells. Transplantation 52:1037–1043.

Platt JL, Fischel RJ, Matas AJ, Reif SA, Bolman RM, Bach FH, (1991b): Immunopathology of hyperacute xenograft rejection in a swine to primate model. Transplantation 52:214–220.

Pober JS, Cotran RS (1990): Cytokines and endothelial cell biology. Physiol Rev 70:427–51.

Practico D, Iuliano L, Alessandri C, Camastra C, Violi F (1993): Polymorphonuclear leukocyte-derived O2-reactive species activate primed platelets in human whole blood. J Physiol 264:1582–1587.

Robson SC, Saunders R, de Jager C, Purves L, Kirsch RE (1993): Fibrin and fibrinogen degradation products with an intact D-domain C-terminal gamma chain inhibit an early step in accessory cell dependent lymphocyte mitogenesis. Blood 81:3006–3014.

Rooney IA, Liszewski MK, Atkinson JP (1993): Using membrane-bound complement regulatory proteins to inhibit rejection. Xeno 1:29–34.

Roth GJ (1992): Platelets and blood vessels: The adhesion event. Immunol Today 13:100–105.

Ruggeri ZM, Ware J (1993): von Willebrand factor. FASEB J 7:308–316.

Savage B, Shattil SJ, Ruggeri ZM (1992): Modulation of platelet function through adhesion receptors: A dual role for glycoprotein IIb-IIIa (integrin alpha IIb beta3) mediated by fibrinogen and gycoprotein Ib-von Willebrand factor. J Biol Chem 267:11300–11306.

Sims PJ, Wiedmer T (1991): The response of human platelets to activated components of the complement system. Immunol Today 12:338–342.

Smyth SS, Joneckis CC, Parise LV (1993): Regulation of vascular integrins. Blood 81:2827–2843.

Starzl TE, Funf J, Tzakis A et al. (1991): Baboon to human liver transplant. Lancet 341:65–71.

Stuhlmeier KM, Cheng Q, Csizmadia V, Winkler H, Bach FH (1994): Alpha globulins selectively inhibit expression of "E-selectin" in endothelial cells. Eur J Immunol 24:2186–2190.

Vanhove B, Bach FH (1993): Human xenoreactive natural antibodies: Avidity and targets on porcine endothelial cells. Transplantation 56:1251–1253.

Vercellotti GM, Platt JL, Bach FH, Dalmaso AP (1991): Enhanced neutrophil adhesion to xenogeneic endothelium via C3bi. J Immunol 146:730.

Walker FJ, Fay PJ (1992): Regulation of blood coagulation by the protein-C system. FASEB J 6:2561–2567.

White DJ, Oglesby T, Liszewski MK et al. (1992): Expression of human decay accelerating factor or membrane cofactor protein genes on mouse cells inhibits lysis by human complement. Transplant Proc 24(2):474.

Winn HJ, Baldamus CA, Jooste SV, Russell PS (1973): Acute destruction by humoral antibody of rat skin grafted to mice: The role of complement and polymorphonuclear leukocytes. J Exp Med 137:893.

Wren SM, Wang SC, Thai NL, Conrad B, Hoffman RA, Fung JJ, Simmons RL, Ildstad ST (1993): Evidence for early Th2 T cell predominance in xenoreactivity. Transplantation 56:905–911.

Zhou WG, Javors MA, Olson MS (1992): Platelet activating factor as an intercellular signal in neutrophil-dependent platelet activation. J Immunol 149:1763–1769.

Zwaginga JJ, Sixma JJ, de Groot PG (1990): Activation of endothelial cells induces platelet thrombus formation on their matrix. Studies of new in vitro thrombosis model with low molecular weight heparin as anticoagulant. Arteriosclerosis 10:49–61.

Chapter 20
The Swine Leukocyte Antigen (SLA) Complex

Joan K. Lunney and David H. Sachs

BACKGROUND

The existence of the swine MHC, or swine leukocyte antigen (SLA) complex, was clearly established in 1970 by Vaiman and Binns and their colleagues (Vaiman et al., 1970; Viza et al., 1970). The SLA complex is now known to consist of a set of linked genes (or haplotype) on swine chromosome 7 (Chardon et al., 1988; Edfors-Lilja et al., 1993; Lunney, 1994). Like the human HLA complex and the mouse H-2 complex, the SLA complex encodes a large number of genes including the class I and class II SLA glycoproteins, complement components, tumor necrosis factor, and heat shock proteins (Fig. 1).

SLA CLASS I REGION

The traditional class I loci are designated SLA-A,B,C and encode 45,000-Da glycoproteins that noncovalently associate with 12,000-Da β_2-microglobulin and that are expressed on the surface of most cells. Serologic evidence clearly proves the existence of two expressed SLA class I gene products and indicates a third in some SLA haplotypes (Chardon et al., 1988; Lunney, 1994). Singer and her colleagues (1982) were the first to clone and express a swine class I gene. Using specific restriction fragment length polymorphisms (RFLP) of genomic DNA from an NIH minipig, her group proceeded to show that one SLA haplotype encoded only 6–8 class I genes as compared to the 15–36 class I genes in other species (Singer et al., 1982, 1988). Even when probed with appropriate nonclassical class I MHC DNA, no more SLA class I genes could

be identified. Only two of Singer's SLA class I genes (PD1, PD14) could be expressed at the protein level in transfected mouse cells while a third (PD6) was detected only at the mRNA level. Vaiman, Chardon, and their colleagues in analyzing DNA from a wide range of SLA haplotyped outbred swine confirmed that there were a limited number of SLA class I genes, although they concluded this number to be 7–10 genes (Chardon et al., 1985).

SLA class I typing alloantisera have been developed in laboratories worldwide; the last international comparative test was reported by Renard et al. (1988). Monoclonal antibodies (MAbs) reactive with SLA class I antigens have been produced; when tested on cells from different swine populations many of these MAbs react with every class I antigen (Lunney, 1994). Other MAb detect SLA class I determinants common to a number of haplotypes and, thus, are designated as broadly polymorphic in their SLA class I reactivity, i.e., they recognize "public" SLA class I specificities. Only a few MAb react with individual, or "private" SLA class I specificities and should be useful for defining specific SLA haplotypes.

SLA CLASS II REGION

The SLA class II loci encode a variety of class II genes, of which only the SLA-DR and SLA-DQ appear to be expressed at the protein level. The expressed proteins consist of 33,000- to 35,0000-Da α (A) chains associated with 27,000- to 28,000-Da β (B) chains. RFLP analyses of SLA class II DNA have revealed at least 3 α chain genes and 5–8 β chain genes for

Transplantation Immunology, pages 339–345
© 1995 Wiley-Liss, Inc.

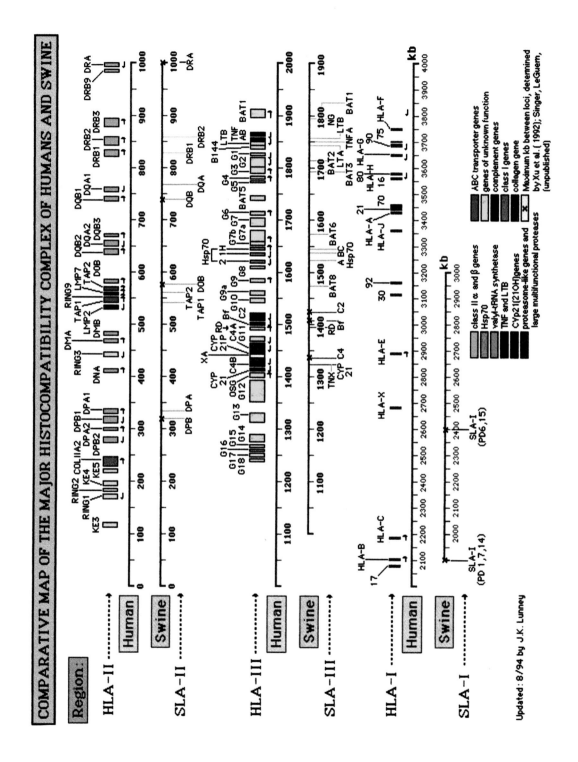

COMPARATIVE MAP OF THE MAJOR HISTOCOMPATIBILITY COMPLEX OF HUMANS AND SWINE

Updated: 8/94 by J.K. Lunney

each chromosome bearing the SLA complex (Sachs et al., 1988). Extensive evidence from LeGuern, Sachs, and colleagues indicates that for each SLA haplotype, there is one monomorphic DRA and two polymorphic DRB genes; one (or more) polymorphic DQA and DQB gene(s); no more than one DPA and one DPB gene, but no evidence for an expressed SLA-DP protein. There is genomic evidence for a DOB and DZA gene but no protein product, and no evidence yet for DX genes (Pratt et al., 1988). cDNA clones have been isolated for DRA and for several alleles of DRB, DQB, and DQA and transfected mouse cell lines produced that express both the SLA-DR and -DQ class II antigens (Gustafsson et al., 1990; Hirsch et al., 1992). Polymerase chain reaction (PCR)-based oligonucleotide primers have been developed to analyze SLA class II expression, sequences, and polymorphism.

At the antibody level, some class II-specific alloantisera have been produced when appropriate SLA recombinant animals have been identified. A few anti-SLA II MAbs have been produced by deliberate immunizations, although most of the useful MAb have been discovered by testing anti-murine, bovine, and human class II MAbs for cross-reactivity on SLA class II antigens (Lunney, 1994). Most of the anti-SLA class II MAb react with monomorphic determinants of class II antigens and, therefore, have limited applicability for use in functional assays. Only recently have Sachs and his colleagues been successful at producing anti-DQ (but not anti-DR) MAb that recognize allelic porcine class II specificities.

There is differential expression of class II antigens on mature swine lymphocytes. B cells and activated macrophages express both SLA-DR and -DQ antigens at similar levels; most peripheral blood monocytes are class II negative or

dull, whereas alveolar macrophages are class II bright. Unexpectedly, many peripheral T cells express class II antigens; SLA-DR is consistently brighter than SLA-DQ. 92% of CD8[+] T cells express SLA-DR antigens whereas only 43% of CD4[+] cells are SLA-DR positive (Lunney and Pescovitz, 1987). The importance/relevance of this unusual class II T cell subset expression has yet to be fully explained. Pescovitz et al. (1984) verified that the pig expresses class II antigens on renal vascular endothelium as has been found for human but not for rodents. This suggests that pigs will be a better model than rodents for transplant studies, particularly for attempts at passive antibody enhancement in class II mismatched grafts. In disease studies, scientists assessing SLA expression after virus inoculation have implicated modulation of expression of SLA class I and class II antigens during infection as a likely factor influencing humoral and cellular antiviral immune responses.

SLA CLASS III REGION

The SLA class III region has been extensively analyzed by Chardon, Vaiman, and their colleagues (Chardon et al., 1988); the steroid 21-hydroxylase (CYP21) and tumor necrosis factor (TNF) genes have been cloned and they, and the complement Bf, C2, and C4 genes, have been mapped to the SLA complex. Recently several other genes have been mapped to this region, including the opposite strand gene (OSG), three heat shock proteins (Hsp70), and BAT1.

SLA MAP

Early mapping of the SLA complex was based on linkage analyses of large numbers of individuals. The use of pulse field gel electrophoretic techniques for the SLA map by Xu et al. (1992) significantly expanded our knowledge. Figure 1 compares an updated version of their map of the SLA complex (Lunney, 1994) to the human HLA complex map. It is clear that the distance from the SLA class I loci to the SLA class III loci is at least 100 kb shorter than for the human genes; similarly, the distance between SLA class III and class II loci is 100 kb shorter. Singer and her colleagues have shown that the 6–10 SLA class I

Fig. 1. Comparative map of the major histocompatibility complex of humans and swine. The HLA map has been compared to the SLA map generated by Xu et al. (1992) and expanded with data from Drs. Chardon, LeGuern, Peelman, Rothschild, Sachs, Singer, Vaiman, and Warner (Lunney, 1994). The three regions of the SLA complex, SLA-I, II, and III, are noted; distances are given in kilobase pairs (kb). Adapted from Campbell and Trowsdale (1993).

genes are separated by no more than 500 kb, indicating that the SLA class I region is compressed when compared to humans or mice. Mapping of the outer limits of the SLA class II region indicates that the SLA-DP gene loci are ∼ 300 kb from SLA-DO and another 150 kb from the SLA-DQ loci. After extensive investigations, it appears that there is only 1 gene each for 210H, C2, and C4, even though other species have 2 or more 210H and C4 genes. Genetic linkage analyses indicate that the SLA complex is tightly linked (Vaiman et al., 1979; Lunney et al., 1986); most recently, linkage studies confirmed that SLA I is 0.8 cM from TNF, which is 0.7 cM from DQB on the short arm of swine chromosome 7 (Edfors-Lilja et al., 1993).

IMPORTANCE OF SLA-DEFINED SWINE

SLA-encoded control of swine immune responses to small antigens were first noted by Vaiman and his colleagues (1978) in SLA-haplotyped outbred swine, and confirmed by Lunney and her colleagues (1986) in the NIH minipigs. Because of the importance of the SLA complex in controlling immune and transplantation responses, herds of swine bred specifically for their SLA haplotypes were independently established in large outbred swine by Binns and his colleagues in England (Viza et al., 1970), by Hruban and his colleagues in Czechoslavokia (Hradecky et al., 1985), and by Smith in the United States in 1993, and in miniature swine (NIH minipigs) by Sachs and his colleagues in the United States (Sachs et al., 1976). These herds have enabled scientists to assess in detail immune responses that regulate organ transplantation and the influences of the SLA genes on animal health following vaccination or infection.

INFLUENCE OF SLA GENES ON TRANSPLANTATION REACTIONS

SLA-defined swine have been used extensively for organ transplantation studies. Starting over 20 years ago with skin and kidney transplants, the pig has now developed into a well-

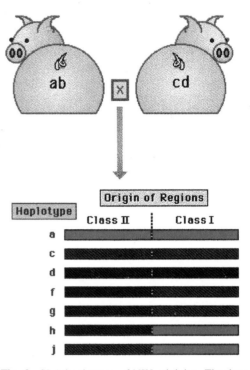

Fig. 2. SLA haplotypes of NIH minipigs. The three original haplotypes (*a, c, d*) and recombinant haplotypes (*f, g, h, j*).

defined large animal model for heart, liver, pancreas, and small bowel organ transplantation as well as for cellular transplantation using bone marrow, hepatocytes, and pancreatic islets (Kenmocji et al., 1994). The availability of three herds of NIH minipigs, each homozygous for a different SLA haplotype (Fig. 2), has provided a model in which organ and tissue transplantation studies can be carried out in similar genetic combinations to those for which transplantation is performed clinically. Transplants within herds or between identical F_1 animals are analogous to transplants between HLA-identical siblings, while transplants between herds are analogous to clinical transplants of unmatched cadaver organs. Genetic disparities of parent to offspring transplants are represented by grafts between different F_1 hybrids, such as SLA^{cd} into SLA^{ac}. Finally, the availability of intra-MHC recombinant strains have made it possible to study the effects of selective differences at class I and/or class II loci on the outcome of tissue and organ

Table I. Effect of SLA Class I and II Genes on Transplant Acceptance[a]

Transplanted tissue	Time in days to tissue rejection due to difference at[b]			
	SLA I and II	SLA I only	SLA II only	Minors only
Heart	7	8	8	31
Kidney	12	20[c]	22	30[c]
Liver	14	ND	ND	>60[c]
Skin	7	11	8	12

[a] Data collected in Sachs' laboratory.
[b] In all cases recipient and donor also differ for minor antigens.
[c] Some animals in these groups became tolerant and showed long-term survival.

transplants (Pescovitz et al., 1984; Rosengard et al., 1992a).

The effects of matching for SLA on the survival of heart, kidney, liver, and skin allografts are shown in Table I. As seen in this table, matching for SLA led to a prolongation of skin graft survival from 7 to 12 days. However, for vascularized grafts the effect of matching was much more striking. Matched liver allografts survived indefinitely (Flye et al., unpublished data), as did approximately one-third of matched kidney allografts (Kirkman et al., 1979a). In the case of kidney allografts, a subsequent backcross analysis indicated that ability to reject MHC-matched allografts was controlled by a non-SLA-linked immune response gene (Pennington et al., 1981). Acceptance of matched vascularized grafts conferred a state of systemic immunologic tolerance to minor transplantation antigens. Thus, skin grafts from the same donor as the kidney showed prolonged survival (> 40 days) when transplanted onto a long-term kidney acceptor, while rejection of a skin graft due to minor antigens at day 11 led to hyperacute rejection of a subsequent kidney allograft from the same donor (Kirkman et al., 1979b).

Recombinant SLA haplotypes made it possible to study the effects of selective class I or class II matching on the same kinds of allografts. As shown in Table I, either class I or class II antigen mismatches (plus minors) were sufficient to cause prompt rejection of skin grafts. However, kidney allografts were uniformly rejected when class II antigen mismatches were present, but showed prolonged or indefinite survival when there was matching for class II and one-haplotype mismatching for class I and minor antigens (Kirkman et al., 1979b). A state of systemic immunologic tolerance to class I plus minors was present in the long-term acceptors, again as indicated by subsequent prolonged survival of grafts from the same donors. Additional studies of the mechanism by which class II-matched grafts induce specific transplantation tolerance are in progress. The data obtained so far indicate that this phenomenon may be the result of a limitation in the level of T cell help available at the time of the first exposure of the immune system to class I plus minor antigens in a vascularized graft. Consistent with this hypothesis are results obtained using cyclosporin A to diminish T cell help at the time of first antigen exposure. A 12 day course has led to the induction of transplantation tolerance in 100% of class II-matched, class I plus minor antigen-mismatched kidney allografts (Rosengard et al., 1992b).

SUMMARY

Structural and functional properties of the SLA complex confirm the similarity of the pig MHC complex to that of humans. The availability of monoclonal antibodies to both class I and class II antigens, of cloned genes from both genomic and cDNA libraries, and of SLA-defined animals makes this species particularly attractive for use as a model for analyzing the influence of MHC genes on transplantation. Some of the properties shared with humans, but distinct from rodents, such as constitutive expression of class II antigens on the vascular endothelium, may explain differences between models in ease of inducing tolerance across MHC barriers. The newer information on the pig genome (Andersson et al., 1993) and the availability of transgenic pigs will further enhance scientists' research to define the genes that regulate transplant success and will potentiate efforts to make the pig the model of choice as universal donor for human xenotransplantation (Sachs, 1994).

REFERENCES

Andersson L, Archibald AL, Gellin J, Schook LB (1993): Report of 1st Pig Gene Mapping Workshop (PGMI). Anim Genet 24:205–216.

Campbell RD, Trowsdale J (1993): Immunol Today 14:349–352.

Chardon P, Vaiman M, Kirszenbaum M, Geoffrotin C, Renard C, Cohen D (1985): Restriction fragment length polymorphism of the major histocompatibility complex of the pig. Immunogenetics 21:161–171.

Chardon P, Geoffrotin C, Vaiman M (1988): Genetic organization of the SLA complex. In Warner CM, Rothschild MF, Lamont SJ (eds): "The Molecular Biology of the Major Histocompatibility Complex of Domestic Animal Species." Ames: Iowa State University Press, pp 63–78.

Edfors-Lilja I, Ellegren H, Wintero AK, Ruohonen-Lehto M, Fredholm M, Gustafsson U, Juneja RK, Andersson L (1993): A large linkage group on pig chromosome 7 including the MHC class I, class II (DQB), and class III (TNFB) genes. Immunogenetics 38:363–366.

Gustaffon K, LeGuern C, Hirsch FS, Germana S, Pratt K, Sachs DH (1990): Class II genes of miniature swine. IV. Characterization and expression of two allelic class II DQB cDNA clones. J Immunol 149:1946–1954.

Hirsch FS, Germana S, Gustaffon K, Pratt K, Sachs DH, LeGuern C (1992): Structure and expression of class II genes in miniature swine. J Immunol 149:841–848.

Hradecky J, Hruban V, Hojny J, Pazdera J, Stanek R (1985): Development of semi-inbred line of Landrace pigs. I. Breeding performance and immunogenetic characteristics. Lab Anim 19:279–283.

Kenmocji T, Mullen Y, Miyamoto M, Stein E (1994): Swine as a allotransplant model. Vet Immunol Immunopathol 43:177–183.

Kirkman RL, Colvin RB, Flye MW, Leight GS, Rosenberg SA, Williams GM, Sachs DH (1979a): Transplantation in miniature swine. VI. Factors influencing survival of renal allografts. Transplantation 28:18–23.

Kirkman RL, Colvin RB, Flye MW, Williams GM, Sachs DH (1979b): Transplantation in miniature swine. VII. Evidence for cellular immune mechanisms in hyperacute rejection of renal allografts. Transplantation 28:24–30.

Lunney JK (1994): Current Status of the swine leukocyte antigen (SLA) complex. Vet Immunol Immunopathol 43:19–28.

Lunney JK, Pescovitz MD (1987): Phenotypic and functional characterization of pig lymphocyte populations. Vet Immunol Immunopathol 17:135–144.

Lunney JK, Pescovitz MD, Sachs DH (1986): The swine major histocompatibility complex: Its structure and function. In Tumbleson ME (ed): "Swine in Biomedical Research." New York: Plenum Press, pp 1821–1836.

Pennington LR, Flye MW, Kirkman RL, Thistlethwaite JR, Williams GM, Sachs DH (1981): Transplantation in miniature swine. X. Evidence for non-SLA-linked immune response gene(s) controlling rejection of SLA-matched kidney allografts. Transplantation 32:315–320.

Pescovitz MD, Sachs DH, Lunney JK, Hsu S-M (1984a): Localization of class II antigens on porcine renal vascular endothelium. Transplantation 37:617–630.

Pescovitz MD, Thistlethwaite JR Jr., Auchincloss H, Ildstad ST, Sharp TG, Terrill R, and Sachs DH (1984b): Effect of class II antigen matching on renal allograft survival in miniature swine. J Exp Med 160:1495–1508.

Pratt K, Sachs DH, Germana S, El-Gamil M, Hirsch F, Gustafsson K, LeGuern C (1988): Class II genes of miniature swine. II. Molecular identification and characterization of beta genes from the SLA[c] haplotype. Immunogenetics 28:22–29.

Renard C, Kristensen B, Gautche C, Hruban V, Fredholm M, Vaiman M (1988): Joint report of the first international comparison test on swine lymphocyte alloantigens (SLA). Anim Genet 19:63–72.

Rosengard BR, Ojikutu CA, Fishbein J, Kortz EO, Sachs DH (1992a): Selective breeding of miniature swine leads to an increased rate of acceptance of MHC-identical but not of class-I disparate, renal allografts. J Immunol 149:1099–1103.

Rosengard BR, Ojikutu CA, Guzzetta PC, Smith CV,

Sundt TM III, Nakajima K, Boorstein SM, Hill GS, Fishbein JM, Sachs DH (1992b): Induction of long-term specific tolerance to class I disparate renal allografts in miniature swine with a short course of cyclosporine. Transplantation 54:490–497.

Sachs DH (1994): The pig as a potential zenograft donor. Vet Immunol Immunopathol 43:185–191.

Sachs DH, Leight G, Cone J, Schwarz S, Stuart L, Rosenberg S (1976): Transplantation in miniature swine. I. Fixation of the major histocompatibility complex. Transplantation 22:559–567.

Sachs DH, Germana S, El-Gamil M, Gustaffson K, Hirsch F, Pratt K (1988): Class II genes of miniature swine. I. Class II gene characterization by RFLP and by isolation from a genomic library. Immunogenetics 28:22–29.

Singer DS, Camerini-Otero RD, Satz ML, Osborne B, Sachs D, Rudikoff S (1982): Characterization of a porcine genomic clone encoding a major histocompatibility antigen: Expression in mouse L cells. Proc Natl Acad Sci USA 79:1403–1407.

Singer DS, Ehrlich R, Golding H, Satz L, Parent L, Rudikoff S (1988): Structure and function of Class I MHC genes in the miniature swine. In Warner CM, Rothschild MF, Lamont SJ (eds): "The Molecular Biology of the Major Histocompatibility Complex of Domestic Animal Species." Ames: Iowa State University Press, pp 53–62.

Trowsdale J, Ragoussis J, Campbell RD (1991): Map of the human MHC. Immunol Today 12:443–447.

Vaiman M, Renard C, Lafage P, Amateau J, Nizza P (1970): Evidence of a histocompatibility system in swine (SL-A). Transplantation 10:155–161.

Vaiman M, Metzger J, Renard C, Vila J (1978): Immune response gene(s) controlling the humoral antilysozyme response (Ir-Lys) linked to the major histocompatibility complex SL-A in the pig. Immunogenetics 7:231–238.

Vaiman M, Chardon P, Renard C (1979): Genetic organization of the pig SLA complex. Studies on nine recombinants and biochemical and lysostrip analysis. Immunogenetics 9:353–362.

Viza D, Sugar JR, Binns RM (1970): Lymphocyte stimulation in pigs. Evidence for existence of a single major histocompatibility locus: PL-A. Nature (London) 227:949–951.

Xu Y, Rothschild MF, Warner CM (1992): Mapping of the SLA complex of miniature swine: Mapping of the SLA gene complex by pulsed field gel electrophoresis. Mam Genome 2:2–10.

Chapter 21
Molecular Biology for the Clinician

Hans Winkler and Fritz H. Bach

Molecular biology has allowed an enormous leap forward in the study and understanding of biology. From the premolecular biology era, at which time we had little understanding of individual genes and their regulation, to the present time, we have been given the opportunity to isolate and study individual genes, express those genes so that large amounts of the protein product can be obtained for analytical or therapeutic purposes, and introduce genes into cells *in vitro* and well as *in vivo,* either to express that gene of interest in its new cell or to turn off a gene normally expressed in that cell.

For transplantation biology, as for so many other fields, the techniques of molecular biology have provided new information on many fronts. Equally important, techniques are available, and being developed, that will allow us to use the information gained to "correct" defects or potentially manipulate a response for the benefit of the patient using methods of genetic engineering.

It is our purpose in this chapter to introduce the reader, at a rather elementary level, to the techniques of molecular biology as they may, and in many cases are, being used in relationship to transplantation. Especially with the advent of a renewed interest in xenotransplantation, these techniques are invaluable and offer the hope that we shall be able, by genetic engineering, to dampen unwanted responses to a xenograft. It is not our purpose to be comprehensive, either in the concepts and techniques discussed, or in cataloging the multiple problems that will no doubt emerge as ones in which molecular biological techniques will find application. Rather, we hope to provide the reader with sufficient basic information, some even repeated in different sections, to allow them to proceed further as their interest dictates.

One of the major revolutions in biology has concerned itself with our increased understanding of the genetic material, the *DNA.* It was only 50 years ago that we first realized that the genetic material is what we now know as DNA; only 40 or so years ago that Watson and Crick published the structure of DNA, which explained so much; and only a little more than 30 years since we learned that there are 46 chromosomes, as opposed to 48, as had been thought before that. In those 30 years, from knowing about the number of chromosomes, we have moved to having an intimate knowledge of individual genes, their structure at the level of the DNA, and something of what regulates their expression, i.e., the productive transcription of the gene and the subsequent synthesis of the corresponding protein (Fig. 1).

Even as we learned these facts, the sequence of events that led from use of the genetic material to synthesis of the proteins that are the centers of biological function was being elucidated. We learned that the sequence of *bases* [thymidine (T), adenine (A), cytosine (C) and guanine (G)] in the DNA provided the information from which the *messenger RNA (mRNA)* molecules were produced, a process referred to as *transcription.* mRNA is a single-stranded copy of a gene that is transported from the nucleus to the cytoplasm for protein synthesis. RNA contains three of the same bases as in DNA; however, instead of the T there is uridine (U). We even learned that under some conditions DNA is syn-

Transplantation Immunology, pages 347–401
© 1995 Wiley-Liss, Inc.

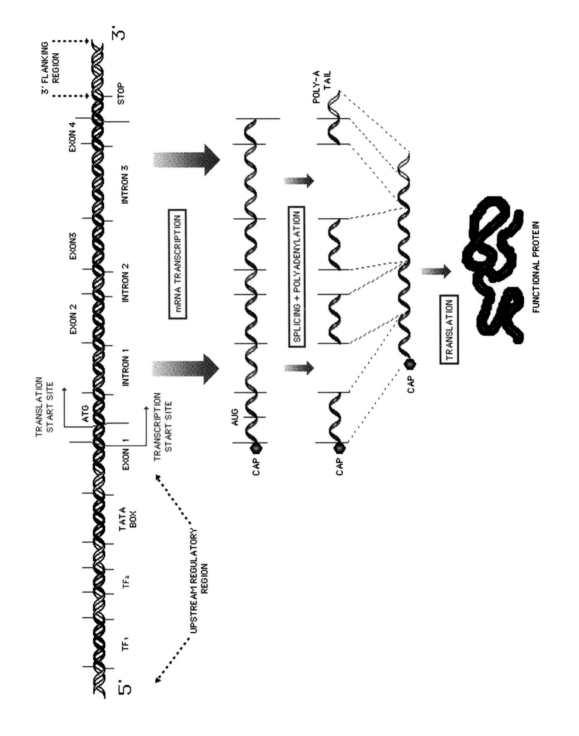

thesized from the information in the RNA, something referred to as *"reverse transcription,"* the enzymatic synthesis of DNA from an RNA template. The RNA, based on the triplet code,[1] is translated into the *protein.*

THE GENETIC MATERIAL

DNA

DNA (deoxyribonucleic acid) is the molecular carrier of genetic information and includes the genes. It is an oriented, linear molecule consisting of four different bases—adenine (A), guanine (G), cytosine (C), and thymine (T)—that are sequentially held together by a sugar–phosphate backbone much like beads on a string (Fig. 2). A single *monomer* in the DNA is composed of a base, a sugar (deoxyribose), and a phosphate, and is called a *nucleotide.* The base is attached to the sugar molecule, which itself has two phosphate groups bound at two positions (3′ and 5′). Each phosphate bridges two sugar molecules (one at the 3′ position and one at the 5′ position) (Fig. 2). This arrangement generates a direction in the DNA molecule (5′ or 3′ or vice versa). A particular sequence of bases in the DNA in one orientation is chemically, and therefore functionally, different from the same sequence in the other direction.

A critical characteristic of the bases is that each of them has a specific affinity to one of the others (A to T and C to G) that allows them to form so-called *base pairs* (bp, Fig. 2). The ability of DNA to form base pairs allows the cell

---

[1]Within the protein-coding part of a gene, three bases in a row, a so-called codon, provide the information of which amino acid will be incorporated into which position in a protein. The sequence of codons on the DNA and mRNA corresponds to the sequence of amino acids in the resulting protein.

Fig. 1. A schematic representation of gene expression. The gene as it exists in the chromosome is transcribed into RNA. The primary transcript is processed, transported to the nucleus, and translated into protein, the final gene product.

actually to contain not only the coding, *"sense"* DNA strand that carries the information from which the mRNA is made, but also a *complementary (antisense)* blueprint of it, in the form of a double-stranded helical DNA molecule. The complementary strand of a certain nucleic acid contains only bases that form base pairs with the original strand. Therefore, in the opposite orientation, there is an A for each T, a T for each A, a G for each C, and a C for each G (Fig. 2). Double strands of DNA are much more stable than single strands and also allow repair of damaged DNA by replacing a missing or modified base on one strand according to its complementary base on the other strand. DNA is often presented as a string of letters (A, G, T, and C) to indicate the sequence of bases of the DNA strand.

RNA

RNA is very similar to DNA from a chemical perspective. It is also a *polymer* assembled from base–sugar–phosphate monomers. It contains adenine, guanine, and cytosine, as does DNA, however, the thymine of DNA is replaced by uracil (U). In addition, the sugar moiety is ribose rather than deoxyribose, which renders RNA chemically less stable, because the presence of ribose allows hydrolysis of the RNA under basic pH conditions. All RNA species in a eukaryotic organism are synthesized by one of three *RNA polymerase* enzymes, which use a double-stranded DNA molecule as a *template,* from which the sense strand of the DNA is copied into a complementary RNA strand. The RNA polymerase incorporates a nucleotide into the nascent RNA molecule only if the base to be incorporated forms a base pair with the template strand of the DNA, with the adenine in the DNA encoding a uracil in the RNA. This process is called *transcription.* In the cell, several forms of RNA can be distinguished according to their structure and function:

Messenger RNA (mRNA) is copied from DNA. mRNA contains the genetic information that is translated into protein in the cytoplasm (see gene expression). Each protein-coding triplet (a *codon,* see footnote 1) of mRNA is responsible for the incorporation of one amino acid into the encoded protein.

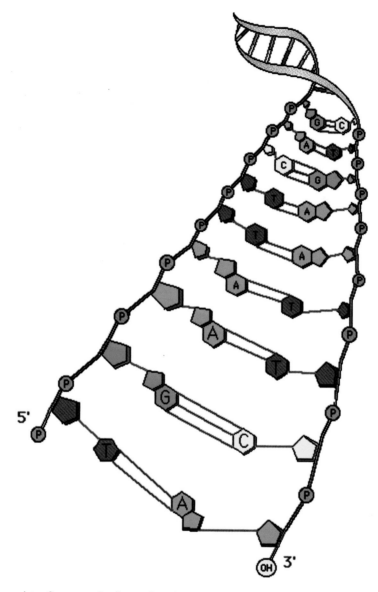

5'

3'

Fig. 2. DNA consists of two strands of opposite orientation. Each strand has a backbone of sugar–phosphate–sugar chains. The sugar (deoxyribose) is indicated as pentagons; the phosphates are shown as circled P. The sequence determining bases (A, G, C, or T) are linked to the sugar moieties as well. This figure was reproduced and modified with kind permission from Raven and Johnson, "Biology," Third edition, Mosby Year Book, Inc., St. Louis, Missouri.

Transfer RNA (tRNA) functions as the carrier of amino acids for protein synthesis. It is the link between mRNA-encoded sequence information and protein sequence. For each amino acid there exists at least one form of tRNA. The special structure of tRNA molecules (Fig. 3) allows them to recognize a sequence element of three bases (one codon) on the mRNA by base pairing (with the *anticodon* on the tRNA molecule. The base pairing between a codon on the mRNA and

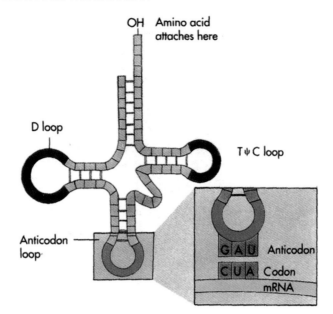

Fig. 3. The structure of a tRNA molecule. A priori, tRNA is single stranded, however, due to intramolecular base-complementarity, the molecule can fold back on itself to create partial double strands. In this case, the double-stranded regions are called stems, the remaining single strands are called loops. A typical tRNA molecule contains five stems and four loops, one of which carries the anticodon, as indicated. This figure was reproduced with kind permission from Raven and Johnson, "Biology," Third edition, Mosby Year Book, Inc., St. Louis, Missouri.

the anticodon of a tRNA molecule leads to the correct incorporation of an amino acid at the right position of a nascent protein chain (Fig. 4).

Ribosomal RNA (rRNA) molecules, together with ribosomal proteins, form *ribosomes,* the organelles on which proteins are synthesized in a process known as *translation.* Some rRNA molecules not only contribute to ribosomal structure but also have catalytic functions in the process of translation, i.e., they facilitate chemical reactions during protein synthesis so that they can occur at the temperature of the cell (usually around 37°C).

Small nuclear RNA (snRNA) refers to RNA molecules that form complexes with proteins (*small nuclear ribonucleoproteins, snRNP*) mainly involved in splicing, the removal of intervening sequences (introns) of the primary RNA molecule to generate mature mRNA (see Fig. 1 and below) from pre-mRNA molecules. The RNA parts of RNPs also have catalytic activity necessary for *splicing.*

Amino Acids—Proteins

Proteins are responsible for two major functions: first, they form most of the structural elements of cells, tissues, and entire organisms and second, in the form of enzymes, they are capable of catalyzing chemical reactions otherwise impossible under conditions sustaining life, such as in an aqueous environment and at low temperature. Like DNA and RNA, proteins are large molecules (*polymers*) derived from smaller ones (*monomers,* in this case amino acids) by linear juxtaposition and chemical bonds between the individual monomers. However, they are built from 20 different monomers, the *amino acids* allowing a much greater diversity of structure as well as function as compared with nucleic acids. There are 20^{100} different possibilities to assemble a protein of 100 amino acids, a number greater than the number of atoms in the universe. Ultimately, the sequence of the amino acids in the protein chain determines the three-

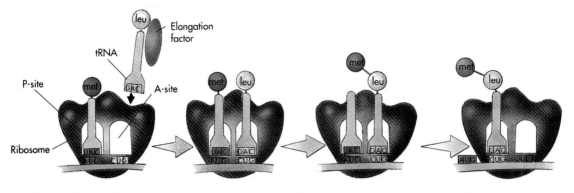

Fig. 4. On the ribosome, at any one time, two tRNA molecules can bind to the mRNA via codon–anticodon base pairing. A peptide bond is formed between the two amino acids linked to the tRNA molecules such that the amino acid from the first tRNA is transferred onto the amino acid that is bound to the second tRNA. Then the ribosome moves three nucle-otides downstream on the mRNA to release the "empty" tRNA and to allow the next amino acid-carrying tRNA molecule to bind. This figure was reproduced with kind permission from Raven and Johnson, "Biology," Third edition, Mosby Year Book, Inc., St. Louis, Missouri.

dimensional structure of the protein, which depends on interactions of the amino acid side chains with each other.

Among themselves, amino acids also show a much higher degree of chemical variation as compared to nucleotides. All amino acids contain a carboxyl group and an amino group on the adjacent carbon atom (the α-carbon atom). This, as with nucleotides, generates a directionality because the amino acids in a *peptide chain* are linked together via their amino and carboxyl groups by *peptide bonds* (Fig. 5). Thus, each peptide chain has a free α-amino group as part of the amino acid at one end (the *amino-* or *N-terminus*) and a free carboxyl group as part of the amino acid at the other end (the *carboxy-* or *C-terminus*). In a peptide, a molecule made up of several to many amino acids, the α-carbon atoms, forms the backbone of the chain whereas the side chains determine the physical and chemical properties.

Progression from DNA to RNA to Protein

The sequence in DNA is transcribed into what is known as a *primary RNA transcript,* which contains both *exons* and *introns.* The exons carry the genetic information that will eventually be translated into protein. This transcript is *processed* in the nucleus during which the introns

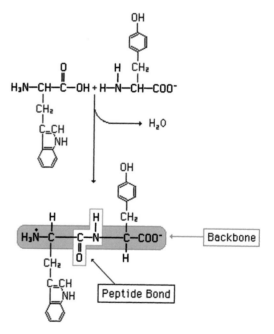

Fig. 5. The peptide bond is formed between the carboxyl (-COOH) group of one amino acid with the α-amino (-NH$_2$) group of the next amino acid. The so formed CO-NH- bond is called a peptide bond.

are removed and the exons are *spliced* together. Moreover, a tail of up to several hundred adenine residues is added to the 3′ end of the mRNA (*polyadenylation*), rendering the mRNA more

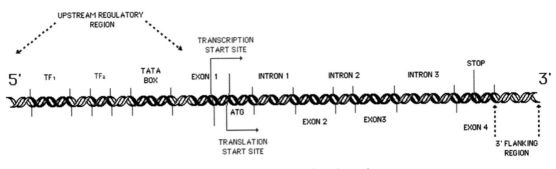

Fig. 6. Graphic representation of a eukaryotic gene.

stable against enzymatic degradation. The resulting mature mRNA molecule is transported to the cytoplasm for *translation* into protein.

The Structure of a Gene

Stretches of DNA on a *chromosome*[2] are called genes if at least part of the region carries the genetic information for a protein (or special types of RNA, e.g., tRNA, rRNA, or snRNA). In this overview, only genes coding for proteins will be described [i.e., genes transcribed by *RNA polymerase II*, one of the three RNA polymerases in eukaryotic cells. This enzyme is capable of synthesizing an RNA copy of DNA sequences containing the right regulatory sequences, i.e., all genes coding for proteins. The product is messenger RNA (mRNA)]. The entity referred to as a gene comprises not only the sequence information for a protein (i.e., the *coding* region), it also contains different types of *regulatory* sequences. In general, a gene can be divided into three parts: (1) the nontranscribed, or flanking regions, (2) the transcribed part (i.e., the *transcript*), and (3) within the transcript, the actual coding region that is translated into protein.

Looking at a gene (Fig. 6) beginning at its 5′ end, the first part encountered is the "*upstream*"

(5′) *regulatory region*. This region is located upstream of the transcription start site. It contains elements (between 6 and 20 bp in length) controlling *transcription*. These sequences are binding sites for specific proteins called *transcription factors*.[3] The binding of a transcription factor to its specific DNA sequence can induce or repress transcription initiation. Tissue-specific expression of a gene, developmental regulation of gene expression, the response of a given gene to external stimuli (inducibility vs. constitutive expression), and the overall level of transcription are all controlled by the combination of transcription factors that binds in the regulatory region.

A part of the regulatory sequences can also be located within the gene or "*downstream*" (3′) of the gene; sometimes they are found up to 50,000 bp away from the transcriptional start site, organized as so-called *enhancers* (see Regulation of Transcription). Other types of sequences regulate transcript maturation (splicing, polyadenylation), mRNA stability, and translation efficiency.

A critical element, present in almost all genes, is the *TATA box;* this element usually contains the sequence TATAAA, hence the name. It is the site where a complex of proteins is assembled that eventually activates the RNA polymerase to

---

[2]The core of a chromosome is a very large molecule of DNA, of up to several hundreds of megabases in length. Bound to this DNA molecule is a multitude of proteins necessary to perform chromosomal functions such as condensation, replication, division, and recombination, to name just a few. Taken together, the chromosomes of a cell contain the entire genetic information of an organism.

[3]The presence and state of activation of special transcription factors determine whether a certain gene is actively transcribed. The binding of a set of properly activated transcription factors to their target sites in the regulatory region of a gene allows them to interact with the general transcription machinery leading to the efficient initiation of transcription.

start RNA synthesis (transcription), which is usually initiated by the polymerase 30 bp downstream of the TATA box. The site at which the polymerase initiates transcription is called the *transcriptional start site*. The protein-coding sequence begins another 100–200 bp downstream from (3' of) the transcriptional start site. The first *base triplet* (a triplet of bases, also called a *codon*, codes for one amino acid in the protein) in the DNA coding for protein is always *ATG*. Which bases are considered the triplets, thus determining the sequence of amino acids in the protein, referred to as the *frame* in which the DNA is read, is determined by the first ATG, which codes for the amino acid *methionine*. The next triplet is then translated into the next amino acid, and so on.

The DNA sequence coding for the entire protein is not contiguous, but is interrupted by noncoding DNA, the *introns*. The number and length of the introns as well as their precise position within the gene are highly variable. Some genes do not have introns (*thrombomodulin*); in other genes introns make up greater than 99% of the sequence of the gene (the transcribed part of the gene responsible for Duchenne muscular

dystrophy covers about 3 million base pairs yet the coding sequence is only a few thousand base pairs in length). Eventually to obtain an mRNA sequence that carries the information for translation and thus synthesis of the protein, the introns are removed from the *primary transcript*, i.e., the RNA molecule that is originally generated by transcription, in a process called *splicing* (Fig. 7). In many cases, the following sequence $^C/_A$ A **G G T** $^A/_G$ A G T (the bold part of the sequence is still part of the previous exon; the underlined sequence is the start of the intron) can be found immediately before and at the start of an intron. The end of an intron is frequently encoded by $(^T/_C) \geqslant {}_{11}N$ $^C/_T$A G **G** (the underlined part of the sequence is intron sequence, the bolded G is the beginning of the next exon; $^C/_A$ refers to C or A). These are the sequences that are recognized in splicing and allow correct joining of the DNA sequences that will remain in the mature messenger RNA (mRNA), which are called *exons*.

All but the first and last exons of a gene are completely translated into protein. The sequence 5' of the translation initiation codon is the *leader sequence* and contains elements necessary for the interaction of mRNA and ribosomes and de-

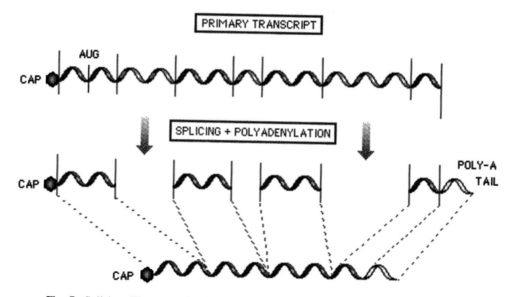

Fig. 7. Splicing. The noncoding introns of the primary transcript are removed and the protein-coding exons are joined together to form the mature transcript (mRNA).

termines the efficiency of translation initiation. The last exon contains the *STOP codon* (UAA, UGA, and UAG signal the end of protein synthesis). STOP codons do not code for an amino acid but lead to the release of the mRNA from the ribosome because there is no tRNA containing an appropriate *anticodon* for these triplets.

Following the STOP codon is the 3′ noncoding sequence. It contains a *polyadenylation signal sequence (AAUAAA)* that is responsible for the addition of a stretch of adenines (up to several hundred) at the 3′ end of the mRNA. Sequences determining the stability of the mRNA may also be present in the 3′ noncoding region. Under certain conditions these sequences (e.g., AUUUA), when present, lead to the rapid enzymatic degradation of the mRNA molecule. The artificial removal of these sequences increases the half-life of the modified mRNA dramatically. The precise point of transcription termination is not well understood, however, some sequences have been identified that can serve as potent transcription terminators.

It becomes obvious from the description above that some regulatory elements are active at the DNA level (e.g., upstream transcription factor binding sites, TATA box, transcription start site), whereas others are recognized on the RNA molecule (the start codon, splicing sites, and control elements, the polyadenylation signal, and the RNA stability-determining elements).

The genes are organized into very long DNA molecules (several million base pairs), the *chromosomes*. In addition to DNA, chromosomes contain proteins (mainly histones), which are necessary for the structural organization into *nucleosomes* and higher order structures that allow such large DNA molecules to be packed into the nucleus. The proteins are also needed for the reproduction of the DNA in the genome during cell divisions (*replication*, i.e., the synthesis of an exact copy of each chromosome preceding cell division). In fact, 70% of the mass of a chromosome is contributed by proteins.

So far, in this chapter, we have presented the basics of genetic information and will now begin to describe particular items important for understanding the power of molecular biology.

Plasmids

Bacteria, in addition to their circular genomic DNA, frequently possess additional extra-chromosomal DNA molecules to supplement their genome. These circular, double-stranded *episomal* DNA molecules are not part of the bulk of the genomic DNA, and are called *plasmids* (Fig. 8). Most bacteria are able to exchange plasmids directly between cells in the process of *conjugation,* during which a bacterial cell transfers a plasmid directly to another bacterial cell and at the same time replicates this plasmid so that a copy remains with the donor bacterial cell. Most plasmids are quite small, containing only 5 to 10 kilobases (*kb*) of DNA. The major function of plasmids is to carry genes conferring resistance to natural antibiotics such as penicillin.

Molecular biologists use plasmids as vehicles or *vectors* to carry pieces of DNA of interest. Usually, since plasmids replicate both to a high number and rapidly, they are used to amplify a gene that is first inserted into the plasmid. Many copies of that gene can be produced by transferring the gene-containing plasmid into bacteria and allowing it to replicate. By this procedure, a few nanograms of DNA can be amplified to yield several milligrams from a large plasmid preparation in about 5 liters of bacterial culture (i.e., a million-fold increase in the amount of DNA).

Several characteristics are desirable in a plasmid vector. Clearly, the number of molecules made in the bacterial cell is important. This is mainly dependent on the *origin of replication (ori;* a special sequence on a DNA molecule where DNA synthesis, i.e., replication starts). Several different *origins* are known, but only one is currently used in all commercially available vectors (colE1). It allows the accumulation of about 100 plasmid molecules per bacterial cell. The second desirable feature of plasmid vectors is to have *selectable marker genes*. Usually these are drug resistance genes that render bacterial cells resistant to ampicillin, tetracycline, or kanamycin. Because only a small fraction of all bacteria are transformed by the procedures, the antibiotic resistance genes are necessary to select bacteria that, in a *transformation* (a procedure to

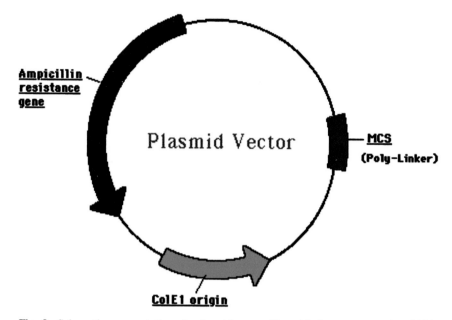

Fig. 8. Schematic representation of a plasmid vector. The critical sequences such as MCS (polylinker), ampicillin resistance gene, and the origin of replication are indicated.

introduce DNA into bacteria), have actually received DNA. By rendering transformed bacteria resistant to an antibiotic like ampicillin, it allows them to grow on the selection media, whereas cells that have not taken up the plasmid cannot survive. A third important aspect of vectors is the number of different sites into which DNA can be integrated by *ligation,* the enzymatic reaction by which two individual DNA molecules are covalently linked into a single molecule. The most advanced plasmid vectors have a *multiple cloning site (MCS, polylinker)*. An MCS is a DNA sequence of about 100 bp containing a number of recognition sites for *restriction enzymes* unique in the entire plasmid; therefore, cutting the plasmid with one of these enzymes will linearize the plasmid at the location of the enzyme recognition site. The MCS allows DNA molecules with a variety of different ends to be ligated into the vector.

In some instances, it is desirable to transfer a plasmid containing a gene of interest into eukaryotic cells after it has been expanded in the bacteria. Vectors for use in eukaryotic systems must include additional selectable markers for such cells.

GENE EXPRESSION AND REGULATION

Transcription

One of the central processes of life is the regulated mobilization of genetic information to generate a distinct phenotype. This requires the transformation of the information encoded by the DNA into protein. Four, and sometimes five, steps can be distinguished in realizing this task. First, the gene to be expressed must be copied into RNA (*transcription*). Second, the primary transcript must be properly *processed* (splicing, polyadenylation). Third, the mature mRNA is transported into the cytoplasm. Fourth, the mRNA is *translated* into a polypeptide chain on the ribosomes. Fifth, in many cases the protein must be *modified posttranslationally,* such as having sugars (carbohydrates) added to it, to exert its function.

Focusing on a single gene, the first step is the production of a blueprint of this gene in the form of a messenger RNA (mRNA) molecule. The process of mRNA synthesis is called *transcription*. The exact conditions under which a certain gene is transcribed depends on the *regulatory sequences* around and within the gene and on the presence of protein *transcription* factors necessary to initiate transcription. RNA polymerase II almost exclusively initiates a transcript about 30 bp downstream (3′) of the TATA box (Fig. 9). The nature of the regulatory sequences determines the rate of transcription initiation and therefore the amount of mRNA synthesized in a certain period of time. Generally, the *rate of transcription initiation* is an important parameter in the regulation of gene expression. After the first, crude copy of the gene is synthesized, extensive processing of the primary transcript takes place in the nucleus. Very early, probably while the transcript is still being extended, the so-called *cap structure* is added at the 5′ end of the RNA. The cap is important for recognition of the mRNA by the ribosome to ensure efficient translation of the transcript. The introns are then spliced out, the poly(A) tail is added, and the mature mRNA is transported to the cytoplasm.

Regulation of Transcription

Genes coding for proteins are transcribed by RNA polymerase II. This enzyme is a multisubunit protein that is not sufficient by itself to initiate transcription of any gene. Rather, additional proteins, belonging to two different groups, are required for the specific regulation of transcription. The first group of proteins belong to the *general transcription machinery,* a group of proteins that assembles around the *TATA box* when the gene is induced. The second group, the gene-specific *transcription factors* are the actual regulatory switches of a given gene. These proteins bind to specific recognition sites within the regulatory region of a gene (Fig. 10) and by interacting with the "general" factors (TATA complex and/or RNA polymerase) regulate the initiation of transcription.

Very rarely, a single specific transcription factor is sufficient to induce transcription of a gene, including assembly of the TATA complex. In such a case, transcription is turned on as soon as the active protein is bound to its recognition sequence in the regulatory region (Fig. 10a). In most cases, however, a number of different factors are required for efficient transcriptional initiation. Therefore, if some essential factors are not bound to the regulatory region, transcription is not initiated (Fig. 10b). Often, all but one of the required factors are active and bound to the regulatory region of a gene and the missing factor (e.g., NFκB) is not present unless it is activated by a specific stimulus (e.g., a cytokine) and in the absence of the stimulus there is no transcription (Fig. 10c). When the cells are stim-

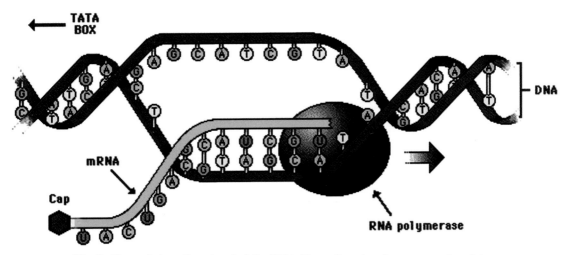

Fig. 9. Transcription. One strand of the DNA (the coding strand) serves as a template. This figure was reproduced and modified with kind permission from Raven and Johnson, "Biology," Third edition, Mosby Year Book, Inc., St. Louis, Missouri.

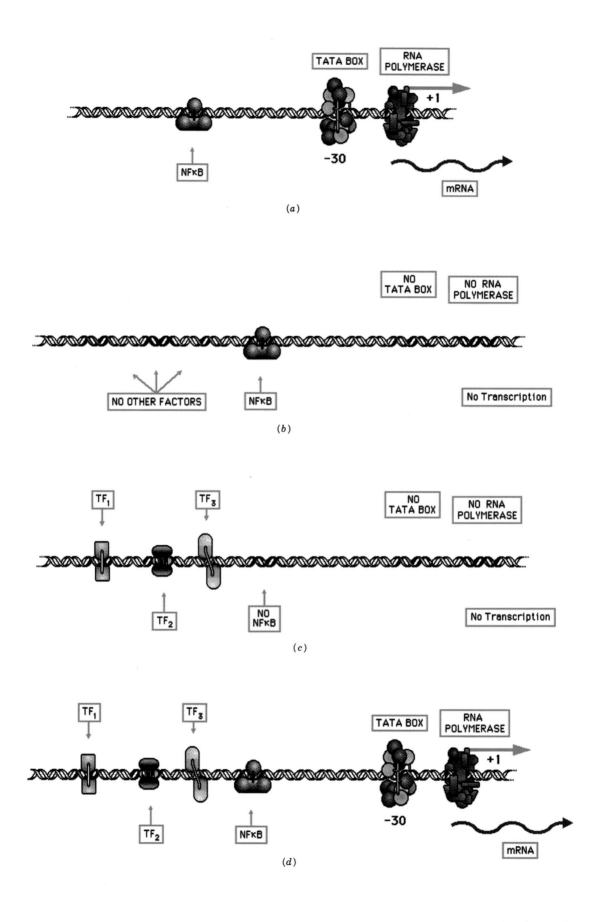

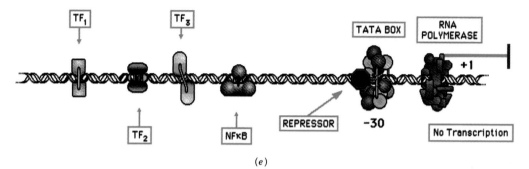

(e)

Fig. 10. (**a**) Transcription from a promoter that only requires one specific transcription factor (NFκB). (**b**) No transcription occurs if additional factors are needed but not present. (**c**) No transcription is possible if all additional factors factor are present but one essential factor is missing. (**d**) Transcription in the presence of all essential factors. (**e**) Transcription is prevented by a repressor even though all essential transcription factors are present.

ulated, however, this factor is activated and acts as a switch to turn on transcription by binding to its recognition site next to the other factors already present (Fig. 10d). Under some circumstances, certain stimuli (glucocorticoids) can cause the activation of a *transcriptional repressor,* which can prevent transcription of a gene, even in the presence of all essential positive transcription factors (Fig. 10e). In many regulatory regions, not all the regulatory elements are also essential for transcription even though they may increase the rate of transcription if the respective factor is bound and active. Therefore, it is assumed that there exists a certain degree of synergism between different regulatory elements and between the proteins that bind to them allowing for subtle modulations in the rate of transcription of a certain gene.

In addition to regulatory elements relatively close to the TATA box there are other types of elements, the enhancers, that function independently of their orientation and location (5′ or 3′) relative to the gene they regulate. They can also be located several kilobases away from the gene. Typically, an enhancer binds several different proteins that, by an as yet unknown mechanism, increase the rate of transcription tremendously, although significant transcription may occur even if the enhancer is not active.

Translation

The process of synthesizing a polypeptide from amino acids in a sequence corresponding to the original DNA sequence is called *translation.*

The sequence information for proteins is encoded in the DNA sequence. Three bases in a row, a so-called *base triplet (codon),* determine the identity of an amino acid. The first amino acid of a protein is always methionine, encoded by AUG on the mRNA. This also sets the *frame* for translation, i.e., the first AUG on the mRNA encodes methionine and each subsequent triplet encodes another amino acid of the protein. The actual connection between mRNA sequence and incorporation of an amino acid corresponding to a certain triplet is made by tRNA (see Fig. 3). This special type of RNA molecule carries a covalently bound amino acid. Each tRNA molecule is capable of recognizing a triplet of bases (*codon*) on the mRNA by virtue of base pairing with the *anticodon* of the tRNA. Thus, translation always starts with methionine-tRNA (met-tRNA^{met}). *met-tRNA* indicates methionine tRNA, i.e., the tRNA molecule that carries methionine. The designation *met-tRNA^{met}* indicates that the methionine tRNA is actually charged with a methionine molecule. The tRNA^{met} carries 5′-CAU-3′ in its anticodon and therefore recognizes an 5′-AUG-3′ codon. There is at least one tRNA for each amino acid. For some amino acids there is more than one base triplet and, therefore, there is more than one type of tRNA, each with different anticodons for one amino acid. For instance, there are 6 codons and 6 different tRNAs for the amino acid serine. This is due to the fact that 3 bases can statistically form 64 different sequences, but there is a need to code for only 20 amino acids and 3 codons are reserved as *STOP* codons (UAA, UAG, and UGA). The process of translation as it occurs on the ribosome is depicted in Figure 4.

Translation is initialized by binding of the mRNA to the small ribosomal subunit. Then the large ribosomal subunit is bound and the first aminoacyl-tRNA, i.e., met-tRNA^{met} binds to the mRNA through base pairing. Next, the second aminoacyl-tRNA (aa$_2$-tRNA^{aa_2}) binds to the second codon of the mRNA and the first peptide bond is formed in that the α-amino group of aa$_2$ reacts with the carboxyl group of aa$_1$. This process includes the detachment of aa$_1$ from its tRNA such that the nascent peptide chain remains bound to aa$_2$. The mRNA moves one codon forward, tRNA^{aa_1} is released from the ribosome and aa$_3$-tRNA^{aa_3} binds to the mRNA at codon 3. The process is repeated until a *STOP codon* is encountered and the mature peptide chain is released from the ribosome. Many steps along the way from transcription initiation to the correctly folded protein can be regulated to either enhance or attenuate expression or even regulate whether the protein will be functionally active or not (e.g., by phosphorylation).

Levels of Regulation of Gene Expression

There are several steps in the process of gene expression that can undergo positive or negative regulation. These steps are (1) transcription initiation, (2) splicing, (3) polyadenylation, (4) mRNA transport, (5) translation initiation, (6) protein transport, and (7) posttranslational modifications.

The first step in the regulation of gene expression is the control of transcription initiation by gene-specific transcription factors. The state of activation of these proteins determines whether a gene is transcribed.

The next step that is sometimes controlled in a cell is the number of introns spliced out of the primary transcript. Depending on the identity of the gene, some introns are spliced out only in a specific cell type and not in others. This results in a different gene product (protein) in the end so that a single gene can encode more than one protein. This overall regulatory strategy used by the cell is called *alternative splicing*.

The addition of the poly(A) tail is also regulated in some genes. The presence of the poly(A) tail influences the stability of the RNA and may also be important for translation efficiency. Whether polyadenylation serves other roles is not known.

The efficiency of translation initiation is another means of controlling gene expression. (1) As long as the mRNA remains in the nucleus it cannot be translated and, therefore, gene expression is not effective. (2) In most cases, the sequence surrounding the AUG on the mRNA is responsible for the efficacy of translation initiation. (3) The rate of translation initiation can be regulated by cofactors such as heme. In erythroid cells, for example, the translation of hemoglobin is positively regulated by heme, an essential cofactor of hemoglobin. A heme-dependent protein kinase phosphorylates a translation initiation factor, which increases the rate of translation initiation. (4) In addition, the 5' end of the transcript, i.e., the nontranslated part of the mRNA (the *leader sequence*), plays a pivotal role in determining the rate of translation initiation. Some leader sequences derived from certain viruses are able to increase translational efficacy tremendously compared to other leader sequences. For this reason such a leader sequence is present in some vectors used for *in vitro* transcription/translation.

Once the polypeptide chain has been synthesized, the protein has to be transported to its site of action. Therefore, the transport process can also be regulated to adjust the level of functional protein at its proper location. Finally, many proteins can be modified, in some cases influencing their activity, by posttranslational modifications such as *phosphorylation* or *glycosylation*. Proteins that are secreted or become membrane-associated proteins contain an additional sequence at their N-terminus, called a *leader sequence* (not to be confused with the leader sequence on mRNA), which is responsible for the trans-membrane migration of the protein, and which is removed from the protein after it has been transported across the membrane.

TOOLS IN MOLECULAR BIOLOGY

Enzymes That Modify DNA and RNA

Restriction enzymes. Technically, molecular biology can be considered a set of tools and methods suitable to manipulate genetic material, i.e., DNA and RNA. To manipulate genes, i.e., DNA, the two most important tools are enzymes to cut and to ligate DNA. Generally, in molecular biology one uses enzymes, referred to as *restriction enzymes,* from bacteria to carry out biochemical reactions in the test tube. When Paul Berg and Hamilton Smith discovered the first restriction enzymes it took the scientific community very little time to realize the potential use of these enzymes. It was the beginning of a revolution in biology, the advent of genetic engineering. Restriction enzymes are part of the bacterial defense system against bacteriophage DNA, which is destroyed by cutting at sites recognized by the bacteria's restriction enzymes. Bacteria producing restriction enzymes protect their own DNA from cutting by also producing a sequence-specific *methylase.* This enzyme methylates the bacterial DNA at the recognition site of the corresponding restriction enzyme. Restriction enzymes, with a few exceptions, do not cut methylated DNA.

Interestingly, the most commonly used restriction enzymes recognize and cut DNA at sequences that are identical in 5′ to 3′ direction on both strands of the DNA such as 5′-GAATTC-3′, i.e., *palindromic sequences* (Fig. 11). The actual "cut" is the hydrolysis of a sugar–phosphate bond between two nucleotides (Fig. 12). Both strands are always cut, either at the same position to generate flush or *blunt ends* or in a staggered position yielding single stranded *overhangs* ("*sticky ends*") after the resulting fragments have been separated (Fig. 12). Recognition sites are usually between 4 and 8 bp in length. The number of base pairs recognized by a particular restriction enzyme also determines the statistical frequency with which a recognition site is likely to occur in a DNA molecule of a certain length. For instance, any particular 4 bp sequence is expected to occur once every 256 bp, whereas a 6 bp sequence should be present every 4,096 bp on the average, and an 8 bp sequence, once every 65,536 bp. These numbers assume a normal distribution of the bases. In fact, bases are not so distributed in all cases.

To date about 500 different restriction enzymes from many bacterial and fungal strains have been identified, recognizing almost as

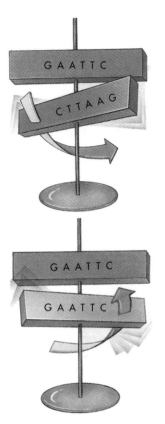

Fig. 11. Two-fold rotational symmetry of palindromic sequences. Both strands have the same sequence (GAATTC) but read in opposite direction. This figure was reproduced with kind permission from Raven and Johnson, "Biology," Third edition, Mosby Year Book, Inc., St. Louis, Missouri.

many different sequences. Therefore, by choosing the appropriate restriction enzyme one can cut DNA at many different, specific sites.

DNA ligase. The second enzyme of importance in molecular biology is *DNA ligase.* The most commonly used DNA ligase is T4 bacteriophage DNA ligase isolated from *Escherichia coli* infected with T4 bacteriophage. More recently the recombinant T4 ligase expressed in *E. coli* from a plasmid containing the T4 ligase gene has become available. This enzyme is able to ligate a broken sugar phosphate bond on one strand of a double-stranded DNA molecule (Fig. 13). Such a break, if it occurs on only one strand, is also called a "*nick.*" To repair a break, DNA ligase requires double-stranded DNA, a 5′-phosphate, a 3′-hydroxyl group, and ATP as a cosubstrate to

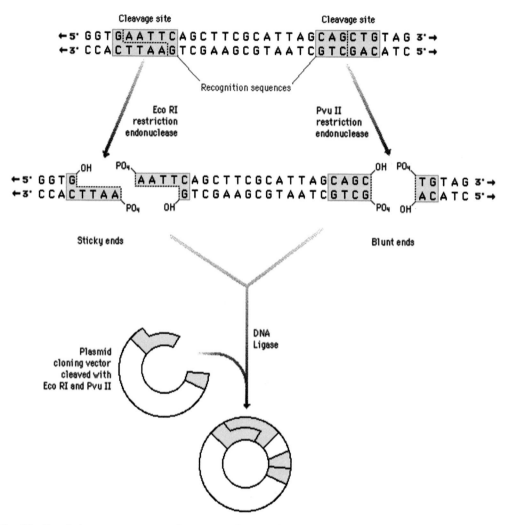

Fig. 12. Restriction enzymes can cut the two strands of DNA in staggered positions (left upper panel) to create overhanging or "sticky" ends. Alternatively, the cut can occur between two nucleotides exactly opposite of each other to generate blunt ends. In any case, a hydroxyl group is left on the resulting 3′-ends whereas the phosphate group is left on the new 5′-ends. This figure was reproduced with kind permission from Lehninger, Nelson and Cox, "Principles of Biochemistry," Second edition, Worth Publishers, Inc., New York, New York.

provide energy for the reaction. Therefore, it is possible to ligate or combine two DNA molecules with either blunt ends or with sticky ends produced by the same enzyme. Sticky ends provide the benefit of being selective, because two different sticky ends cannot be ligated due to the lack of complementarity in the overhangs. In addition, the ligation of two DNA molecules with compatible sticky ends is more efficient because their ends are juxtaposed by hybridization of the complementary single-stranded ends of the molecules (see Fig. 13).

DNA polymerase. Another frequently used enzyme in molecular biology is *DNA polymerase*. A number of different DNA polymerases are currently available.

DNA polymerase is able to synthesize DNA complementary to a single strand of DNA. The enzyme requires a *primer*, i.e., a short molecule

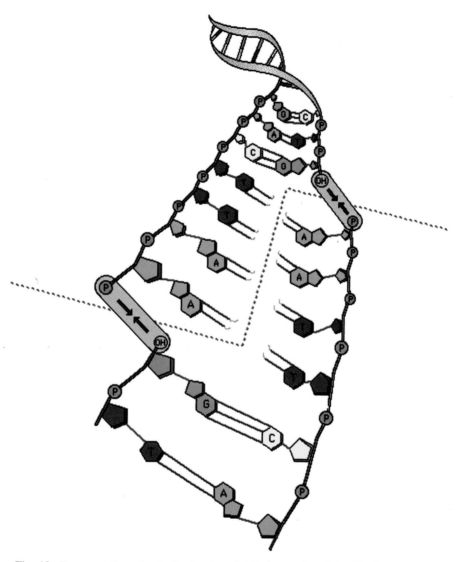

Fig. 13. Representation of a single strand cut (nick) that can be rejoined by DNA ligase. This figure was reproduced and modified with kind permission from Raven and Johnson, "Biology," Third edition, Mosby Year Book, Inc., St. Louis, Missouri.

of DNA hybridized to a complementary single strand of DNA that can be extended in the 3' direction. The primer must have a 3'-hydroxyl group onto which the polymerase can add the next nucleotide. The substrates are deoxynucleotide triphosphates (dNTPs) with the triphosphate group on the 5' end of the sugar. Two phosphates are hydrolyzed away during the reaction to provide for the necessary energy. Most DNA polymerases have two domains, the actual

polymerase domain and a proofreading domain (3'-5'-exonuclease). If, by chance, a nucleotide is incorporated that does not form a base pair with the template, further DNA synthesis is blocked. In this case, the polymerase slides back and the proofreading domain removes the mismatched base (Fig. 14).

The various enzymes are used for different purposes. For instance, in DNA sequencing certain derivatives of bacteriophage T7-derived

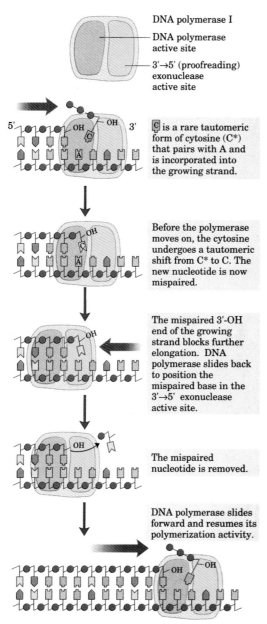

DNA polymerase I

DNA polymerase
active site

3'→5' (proofreading)
exonuclease
active site

C is a rare tautomeric
form of cytosine (C*)
that pairs with A and
is incorporated into
the growing strand.

Before the polymerase
moves on, the cytosine
undergoes a tautomeric
shift from C* to C. The
new nucleotide is now
mispaired.

The mispaired 3'-OH
end of the growing
strand blocks further
elongation. DNA
polymerase slides back
to position the
mispaired base in the
3'→5' exonuclease
active site.

The mispaired
nucleotide is removed.

DNA polymerase slides
forward and resumes its
polymerization activity.

Fig. 14. DNA synthesis and error correction by DNA polymerase. This figure was reproduced with kind permission from Lehninger, Nelson and Cox, "Principles of Biochemistry," Second edition, Worth Publishers, Inc., New York, New York.

DNA polymerase are frequently employed. In addition to its use in sequencing, DNA polymerase is used for incorporation of radioactive nucleotides to generate a "hot" DNA probe for hybridizations. Thermostable DNA polymerases from thermophile bacteria such as *Thermus aquaticus* (*Taq* polymerase) or *Thermococcus litoralis* (Vent® polymerase) are used for *polymerase chain reactions* (*PCR*), a procedure discussed in detail below.

Reverse transcriptase. The function of *reverse transcriptase* is very similar to that of DNA polymerase I and the other DNA polymerases. However, whereas DNA polymerase I is a DNA-dependent DNA polymerase, i.e., makes DNA copies from DNA, reverse transcriptase is an RNA-dependent DNA polymerase. The importance of this enzyme is emphasized by the fact that it earned its discoverers, Howard Temin and David Baltimore, a Nobel Prize. Before it was discovered the central rule of biology stated that the flow of genetic information was strictly directional from DNA to RNA but never vice versa.

The function of the enzyme is to copy single-stranded RNA into a *complementary DNA* (*cDNA*) strand. Reverse transcriptase is not normally present in eukaryotic or prokaryotic cells. Rather, it is derived from a specialized group of viruses, the *retroviruses*. These viruses use RNA rather than double-stranded DNA to store their genetic material, a feature that is associated with high rates of mutation. This general characteristic of RNA viruses bears an evolutionary advantage in that it is more difficult to prepare vaccines against them.

In the laboratory, reverse transcriptase is used to synthesize cDNA from mRNA *in vitro*. Usually, the total mixture of mRNAs from an organ or from cells in culture is reverse-transcribed in bulk and the cDNAs are ligated into a vector (with one cDNA per vector) to generate a *cDNA library* from which individual genes can be selected using a variety of approaches (see also Production of a cDNA Library). The library consists of thousands of vectors, with a given percentage of the vectors containing cDNA inserts. Depending on the number of plaques (each plaque contains a vector, hopefully with an insert cDNA), and the frequency of the message (mRNA) for a given gene, one can locate that gene, in the form of the cDNA, in the library.

IMPORTANT TECHNIQUES
AND PROCEDURES

Gel Electrophoresis

Molecular biologists deal with complex mixtures of molecules, usually composed of DNA fragments of different lengths or RNA molecules isolated from cells. A mixture of RNA molecules isolated from a population of cells is composed of several thousand different molecules of distinct sequence. Each species represents a gene either coding for a protein or for ribosomal RNA etc. The relative amount of a particular mRNA molecule for the most part varies from 0.1 to 0.001% of the total. A common and important way to separate individual molecules partially is *gel electrophoresis*. DNA and RNA molecules can be separated on an *agarose gel* (see below) according to molecular weight. The length or size of a particular molecule determines the velocity with which it is able to move through the agarose gel that contains pores of a certain size. Smaller molecules move faster through the pores than larger ones and are, therefore, able to travel a longer distance in the gel in a certain period of time. The principle of agarose gel electrophoresis relies on the movement of the electrically charged DNA or RNA molecules in an electric field. This results in a separation of the mixture in which the smaller (shorter) molecules will have moved farther along the gel than the longer (larger) molecules at the end of the *electrophoresis* "run."

The size range of molecules that can be effectively separated depends on the concentration of a gel, and thus the pore sizes in that gel. On a 0.8% agarose gel, DNA fragments between approx. 300 and 10,000 bp can be separated from each other. The *resolution* of a gel, i.e., how easily two molecules that are close to one another in size can be separated, depends on the size of those molecules and other factors. The resolution of a 0.8% gel is about 50 bp in the size range of 300 to 3,000 bp. With increasing size of the molecules to be separated, the resolution of a gel decreases. Furthermore, resolution increases with the distance traveled through the gel. Thus, to separate two fragments of 5,000 and 4,500 bp, respectively, a 0.8% agarose gel has to be long enough, and run for a sufficient length of time, to allow the molecules to migrate between 7 and 10 cm. To separate a 500-bp fragment from a 1000-bp fragment takes a run of only about 1 to 2 cm.

Practically, gels are prepared as slabs of about 0.5 cm thickness and varying sizes by dissolving agarose in boiling buffer and casting the hot solution into a mold including a "comb" to form wells (Fig. 15). Upon cooling, the mixture solidifies to form the gel and the samples to be analyzed are loaded into the individual wells formed by the comb. After electrophoresis, the gel is soaked in a solution of ethidium bromide and the DNA fragments can then be visualized under UV light. All molecules of a certain length appear as a fluorescent band in the gel (see Fig. 15). This is because the ethidium bromide *intercalates* between the bases of the DNA or RNA and only when it is intercalated does it fluoresce under UV light. Intercalation is possible because the ring structure of the four bases is planar due to its degree of aromaticity. In a DNA or RNA molecule, the bases are positioned parallel to each other, a conformation also known as "stacking." The equally planar ethidium molecule inserts between the stacked bases. The amount of ethidium bromide intercalated into a certain fragment, i.e., the intensity of a band, depends on the length of the fragment. For that reason, the minimal detectable number of molecules is also dependent on size. Generally, about 20 ng of a 100-bp fragment can still be detected on an agarose gel.

The second type of gel electrophoresis commonly applied in molecular biology is *polyacrylamide gel electrophoresis (PAGE)*, which is used to separate proteins. If the proteins are first dissolved in *sodium dodecyl sulfate (SDS)*, which essentially linearizes them, subsequent analysis in SDS-PAGE gels will separate the proteins on the basis of size, by the same criteria discussed above for separation of DNA or RNA. The smaller the molecule in its extended form, the further it will travel through the pores of the gel. Proteins can also be separated by charge, in which case they are exposed in the gel to a charge gradient; under these conditions the proteins are allowed to travel to a position in the gel at which they have no charge, their *isoelectric point (pI)*.

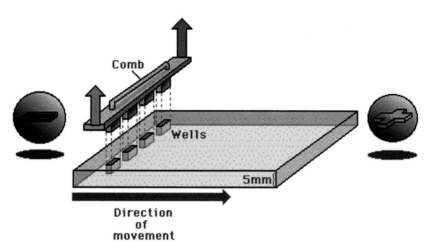

Fig. 15. Agarose slab gel. The − and + sign indicate the polarity of the electric field that is applied to the gel.

A special kind of PAGE is used to separate single-stranded DNA molecules, e.g., for sequencing. With this type of gel, DNA molecules differing by a single base in length can be separated.

Isolation of DNA Fragments from Gels

It is important to be able to isolate DNA fragments from agarose gels. A technique to achieve this uses positively charged paper that is inserted into a slot that is cut into the gel immediately in front of the band to be isolated. Diethylaminoethyl-derivatized (DEAE) cellulose paper is used. Under the buffer conditions used in gel electrophoresis, the DEAE residues carry a positive charge to which the negatively charged phosphate groups of the DNA bind.

The DNA fragments are first separated by electrophoresis [(Fig. 16(1)] and then the paper is placed in front of the band to be isolated [(Fig. 16(2)]. Electrophoresis is then continued and the DNA is "electrophoresed" onto the paper strip [(Fig. 16(3)]. The paper can then be removed from the gel together with the DNA from the band of interest now bound to the paper. At high salt concentrations, the DNA can be subsequently eluted from the paper and can then be used for further experiments as a purified fragment of DNA, i.e., a mixture of identical DNA molecules. Usually about 100 ng to several mi-

crograms of DNA fragments can be purified in this way.

DNA fragments separated in polyacrylamide gels are isolated from the gel either by diffusion, if the fragment is very short (up to about 50 bp), or, if the fragments are larger, by electrophoresis onto DEAE-paper. In this case the band is cut out from the gel and then placed in an agarose gel in which it is "electrophoresed" onto the paper as described above. An agarose gel is used instead of the acrylamide gel to allow easier insertion of the paper.

Polymerase Chain Reaction (PCR)

First thought of in 1984, this technique has conquered the hearts of every molecular biologist because it is one of the most beautiful examples of making use of naturally occurring enzymes in an *in vitro* system. For that reason its inventor, Karl Mullis, has been awarded the 1993 Nobel prize. The method, in its original application, employs DNA polymerase to amplify a DNA fragment geometrically *in vitro*. Amplification is achieved by repeatedly synthesizing copies of the original fragment yielding a maximum 1×10^{10} to 1×10^{12}-fold multiplication of the original DNA molecules with that sequence. The overall reaction can be divided into several steps (Fig. 17). First, the template DNA, which can be very few molecules or even

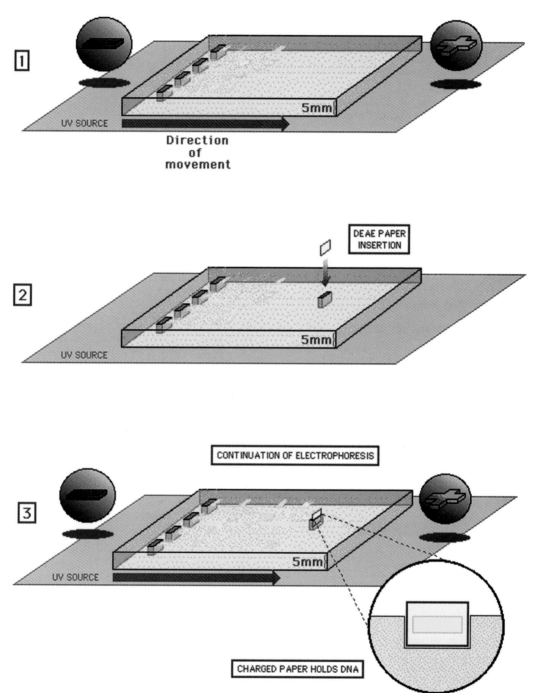

Fig. 16. (1) Electrophoresis of DNA in the gel. (2) Insertion of the DEAE paper in front of the band to be isolated. (3) Continuation of electrophoresis until the band has moved onto the paper.

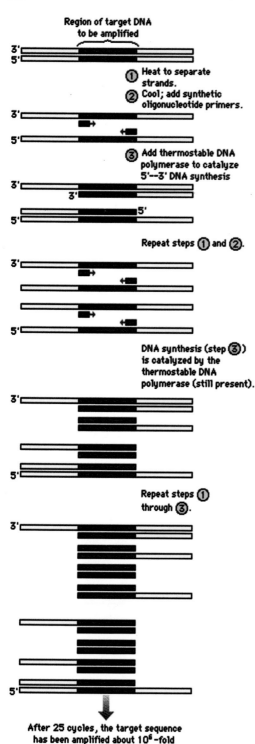

Region of target DNA to be amplified

① Heat to separate strands.
② Cool; add synthetic oligonucleotide primers.

③ Add thermostable DNA polymerase to catalyze 5'–3' DNA synthesis

Repeat steps ① and ②.

DNA synthesis (step ③) is catalyzed by the thermostable DNA polymerase (still present).

Repeat steps ① through ③.

After 25 cycles, the target sequence has been amplified about 10^6-fold

a single molecule, is completely *denatured*. In the case of DNA, denaturation is the separation of the complementary strands. Then, two single-stranded oligonucleotides, the primers for the subsequent DNA synthesis, are allowed to hybridize to the template DNA at the ends of the segment to be replicated by adjusting to the required temperature. The primers must fulfill the following requirements. Each primer must hybridize to one of the template strands; the distance between the primer hybridization sites determines the length of the amplification product. The primers must be designed such that their 3'-ends point toward each other, i.e., synthesis from one primer extends in the direction of the other, and vice versa. The base on the very 3'-end of each primer must be complementary to the template. After a short incubation period for hybridization, the temperature is adjusted for DNA synthesis (72°C for *Taq* polymerase). A certain length of time is allowed for DNA synthesis after which the cycle is completed and the next cycle can be started with DNA denaturation at 94°C. (One cycle, thus, includes denaturation, annealing of the primers, and second strand DNA synthesis.) Usually, 25 to 45 cycles are carried out to obtain the degree of amplification discussed above.

Considering these steps, it becomes obvious that the availability of thermostable DNA polymerases is a great advantage. Using a thermostable polymerase allows one to carry out all the cycles in one reaction tube without changing or adding any of the components during cycling; it is necessary only to be able to change the temperature as quickly as possible and then hold a certain temperature for a period of time. The half-life of *Taq* polymerase at 94°C is about 45 min. If in each cycle denaturation is carried out at 94°C for 1 min about 50% of the original enzyme activity is lost during the complete PCR

Fig. 17. Polymerase chain reaction. The different steps of the amplification cycle are depicted. This figure was reproduced with kind permission from Lehninger, Nelson, and Cox, "Principles of Biochemistry," Second edition, Worth Publishers, Inc., New York, New York.

reaction. At present, commercially available, programmable PCR machines are capable of fast and exact temperature control between 0 and 100°C.

Radioactive Labeling of DNA Fragments

The fact that complementary DNA strands bind to each other with considerable affinity, and thus specificity, is often exploited in molecular biology to identify a specific DNA or RNA sequence within a complex mixture of sequences (see "blotting" techniques below). The DNA probes used to identify sequences in this way must be somehow "labeled" to visualize them. The most sensitive label, allowing the detection of minimal quantities of DNA or RNA in a sequence-specific manner, is radioactivity. The most effective radioactive isotope for labeling DNA or RNA is ^{32}P. The starting material is radioactively labeled deoxynucleoside triphosphates, the substrates of DNA polymerase for incorporation into newly synthesized DNA. The phosphate group linked to the sugar moiety (the α-phosphate) contains the ^{32}P atom. The labeling procedure is as follows. First, ca. 50–100 ng of the purified DNA fragment (the "template") is denatured, i.e., turned into single strands, by heating to 98°C and cooling quickly. Quick-cooling does not allow the single strands to renature because at 0°C there is not enough energy present for the strands to renature. Then, a large excess of a mixture of single-stranded random nonanucleotides is added. These are single-stranded DNA molecules, nine nucleotides long with a random sequence, generated by the non-enzymatic synthesis of 262,144 different molecules by sequentially adding randomly one of the four possible nucleotides onto a growing chain of DNA nine times. Because of the randomness of their sequences, some of the nonamers must be complementary to a stretch of nine bases on the DNA fragment to be labeled and will therefore hybridize to it (Fig. 18). The result is that practically all single-stranded template molecules will have a nonamer hybridized to it somewhere. This primer is then extended by adding DNA polymerase and deoxynucleotide triphosphates (dNTPs). One or more of the dNTPs is

radioactive and thus the newly synthesized DNA will also be radioactive. The resulting radioactive DNA is a mixture of fragments of different lengths depending on how far from the 5'-end of the template a given nonamer hybridized.

Southern Blotting

Named after its inventor, E.M. Southern, this technique is used to identify, and sometimes also quantify, certain DNA fragments in a mixture of fragments. The fragments are first separated by gel electrophoresis. Then, a fragment(s) that has migrated to a given positions in the gel and that contains a specific and known sequence, e.g., a part of a gene, can be identified as follows. The principle of the method is to use a labeled (usually with radioactivity) *probe* that has a sequence complementary to the molecule one wishes to identify, and allowing that probe to hybridize to any DNA fragments of interest in the gel.

First, the DNA fragments to be analyzed, e.g., genomic DNA from a particular organism, or cell, are separated in an agarose gel after being cut with a restriction enzyme. To be able to hybridize this DNA with a known, radioactive fragment, the content of the gel must be transferred to, and immobilized on, a solid support, usually a nitrocellulose filter. Before transfer, the DNA is denatured by soaking the gel in a sodium hydroxide solution. Transfer is achieved by capillary forces. The nitrocellulose filter is put on top of the gel. A stack of paper towels is piled on top of that and a small weight is used to gently press the stack together. The capillary forces of the paper towels will force most of the liquid contained in the gel through the nitrocellulose filter to be soaked up by them. During this process, the DNA that is carried with the liquid binds to the nitrocellulose membrane because it cannot pass through it. The transfer is usually done overnight after which the nitrocellulose membrane is baked *in vacuo* at 80°C covalently and irreversibly to link the DNA to the membrane. The membrane is now ready for hybridization.

To test whether a certain DNA sequence is present in the mixture previously run on the gel, and whether this sequence is also contained in a

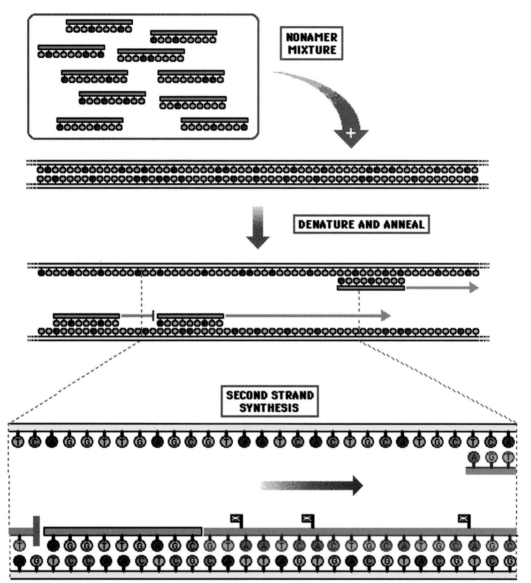

Fig. 18. Radioactive labeling of DNA. A selection of random nonamers is shown in the upper boxed panel. The nonamers are mixed with the template DNA and after denaturation, they are annealed to the template. During synthesis of the second strand, radioactive nucleotides (flags) are incorporated.

fragment of the expected size (predicted based on the restriction enzyme used to obtain the fragment), a purified, radioactively labeled DNA fragment (*probe*) containing only a sequence complementary to the one of interest can be hybridized to the DNA on the membrane (Fig. 19). The probe is denatured and mixed into a hybridization solution that contains components facili-

Fig. 19. (**a**) Graphic representation of a device used for Southern blotting. The arrows indicate the flow of the buffer that carries the DNA from the gel onto the membrane. (**b**) Pictorial representation of the probe (radiolabeled DNA fragment) hybridizing to the filter. The result is an autoradiograph (bottom) showing bands for each fragment that hybridized with the probe.

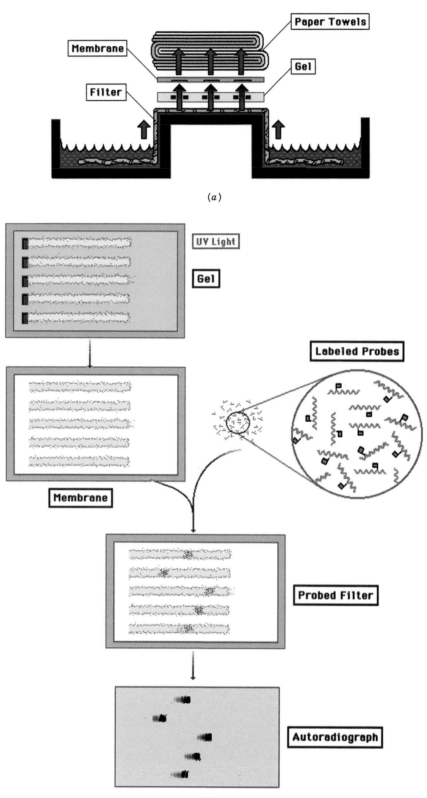

Paper Towels

Membrane

Gel

Filter

(a)

UV Light

Gel

Labeled Probes

Membrane

Probed Filter

Autoradiograph

(b)

tating hybridization. It is then added to the membrane and incubation is carried out overnight at about 55–60°C. During this period of time, the radioactive DNA fragment will hybridize only to sequence(s) on the membrane complementary to it. After washing, a film is put on the membrane and wherever the radioactive fragment is specifically hybridized to the DNA on the filter will be recorded on the film. After developing the film, a band is visible at the position of the corresponding DNA fragment on the membrane.

Southern blotting can be used for the analysis of genomic DNA clones to find a given DNA sequence for which the cDNA has previously been isolated. A short cDNA fragment is used as a radioactive probe to find out which fragment(s) of a particular genomic DNA clone, usually 10–20 kb in length, contain this particular sequence. Moreover, a particular blot can be "stripped," i.e., the cDNA probe can be removed, which allows hybridization of the blot with a different probe. The procedure can be repeated several times, which increases the efficacy of this method considerably.

One particular application of Southern blotting is to characterize the length of restriction fragments associated with a given gene(s). (A restriction fragment refers to the length of DNA between two identical restriction sites cut by a given restriction enzyme.) The rationale for this is that sequences within (introns) or around (5' and 3' flanking regions) a particular gene may vary significantly between different individuals; thus, the restriction fragments isolated in association with that gene, using a given restriction enzyme, will vary in length. This difference is called *restriction fragment length polymorphism (RFLP)*. As described in Chapter 19 on xenotransplantation, RFLP analysis can be used to define the particular genes carried by any one individual at one of the HLA class II loci, based on the fact that a given allele of that locus is to a large extent associated with the same introns and flanking sequences in all individuals of that population. On the other hand, a different allele of that locus will be associated with different sequences, and thus with different RFLP patterns. This technique is now often used for prenatal diagnosis of

genetic disorders for which RFLPs have been established (Fig. 20).

Northern Blotting

This method, a variant of the Southern blot, is used to obtain semiquantitative information on the amount of a specific mRNA, corresponding to a gene of interest, in a complex mixture of mRNAs present in a cell. Usually, total RNA isolated from cultured cells or from tissue is separated on an agarose gel containing formaldehyde and formamide to prevent formation of secondary structures in the RNA molecules. The formation of intramolecular double strands must be avoided to ensure that separation is by size only. If, for some reason, a secondary structure is formed, two molecules of different size can move with the same mobility on the gel because of their different structure. The blotting and hybridization procedure is very similar to the one applied for Southern blotting. A Northern blot provides information about both the size and the identity of a particular RNA molecule in a complex mixture of RNA molecules. In addition, one can obtain an estimate of the relative abundance of those mRNA molecules by comparing them to internal standards.

This technique is frequently used to assess whether a gene of interest is expressed in a given cell, or whether it is induced in response to various stimuli in that population of cells. The level of mRNA that is detected for a given gene on a Northern blot is referred to as the *"steady-state"* mRNA level, which reflects two factors: first, the rate of transcription of that gene, i.e., how many copies of the mRNA are being produced from the gene in a given period of time, and second, the amount of degradation of the mRNA that takes place. It does not follow that the amount of mRNA present will predict the level of protein found; regulation also occurs at the level of translation.

As with Southern blots, the probe can be "stripped" from a Northern blot and rehybridization with another probe is possible. Also, if the sizes of the mRNAs for several genes are known and significantly different, then a single blot can be probed at one time with several probes. Thus,

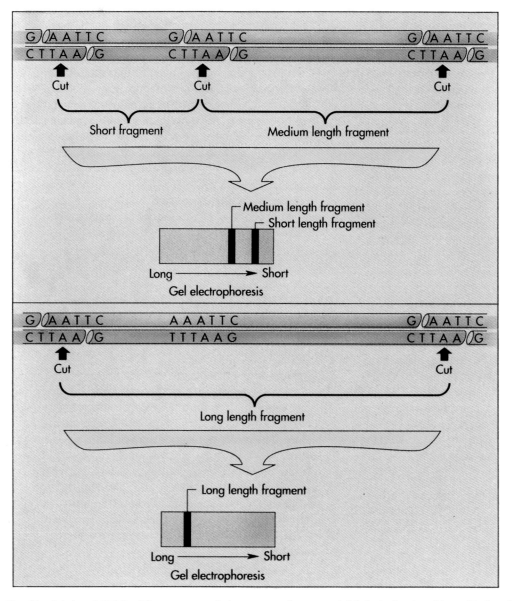

Fig. 20. Origin of RFLPs. The upper panel shows one allele with three *Eco*RI recognition sites in the region to be analyzed. Using that enzyme results in two fragments that are visible in the Southern blot. The bottom panel shown an altered allele in which one of the *Eco*RI sites is mutated. As a result, there is only one fragment visible in the Southern blot and its length is the sum of the two fragments found in the other allele. This figure was reproduced with kind permission from Raven and Johnson, "Biology," Third edition, Mosby Year Book, Inc., St. Louis, Missouri.

several genes can be analyzed on a single membrane.

RNase Protection Assay

RNase protection is a more sensitive and quantitative procedure to measure mRNA levels in cellular extracts than are Northern blots. Here, the mRNA of interest is detected by hybridization with a radiolabeled probe of the complementary sequence, an *antisense* probe. Such a probe is usually generated by *in vitro* transcription from a plasmid containing the cDNA of the gene for which the mRNA is to be measured (Fig. 21). The "hot" probe is incubated with total RNA in solution at a temperature that allows the rapid formation of hybrids. The probe is in large excess compared to the mRNA and therefore "drives" the hybridization reaction to completion, i.e., at the end, all mRNA molecules complementary to the probe should exist as hybrids with the probe. After hybridization is complete, single-stranded RNA is removed by *ribonuclease (RNase)* treatment (Fig. 22). The RNases used are specific for single-stranded RNA and thus all the hybrids remain intact whereas the single-stranded excess probe and other mRNA is degraded. Nucleic acids are then precipitated from the resulting mixture and loaded onto a

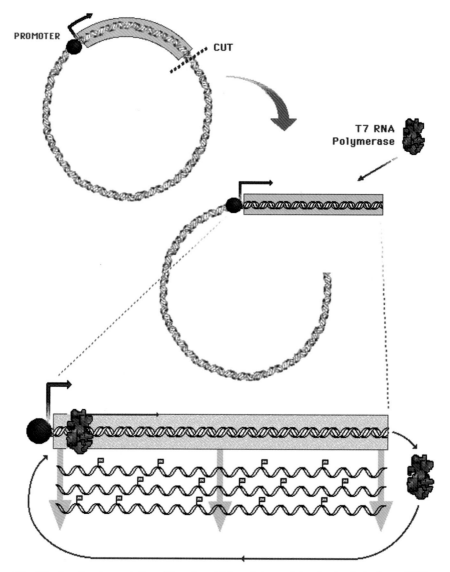

Fig. 21. *In vitro* transcription. The plasmid template contains the bacteriophage DNA polymerase promoter immediately upstream of the fragment to be transcribed. The resulting RNA is labeled (flags) if radioactive ribonucleoside triphosphates are used in the transcription reaction.

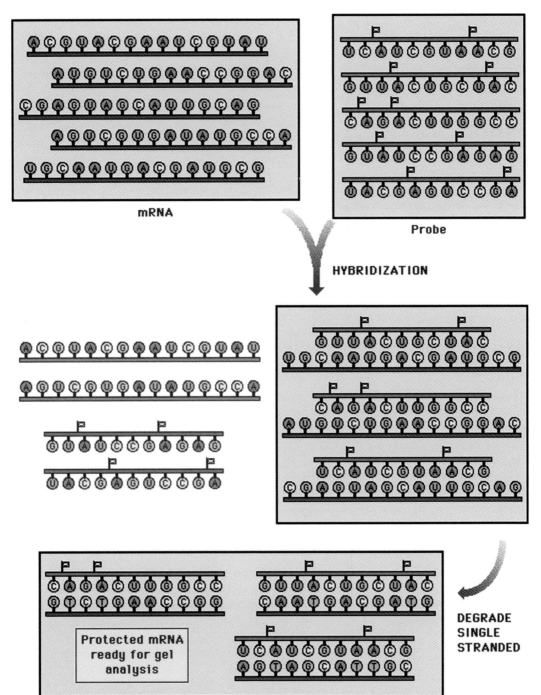

Fig. 22. RNase protection. The steps of the procedure are shown. The formation of double-stranded RNA leads to resistance from RNase degradation and to the formation of a protected fragment that is different in size from the original probe.

sequencing gel. The size of the protected radio-active fragment can be determined and confirms the identity of the mRNA analyzed. In addition, the amount of radioactivity in the observed band can be used to estimate the amount of mRNA present in the extract.

RNA Stability Assay

To determine the stability of a specific mRNA, cultured cells are induced with a stimulus known to increase the steady-state level of the respective mRNA. Treatment with the stimulus is carried out for a period of time sufficient to reach high mRNA levels. At this point, acti-nomycin D is added to the cells to stop transcription. Actinomycin D is a potent inhibitor of RNA polymerase II; in the presence of actinomycin D, transcription is stopped. Aliquots of cells are harvested at about 15 min, or shorter, time intervals and RNA is prepared from these cells. RNAs are analyzed on a Northern blot, which allows determination of the half-life of the mRNA.

In situations in which the mRNA is present constitutively, this approach also allows determination of whether the stimulus changes the stability of the message by comparing the relative amounts of mRNA from the unstimulated cells with mRNA from induced cells over the time course. If there is increased instability, the signal intensity on the Northern blot would diminish faster with the RNAs from the stimulated cells. If the stimulus does not influence mRNA stability, mRNAs from both stimulated and unstimulated cells should decay at the same rate.

Reverse Transcription-Polymerase Chain Reaction (RT-PCR)

RT-PCR is the most sensitive method to detect mRNA in cellular extracts. The first step involves reverse transcription (cDNA synthesis) of the RNA extract. The primer for the cDNA synthesis is chosen to be specific for the gene for which the mRNA level should be determined. The cDNA of interest is amplified by PCR using two primers specific for the gene of interest. The resulting PCR fragment is subsequently analyzed on an agarose gel. Although there are

approaches that allow semiquantitative evaluation of RT-PCR results, this method is not particularly suitable for quantitating the amount of mRNA present but rather is used to determine if there is any mRNA at all. The sensitivity of this method allows one mRNA molecule per cell to be detected.

Western Blotting

To identify proteins, usually according to their molecular weight, and based on their reactivity with a specific antibody, the proteins are first separated according to molecular weight on a denaturing polyacrylamide gel and electro-transferred[4] to a membrane. As with RNA, the proteins have to be forced into a uniform conformation to achieve separation by size only. This is done by denaturing (i.e., destroying the three-dimensional structure of the protein) them in a detergent, *sodium dodecyl sulfate* (*SDS*), so that they assume an approximately rod-shaped conformation.

To identify a particular protein on the blot, an antibody specific for the protein of interest is used. After the specific antibody is bound to the corresponding protein on the membrane, it is visualized by using yet another, second, antibody recognizing the *Fc* portion of the first antibody. The second antibody is covalently linked to an enzyme that is able to generate a colored precipitate in the presence of the appropriate substrate (Fig. 23). *Phosphatase* is the classical enzyme used in this respect. The most advanced substrates employed are converted into chemiluminescent products by phosphatase allowing the detection of minimal quantities of protein on the membrane. Since the enzyme is localized only at the spot on the membrane where the first antibody originally bound, only this spot will be stained at the end of the reaction. Western blot-

---

[4]Proteins cannot be transferred to a membrane by capillary forces. In this case the membrane is put on top of the gel and this stack is placed between two planar graphite electrodes at least the size of the gel. The assembled "sandwich" is immersed into a buffer tank and an electric field is applied via the two electrodes, which leads to electrophoresis of all the proteins in the gel onto the membrane where they become immobilized.

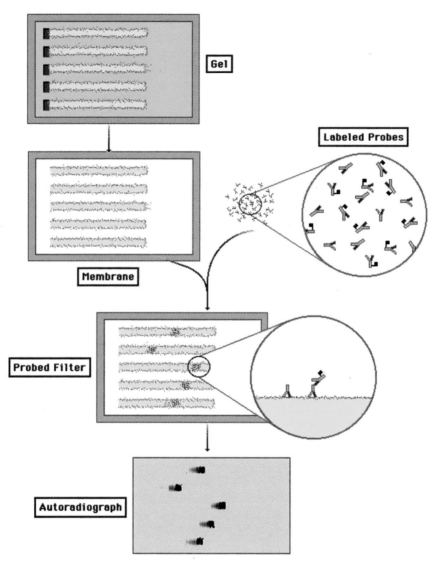

Fig. 23. Western blotting. The steps of this procedure include the electrotransfer of the proteins from the gel onto a membrane. The membrane is then treated with the specific antibody that is covalently linked to an enzyme (flags). After the excess antibody is washed away, the substrate is added and the colored reaction product precipitates at the site where the antibody is bound to the protein resulting in colored bands on the membrane.

ting is frequently used to analyze cell extracts for the presence of a particular protein.

Production of a cDNA Library

One of the most powerful techniques of molecular biology allows one to prepare a "library" that contains all, or almost all, of the genes that are expressed, i.e., that are transcribed, in a given cell or tissue. Such a library is referred to as a cDNA library since it is a reflection of the mRNAs that are present in a given cell/tissue, and that are reverse-transcribed to yield cDNAs. A cDNA library is a collection of such DNA fragments inserted in a vector plasmid, with each fragment being contained in its own plasmid. It is, therefore, a rather complex mixture of genes, whose representation in the library depends mostly on the amount of mRNA present in the cells.

The first step in the construction of a cDNA library is the isolation of poly(A) RNA (i.e., mRNA) from about 1×10^7 cells. The mRNA is reverse-transcribed into complementary DNA (cDNA) by reverse transcriptase. The reaction must be primed using either oligo(dT) or random primers, such as used for labeling reactions. Oligo(dT) hybridizes to the poly(A) tail of all mRNA molecules and can then be extended toward the 5'-end of the mRNA molecule. By using oligo(dT) primers one rarely obtains full length cDNA because reverse transcription *in vitro* tends to be terminated prematurely due to RNA secondary structure. Random primers, in contrast, "prime" and start transcription at several locations in the mRNA; thus, there is a good chance that the entire mRNA will be copied.

After second strand synthesis, the double-stranded cDNA is ligated into a *bacteriophage* vector. The genome of bacteriophage λ is frequently used as a vector to allow efficient introduction of the cDNA produced from a total mRNA preparation into bacteria for amplification. This allows the rather minute amounts of total cDNA, which is a mixture of all the different cDNAs, to be amplified in the bacteria. After ligation, the cDNA (now inserted into the bacteriophage DNA) is packaged into a bacteriophage protein shell to produce infectious bacteriophage particles using a packaging extract (Fig. 24).[5] The mixture of bacteriophage, now each containing a cDNA, represents a library of expressed genes of a given cell type; the number of bacteriophage containing a given gene in the library depends mostly on the number of mRNA molecules for that gene present in the cell from which the initial mRNA was isolated. The bacte-

riophage pool (and several dilutions of them) is then used to infect appropriate host bacteria. Only one phage particle infects one bacterial cell. The mixture is transferred onto agar plates with a soft agar overlay. When the plates are incubated at 37°C, the bacteria (in an excess of phage) begin to divide and form a confluent bacterial "lawn." Infected bacterial cells are lysed after the single phage particle has multiplied several thousand fold within the bacterial cell. The released phage, in turn, infect the surrounding bacterial cells and after several rounds of infection and lysis, clear spots (*plaques*) become visible in the bacterial lawn. Each plaque contains a few million phage particles, all of which theoretically carry the same gene because the phage of a plaque are all derived from a single original phage. The phage of a single plaque are therefore called a *clone* (a number of identical cells or molecules derived from a single precursor by identical duplication). Approximately 1×10^5 plaque-forming units are usually derived to optimize the probability that essentially all expressed genes of the cell are represented in the library. The rationale for this procedure is to separate all expressed genes from each other and to have them in a sufficient number for further analysis.

A given gene in the library is found in one of two ways. The plaques are first transferred onto a membrane. That membrane, in analogy with Southern and Western blotting, is then probed either with a nucleic acid probe or with an antibody. In the latter case, it is important to have the cDNAs in the library placed in *expression vectors* that actually lead to production of small amounts of the protein encoded by the gene in that phage. That protein associated with a plaque is then detected with the antibody.

Nuclear Run-Off Analysis

As mentioned above, Northern blotting can determine only the steady-state concentration of mRNA for a gene of interest. However, it is often important to know whether gene expression is regulated on the transcriptional or posttranscriptional level (i.e., the regulation of splicing, mRNA stability, or translation). To measure

---

[5]Protein extracts from bacteria infected with the appropriate phage are prepared from a stage in infection when all phage protein have been synthesized but not yet been assembled into phage particles. Mixing these extracts with phage DNA leads to the assembly of infectious phage particles. Packaging extracts are commercially available.

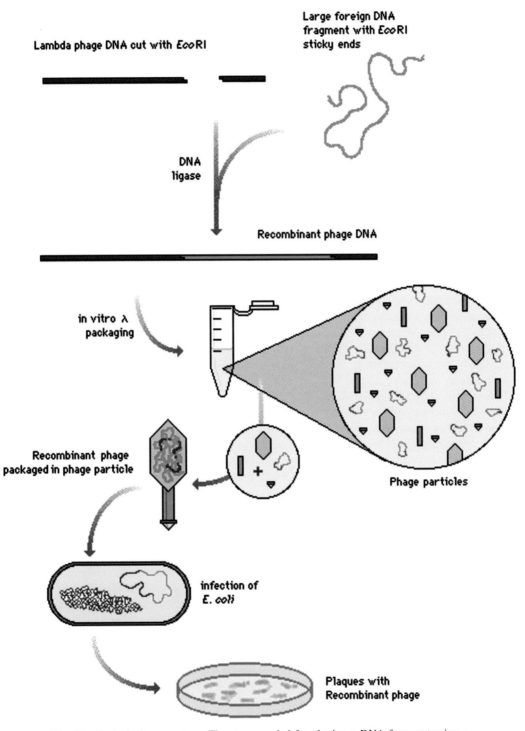

Fig. 24. Bacteriophage vectors. The steps needed for cloning a DNA fragment using a bacteriophage vector are shown. In particular, the packaging of the vector DNA into a phage particle is illustrated.

transcriptional rate, the incorporation of labeled nucleotides into mRNA within a certain period of time must be assayed. Technically, nuclei are isolated from cells in which the expression of a certain gene is to be studied. The nuclei are then incubated for a certain period of time with radioactive UTP, which is incorporated only into RNA. Total RNA is then prepared from these nuclei.

To identify a particular mRNA corresponding to a certain gene of interest, a membrane hybridization technique is used. First, a relatively large quantity of denatured cDNA, specifically of the gene of interest, is bound to a membrane by spotting it on the membrane or by using a slot blotting device. Then, the membrane is incubated with the radioactive RNA under hybridization conditions similar to those used in Northern blotting. The radioactivity specifically hybridizing to the membrane, reflecting the mRNA synthesized by the gene of interest, can be quantified and is directly proportional to the rate of transcription of the gene of interest.

Usually the nuclei are prepared from a number of batches of cells kept under inducing or repressing conditions and the different transcriptional rates are compared. Moreover, a constitutively expressed gene is included in the analysis as an internal standard. The gene coding for glyceraldehyde phosphate dehydrogenase (GAPDH), a key enzyme in glycolysis, is often used. The gene for this enzyme is expressed in all cells and its transcriptional rate remains constant under almost any circumstance.

Transformation of Bacterial Cells

The introduction of DNA into bacterial cells is called *transformation*. Plasmids are used to introduce genes because plasmids can be maintained as double-stranded, circular DNA molecules in the form of *episomes* (i.e., genetic elements that are maintained independently of the bacterial genome) in bacteria. The major obstacle to getting DNA into bacterial cells is the bacterial cell wall. For that reason, the cells to be transformed are obtained from a very fast growing culture that does not allow for much cell wall synthesis between two cell divisions. In addi-

tion, the cells are treated with calcium chloride ($CaCl_2$), which leads to a swelling of the proteoglycan containing cell wall. Bacterial cells manipulated to allow entry of the plasmids are called "*competent.*" The plasmid to be introduced is added to the competent cells and the mixture is incubated on ice. A short heat shock ensures efficient DNA uptake before liquid medium is added to allow regeneration of the weakened cell wall. The cells are then spread on a plate containing selective medium to permit only growth of cells harboring a plasmid.

Transfection of Tissue Culture Cells

For genetic manipulation of eukaryotic cells at the molecular level, the introduction of DNA into the cells in culture is of vital importance. During the past 10 years or so, a number of different approaches have been developed, some for quite special purposes. The basic requirements for a useful transfection technique must allow one to target the DNA of interest to the cell and to promote its uptake into the cell.

One of the first techniques described uses *calcium phosphate precipitation*. The DNA to be introduced into the cell is mixed with calcium chloride and sodium phosphate and added to the cells. Small particles of DNA and calcium phosphate [$Ca_3(PO_4)_2$] precipitate onto the cells and are eventually taken up into the cells by endocytosis. Once the DNA has entered the cells it can also enter the nucleus, the only location in the cell where the exogenous genes can be transcribed. This probably happens by passive diffusion and incorporation into newly formed nuclei after cell division. Usually, only about 1–5% of the cells are transfected by this technique.

If stable expression of an introduced gene is needed, the vector is linearized before transfection to increase the probability of integration into a random location on any chromosome. Considering the low efficiency of transfection, and the even lower efficiency of integration, it is evident that positive selection is needed to isolate stably transfected clones. With selection, about 0.001 to 1% of the transfected cells actually integrate the plasmid. Selection is usually accomplished by including an antibiotic resistance gene in the vector and using selective medium to allow only cells that stably express the resistance gene to proliferate. The level of expression and the function of included regulatory sequences are strongly dependent on the site of integration. If integration occurs into transcriptionally silent chromatin, even the presence of otherwise strong *enhancers* (see Regulation of Transcription) in the vector may not lead to any detectable transcription of the introduced gene. On the other hand, if the DNA is integrated close to a naturally active, strong enhancer in the genome, expression of the introduced gene may become independent of regulatory elements included in the transgene (i.e., genes introduced stably into cells of an organism; the recipient animals are called "transgenic animals").

In attempts to increase the efficiency of introducing DNA into cells, additional methods have been developed. In analogy to bacteriophage vectors, viral vectors are used to introduce DNA constructs into cells in culture efficiently. *Retroviruses* are especially useful because they practically infect 100% of the target cells and, in addition, stably integrate their genome into one of the host's chromosomes. There are, however, important limitations[6] to the application of retroviruses. From the technical point of view, the construction of a retroviral *vector* is much more tedious than preparing a vector for $Ca_3(PO_4)_2$ precipitation. The reason for that is as follows. After the gene of interest has been inserted into the DNA of a suitable retroviral vector, retroviral particles have to be produced in a so-called packaging cell line. The retroviral vector is introduced into the packaging line by a conventional method, such as $Ca_3(PO_4)_2$-mediated transfection. The packaging line produces retroviral particles containing the genetic material introduced

---

[6]A key biological limitation is the fact that integration of the retroviral DNA into the host genome may have drastic effects on the cell. For example, if the point of integration is close to a growth regulatory gene that is normally not expressed in differentiated cells, tumor transformation of the cell may be the result. This is due to strong enhancer elements located at the ends of the viral DNA. These enhancers can take control over gene expression in their vicinity and lead to the constitutive, high level expression of nearby genes.

into the cells previously. These particles are very efficient in infecting cells, although the cells have to be dividing. The retroviral vectors are designed to be replication deficient to prevent them from replicating in a cell and killing that cell after they are introduced. This guarantees stable integration of the DNA into the host's genome (Fig. 25).

Methods for the Transfer of Genes into Cells *in Vivo*

DNA transfer methods that permit introduction of genes into cells *in vivo* in the grown organism/individual are now being developed. In many cases, the cells into which one would like to introduce a gene are not dividing, and thus retroviral gene transfer is not applicable. *Adenovirus* vectors are promising candidates in this respect. These viruses have a broad host range and do not integrate their genome into host chromosomes. Although expression from the *episome* is detectable for several weeks, the episome will eventually be lost in dividing cells because it is not replicated by the cellular replication machinery. Moreover, the adenoviruses must be 100% replication deficient, otherwise the replication competent viruses will destroy the target tissue.

Positively charged *liposomes* have also been used to introduce genes into cells *in vivo* as well as *in vitro*. These lipid vesicles are assembled *in vitro* from a mixture of positively charged and neutral lipids. Due to the positive charge, any DNA molecule will adhere to the liposomes both inside and outside. The hydrophobic nature of the vesicles generates an affinity to other lipid environments such as the plasma membrane of cells. Once the liposomes get into contact with the plasma membrane, the two lipid bilayers fuse, leading to the eventual release of the attached DNA into the cytoplasm of the cell. Again, as with any other nonretroviral method, the stability of the introduced DNA is limited, i.e., if the exogenous DNA is not integrated and replicated with the rest of the genome it will eventually be·lost due to dilution. Naturally, selection of integrants is not applicable for *in vivo* experiments since the target cells are not divid-

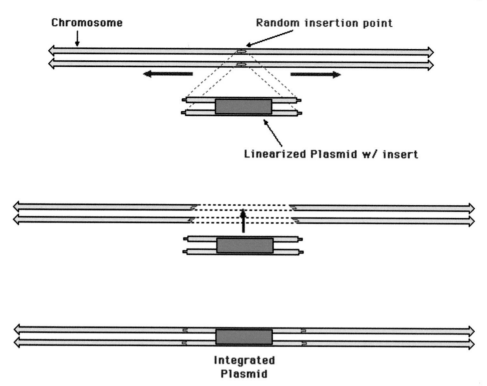

Fig. 25. Schematic representation of an integration event. At the random insertion point there is a single double-strand break and the ends of the fragment are joined with the ends of the chromosome after the break.

ing as they do *in vitro* (see also Nabel et al., 1990).

One additional method that allows introduction of DNA into nondividing cells *in vivo* is *receptor-mediated gene transfer,* or *"transferrinfection"* (Zenke et al., 1990). This method makes use of the existence on the surface of a cell of a receptor for a given ligand (such as transferrin), and the ability of the cell to internalize the receptor–ligand complex. A gene of interest is attached to transferrin, and this complex added to the cells. Certain adenovirus components that help the transferrin–gene complex to break out of intracellular vesicles can also be added to the complex.

DNA Sequencing

A major goal of genetic engineering is to manipulate genetic information. To do that, it is imperative to be able readily to decipher the

DNA code, i.e., determine the nucleotide sequence without great effort. The use of naturally occurring enzymes and *in vitro* engineered derivatives of them allows us to sequence long stretches of DNA (ca. 400 bases) in one run, and even to automate the process of data acquisition and analysis after the enzyme reaction has been carried out. The principle of the method is outlined in Figure 26.

Sequencing reactions are carried out by extending a previously annealed single-stranded primer on the unknown DNA molecule using DNA polymerase. To obtain the sequence, the primer extension reaction is performed in four different reactions. Each reaction contains dATP* (radioactively labeled), dGTP, dCTP, and dTTP. In addition there is *dideoxy-ATP* (*ddATP*) in the reaction mixture that determines the sequence of A-residues, ddCTP for the sequence of C residues, ddGTP for G residues, and ddTTP for T residues. The amount of dideoxy-

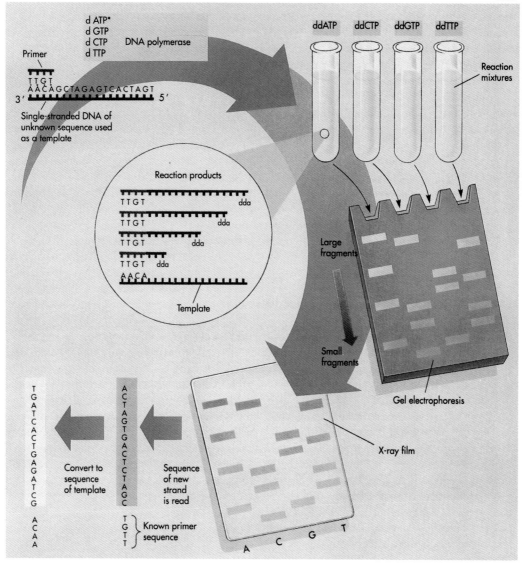

Fig. 26. Steps in DNA sequencing. A short primer is annealed to the known end of the otherwise unknown fragment. After the short labeling reaction using radioactive dATP (indicated by the *) the reaction is divided into four tubes containing dideoxy-ATP, dideoxy-CTP, dideoxy-GTP, and dideoxy-TTP, respectively. The reaction product of one vial is shown (circle). The products of each reaction are loaded into a different well of the sequencing gel. After autoradiography of the gel, the sequence can be read (see accompanying text). This figure was reproduced with kind permission from Raven and Johnson, "Biology," Third edition, Mosby Year Book, Inc., St. Louis, Missouri.

GTP in the "G reaction," for example, is small enough to allow extension of the newly synthesized DNA up to about 1 kb with only sporadic incorporation of the ddGTP at random G residues. The same is true for all four reactions. Whenever a ddNTP is incorporated the extension of the new DNA strand is terminated. Therefore, all newly synthesized molecules in the "G reaction" that have incorporated ddGTP end at a G residue, all molecules in the C reaction that have ddCTP incorporated end at a C residue, and so on. Since dNTP incorporation is sporadic and random, at the end of the reaction, there will be a number of molecules, for instance in the G reaction, that were terminated at each G residue between the primer and about 1000 nucleotides downstream of the primer. The incorporation of the radioactively labeled dATP in all reactions allows the detection of the newly synthesized DNA molecules.

At this point, the synthesis products are separated by size on a denaturing polyacrylamide gel ("*sequencing gel*"). The gels are especially designed for the separation of single-stranded DNA of 50 to about 500 base pairs at a one nucleotide resolution. Each of the four reactions is denatured by heating and quick cooling and loaded onto the gel. Each band in a lane represents an extension product. Considering the "A lane," the lane in which the "A reaction" was loaded, the lowest band, i.e., the one with the highest mobility, represents an A residue close to the primer. The next slower band corresponds with the next A residue in the sequence, and so on.

The complete sequence is then read. The starting point, i.e., the 5'-end of the new sequence, is the lowest band visible on the film (nucleotide n). The lane in which it is found determined its identity (A, C, G, or T). Then the band representing nucleotide $n + 1$ is identified (in one of the four lanes) by searching for the next larger band, and its identity is recorded according to the lane in which it is found. The process is continued until a region of the film is reached where the resolution does not allow the distinction of two subsequent bands.

During the last few years a number of automated sequencing apparatuses have been offered commercially. Some of these machines allow the accumulation of sequence information about thousands of bases of a given gene in a single day.

In Vitro Transcription/Translation

When the cDNA of a gene has been cloned, it is often desirable to obtain the gene product, i.e., the protein encoded by the gene. Since it is usually very difficult to purify the protein of interest, for instance from all the proteins in a whole cell, a method has been developed that allows the

production *in vitro* of very small quantities of protein, but sufficient for certain analyses, using the gene that has been isolated. This is achieved by transferring the processes of transcription and translation into an *in vitro* system.

Special vectors are available to allow *in vitro* transcription of a DNA sequence cloned into the vector. The critical characteristic of such a vector is the presence of a very strong bacteriophage promoter, such as the promoters of bacteriophage SP6 and T7. Their function is to bind the corresponding bacteriophage RNA polymerase, which, once it is bound, initiates transcription from a point very close downstream of the promoter. When such a vector is incubated in the presence of ribonucleotide triphosphates (rNTPs) and the appropriate RNA polymerase, about 10 mg of RNA per μg of template DNA can be transcribed in 30 min. The plasmid is cut at a given location to determine the length, and thus the 3'-end, of the transcript.

RNA synthesized *in vitro* can be translated into protein in a cell-free translation system. Cytoplasmic extracts, either from rabbit reticulocytes or wheat germ, are depleted of endogenous mRNA and enriched with ribosomes and amino acids. Thus, 99% of the protein translated in such a system is derived from the RNA added. Including radioactively labeled amino acids allows the synthesis of radioactive proteins for more sensitive detection.

In Situ Hybridization

For the study of gene expression in whole organisms or cells of an organ, it is often important to be able to localize expression of a certain gene to particular cell types or tissues. If the protein that is the gene product is reasonably abundant, immunocytochemistry on thin sections is able to localize the protein. If the protein is present only in low concentration or an antibody is not available, it is possible to detect the mRNA of the gene (also dependent on the number of mRNA molecules per cell) in thin sections of the tissue of interest.

The procedure includes hybridizing a single-stranded probe, complementary to the mRNA of interest, to fixed thin sections. Usually, *in vitro* transcribed and radioactively labeled RNA is used as a probe because that allows the removal of unhybridized RNA by single-strand-specific RNases that do not degrade RNA–RNA hybrids. The RNase treatment after hybridization reduces the otherwise observed nonspecific background significantly. The double-stranded hybrid RNA, which indicates the presence of specific mRNA in the cells, is then detected by immersing the sample into film emulsion. After developing, the silver grains formed can be detected under the microscope.

A different approach to *in situ* detection of specific mRNA makes use of reverse transcription and PCR performed on tissue sections. This is a relatively new technique. First, the section is incubated in the presence of reverse transcriptase to synthesize cDNA of all mRNA molecules in the sample. The primer for reverse transcription is oligo(dT), a single-stranded DNA molecule consisting of 18 to 25 thymidine residues that hybridizes to the poly(A) tail of mRNA molecules. Then, a PCR reaction using two primers carrying fluorescent labels is performed. After washing away unincorporated primers, the PCR product can be visualized under the fluorescence microscope. This technique is still too new to predict its overall usefulness.

EXAMPLE ANALYSES

Analysis of Gene Expression

Studying the expression of genes in certain tissues in response to various stimuli has been a major interest of molecular biologists for the past 20 years. Usually a specific cell type, e.g., endothelial cells, is studied *in vitro* to determine which stimuli are able to induce which genes. For instance, by growing endothelial cells *in vitro,* it has been possible to find a panel of genes that is induced concomitant with "endothelial cell activation." To determine if a gene is induced transcriptionally, a nuclear run-off experiment must be carried out. In addition, the stability of the specific mRNA of interest should be determined in the absence and presence of stimulus. This procedure has been described (see RNA Stability Assay).

To measure specific mRNA accumulation *in vivo* tissue sections must be analyzed by *in situ* hybridization (see *In Situ* Hybridization). A labeled probe for a given gene is hybridized to the tissue section by techniques that optimize hybridization to mRNA. The technique has the advantage of localizing the cells producing the mRNA in question (since one will visualize the labeled probe associated with given cells), as well as allowing some measure of quantitation. While not used to date in transplantation studies to any degree, *in situ* hybridization data provide information about temporal and spatial expression patterns of genes, as it has been used with small animals like *Drosophila* and mice where whole body sections can be analyzed.

Function of the Gene Product

The determination of the function of a certain gene product (almost always a protein) is of major importance. There are many ways to identify and isolate new genes that do not provide any information about the function of the gene product.

Molecular biologists make use of this type of approach by trying to inhibit expression of the gene of interest completely. If this can be achieved, it is the equivalent of generating a mutation in the classical sense. The resulting "mutant" phenotype is called a "*phenocopy.*"

There are, to date, two technical approaches to generate phenocopies: first, the deletion, and therefore functional inactivation, of both alleles of the gene of interest, a procedure that, due to technical reasons, is now feasible *in vivo* only in mice, since embryonic stem cells are available in only some strains of mice.

This rather tedious procedure, frequently called "gene knock-out," requires the isolation of embryonic stem cells of the organism in which the gene is to be destroyed. These stem cells are then cultured *in vitro* and injected with a DNA construct containing a partial sequence of the gene to be deleted and a selectable marker gene. The construct is engineered in such a way that upon selection, the only surviving cells are ones that have integrated the construct at the locus of the endogenous gene (by *homologous recom-*

bination) that destroys the gene (Fig. 27). In the process of homologous recombination, two recombinational events take place that allow the DNA segment to replace the endogenous gene, or some part thereof. The surviving cells, having deleted one allele, are propagated and after a sufficient number of cells is reached, the procedure can be repeated with a construct contain-

ing a different selectable marker to destroy the second allele of the gene. Then, embryonic stem cells carrying the deletion are injected into early mouse embryos and the embryos are implanted into pseudopregnant mice. The resulting litter will not carry the deletion in all of their cells. The goal of the procedure is, however, to achieve germline transmission of the deletion so that ho-

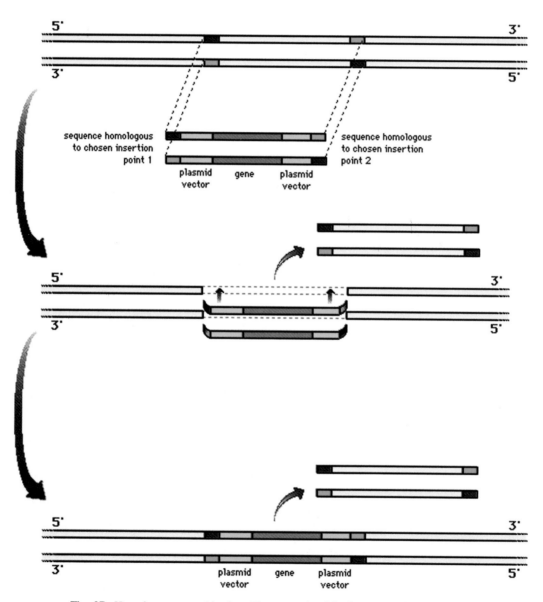

Fig. 27. Homologous recombination. The two ends of the fragment to be integrated into the host genome induce a separate double-strand break in the chromosome. The part of the chromosome between the two integration points is deleted.

mozygous animals can be derived by appropriate breeding. Such homozygous mice can then be analyzed in detail to determine the exact phenotype of the deletion.

Second, *antisense* RNA constructs coding for RNA complementary to the endogenous mRNA of the gene to be inhibited can be introduced, for instance, by using retroviral vectors. Antisense expression plasmids contain cDNA inserts in the "opposite orientation" (i.e., antisense). Transcription of such a construct results in the synthesis of a sequence complementary to the endogenous mRNA. The RNA transcribed from the antisense construct is therefore able to hybridize to the endogenous mRNA and can thus prevent translation of that mRNA, resulting in a missing gene product, equivalent to a classical mutation. The extent to which the gene must be inhibited to yield a phenotype that is analyzable varies. Alternatively, especially in tissue culture, short antisense oligonucleotides, performing the same function, have been employed successfully to generate phenocopies.

Studies of Regulation of Gene Expression

Reporter constructs. Understanding how cells function, and what determines the identity of a certain cell type, is eventually possible only if one is able to understand the "molecular program" of a certain cell. This "molecular program" can be described as the expression of different sets of genes related to time and circumstance. The ability to express a certain group of genes at a certain time, and to react to certain stimuli by inducing or repressing some genes, determines the identity of a cell. For this reason, it is of major import to study the regulation of genes in specific cell types.

The primary goal in analyzing the regulation of a certain gene is to identify DNA elements around (5′ or 3′ in relationship to the gene itself) or within the gene (e.g., in introns) that are able to influence transcriptional activity of the gene. Usually, the 5′-flanking region is the first target of investigation. The most common approach to analyzing regulatory elements is by linking them to a reporter gene (Fig. 28). The reporter construct used is a plasmid that consists of the regulatory region of DNA to be analyzed fused to the 5′-end of the reporter gene. The regulatory region is the only sequence driving transcription of the reporter gene. The reporter gene codes for an enzyme so that the amount of protein of that enzyme synthesized can easily be determined. Since mRNA stability and translational efficiency of the reporter gene should be constant and independent from the regulatory region of the gene to be analyzed, the amount of reporter protein in the cells directly reflects the activity of the regulatory region fused to it. The regulatory region can be manipulated by deleting, mutating,

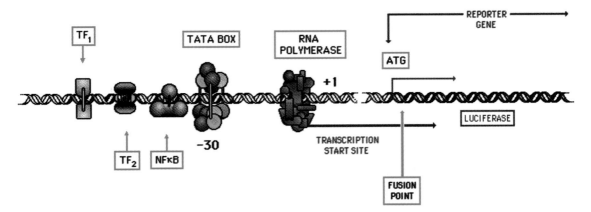

Fig. 28. Schematic representation of a reporter plasmid. The regulatory region to be analyzed is shown fused to the coding region of luciferase, an enzyme whose activity can easily be measured.

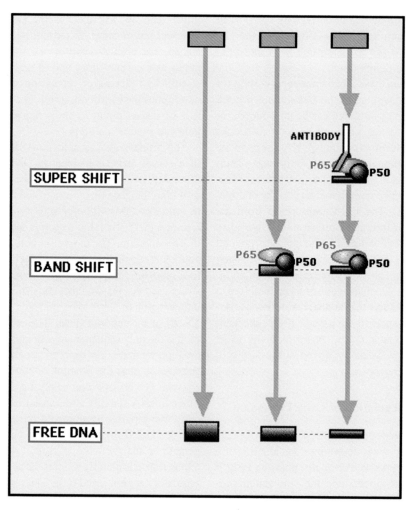

Fig. 29. Electrophoretic mobility shift assay. The first lane represents free DNA only. The next lane shows an additional slower migrating band that represents the complex between the DNA and the protein bound to it (NFκB). The third lane depicts a situation where in addition to the DNA and the binding factor, a specific antibody recognizing NFκB is included. This results in a third, even slower, band, representing the ternary complex of DNA, NFκB, and antibody.

or adding sequences from the original regulatory region. Comparing the relative amounts of reporter protein produced with the different regulatory region variants allows one to deduce the relative importance of certain sequences for transcriptional activation.

Protein–DNA interactions. Once important elements (usually 6–25 bp per element) in the regulatory region have been identified, it is of interest to identify proteins (transcription factors) that bind to such DNA sequences. Several methods have been developed to analyze protein–DNA interactions *in vitro* and *in vivo*. The two most widely used methods for *in vitro* analysis of protein–DNA interactions are electrophoretic mobility shift assays (EMSA) and DNase I footprinting.

Electrophoretic mobility shift assay (EMSA). EMSAs are carried out by combining a known DNA sequence that is a short (usually around 20 bases long), radioactively labeled, double-stranded oligonucleotide, with protein extracts isolated from the nucleus of the cells of interest.

In case the specific transcription factor(s) recognizing the DNA sequence being studied is present and active in the extract, it (they) will bind to the DNA molecule. When the mixture is separated on a polyacrylamide gel, the protein–DNA complexes move more slowly on the gel than the free DNA molecules. After autoradiography of the gel, the position of radioactive bands allows one to determine whether such a protein–DNA complex was present and resulted in a "band shift." To identify proteins binding to a certain DNA sequence one can include specific antibodies in the protein/DNA binding reaction. In case the antibody binds a protein that also binds to the DNA fragment, the resulting trimeric complex of DNA, protein, and antibody will migrate even slower through the gel, a phenomenon called "super shift" (Fig. 29).

DNase I footprinting. Another method to analyze *in vitro* protein–DNA interactions is DNase I footprinting. This method is mainly employed to determine the exact binding site of proteins on a larger (up to 400-bp) DNA fragment. The radioactively end-labeled[7] DNA fragment is treated with DNase I (catalyzes the hydrolysis of phosphodiester bonds between nucleotides in a random, sequence-independent manner) in the presence and absence of nuclear proteins extracts known (e.g., by EMSA) to contain a protein(s) binding to this DNA fragment. Under the appropriate conditions each DNA molecule is randomly cleaved by DNase I only once on one strand. In the case of free DNA molecules (without any proteins bound to them), the result is a mixture of DNA molecules cleaved once at a random position between the radioactive label and the other end. Since the end-labeling incorporates radioactivity into only one strand, separation of the denatured, single-stranded fragments on a sequencing gel ideally generates a ladder of bands where each band

corresponds to a fragment cut at a different position by the DNase I. Two neighboring bands correspond to two fragments cut at adjacent nucleotides.

In case a protein (a transcription factor) is bound to the DNA molecule when DNase I is added, the part of the DNA molecule to which the protein is bound (covering approximately 20 bp) is not accessible to DNase I, i.e., the enzyme cannot cut within that protected region. Thus, fragments corresponding to DNA molecules cut in this region are not present in the mixture, and therefore do not appear on the autoradiograph, leaving a section of the ladder blank (the "footprint" of the protein on the DNA; Fig. 30).

Methylation interference. Analysis of the sequence-specific interaction of proteins with DNA involves the determination of the bases in close contact with the protein. Usually, of the 10 to 20 bp protected in a DNase I footprint, only a few are actually in very close proximity to the protein. Methylation interference analysis allows the detection of such contact points.

As with DNase I footprinting, the probe is end-labeled and thus only one strand carries a radioactive label, and only that strand will be visible on the gel at the end of the experiment. Before allowing the protein to bind to the DNA *in vitro,* the probe is methylated at G and A residues. The methylation reaction is carried out under conditions such that only one methyl group is introduced per DNA molecule. Since the methylation occurs at random, each G residue will be methylated in the population of DNA molecules. The protein is then allowed to bind to the fragment and DNA molecules with and without attached protein are separated on a preparative EMSA gel using 5 to 10 times more material than in a regular EMSA. This is done to be able to recover enough material from the gel after electrophoresis for further analysis. After electrophoresis and autoradiography, the parts of the gel containing the free and bound DNA are cut out of the gel and the DNA is eluted from the gel slice. The DNA can then be cleaved specifically at methylated G residues to generate DNA molecules extending from one end to the next methylated G (Fig. 31). Separating the cleaved products of the free DNA on a sequencing gel results

---

[7]End-labeling of a DNA fragment can be achieved by either filling in 5′ overhanging, single-stranded ends with DNA polymerase using radioactive nucleotides or by removing the 5′ phosphate and replacing it with a radioactive one. If only one end should be labeled, restriction digest close to the end not to be labeled can be used to remove the label previously added. This leaves only one end with a label.

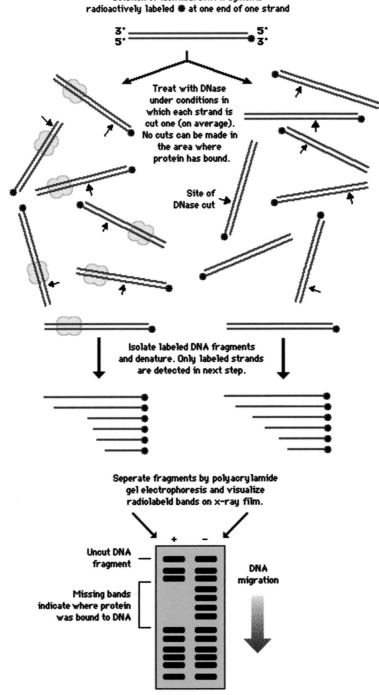

Fig. 30. Footprinting analysis of the binding site of a protein on a DNA fragment. Separate experiments are carried out in the presence (+) and absence (−) of the protein. This figure was reproduced with kind permis- sion from Lehninger, Nelson, and Cox, "Principles of Biochemistry," Second edition, Worth Publishers, Inc., New York, New York.

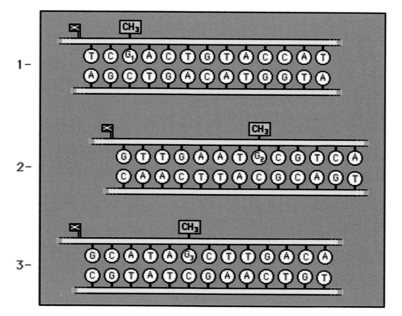

(a)

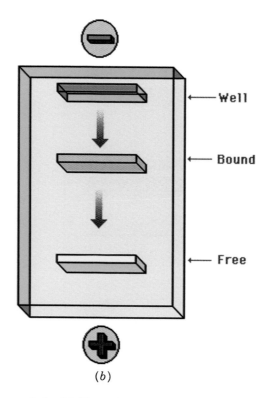

(b)

Fig. 31. Methylation interference analysis. (**a**) The end-labeled (flags) DNA fragment to be used is methylated at random G residues (-CH$_3$). (**b**) The DNA is mixed with the binding protein and free and bound DNA are separated on an EMSA gel. After electrophoresis, the free and bound DNA is isolated from the gel. (**c**) The free DNA is cleaved at methylated G residues. Molecules carrying a label are shown on the right, sorted according to length. (**d**) The bound DNA is also cleaved at methylated G residues. The labeled molecules, sorted according to length, are shown on the right. (**e**) Representation of an autoradiograph of a sequencing gel on which the cleaved free and bound DNA was separated. On the right, the molecules corresponding to the bands on the gel are depicted.

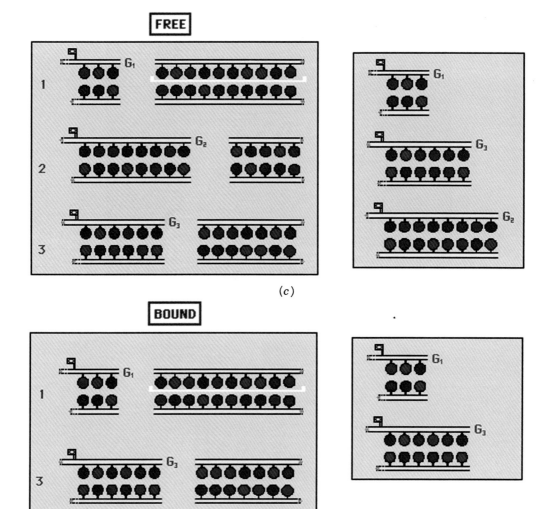

(c)

(d)

Fig. 31. (*Continued*)

in a ladder of bands in which the shortest band corresponds to the first G after the radioactively labeled end. Each larger fragment corresponds to another G farther away from the label. The sequence of bands on the gel therefore corresponds to the sequence of G residues in the DNA.

If a certain G residue is normally in close contact with the bound protein, methylation of such a G residue interferes with binding of the protein and, thus, bands corresponding to such a G residue will not be present in the DNA isolated from the retarded band (containing protein-bound DNA) in the gel. Therefore, any cleavage products present in the free DNA but absent from the DNA to which a protein is bound indicate that methylation of that particular G residue in the fragment interfered with protein binding, which in turn is interpreted as representing a close contact point between the G residue and the protein.

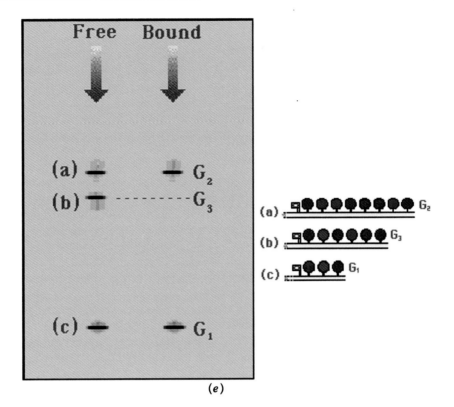

Fig. 31. (*Continued*)

EXAMPLE APPLICATIONS

This section gives examples of areas of research in transplantation biology that use the tools of molecular biology. The examples given are a relatively random selection of all those that could be listed.

Cells and Their Functions in Rejection

One problem that faces us in transplantation immunology is to try to relate cells that invade a graft (undergoing rejection or that is tolerated) to cytokines that are produced in the tissue. We have learned a great deal about the types of T lymphocytes that infiltrate rejecting grafts, and have identified the subsets of cells involved based largely on cell surface markers. However, a major level of analysis that had been possible *in vitro* but not *in vivo* is to study the cytokines produced by those T cells. It is appreciated now that CD4+ helper T cells (Th1 cells) make a different set of cytokines [e.g., interleukin 2 (IL-2) and interferon γ (IFN-γ)] than do CD4+ T cells (TH2) that may function to suppress the immune response (e.g., IL-4 and IL-10). Using tools of molecular biology, sections of tissue from an organ of interest that has been transplanted can be studied in two ways. First, the messenger RNA (mRNA) can be extracted and studied in a semiquantitative manner (Northern blotting, RNase protection assay). By having the appropriate "molecular probes" for the mRNA of each of the cytokines, it is possible, in a semiquantitative manner, to assay which of the cytokines are being produced by cells in that tissue. Second, one can use similar probes for the cytokines and actually look at the site of production, i.e., associate cytokine production with a particular cell (*in situ* hybridization).

Genetic Manipulation of Cells

To manipulate cells on the genetic level (e.g., by either expressing "foreign" genes ectopically or by turning off certain genes) it is first necessary to isolate the gene of interest and amplify it so that it can be appropriately engineered *in vitro* before being used to manipulate cells, organs, or whole animals. We shall use the example of searching for a gene that codes for a protein that inhibits complement.

Isolation of the gene. The isolation of the DNA coding for a certain gene of interest requires a tool to identify this gene selectively and unambiguously in a complex mixture of genes from a certain cell type. Let us assume that in our case a specific antibody recognizing the gene product (the protein encoded by the gene) is available. That means the protein was isolated, purified to homogeneity, and mice or rabbits were immunized with the purified protein. In the case of immunizing rabbits, the resultant antiserum is usually further purified by affinity purification on the immunizing protein immobilized on a chromatography matrix. The purified reagent is referred to as an "antibody."

One approach is to prepare a cDNA expression library and then to identify the plaque(s) of that library that contain the phage carrying the gene of interest. In our case, a bacteriophage vector was chosen that contains regulatory sequences that allow the "foreign" gene inserted in the vector to be expressed as a protein in the bacterial host cells. Therefore, each plaque also contains the protein encoded by the cloned gene. To preserve the library, a replica is made by transferring a part of each plaque onto a membrane filter that tightly binds proteins. Now the filter can be treated with the antibody against the sought-for gene product. The bound antibody can be visualized by using a second, enzyme-coupled antibody and performing a colored product-generating enzyme reaction (Fig. 23). The plaque(s) on the "master" plate corresponding to the colored spot on the replica membrane is thus identified as containing the phage clone carrying the gene of interest.

After identification of the plaque representing the gene of interest, it is necessary to obtain a larger quantity of the phage. This is done by using phage derived from the plaque to infect more bacteria to produce a high titer stock.

Phage particles are not the ideal starting material for preparing significant amounts of DNA (e.g., for sequencing etc.) because the inserted DNA is much shorter than the phage genome (10–20% for cDNA). Therefore, it is desirable to subclone the insert DNA into a much smaller plasmid. Modern phage vectors allow the conversion from linear phage to circular plasmid simply by infecting special host bacteria, which, rather than replicating the infecting phage, excise the insert and some flanking sequences and generate a circular, double-stranded plasmid. Now, almost unlimited amounts (milligrams) of the plasmid can be produced in bacteria. For one sequencing reaction, about 5 μg of DNA is needed, and thus 50–100 μg is sufficient to obtain a complete sequence for most genes.

Cloning into expression vector and transfection into cultured cells. Computer analysis of the obtained DNA sequence allows the localization of all restriction enzyme recognition sites in the insert DNA. This information is used to cut out the insert from the original plasmid and ligate it into a special eukaryotic expression vector. Such a vector must contain all necessary regulatory sequences to ensure stable, high level expression of the inserted gene in mammalian cells. These sequences include enhancers, polyadenylation signals, and a selectable marker gene. The expression plasmid plus insert is again amplified in bacteria because 300 to 500 μg of highly purified expression plasmid is needed for introducing the plasmid (transfection) into endothelial cells (EC), for example.

After transfection, the EC are grown in a selective culture medium allowing only cells expressing the marker gene (which therefore have received the entire plasmid) to survive. Two weeks later, when colonies of cells containing the plasmid have grown up, the cells are subcultured and the presence of the "new" gene is tested by Southern blotting. Clones proving positive for the gene are now tested for appropriate expression of the gene by Northern blot analysis. Those with high levels of expression are selected for a functional analysis, in our case the effective inhibition of complement activity.

Finding new genes of interest. We are gaining an increased appreciation of how important the endothelium, and the endothelial cells, are in transplantation. This is evident in a major way in xenotransplantation, but also applies to allotransplantation; in both situations the endothelial cells are "activated." One question that arises is what new genes are induced with EC activation, and thus what new protein products are expressed by the activated EC. There are several approaches to finding such new genes, that are referred to as "activation" genes. One particularly elegant approach involves the following. One can make what is known as a "cDNA library" of the genes that are expressed in activated EC. Such a library has in it DNA copies of all the genes that are transcribed only in the activated EC, i.e., genes for which an mRNA copy is present in the activated EC.

Differential Library (Δ-Library, Subtraction Library, Delta Library)

To find genes that are present in activated EC, but not in resting EC (i.e., before activation), one can mix the single-stranded cDNA (generated by reverse transcription of mRNA) from the activated EC with an excess of mRNA from the resting EC. For each gene that is expressed in both the resting and the activated EC, the mRNA from the resting EC will combine with the DNA for those genes from the activated cells, forming mRNA–DNA hybrids. The only DNA from the activated cells that will remain as single-stranded DNA is from those genes that are not expressed in the resting EC, i.e., for which there is no mRNA in those cells (Fig. 32). It is possible to separate the mRNA–DNA hybrids from the single-stranded DNA, and, thus, by a variety of techniques, those single-stranded DNA molecules that are left after subtracting shared genes can be studied after second strand synthesis and ligation into a plasmid vector for amplification in bacteria.

Production of Recombinant Proteins

For both experimental and potentially therapeutic purposes, it is important to make antibodies to certain molecules of interest. In some cases, such as the situation just described to find new genes that are present in activated EC, we have the gene in hand but not the protein. The availability of a cDNA clone allows one to produce large quantities of the protein encoded by that cDNA eventually to obtain an antibody against that protein. The protein can also be used for biochemical and functional analyses. If posttranslational modification, such as glycosylation or phosphorylation, is not expected to be important for the function of the protein, the simplest way is to express the cDNA in bacteria. A variety of vectors are available that allow high level expression of the inserted cDNA in *E. coli*. A good expression system can produce the protein of interest so that it will constitute up to 5% of the total bacterial protein. Many times the vectors contain extra sequences expressed either at the C- or N-terminus of the recombinant protein so the produced protein can be purified on an affinity column binding to the portion of the protein encoded by that extra sequence.

Other methods are available to produce a recombinant protein that is modified posttranslationally, and where that modification is of importance, to optimize the probability that those modifications will take place. These methods include expression in mammalian cells as well as baculovirus (Miller, 1988).

Producing a Transgenic Animal

A key area of interest to the investigators in xenotransplantation involves the introduction of new genes into cells of the graft. It seems likely that by using other techniques, introduction of genes into certain cells of humans will also be used. Two potential goals exist for introducing new genes: either to express the gene of interest so that the protein encoded by the gene is now present and functional in the cell, or to turn off a gene that is normally expressed in that cell. One example of this, discussed in Chapter 19 on xenotransplantation, it to introduce a human gene into the endothelial cells of a pig organ that would be transplanted to a human. One such gene codes for a membrane-associated inhibitor of complement (e.g., "decay accelerating factor," DAF). Thus, pig EC that express this inhibitor would be more resistant to the action of human complement, and might have less of a

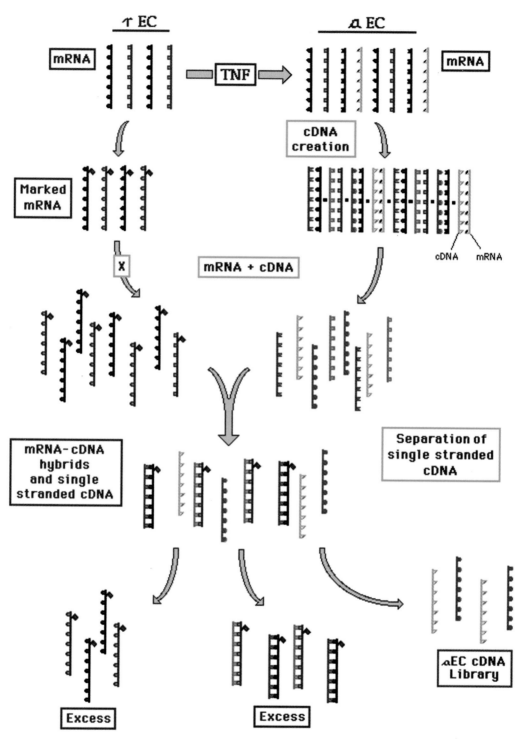

Fig. 32. Steps involved in producing a Δ-library. An excess of mRNA from resting EC (rEC) and cDNA from activated EC (aEC) are shown. The flags on the RNA molecules from the rEC indicate biotinylation.

reaction to the factors, including complement, that incite rejection in such situations. Pigs expressing one of these complement-inhibiting genes have already been derived. They are said to carry the human "*transgene*" and are referred to as "*transgenic*" *pigs*. The tools of molecular genetics, which were discussed in the previous section, allow this kind of gene transfer, with subsequent expression of the gene in its new host cell, not only in tissue culture, but also *in vivo*.

To derive a transgenic animal, the cDNA of the gene to be introduced has to be cloned into a eukaryotic expression vector, much as for expression in cultured cells. This construct is then microinjected into the male pronucleus of fertilized oocytes isolated from the animal species of choice, in our case pigs. The oocytes are then reimplanted into the pig, which is then left to continue pregnancy to full term. Between 0.5 and 4% of pigs can be expected to carry a transgene in successful experiments. The resulting progeny are then analyzed in several ways.

First, peripheral leukocytes are tested by Southern blot to determine which individuals have stably integrated the construct. Next, the positive individuals are tested for expression of the mRNA for the "foreign" gene, and for the protein encoded by that mRNA. Here, it is often observed that expression of the gene is dependent on the tissue analyzed, i.e., one should analyze the tissue where one would like to see the expression of the gene, in our case endothelial cells. Finally, the transgenic animals are bred to produce offspring homozygous with respect to the transgene. Once a sufficient number of homozygous transgenic animals have been obtained, organs of these can be used for the ultimate test—the function of the transgene *in vivo*. In our case that would mean to transplant a heart from a transgenic pig into a primate to evaluate the effect of human DAF expression on hyperacute rejection of the organ.

Turning off a Gene

In many experimental, and again therapeutic, situations, it is desirable to turn off a given gene. As reviewed previously, mRNA has to be made as a part of the process that leads to gene expression. A technique of molecular biology, called "*antisense,*" can be used to prevent the production of protein by a given gene. Short stretches of nucleic acids (*oligonucleotides*) that are complementary to (the antisense base sequence) and thus bind the region of the mRNA around the *translation* start site are introduced into the cell. These introduced oligonucleotides ("oligos") bind to the *mRNA* in question and prevent that mRNA from being translated. In some cases, investigators have even introduced genetic constructs that have base sequences in them from which very large amounts of a given antisense RNA can be synthesized continuously within the cell and thus permanently prevent translation of the gene in question.

It is obvious from this very short review that the possibilities to develop new therapies in many fields of medicine have significantly increased with the advent of molecular biology. However, it must also be considered that practically all of the described techniques are quite elaborate, time-consuming, and expensive. Furthermore, the feasibility of a certain approach in one species does not necessarily mean that it can be applied to another species. For instance, it is about 10 times less efficient to derive a transgenic pig than it is to derive a transgenic mouse, and considerable effort was spent to adapt the procedure to the new species. Therefore, one should be cautious in predicting how long it will take until safe genetic manipulation of different species, including humans, will be commonplace in day-to-day medical procedure, although a theoretical basis has been well established.

REFERENCES

Miller LK (1988): Baculoviruses as gene expression vectors. Annu Rev Microbiol 42:177–200.

Nabel EG, Plautz G, Nabel GJ (1990): Site-specific gene expression *in vivo* by direct gene transfer into the arterial wall. Science 249:1285–1288.

Zenke M, Steinlein P, Wagner E, Cotten M, Beug H, Birnstiel ML (1990): Receptor-mediated endocytosis of transferrin-polycation conjugates: An efficient way to introduce DNA into hematopoietic cells. Proc Natl Acad Sci USA 87:3655–3659.

GLOSSARY

Actinomycin D: Inhibitor of eukaryotic RNA polymerase II. Inhibits transcription of mRNA.

Adenovirus: Eukaryotic DNA virus. Can be used for transfection of cells *in vivo*.

Agarose: Polysaccharide derived from blue-green algae. Mixed with water (up to 2% agarose) it forms a gelous matrix that allows the separation of DNA and RNA molecules according to size in an electric field.

Alternative Splicing: The removal of different introns from a primary transcript in different tissues leading to a different gene product in the different tissues.

Amino Acid: Chemical component of proteins containing at least one carboxyl group (-COOH) and an amino group ($-NH_2$) on the carbon atom (-C) adjacent to the carboxyl group (α-carbon).

Anticodon: A group of three adjacent bases on a tRNA molecule that are able to recognize, by base pairing, a codon on an mRNA molecule when bound to a ribosome.

Antisense: A sequence complementary to a coding sequence.

Bacteriophage: A prokaryotic DNA virus that infects bacteria. Used as a vector for efficient transformation of bacterial cells.

Bases: The critical chemical components of DNA and RNA. DNA contains adenine (A), guanine (G), cytosine (C), and thymine (T). RNA contains uracil (U) instead of thymine.

Base Pair: Two complementary nucleotides that interact through hydrogen bonds. Only G-C (or C-G) and A-T (or T-A) base pairs are possible.

Base Triplet: A group of three sequential bases on an RNA or DNA molecule. Also called codon.

Blunt Ends: The end of a double-stranded DNA molecule when both strands are of equal length and have no single-stranded overhangs.

C-Terminus: One end of a polypeptide or protein chain containing a free carboxyl group.

Cap Structure: A special, inverted, methylated guanosine triphosphate that is added onto the 5'-end of a primary transcript during mRNA maturation.

cDNA: DNA that has been generated by reverse transcribing mRNA using *reverse transcriptase*.

cDNA Library: A collection of *cDNAs* representing all expressed genes of a certain cell type or tissue.

Clone: A number of identical DNAs, cells, or organisms that are derived from a single progenitor by identical replication.

Coding Region: The part of a gene or an mRNA that codes for a polypeptide or protein.

Codon: Three consecutive nucleotides on an mRNA or DNA that are within the coding region.

Competent: Bacterial cells that have been treated to allow them to take up DNA from the environment.

Complementary: A nucleotide sequence is complementary to another if it contains, in opposite direction, a T residue for every A residue in the other sequence (and vice versa) and for every G residue it contains a C (and vice versa).

Conjugation: A process during which two bacterial cells exchange genetic information (i.e., DNA).

Delta Library: A library of cDNAs from which a subset of sequences has been subtracted by hybridization.

Denaturation: With respect to proteins, denaturation describes the destruction of the native, tertiary, conformational structure. Denaturation of DNA is the separation of the two strands. Partial double-stranded parts of an RNA molecule (stems) can also be denatured.

DNA (Deoxyribonucleic Acid): The carrier of genetic information. A polymer containing a sugar–phosphate backbone to which the bases are attached via the sugar molecule to form structure.

DNA Ligase: An enzyme that allows the rejoining of two DNA molecules by building a sugar–phosphate bond between the terminal 3'-hydroxyl (-OH) group in one molecule and the terminal 5'-phosphate in the other molecule. The bonds are formed on both strands.

DNA Polymerase: An enzyme that is able to synthesize a complementary DNA strand provided that a template strand is present to which a short second strand is annealed. The short second strand (the primer) must contain a 3'-hydroxyl (-OH) onto which the first nucleotide can be added. Only nucleotides complementary to the template strand are added.

DNA Sequencing: The determination of the base sequence of a DNA molecule.

DNase I Footprinting: The mapping of a protein-binding site on a DNA molecule based on the protection of the binding site by the protein from DNase I digestion.

Electrophoretic Mobility Shift Assay (EMSA): Analytical method to study protein–DNA interactions. The principle of the method is the different mobility of DNA and DNA–protein complexes in a polyacrylamide gel.

Embryonic Stem Cells (ESC): Undifferentiated cells derived from early embryos that can be cultured *in vitro*. After genetic manipulation, ESC can be reimplanted into developing embryos and will eventually become part of the whole organism that will then carry the genetic alteration in most of its cells.

Enhancer: A regulatory DNA element that increases transcriptional rate. By definition, enhancers function independently from their position (3' or 5') relative to the gene. They are also active over a long range (several kilobase pairs).

Episomal: Genetic information that exists independently from the overall genome of an organism and is therefore not part of a chromosome is called episomal.

Exon: The parts of the coding region of a gene that remains in the mature mRNA after *splicing* and is eventually translated into protein.

Expression: In genetics the expression of genes is the manifestation of genetic information as a phenotype.

Expression Vector: A cloning vector that is designed to allow transcription in bacteria of the inserted gene. A strong bacterial promoter is placed immediately upstream of the point of the cloning site.

Gel Electrophoresis: The separation of charged molecules according to size or charge in a gel matrix.

General Transcription Machinery: A number of proteins essential for transcription of every protein-coding gene. These proteins include the RNA polymerase II subunits, initiation factors that assemble on the TATA box, and elongation factors that bind to the polymerase after the initiation of transcription.

Glycosylation: The posttranslational addition of carbohydrates to a polypeptide chain. Depending on the type of glycosylation it can occur either in the endoplasmic reticulum or in the Golgi.

Homologous Recombination: The recombination of to DNA molecules at sites of sequence homology. The frequency of homologous recombination is approximately 10^{-7} to 10^{-8}.

***In Situ* Hybridization:** A method to determine qualitatively the presence of a certain mRNA in a tissue section.

Intercalation: The insertion of planar molecules between two consecutive bases of one strand of DNA or RNA.

Intron: A sequence within the transcribed part of a gene that is removed from the primary transcript in a process called splicing.

Isoelectric Point (pI): The pH value at which the number of positive charges of a multivalent molecule equals the number of negative charges; thus the net charge of a molecule at its pI is zero.

Leader Sequence: The sequence on a mRNA molecule that is 5' to the translation start.

Ligation: The enzymatic creation of a phosphodiester bond between two DNA (or RNA) molecules.

Liposomes: Lipid vesicles created *in vitro* by sonicating different lipids.

Messenger RNA (mRNA): RNA that codes for and is translated into a protein in the cytoplasm.

Methylase: An enzyme that is part of the restriction/methylation system of bacteria. The enzyme adds a methyl (-CH$_3$) group to bases in all recognition sites of the corresponding restriction enzyme. This protects the bacteria's own genome from degradation by the restriction enzyme that is directed against infectious bacteriophage DNA.

Methylation Interference: A method to determine the close contact points of a bound protein on DNA. The method is based on the fact that methylation of a base that is normally in close contact with the protein prevents binding of the protein.

Multiple Cloning Site (MCS, or polylinker): A part of a cloning vector that contains a number of different restriction enzyme recognition sites adjacent to each other. Each of these sites is unique in the entire vector.

N-Terminus: One end of a polypeptide core protein chain that contains a free α-amino group.

NFκB: A transcription factor that exists in an inactive state in the cytoplasm and can be rapidly activated (e.g., by cytokines, phorbol esters, endotoxin).

Northern Blotting: A method to determine semiquantitatively the relative amount of mRNA in a certain cell type or tissue.

Nuclear Run-off Analysis: A method to determine the relative rate of transcription for a specific gene in a certain cell type or tissue.

Nucleotide: The monomeric component of DNA and RNA. It consists of a sugar (ribose or deoxyribose) to which a phosphate and a base are bound at different carbon atoms.

Oligonucleotides: A small single-stranded DNA or RNA molecule.

Origin of Replication: A specific sequence on plasmids at which replication of the plasmid *in vivo* is initiated.

Palindromic Sequence: A sequence that is identical on both strands of a double-stranded molecule when read in opposite direction on the two strands.

Peptide: A small number of amino acids linked by peptide bonds (i.e., a very small protein).

Peptide Bond: The chemical bond between individual amino acids in a peptide chain. It is an amide linkage (-CO-NH-) between the carboxyl group (-COOH) of one amino acid and the α-amino group (-NH$_2$) of the other.

Phenocopy: The inactivation of both alleles of a gene or the prevention of its expression resulting in the same effect as a mutation.

Phosphorylation: The posttranslational addition of one or more phosphate groups onto a protein on the hydroxyl groups of serine, threonine, or tyrosine.

Plaques: Clear spots on a bacterial lawn due to lysis of the bacteria by bacteriophage.

Plasmid: A circular, double-stranded DNA molecule derived from bacteria.

Poly(A) Tail: A number of A residues added to the 3'-end of an mRNA molecule.

Polymerase Chain Reaction (PCR): Enzymatic amplification of DNA *in vitro*. The procedure involves repeated cycles of denaturation, annealing of primers, and extension of the primers by a thermostable DNA polymerase.

Primer: A short single-stranded DNA molecule that is annealed to another strand of DNA and can be extended in the 3' direction by DNA polymerase.

Probe: A labeled molecule of DNA or RNA that can be used to hybridize to a membrane of a Southern or Northern blot to detect a specific band of DNA or mRNA.

Protein Synthesis: See **Translation.**

Replication: The identical duplication of DNA and also whole genomes.

Repressor: A negative transcription factor whose binding to a certain sequence in the regulatory region of a gene can prevent transcription.

Restriction Enzymes: Endonucleases that recognize specific sequences (palindromic) on double-stranded DNA and cut the DNA on both strands.

Restriction Fragment Length Polymorphism (RFLP): Allelic differences observed as different length restriction fragments derived from genomic DNA from different individuals and hybridized with the same probe.

Retrovirus: A eukaryotic RNA virus that reverse-transcribes its RNA genome in the host cell and integrates it into the host genome.

Reverse Transcriptase: RNA-dependent DNA polymerase that is able to synthesize DNA from an RNA template.

Ribonuclease (RNase): Enzyme that degrades RNA.

RNA Polymerase: An enzyme that synthesizes RNA to form a double-stranded DNA template.

RNA Stability Assay: A method to determine the half-life of a specific mRNA in a cell.

RNase Protection Assay: A sensitive method to measure steady-state mRNA levels.

Selectable Marker Genes: Genes present on vectors that allow the positive selection of cells having received the vector (e.g., antibiotic resistance genes).

Sequencing Gel: A special type of polyacrylamide gel containing urea that is used for sequencing DNA. The resolution is high enough to be able to see the difference in mobility of two single-stranded molecules that differ by only one nucleotide in length.

Small Nuclear RNA (snRNA): RNA species in the nucleus that are part of ribonucleoproteins and fulfill a function in splicing.

Sodium Dodecyl Sulfate (SDS): A strong detergent used to denature proteins for gel electrophoresis separation according to size.

Southern Blotting: A method to detect a certain DNA molecule in a complex mixture of DNA (e.g., complete genomic DNA).

Splicing: The process in mRNA maturation by which introns are removed.

Sticky Ends: Single-stranded overhangs (ca. 2–4 bases) generated by certain restriction enzymes that cut the two strands of their target DNA at staggered positions.

TATA Box: A regulatory element present in almost all mRNA coding genes. The assembly of a protein complex on the TATA box is essential for the initiation of transcription.

Template: A sequence to which a complementary strand is synthesized.

Transcription Factor: Proteins that can influence transcription either positively or negatively.

Transcriptional Start Site: The nucleotide on the DNA of a gene at which RNA polymerase starts to synthesize RNA. For RNA polymerase II genes it is ca. 30 bp 3' of the TATA box.

Transfection: The introduction of DNA into higher eukaryotic cells either *in vitro* or *in vivo*.

Transfer RNA (tRNA): The RNA type that carries amino acids to the ribosome and also recognizes the codons on the mRNA.

Transferrinfection: A method to introduce DNA into eukaryotic cells by linking it to a protein (transferrin) that is bound by a receptor on the target cell surface and subsequently internalized. Also called receptor-mediated gene transfer.

Transformation: Introduction of DNA into bacterial cells.

Transgene: A "foreign" gene stably integrated into the genome.

Translation: The synthesis of protein on a ribosome.

Vector: A DNA molecule (plasmid or phage) used to clone a certain fragment of DNA or to generate a library.

Western Blotting: The transfer of proteins separated on an polyacrylamide gel to a membrane and detection of certain proteins on the membrane using a specific antibody.

Index